Gastroenterology and Nutrition: Neonatology Questions and Controversies

Gastroenterology and Nutrition

Neonatology Questions and Controversies

Series Editor

Richard A. Polin, MD
Professor of Pediatrics
College of Physicians and Surgeons
Columbia University
Director, Division of Neonatology
Morgan Stanley Children's Hospital of New York – Presbyterian
Columbia University Medical Center
New York, New York

Other Volumes in the Neonatology Questions and Controversies Series

Cardiology

Hematology, Immunology and Infectious Disease

Nephrology and Fluid/Electrolytes Physiology

Neurology

The Newborn Lung

Gastroenterology and Nutrition
Neonatology Questions and Controversies

Josef Neu, MD
Professor of Pediatrics
University of Florida College of Medicine
Gainesville, Florida

Consulting Editor

Richard A. Polin, MD
Professor of Pediatrics
College of Physicians and Surgeons
Columbia University
Director, Division of Neonatology
Morgan Stanley Children's Hospital of New York – Presbyterian
Columbia University Medical Center
New York, New York

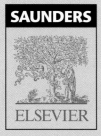

SAUNDERS

ELSEVIER

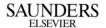

1600 John F. Kennedy Blvd.
Ste 1800
Philadelphia, PA 19103-2899

GASTROENTEROLOGY AND NUTRITION: Neonatology Questions and Controversies   ISBN: 978-1-4160-3160-4
Copyright © 2008 by Saunders, an imprint of Elsevier Inc.

Library of Congress Cataloging-in-Publication Data

Gastroenterology and nutrition: neonatology questions and controversies/[edited by] Josef Neu; consulting editor, Richard A. Polin.—1st ed.
   p. ; cm.
  Includes bibliographical references.
  ISBN 978-1-4160-3160-4
  1. Pediatric gastroenterology. 2. Newborn infants—Diseases. I. Neu, Josef. II. Polin, Richard A, (Richard Alan), 1945-
  [DNLM: 1. Gastrointestinal Diseases. 2. Infant, Newborn, Diseases. 3. Infant Nutrition Physiology. 4. Infant, Newborn. WS 310 G2555 2008]
  RJ446.G363 2008
  618.92′33—dc22

                                  2007044201

ISBN: 978-1-4160-3160-4

Publishing Director: Judith Fletcher
Developmental Editor: Lisa Barnes
Associate Developmental Editor: Bernard Buckholtz
Senior Project Manager: David Saltzberg
Design Direction: Karen O'Keefe-Owens

Printed in China

Last digit is the print number: 9 8 7 6 5 4 3 2

Contents

Section III
SELECT CLINICAL ENTITIES, 279

Contributors

Kjersti Aagaard-Tillery, MD, PhD
Assistant Professor
Obstetrics and Gynecology
Department of Obstetrics and Gynecology
Division of Maternal-Fetal Medicine
Baylor College of Medicine
Houston, Texas
  Adult Consequences of Neonatal and Fetal Nutrition: Mechanisms

Joel M. Andres, MD
Professor of Pediatrics
  Fellowship Program Director of Pediatric Gastroenterology,
Hepatology and Nutrition
Division of Pediatric Hepatology
Department of Pediatrics
University of Florida College of Medicine
Gainesville, Florida
  Cholestasis in Neonates and Infants

Tracy Gautsch Anthony, PhD
Assistant Professor
Department of Biochemistry and Molecular Biology
Indiana University School of Medicine
Evansville, Indiana
  Regulation of Protein Synthesis and Proteolysis in the Neonate by Feeding

Nancy Auestad, PhD
Director, Nutrition Science
Kellogg Company
Battle Creek, Michigan
Adjunct Professor
Department of Human Nutrition
Columbus, Ohio
  Diverse Roles of Lipids in Neonatal Physiology and Development

Carol Lynn Berseth, MD
Director Medical Affairs, North America
Mead Johnson Nutritionals
Evansville, Indiana
  The Intestine as a Neuroendocrine Organ

Douglas G. Burrin, PhD
Associate Professor
USDA-ARS Children's Nutrition Research Center
Department of Pediatrics
Baylor College of Medicine
Houston, Texas
Trophic Factors in the Neonatal Gastrointestinal Tract

Ricardo A. Caicedo, MD
Clinical Instructor
Pediatric Gastroenterology and Nutrition
Wake Forest University Baptist Medical Center
Winston Salem, NC
Intestinal Barrier Function: Implications for the Neonate and Beyond

Mike K. Chen, MD
Associate Professor of Surgery and Pediatrics
University of Florida College of Medicine
Gainesville, Florida
Short Bowel Syndrome and Intestinal Tissue Engineering

Erika C. Claud, MD
Assistant Professor
Department of Pediatrics
Section of Neonatology
The University of Chicago
Chicago, Illinois
The Intestinal Microbiota and the Microbiome

Dominique Darmaun, MD, PhD
Professor of Nutrition
Human Nutrition Research Center
University of Nantes
Attending Physician
Hotel-Dieu Hospital
Nantes, France
Noninvasive Techniques to Monitor Nutrition in Neonates

Michael K. Davis, MD
Fellow Pediatric Gastroenterology
Pediatric Gastroenterology
University of Florida College of Medicine
Gainesville, Florida
Cholestasis in Neonates and Infants

Clotilde desRobert
Neonatal Intensive Care Unit
University Hospital of Nantes
Nantes, France
Adult Consequences of Neonatal and Fetal Nutrition: Mechanisms

Martha Douglas-Escobar, MD
Fellow of Neonatology
Department of Pediatrics
University of Florida College of Medicine
Gainesville, Florida
> *Necrotizing Enterocolitis: Pathogenesis, Clinical Care and Prevention, and Intestinal Barrier Function: Implications for the Neonate and Beyond*

Frank R. Greer, MD
Professor of Pediatrics
University of Wisconsin School of Medicine and Public Health
Madison, Wisconsin
> *Macro and Micronutrients*

William W. Hay, Jr
Professor of Pediatrics
Director, Neonatal Clinical Research Center
Scientific Director, Perinatal Research Center
University of Colorado School Of Medicine
University of Colorado Denver
Denver, Colorado
> *Nutritional Requirements of the Very Low Birth Weight Infant*

Michael Janeczko, MD
Postdoctoral Fellow
Neonatology Section
Department of Pediatrics
Baylor College of Medicine
Houston, Texas
> *Trophic Factors in the Neonatal Gastrointestinal Tract*

Robert H. Lane, MD
Associate Professor
Associate Division Chief, Division of Neonatology
Director, Neonatal – Perinatal Fellowship
Director, Neonatal – Perinatal Research
University of Utah School of Medicine
Department of Pediatrics
Division of Neonatology
Salt Lake City, Utah
> *Adult Consequences of Neonatal and Fetal Nutrition: Mechanisms*

Nan Li, MD
Assistant Scientist
Department of Pediatrics
University of Florida College of Medicine
Gainesville, Florida
> *Intestinal Barrier Function: Implications for the Neonate and Beyond*

Patricia W. Lin, MD

Assistant Professor of Pediatrics
Division of Neonatal Perinatal Medicine
Department of Pediatrics
Emory University School of Medicine
Atlanta, Georgia

Innate Immunity and Epithelial Biology: Special Considerations in the Neonatal Gut

Alan Mayer, MD

Associate Professor of Pediatrics
Department of Pediatrics
Medical College of Wisconsin
Children Hospital of Wisconsin
Milwaukee, Wisconsin

The Exocrine Pancreas

Nichole Mitchell, MD

Fellow of Neonatology
Department of Pediatrics
Division of Neonatology
University of Utah School of Medicine
Salt Lake City, Utah

Adult Consequences of Neonatal and Fetal Nutrition: Mechanisms

Susan Hazels Mitmesser, PhD

Manager, Global Medicine Communications
Medical Affairs
Mead Johnson Nutritionals
Evansville, Indiana

Regulation of Protein Synthesis and Proteolysis in the Neonate by Feeding

Robert K. Montgomery, PhD

Instructor
Division of Gastroenterology and Nutrition
Children's Hospital
Boston, Massachussetts

Gastrointestinal Development: Morphogenesis and Molecular Mechanisms

Andrew S. Neish

Associate Professor in Pathology and Laboratory Medicine
Epithelial Pathobiology Unit
Department of Pathology and Laboratory Medicine
Emory University School of Medicine
Atlanta, Georgia

Innate Immunity and Epithelial Biology: Special Considerations in the Neonatal Gut

Josef Neu, MD
Professor of Pediatrics
University of Florida College of Medicine
Gainesville, Florida

Necrotizing Enterocolitis: Pathogenesis, Clinical Care and Prevention, and
Intestinal Barrier Function: Implications for the Neonate and Beyond

J. Marc Rhoads, MD
Professor of Pediatrics
Director, Division of Gastroenterology
University of Texas Health Science Center
Houston, Texas

Short Bowel Syndrome

Jean-Christophe Rozé, MD
Professor of Pediatrics
Director of the PICU and the NICU
Department of Neonatology and Pediatric Intensive Care
Hôpital Mère-et-Enfant
Professor of Pediatrics
University of Nantes
Nantes, France

Noninvasive Techniques to Monitor Nutrition in Neonates

Ian. R. Sanderson, MD, MSc, FRCP, FRCPCH
Professor of Pediatric Gastroenterology
Barts and The London
Queen Mary, University of London
London, United Kingdom

Dietary Regulation of Gene Expression

Patti J. Thureen, MD
Professor of Pediatrics
The University of Colorado School of Medicine
Professor of Pediatrics
The University of Colorado Hospital
Professor of Pediatrics and Neonatologist
The Children's Hospital
Aurora and Denver, Colorado

Nutritional Requirements of the Very Low Birth Weight Infant

W. Allan Walker, MD

Director, Mucosal Immunology Laboratory
Pediatric Gastroenterology & Nutrition Unit
Massachusetts General Hospital for Children
Conrad Taff Professor of Nutrition
Professor of Pediatrics
Director, Division of Nutrition
Harvad Medical School
Boston, Massachusetts

The Intestinal Microbiota and the Microbiome

Steven L. Werlin, MD

Professor of Pediatrics
The Medical College of Wisconsin
The Children's Hospital of Wisconsin
Milwaukee, Wisconsin

The Exocrine Pancreas

Series Foreword

"Learn from yesterday, live for today, hope for tomorrow. The important thing is not to stop questioning."

ALBERT EINSTEIN

"The art and science of asking questions is the source of all knowledge."

THOMAS BERGER

In the mid-1960s W.B. Saunders began publishing a series of books focused on the care of newborn infants. The series was entitled *Major Problems in Clinical Pediatrics*. The original series (1964–1979) consisted of ten titles dealing with problems of the newborn infant (*The Lung and its Disorders in the Newborn Infant* edited by Mary Ellen Avery, *Disorders of Carbohydrate Metabolism in Infancy* edited by Marvin Cornblath and Robert Schwartz, *Hematologic Problems in the Newborn* edited by Frank A. Oski and J. Lawrence Naiman, *The Neonate with Congenital Heart Disease* edited by Richard D. Rowe and Ali Mehrizi, *Recognizable Patterns of Human Malformation* edited by David W. Smith, *Neonatal Dermatology* edited by Lawrence M. Solomon and Nancy B. Esterly, *Amino Acid Metabolism and its Disorders* edited by Charles L. Scriver and Leon E. Rosenberg, *The High Risk Infant* edited by Lula O. Lubchenco, *Gastrointestinal Problems in the Infant* edited by Joyce Gryboski and *Viral Diseases of the Fetus and Newborn* edited by James B. Hanshaw and John A. Dudgeon. Dr. Alexander J. Schaffer was asked to be the consulting editor for the entire series. Dr. Schaffer coined the term "neonatology" and edited the first clinical textbook of neonatology entitled *Diseases of the Newborn*. For those of us training in the 1970s, this series and Dr. Schaffer's textbook of neonatology provided exciting, up-to-date information that attracted many of us into the subspecialty. Dr. Schaffer's role as "consulting editor" allowed him to select leading scientists and practitioners to serve as editors for each individual volume. As the "consulting editor" *for Neonatology Questions and Controversies*, I had the challenge of identifying the topics and editors for each volume in this series. The six volumes encompass the major issues encountered in the neonatal intensive care unit (newborn lung, fluid and electrolytes, neonatal cardiology and hemodynamics, hematology, immunology and infectious disease, gastroenterology, and neurology). The editors for each volume were challenged to combine discussions of fetal and neonatal physiology with disease pathophysiology and selected controversial topics in clinical care. It is my hope that this series (like *Major Problems in Clinical Pediatrics*) will excite a new generation of trainees to question existing dogma (from my own generation) and seek new information through scientific investigation. I wish to congratulate and thank each of the volume editors (Drs. Bancalari, Oh, Guignard, Baumgart Kleinman, Seri, Ohls, Yoder, Neu and Perlman) for their extraordinary effort and finished products. I also wish to acknowledge Judy Fletcher at Elsevier who conceived the idea for the series and who has been my "editor and friend" throughout my academic career.

Richard A. Polin, MD

Preface

In the past 4 decades, neonatology – collaborating with fetal maternal medicine, pediatric surgery and other pediatric subspecialties – has been remarkably successful in improving the survival of critically ill newborns. Unfortunately, the genetic potential for both optimal physical health and neurodevelopment of too many of these survivors remains unmet, partially due to the long-term effects of preventable stresses occurring in early neonatal life.

Despite burgeoning knowledge that nutritional optimization is a modulator of many of these stresses, nutritional management during the most stressful periods has continued to be overshadowed by other "more critical" aspects of care in the neonate. The major "hot topics" in neonatology continue to focus on lung development, respiratory support measures, neuroprotection of asphyxiated infants, pharmacologic management strategies for infections, and bilirubin metabolism. However, small but important steps are beginning to be made in early initiation of parenteral and enteral feedings in these infants. Nevertheless, we have a long way to go in understanding the actual metabolic capabilities of the critically ill neonate, as well as the digestive absorptive and other physiologic potential of the neonatal gastrointestinal tract.

The recognition that the gastrointestinal tract is much more than an organ of digestion and absorption – also a major conduit of immunologic and endocrine signals that can become "hard wired" into adult life and even into next generations – requires considerable further elucidation. The recent discovery of a "new organ" – the intestinal microflora (or "microbiome"), which is an integral part of the ecosystem that the largest part of the human surface area interacts with – has major implications for optimal nutrition, development and immunologic defenses as well as tolerance.

This unique book incorporates clinical neonatal gastroenterology and nutrition with up-to-date research. It provides the reader with a better understanding of the developmental biology of the gastrointestinal tract, nutritional needs of the premature infant, and methods for supporting these needs. It discusses pathophysiology and treatment of diseases such as necrotizing enterocolitis, cholestatic liver disease, and short bowel syndrome. It also provides a primer for exciting research directions, including the intestinal microbiome, the relationship of intestinal inflammation and barrier dysfunction to intestinal and more generalized disease, tissue engineering, and epigenetic mechanisms of developmental origins of adult health and disease.

Josef Neu, MD

Section I

Scientific Overview and Developmental Perspectives

Chapter 1

Gastrointestinal Development: Morphogenesis and Molecular Mechanisms

Robert K. Montgomery, PhD

Morphogenesis

Molecular Mechanisms

Organ Development

Conclusions

Survival of the newborn human infant depends on a successful transition from the intrauterine to the extrauterine environment. A major factor is the maturation of sufficient gastrointestinal function to provide for adequate nutrition. At birth the gastrointestinal tract is uniquely adapted to the absorption of breast milk and its nutrient components, exclusion of foreign antigens, pathogens, and some xenobiotics, adaptation to the intestinal microflora, and, with the kidney, maintenance of water balance. In the full-term infant, these processes are integrated and support normal growth and development.

Many essential mechanisms are mature at birth, but some, such as bilirubin conjugation and excretion, and hepatic drug metabolism, are only completed in the early post-natal period. The interaction between the initially sterile gastrointestinal tract and the microbiota that colonize it after birth is increasingly being recognized as a crucial component of postnatal development (1, 2). Other mechanisms develop later in the post-natal period, such as esophageal sphincter function and motility, gastric acid and intrinsic factor secretion, gastric motility, intestinal glucose absorption, vitamin B12 and bile salt absorption, synthesis of bile acids and the expansion of the bile acid pool, and the secretory response to bacterial toxins. Pancreatic exocrine function is completed after approximately 6 months of age and endocrine function characterized by insulin release after feeding is also delayed, but for not quite as long.

Detailed descriptions of the morphogenesis of the human gastrointestinal tract are available in standard texts. More extensive discussion of gastrointestinal tract development is provided in several reviews (3–8). This chapter will provide an overview of morphogenesis and focus on the current understanding of the molecular mechanisms of gastrointestinal development. Selected milestones in the anatomic and morphological development of the human gastrointestinal tract are summarized in Table 1-1.

Table 1-1 Developmental Milestones

Event	Time of first expression
Gastrulation	week 3
Gut tube largely closed; liver and pancreas buds	week 4
Growth of intestines into cord	week 7
Intestinal villus formation	week 8
Retraction of intestines into abdominal cavity	week 10
Organ formation complete	week 12
Parietal cells detectable, pancreatic islets appear, bile secretion intestinal enzymes detectable	week 12
Swallowing detectable	week 16–17
Mature motility	week 36

MORPHOGENESIS

Proliferation of cells from the fertilized egg gives rise to the blastocyst. The embryo proper will develop from a compact mass of cells on one side of the blastocyst, called the inner cell mass. It splits into two layers, the epiblast and hypoblast, which form a bilaminar germ disc from which the embryo develops. At the beginning of the third week of gestation, the primitive streak appears as a midline depression in the epiblast near the caudal end of the disc. During gastrulation, epiblast cells detach along the primitive streak and migrate down into the space between the two germ layers.

The process of gastrulation generates the endoderm cells which will form the epithelia lining the gastrointestinal tract. Some of the cells migrating inward through the primitive streak displace the lower germ layer (hypoblast) and form the definitive endoderm. Gastrulation establishes the bilateral symmetry and the dorsal/ventral and craniocaudal axes of the embryo. Formation of the three germ layers brings into proximity groups of cells, which then give rise to the organs of the embryo through inductive interactions. As described below, the molecular mechanisms of many of these processes are now being elucidated.

The gut tube is formed by growth and folding of the embryo. The tissue layers formed during the third week differentiate to form primordia of the major organ systems. A complex process of folding, driven by differential growth of different parts of the embryo, converts the flat germ disc into a three-dimensional structure. As a result, the cephalic, lateral, and caudal edges of the germ disc are brought together along the ventral midline, where the endoderm, mesoderm, and ectoderm layers fuse to the corresponding layer on the opposite side, converting the layers into the gut tube.

Folding of the embryo first forms a closed gut tube at both the cranial and caudal ends. The anterior and posterior ends of the developing gut tube where the infolding occurs are designated the anterior and posterior (or caudal) intestinal portals. Initially, the gut consists of blind-ending cranial and caudal tubes, the foregut and hindgut, separated by the future midgut, which remains open to the yolk sac. As the lateral edges continue to fuse along the ventral midline, the midgut is progressively converted into a tube, while the yolk sac neck is reduced to the vitelline duct. Remnants of this duct occasionally fail to regress and form Meckel's diverticulum.

Three pairs of major arteries develop caudal to the diaphragm to supply regions of the developing abdominal gut. The regions of vascularization from these three arteries provide the anatomical basis for dividing the abdominal gastrointestinal tract into foregut, midgut, and hindgut. The celiac artery is the most superior of the three. It develops branches that vascularize the foregut from the abdominal esophagus to the descending segment of the duodenum, as well as the liver, gall bladder, and pancreas, which are derived from the foregut. The superior mesenteric artery supplies the developing midgut, the intestine from the descending segment of the duodenum to the transverse colon. The inferior mesenteric artery vascularizes the hindgut – the distal portion of the transverse colon, the descending and sigmoid colon, and the rectum. The separately derived inferior end of the anorectal canal is supplied by branches of the iliac arteries.

During the early part of the fourth week, the caudal foregut just posterior to the septum transversum expands slightly to initiate formation of the stomach. Continued expansion gives rise to a spindle-shaped or fusiform region. The dorsal wall of this fusiform expansion of the foregut grows more rapidly than the ventral wall, producing the greater curvature of the stomach during the fifth week. The fundus of the stomach is formed by continued differential expansion of the superior portion of the greater curvature. A rotation of 90° around a craniocaudal axis during the seventh and eighth weeks makes the original left side the ventral surface and the original right side the dorsal surface of the fetal stomach. Thus, the left vagus nerve supplies the ventral wall of the adult stomach and the right vagus innervates the dorsal wall. Additional rotation about a dorsal/ventral axis results in the greater curvature facing slightly caudal and the lesser curvature slightly cranial.

By about the third week of gestation, the gut is a relatively straight tube demarcated into three regions: the foregut, which will give rise to the pharynx, esophagus, stomach, and proximal duodenum; the midgut, which is open ventrally into the yolk sac and will produce the remainder of the duodenum, small intestine and proximal colon; and the hindgut, which will develop into the distal colon and rectum. The hepatic and pancreatic primordia arise at the junction between the foregut and midgut.

The rapid growth of the midgut causes its elongation and rotation. By 5 weeks, the intestine elongates and begins to form a loop which protrudes into the umbilical cord. Shortly thereafter, the ventral pancreatic bud rotates and fuses with the dorsal pancreatic bud. At 7 weeks, the small intestine begins to rotate around the axis of the superior mesenteric artery, moving counterclockwise (viewing the embryo from the ventral surface) approximately 90°. From 9 weeks onward, growth of the intestine forces it to herniate into the umbilical cord. The midgut continues to rotate as it grows, then returns to the abdominal cavity. By about 10 weeks, rotation has completed approximately 180°. By about 11 weeks, rotation has continued an additional 90° to complete 270°, and then the intestine retracts into the abdominal cavity, which has gained in capacity not only by growth, but by regression of the mesonephros and reduced hepatic growth. The control of re-entry has not been elucidated, but it occurs rapidly, with the jejunum returning first and filling the left half of the abdominal cavity, and the ileum filling the right half. The colon enters last, with fixation of the cecum close to the iliac crest and the upward slanting of the ascending and transverse colon across the abdomen to the splenic flexure. Later growth of the colon leads to elongation and establishment of the hepatic flexure and transverse colon. The position of the abdominal organs is completed as the ascending colon attaches to the posterior abdominal wall. This process gives rise to the complex relations of nervous and vascular supply to the adult organs of the gastrointestinal tract. It is essentially completed by 12 weeks of gestation.

The cloaca gives rise to the rectum and urogenital sinus. Early in embryogenesis, the distal hindgut expands to form the cloaca. Between the fourth and sixth weeks, the cloaca is divided into a posterior rectum and anterior primitive urogenital sinus by the growth of the urorectal septum. Thus, the upper and lower parts of the anorectal canal have distinct embryological origins. The original cloacal membrane is divided by the urorectal septum into an anterior urogenital membrane and a posterior anal membrane. The anal membrane separates the endodermal and ectodermal portions of the anorectal canal. The former location of the anal membrane, which breaks down during the eighth week, is marked by the pectinate line in the adult. The distal hindgut gives rise to the upper two-thirds of the anorectal canal, while the ectodermal invagination called the anal pit represents the source of the inferior one-third of the canal. A number of structural anomalies, such as imperforate anus, arise from developmental errors during this process. The pectinate line also marks the separation of the vascular supply of the upper and lower segments of the canal. The upper anorectal canal superior to the pectinate line is served by branches of the inferior mesenteric artery, and veins draining the hindgut. By contrast, the region inferior to the pectinate line is supplied by branches of the internal iliac arteries and veins. The innervation of the anorectal canal also reflects the embryologic origins of the upper and lower portions. The superior portion of the canal is innervated by the inferior mesenteric ganglia and pelvic splanchnic nerves, while the inferior canal is supplied from the inferior rectal nerve.

The liver diverticulum arises as a bud from the most caudal portion of the foregut. During embryogenesis, specification of the liver, biliary tract and pancreas occurs in a temporally regulated pattern. The liver, gall bladder, and pancreas, and their ductal systems, develop from endodermal diverticulae that bud from the duodenum in the fourth to sixth weeks of gestation.

At about 30 days of embryogenesis, the pancreas consists of dorsal and ventral buds which originate from endoderm on opposite sides of the duodenum. The dorsal bud grows more rapidly, while the ventral bud grows away from the duodenum on the elongating common bile duct. As the duodenum grows unequally, torsion occurs and the ventral pancreas is brought dorsad so that it lies adjacent to the dorsal pancreas in the dorsal mesentary of the duodenum; the two primordia thus fuse at about the 7th week. The head and uncinate process of the mature pancreas stem from the ventral primordium, whereas the remainder of the body and tail is derived from the dorsal primordium. Subsequently, the ducts originally serving each bud join to form the duct of Wirsung, although the proximal original duct of the dorsal bud often remains as the accessory duct of Santorini. Structural variants, such as annular pancreas, arise from developmental anomalies during this process.

The prevertebral sympathetic ganglia develop next to the major branches of the descending aorta. The postganglionic sympathetic axons from these ganglia grow out along the arteries and come to innervate the same tissues that the arteries supply with blood. The postganglionic fibers from the celiac ganglia innervate the distal foregut region from the abdominal esophagus to the entrance of the bile duct into the duodenum. Fibers from the superior mesenteric ganglia innervate the midgut, the remaining duodenum, jejunum, ileum, ascending colon, and two-thirds of the transverse colon. The inferior mesenteric ganglia innervate the hindgut, the distal third of the transverse colon, the descending and sigmoid colon, and the upper two-thirds of the anorectal canal.

The vagus nerve and the pelvic splanchnic nerves provide preganglionic parasympathetic innervation to ganglia embedded in the walls of visceral organs. Unlike the sympathetic ganglia, parasympathetic ganglia form close to the organs they innervate and produce only short postganglionic fibers. The central neurons of the parasympathetic pathways reside in either the brain or the spinal cord. Preganglionic parasympathetic fibers associated with cranial nerve X form the vagus nerve, which extends into the abdomen, where these fibers synapse with the parasympathetic ganglia in target organs, including the liver and the gastrointestinal tract proximal to the colon. Parasympathetic preganglionic fibers arising from the spinal cord form the pelvic splanchnic nerves, which innervate ganglia in the walls of the descending and sigmoid colon and rectum. Neural crest cells that migrate into the developing intestinal tract beginning at week seven form a critical component of the enteric nervous system. Genetic abnormalities in this process can lead to the development of Hirschsprung's disease, as described below.

MOLECULAR MECHANISMS

There are three major developmental milestones in formation of the gastrointestinal tract. First is the initial specification of the endoderm. Second is formation and patterning of the gut tube that establishes the anterior-posterior axis and the boundaries between different organs. Third is the initiation of formation of organs that are outgrowths of the gut tube, such as liver and pancreas. Experiments in model organisms have identified families of genes involved in endoderm specification that are highly conserved in evolution, while other genes may be specific to vertebrate gut development. The epithelium of the gastrointestinal tract is derived from the endoderm, one of the three embryonic germ layers that originate during gastrulation of the embryo. Studies in model organisms such as *C. elegans*, *Drosophila*, *Xenopus*, zebrafish, and mice have identified some of the critical molecular regulators of endoderm formation (6–9). Mouse models in which the identified genes have been knocked out now suggest the basis for developmental disorders of the human gastrointestinal tract such as pyloric stenosis, atresia, and imperforate anus (10).

Specification of the Endoderm

Specification of the endoderm can be traced to the earliest stages of embryo formation. Classical experiments demonstrated that explants of chick embryos prior to gastrulation were capable of gastrointestinal development, indicating that their fate had already been specified. Chick endoderm explanted prior to formation of the gut tube expresses in vitro the molecular markers that would normally develop in vivo, consistent with early specification (11). Evidence is accumulating in support of the hypothesis that the original patterning of the endoderm is cell autonomous, but that full development of the organs requires a reciprocal interaction between the endoderm and mesoderm. Gene families that act to specify endoderm have now been identified in a number of model organisms. One class of genes encodes transcription factors that directly activate target genes. A second class encodes signaling molecules that mediate cellular interactions. At least some of the transcription factors involved in specification of the endoderm continue to be expressed in the gastrointestinal tract throughout development, such as the forkhead-related factors (*Fox* genes) and GATA factors. Signaling pathways, such as those mediated by members of the TGFβ superfamily of growth factors, including TGFβ and the bone morphogenetic proteins (BMP), and the hedgehog pathways, act at different times and in different locations to regulate GI development. The transcription factor sox-17 has also been shown to be critical for the early development of endoderm in mice, although its later role is unknown (12). Recently, Notch signaling has emerged as an important regulator in gastrointestinal development.

It remains unclear whether a single 'master gene' initiates the formation of the endoderm, setting in motion the process of gastrointestinal development. In some of the model systems, genes have been identified that appear to be both necessary and sufficient to specify endoderm, for example the *mixer* gene in *Xenopus* (13). The mouse gene *mixl1* has a critical role in differentiation of embryonic cells into definitive endoderm (14). In other model organisms, genes have been identified that are necessary, but may not be sufficient.

Studies in model systems have identified early steps in the induction of endoderm. Mouse endoderm is derived from the anterior primitive streak of the epiblast.

An early critical regulator of endodermal development is nodal, a ligand of the TGFβ superfamily. Nodal is expressed at the mouse organizing center, or node, in the blastoderm. Embryos lacking nodal fail to gastrulate or form the definitive endoderm. Similarly zebrafish embryos lacking nodal homologues fail to form endoderm (15). Conversely, expression of a constituitively active TGFβ receptor drives embryonic cells to become endoderm. TGF signaling is transmitted through a conserved set of intermediary proteins, the Smad proteins. Smad2 is essential for endoderm development, as germ line knockouts fail to form hindgut endoderm (16), while mutant forms give rise to various foregut defects (17). FoxA2, also essential for normal endoderm development, is a downstream target of nodal signaling via Smad2. Smad2 and Smad3 coordinately regulate development of the mouse endoderm, with differential effects on foregut and hindgut development. This Smad signaling is also required for liver development, as studies suggest that the critical liver gene Hex is a direct target, whose expression is reduced or absent in animals with defective Smad expression (17).

From its earliest stages, the endoderm is in close apposition to mesoderm throughout the gastrointestinal tract. Tissue recombination experiments have shown that patterning of the endoderm and its differentiation into separate organs results from signaling between the mesoderm and the endoderm (18). The earliest identified step in anterior/posterior patterning in mouse endoderm requires signaling from mesoderm to endoderm by fibroblast growth factor 4 (FGF-4) (19). Other members of the FGF family and their receptors are critical in liver development. Three other important gene families critical for mesoderm/endoderm signaling are the hedgehogs, the BMPs, and the *hox* genes.

Two GATA transcription factor genes are essential in specification of the cells which give rise to the intestinal epithelium of *C. elegans*, while a *Drosophila* GATA factor is encoded by the gene *serpent*, previously demonstrated to be required for differentiation of gut endoderm. Three members of the GATA family are expressed in vertebrate intestine. Distinct functions for GATA-4, -5, and -6 in intestinal epithelial cell proliferation and differentiation have been suggested, but their role in early development of the mammalian intestine remains unresolved. In addition to the GATA factors, members of the forkhead-related (*Fox*) family and members of the Wnt/Tcf signaling pathway are critical regulators of endoderm formation. Members of the TGFβ superfamily critical in the initiation of endoderm formation have been identified in vertebrates. A scaffolding molecule important in the TGF pathway, ELF3, is also required, as null mice completely lack intestinal endoderm (20).

Many transcription factors initially identified as liver-specific have key roles in the intestine. When analyzed in mouse development, several of these transcription factors have been found to be expressed in patterns suggesting that they may also regulate intestinal development. For example, Hepatic Nuclear Factor 3β (HNF3β–now FoxA2) has been shown to be critical for the earliest differentiation of the gastrointestinal tract and continues to be expressed in the adult progeny of the endoderm (21). Homozygous null mutants of HNF3β do not form a normal primitive streak which gives rise to the gut tube and other structures. HNF3β is critical to formation of the foregut and midgut, but not the hindgut (22). Multiple members of this family have been identified, some of which display intestine-enriched or intestine-specific expression. One of the family members *Foxl1*, normally expressed in the intestinal mesoderm, is a critical mediator of epithelial/mesenchymal interactions. Its elimination led to abnormal epithelial cell proliferation and aberrant intestinal development (23). Its action is mediated through expression of proteoglycans that act as co-receptors for WNT and thus activate the WNT/β-catenin pathway regulating cell proliferation (24). Zaret and co-workers have presented a model in which FoxA2 and GATA act to open up endodermal DNA, making binding sites accessible in preparation for later binding of the transcription factors that regulate cell-specific genes (25). Thus, it appears likely that during intestinal development multiple members of the *Fox* family interact in a complex mechanism which remains to be elucidated.

Several mouse homeobox genes related to *Drosophila caudal* are expressed specifically in the intestine. One, *Cdx-1*, is restricted to the adult intestine, but is expressed widely in the developing embryo. Another, *Cdx-2*, is expressed in visceral endoderm of the early embryo, but restricted to the intestine at later stages. Forced expression of *Cdx-2* will induce differentiation in an intestinal cell line that does not normally differentiate (26), while ectopic expression of *Cdx-2* in stomach tissue results in development of intestine-like tissue (27). *Cdx-2* is clearly a critical intestine-specific differentiation factor, but its role in early development of the intestine remains unclear.

Formation of the Gut Tube

The gut tube is formed from a layer of endoderm by a process of folding that begins at the anterior and posterior ends of the embryo. Reciprocal signaling between endoderm and mesoderm continues to be critical to the developmental process.

A key mechanism that has emerged as a mediator of endoderm/mesoderm interactions in the organization of the gastrointestinal tract involves the sonic (Shh) and Indian hedgehog (Ihh) signaling proteins. Both Shh and Ihh play critical roles in anterior/posterior patterning and concentric patterning of the developing gastrointestinal tract, at least in part through their role in development of muscle from the mesoderm (28). One target of this signaling pathway is a second family of signaling molecules, the BMPs (29, 30).

Shh is first detectable in the primitive endoderm of the embryo, later in the endoderm of the anterior and posterior intestinal portals, and subsequently throughout the gut endoderm and in the adult crypt region. BMP4 is expressed in the mesoderm adjacent to the intestinal portals and can be induced ectopically in the visceral mesoderm by Shh protein. The endoderm of the intestinal portals is the source of Shh; the portal regions can act as polarizing centers if transplanted. Shh also induces the expression of *hox* genes. Producing abnormal epithelial cell proliferation later in development probably has its effect through reduced expression of BMP-2 and BMP-4. Shh is a critical regulator of both foregut and hindgut development, as null mice display foregut anomalies such as esophageal atresia and tracheo-esophageal fistula and hindgut anomalies such as persistent cloaca (31, 32). Furthermore, the transcription factors Gli2 and Gli3, which are transducers of Shh signaling, also are required. Mice in which Gli3 expression is reduced on a Gli2 null background display esophageal atresia and tracheo-esophageal fistula (31). It has also been demonstrated that mutant mice that lack Gli2 or Gli3 exhibit imperforate anus with recto-urethral fistula and anal stenosis (33). The patterning role is apparently completed by mid-gestation in mice, as hedgehog antibody blocking experiments initiated at embryonic day 12.5 did not affect intestinal morphology. However, crypt proliferation and lipid metabolism were disrupted, indicating additional roles for hh at later stages of development (34).

ORGAN DEVELOPMENT

Patterning

In *Drosophila*, the large family of homeotic genes is expressed in the body in a precise anterior to posterior order. The homeotic genes encode transcription factors, incorporating a conserved homeobox sequence, which regulate segmentation and pattern formation. Vertebrates have homologous *hox* genes which play important roles in the formation of distinctly delineated regions of the brain and skeleton. There are four copies of the set of vertebrate genes, *hoxa, b, c,* and *d,* which form groups of paralogues, e.g., *hoxa-1, hoxb-1,* and *hoxd-1.* Within each group, the genes are expressed in the embryo in an anterior to posterior sequence of regions with overlapping boundaries, e.g., *hoxa-1* in the occipital vertebrae to *hoxa-11* in the caudal vertebrae.

A detailed study of the developing chick hindgut demonstrated a correlation between the boundaries of expression of *hoxa-9, -10, -11,* and *-13* in the mesoderm and the location of morphologic boundaries. Regional differences in expression of homeobox genes in the developing mouse intestine have also been demonstrated (35). Interference with the expression of specific *hox* genes produces organ-specific gastrointestinal defects. Disruption of *hoxc-4* gave rise to esophageal obstruction due to abnormal epithelial cell proliferation and abnormal muscle development (36). Alteration of the expression pattern of *hoxc-8* to a more anterior location caused distorted development of the gastric epithelium (37). Loss of mesenchymal *hoxa-5* alters gastric epithelial cell phenotype (38). Mice with disrupted *hoxd-12* and *hoxd-13* genes display defects in formation of the anal musculature (39). A more extensive deletion of a complex of *hoxd* genes (*hoxd-4, d-8, d-9, d-10,* and *d-11*) eliminated the ileocaecal valve (40). Expression of the human homologues of a number of homeobox genes has also been shown to be region-specific (41). These data indicate that the *hox* genes are critical early regulators of proximal to distal, organ-specific patterning. Ectopic expression of *hox* genes in chicken has suggested that morphology of the intestine may be altered (29, 30). The *caudal* genes are members of a divergent homeobox gene family and regulate the anterior margins of *hox* gene expression as well as having gastrointestinal-specific roles. Almost all of the *hox* genes analyzed are expressed in mesodermal tissue, probably affecting endodermal development via epithelial/mesenchymal interactions (42).

Regional Specification

Organs such as the stomach are first identifiable by thickening in the mesodermal layer. Early in the process of patterning, BMP4 is expressed throughout the mesoderm. Sonic hedgehog is expressed in the endoderm and is an upstream regulator of BMP4. The patterning of BMP4 expression in the mesoderm regulates growth of the stomach mesoderm and determines the sidedness of the stomach. Location of the pyloric sphincter is dependent upon the interaction of BMP4 expression and inhibitors of that expression (43). BMP signaling independently regulates the genes *Sox9* and *Nkx2.5* to specify the pyloric sphincter (44). Patterning of the concentric muscle layer structure is dependent upon Shh signaling that induces formation of lamina propria and submucosa, while inhibiting smooth muscle and enteric neuron development near the endoderm (28, 45).

Esophagus

Morphogenesis and Differentiation

The human esophagus can be identified as a distinct structure early in embryogenesis (4 weeks), and elongates during subsequent development relatively more rapidly than the fetus as a whole (46). At 10 weeks, ciliated columnar epithelium appears in the esophagus. Stratified squamous epithelium replaces it around 20–25 weeks, a process which begins in the mid-esophagus and proceeds both caudad and cephalad (47).

Hitchcock et al. have studied the esophageal musculature and innervation of the esophagus in fetuses of 8–20 weeks gestation, and in infants 22–161 weeks of age (48). The circular muscle is present at 8 weeks, but the longitudinal muscle does not become apparent until approximately 13 weeks of gestation. In fetuses, the thickness of the muscularis externa increases linearly from 8 weeks to term (40 weeks), then growth slows postnatally.

Cellular proliferation occurs in the basal zone of the esophagus, from which cells move toward the lumen and differentiate. Based on their proliferative characteristics, candidate stem cells have been tentatively identified in the basal layer, although there are no specific markers and the cells have not been isolated or further characterized (49). Early progenitor cells of the esophagus express the p53-related protein p63. Targeted deletion of p63 indicates that it plays a critical role in the development of normal esophageal epithelia and controls the commitment of early stem cells into basal cell progeny and the maintenance of the basal cells (50). The homeodomain transcription factor Nkx2.1 is expressed in the anterior foregut along the dorsoventral boundary which will separate the esophagus and trachea. In null mice, there is a failure of septation, leading to the formation of a common lumen connecting the pharanx to the stomach, a condition similar to tracheoesophageal fistula (51).

Stomach

Morphogenesis

The morphological and histological development of the stomach is complete at term. The fetal stomach grows in a linear fashion from 13 to 39 weeks, and the characteristic anatomical features (greater curvature, lesser curvature, fundus, body and pylorus) can be identified by 14 weeks. Abnormal ultrasound images can identify the presence of congenital anomalies. Failure to delineate the fetal stomach ultrasonographically in the second trimester indicates esophageal atresia, and an enlarged fetal stomach may herald the presence of gastric outlet obstruction or duodenal atresia (52). Pyloric stenosis is an anomaly of stomach development. Vanderwinden et al. (53) suggested that infantile hypertrophic pyloric stenosis (IHPS) is associated with abnormal neuronal nitric oxide synthase-1. A mouse model was consistent with this hypothesis (54), but a genetic basis has not yet been established. Recent studies have found an increased risk of stenosis in carriers of a polymorphism in the promoter of nitric oxide synthetase (55).

Both the Wnt signaling pathway and hedgehog signaling regulate stomach development. The divergent homeobox gene *Barx1* is strongly expressed in the mesenchyme of the prospective stomach during organogenesis. Barx1 directs expression of two antagonists of Wnt signaling. Inhibition of the Wnt signaling pathway allows development of stomach specific epithelium. In the absence of Barx1, the epithelium takes on more intestine-like characteristics (56). GATA4 deficiency is associated with impaired differentiation into glandular, but not squamous epithelium, reflected in an increased expression of Shh in GATA4-deficient cells. GATA4 may be involved in the gastric epithelial response to BMP signaling (57). An orphan member of the steroid receptor superfamily, COUP-TFII, is required for radial and anteroposterior patterning of the developing stomach. COUP-TFII is a downstream target of hedgehog signaling, a previously identified regulator of gastrointestinal patterning (58).

Detailed studies of the development of the mouse stomach from Leblond and co-workers have established that the epithelial cells of the gastric pits arise from stem cells located in the neck region. As these stem cells divide, they produce cell populations which move upward and populations which move downward (59, 60). Parietal cell lineage ablation experiments suggested that the balance between parietal, pit, and zymogen cells is maintained by interactions among the cell lineages (61). Progenitor cells have also been identified in the human stomach epithelium (62). Expression of Musashi1, previously suggested to be a marker for small intestinal stem cells, has also been implicated as a marker for the progenitor cells of the human antrum (63).

Liver

Morphogenesis

The liver diverticulum emerges from the most caudal portion of the foregut just distal to the stomach about the fourth week of gestation. It is first detectable as a thickening of the ventral duodenum. Hepatogenesis is initiated through an instructive induction of ventral foregut endoderm by cardiac mesoderm. A series of elegant experiments have identified a number of signaling pathways involved in the complex process of development of the liver (5). The appearance of mRNA for the liver-specific protein albumin in endodermal cells of the liver diverticulum is one of the earliest indications of hepatocyte induction. The immediate signal is provided by fibroblast growth factors from the cardiac mesoderm that bind to specific receptors in the endoderm (64). In fact, cultured endoderm can be induced to form primitive hepatoblasts in vitro by incubation with FGF (64). Response to the inductive FGF factors requires the establishment of competence in the endoderm. The onset of *Foxa* gene expression in the endoderm precedes hepatic induction by FGF. Specification by *Foxa1* and *Foxa2* has now been shown to be an essential step in the initiation of liver development; in the absence of both *Foxa1* and *Foxa2* in the enterocytes, the liver bud does not form, although the cardiac mesenchyme is normal (65). After formation of the liver bud, hepatocyte growth factor is required for continued hepatocyte proliferation (66). The hepatic diverticulum grows into the septum transversum and gives rise to the liver cords, which become the hepatocytes. During this process, a combination of signals from the mesodermal cells of the septum transversum, including BMP, is necessary for liver development (67). During migration of the liver endoderm cells into the septum transversum, they are surrounded by endothelial precursor cells which provide another critical factor. In the absence of blood vessel formation, the growth of liver epithelium is impaired, demonstrating that liver morphogenesis requires this interaction with blood vessel endothelium. The effect is due to the endothelial cells themselves, not circulating factors in the blood (68).

Biliary epithelial cells are thought to originate from bipotential hepatoblasts capable of differentiation into hepatocytes or biliary cells, but their origin has been much debated. Transplantation experiments and isolation of multipotential stem cells from fetal mouse liver are consistent with a hepatoblast origin, but definitive lineage analysis remains to be done (69). Morphogenesis of the intrahepatic bile ducts is similar in humans and in rodent models. Initially, a subset of hepatoblasts, considered to be biliary precursor cells, located close to the portal vessel mesenchyme express biliary-specific cytokeratins. A single layer of these cells then forms a continuous ring, called the ductal plate, around the portal mesenchyme. The ductal plate becomes partly bilayered and focal dilatations appear in the bilayer, giving rise to the bile ducts. The remainder of the ductal plate regresses. In humans, the ductal plate appears to regress by apoptosis (70). The formation of the bile ducts occurs along a gradient from the hilum to the periphery of the liver. The human liver primordium that emerges from the endoderm consists of a cranial and a caudal portion. The caudal portion gives rise also to the extrahepatic bile ducts and gallbladder (69). Secretion of bile into the duodenum begins during the fourth month.

Delineation of the molecular regulation of ductal plate formation has identified a number of key factors. The transcription factor HNF6 regulates the number of cells entering the biliary epithelial cell pathway, as well as their location near the portal mesenchyme (71). A mesenchymal transcription factor, FoxF1, is required for gallbladder development (72). Targeted deletion of HNF1β causes developmental abnormalities in the intrahepatic bile ducts (71). There are a number of human diseases called ductal plate malformations. Anomalies of portal mesenchyme and portal blood vessels in these diseases suggest a functional interaction among the components of the portal tract. Alagille syndrome, associated with haploinsufficiency of Jagged-1, a Notch receptor ligand, provides evidence for such an interaction. Liver histopathology demonstrates intrahepatic duct paucity and cholestasis. An increased number of arteries and fibrosis are observed in portal tracts devoid of bile ducts. Mouse models do not completely recapitulate the human syndrome, but a homozygous Notch2 null mouse does display a spectrum of abnormalities similar to the human disease (73). These data indicate that development of the biliary tract is a complex interaction among mesenchyme, ducts, and blood vessels.

Pancreas

Morphogenesis

Morphogenesis of the human pancreas begins at about 30 days of gestation. Formation of the pancreas is initiated by the emergence of dorsal and ventral pancreatic buds on opposite sides of the foregut. As these epithelial buds enlarge, a treelike ductal system develops by growth and branching. As the gut tube grows and rotates, the two pancreatic buds come together and fuse at about the seventh week of gestation. Individual endocrine cells are identifiable initially, with islets becoming established later. Around 20 weeks gestation, enzyme activity is detectable in the exocrine pancreas and secretion begins around the fifth month, with each enzyme developing in an individual pattern (74).

Development of the pancreas has provided one of the classic examples of epithelial-mesenchymal interactions. Previous investigations showed that growth and differentiation of the pancreas required the presence of mesenchyme, although both endocrine and exocrine cells develop from the foregut endoderm. Analysis of the development of separated endoderm and mesenchyme under different conditions indicated that the 'default pathway' of pancreatic differentiation leads to endocrine cells, while a combination of extracellular matrix and mesenchymal factors is required for complete organogenesis (75).

The dorsal pancreatic bud arises in an area where Shh expression is repressed by factors from the notochord (76). Competence to respond to instructive signals depends on the prior expression of endoderm factors, such as HNF1β, HNF3a and β (FoxA1 and A2), HNF4a, HNF6 and GATA4, 5, and 6 (77). Several of these factors directly control Pdx-1 expression. The prepancreatic endoderm expresses two parahox genes, *pdx-1* and *hlx9*. Expression of the *pdx-1* gene in cells of the pancreatic bud is one of the earliest signs of pancreas development, and *pdx-1*-expressing progenitor cells give rise to all pancreatic cells. Indicating that different factors control dorsal and ventral pancreatic specification, *hlx9* expression precedes pdx-1 in the dorsal prepancreatic endoderm. In Hlx9 null mice, the dorsal prepancreatic endoderm does not express Pdx-1, and formation of the dorsal bud is never initiated. The ventral lobe generates all four types of hormone-producing cells in islets of Langerhans, but in significantly reduced numbers (78, 79).

The PDX-1 protein was found to be expressed in the epithelium of the duodenum immediately surrounding the pancreatic buds, as well as in the epithelium of the buds themselves. Examination of an initial *pdx-1* knockout mouse indicated that while development of the rest of the gastrointestinal tract and the rest of the animal was normal, the pancreas did not develop. A second group, which independently made a *pdx-1* null mouse, found that the dorsal pancreas bud did form, but its development was arrested (80). The defect due to the *pdx* knockout was restricted to the epithelium, as the mesenchymal cells maintained normal developmental potential. In addition, the most proximal part of the duodenum in the null mice was abnormal, forming a vesicle-like structure lined with cuboidal epithelium, rather than villi lined by columnar cells, indicating that *pdx-1* influences the differentiation of cells in an area larger than that which gives rise to the pancreas, consistent with the earlier delineated domain of expression. A case of human congenital pancreatic agenesis has been demonstrated to result from a single nucleotide deletion in the human *pdx-1* gene (81).

Notch signaling determines which cells will differentiate into endocrine cells. Endocrine cell precursors transiently express neurogenin3 (ngn3), which is inhibited by Notch signaling. Mice lacking ngn3 fail to form any endocrine cells, while overexpression of ngn3 causes the differentiation of the entire pancreas into endocrine cells. Cells in which ngn3 is extinguished by Notch signaling can become exocrine cells. An additional factor, P48, is required to determine an exocrine fate. In mice lacking P48 the exocrine pancreas is absent although islets form. Expression of ngn3 determines an exocrine cell fate, but the timing and interaction of other critical factors that determine the four endocrine cell types remain unclear (77). A more detailed description of current understanding of the molecular mechanisms of pancreatic development is presented in several review articles (4, 77, 79).

Small Intestine

Morphogenesis and Differentiation

The ontogeny of the small intestine can be thought of as proceeding through three successive phases: morphogenesis and cell proliferation, cell differentiation, and cellular and functional maturation (82). By 13 weeks of gestation, organogenesis of the human intestine is complete (83).

It is well established that, by morphological and biochemical criteria, the human fetal intestine is more mature at term than that of commonly examined mammalian models. In contrast to the well-studied rodents, development of the human intestine is largely completed well before birth, around the end of the first trimester, and by the 22nd week the absorptive epithelial cells resemble those of the adult intestine. Human absorptive cells at mid-gestation resemble those of the 5–15 day suckling rat, while the proximal human absorptive cells at 22 weeks resemble those of the weaned rat (84).

The process of morphogenesis occurs in human fetal intestine very much as it does in the rat (84). Mucosal remodeling and villus formation proceed in a cranial-caudal direction, beginning at 9–10 weeks. The earliest indication is the appearance of subepithelial aggregations of mesenchymal cells associated with projections into the central lumen of the overlying stratified epithelium. Studies of mouse PDGF and PDGF receptor knockouts suggest the presence of an organizing center in the mesoderm of the nascent villi that may regulate their formation (85). Distinctive junctional complexes appear between cells in the deeper layers of the stratified epithelium during the period of villus formation. Within the mesenchymal invaginations, smooth muscle cells and blood vessels appear as development progresses. Smooth-muscle-specific protein markers have been reported in the human fetal jejunum as early as 8 weeks (86). There are few data on human muscle development. The available information on intestinal muscle development has been reviewed by McHugh (87). Apparent abnormalities of muscle morphogenesis in children have been reported (88). Columnar epithelium initially lines only the apices of the developing villi, but appears along the sides as the villi mature. After 10 weeks, only the intervillus epithelium remains stratified. In all levels of the stratified epithelium, mitotic figures are abundant. Occasional mitoses are seen on villi until 16 weeks, but by 10–12 weeks most mitotic figures are restricted to the intervillus regions and developing crypts. Crypts first appear as solid cords of epithelial cells, but by 12 weeks display a small lumen lined by undifferentiated simple columnar cells. Between 17 and 20 weeks, the first indications of muscularis mucosa develop near the base of the crypts (83). Little information is available on mechanisms of vascularization. Analysis of mice with a targeted gene disruption has demonstrated that a chemokine receptor is necessary for normal vascularization of the gastrointestinal tract (89). Prior to villus formation at 9–10 weeks, the stratified epithelium contains undifferentiated absorptive cells, goblet cells, and enteroendocrine cells. Paneth cells are observed at the base of developing crypts at 11–12 weeks. Paneth cells provide elements of innate immunity in the intestine. The defensins secreted by Paneth cells are important in host defense from microbial pathogens; their deficiency may play a role in the pathophysiology of Crohn's disease (90). All other epithelial cell types known to occur in adult human intestine appear by the beginning of the second trimester (83). By 12 weeks, 13 morphologically distinctive types of enteroendocrine cells are identifiable (83). In addition to the four major cell lineages, M cells, unique cells restricted to domes of epithelium overlying lymphoid follicles of maturing Peyer's patches, are present by 17 weeks (83). Available data indicate that M cells arise from the same intestinal stem cells as the other lineages (91). Caveolated or tuft cells are identified by 16 weeks of gestation.

Stem Cells

Since the definitive study by Cheng and Leblond in 1974 (92), it has been accepted that the small intestinal crypts contain stem cells that give rise to the four cell lineages present in the intestinal epithelium (93, 94). Proliferative cells are restricted to crypts early in development of the intestine. Presumably a subset of these cells represents the stem cell compartment, but little is known of the early stages of stem cell development. Studies using irradiation to measure the regenerative capacity of the gut have led to the estimated location of the stem cell at cell position four above the murine crypt base and an estimated number of 3–5 stem cells per crypt. The stem cells produce a transit cell population which, after additional divisions, gives rise to all of the cell lineages (95, 96). An analysis by Bjerknes and Cheng indicated that the crypts in mouse intestine contained a population of short-lived lineage-committed progenitor cells (lasting for days) and a population of long-lived progenitor cells (lasting months), as well as pluripotential stem cells (97). It is unclear when the definitive stem cells become established during development. In mice and humans crypts that originally are polyclonal become monoclonal, that is, all the descendent cells within the crypt arise from a single stem cell during subsequent development for reasons as yet unclear (98, 99). As the intestine increases in size during development, crypts increase in numbers by fission, probably as a result of reaching a limiting size, a process that continues more slowly during adult life.

Considerable progress has been made in recent years in understanding regulation of the small intestinal stem cell and of cell fate determination. Although several studies suggested that multipotent stem cells from other tissues, especially the bone marrow, could contribute to the epithelium of the small intestine (100), careful analysis indicates that, at best, this is an extremely rare event, if it occurs at all (101). However, what does occur is incorporation of cells originating from transplanted bone marrow cells into the pericryptal fibroblast population (102). Thus, it is possible that such transplanted cells influence intestinal stem or progenitor cells through epithelial/mesenchymal signaling.

ROLE OF WNT SIGNALING

Elucidation of the molecular basis of stem cell regulation and subsequent cell lineage allocation began with knockout of the *Tcf-4* gene, an important mediator in the intestinal Wnt signaling pathway. Wnt proteins are secreted glycoproteins with roles in differentiation and organogenesis of numerous tissues (103). Tcf-4 null mice lost proliferating epithelial cells late in gestation, demonstrating that Tcf-4 was a critical stem cell regulator (104, 105). When cells bind Wnt, β-catenin is released from an intracellular complex with APC and activates Tcf-4, resulting in cell proliferation. In the absence of Wnt signal, Tcf-4 acts as an inhibitor and cells differentiate. Two groups have examined the effects of inhibiting Wnt signaling using the inhibitor *dickkopf* (DKK) to block the cell surface receptor, either in transgenic mice or using a viral vector. If Wnt signaling is blocked by expression of DKK, proliferation ceases and crypts disappear. If the inhibitor is removed, proliferation resumes, and crypts regenerate (106). This suggests that Wnt signaling regulates stem cell proliferation, but is not necessary for stem cell survival, at least in the short term. Conversely, elimination of APC, which normally sequesters β-catenin in the cytoplasm, in conditional knockout mice led to nuclear localization of β-catenin, resulting in activation of Wnt signaling throughout the epithelium. All of the epithelial cells of both crypt and villus were transformed into proliferating, undifferentiated cells. Furthermore, expression of extracellular matrix components by the mesenchyme was also affected by the loss of APC in the epithelium (107). A recent paper in which APC was inactivated using a somewhat different approach, also found that the proliferative compartment was dramatically expanded at the expense of differentiated villus cells. In addition, the Paneth cell compartment was expanded, with increased expression of defensin genes driven by Wnt signaling (108). A similar function of Wnt signaling was reported by van Es et al. (109). These observations suggest that Wnt signaling separately drives both a stem cell program and, in addition, a Paneth cell maturation program. The mechanism, however, is unclear, as the available data suggest that the goblet and Paneth cells are derived from the same lineage (110).

The crypt epithelium itself secretes Wnt-6 and -9b. An extensive analysis of mRNA expression patterns revealed the receptors frizzled-5 and -6 in crypt epithelium, while the surrounding mesenchyme synthesized the receptor antagonist sFRP-1. Cells in the villus lamina propria expressed mRNA for Wnt-2b, -4, and -5a (111). Clevers and co-workers have suggested a model in which the crypt epithelium maintains a gradient of Wnt factors, inducing cell proliferation, and, as the cells migrate upward, levels of Wnt factor decrease, leading to a cessation of cell proliferation and entrance into the differentiation pathways (112). The recent data are consistent with this model, in which a complex array of Wnts, Wnt receptors, and Wnt antagonists regulates the small intestinal stem cells and proliferation and differentiation of epithelial cells.

In addition, numerous cellular proteins, whose roles are still being elucidated, are involved in the Wnt signaling process (103). EphB2 and EphB3 were identified as downstream targets of Tcf-4 and shown to be critical for regulation of epithelial cell migration. The Eph and ephrin proteins are transmembrane signaling proteins important in cell-cell adhesion and repulsion. In mice null for both EphB2 and EphB3, Paneth cells migrate up the villi, rather than moving to the crypt base. Consistent with this observation, when β-catenin, upstream of EphB3, is knocked out, the Paneth cells are also mislocalized (113). These data suggest that maturation of Paneth cells is cell autonomous and not a result of their position in the crypts, which depends upon Eph/ephrin signaling. Apparently, the lack of proper signaling does not disrupt the overall cytodifferentiation and villus formation during fetal development, suggesting that this process is dependent upon other mechanisms.

BMP SIGNALING PATHWAY

At least two members of the bone morphogenetic protein family of TGFβ-related factors, BMP4 and BMP2, have been implicated in development of the intestine at different times (114). They are synthesized by mesenchymal cells and act through the BMP receptor 1 (BMPR1). Mesenchymal cells in the adult lamina propria secrete BMP4 (45). During villus formation, a high level of *bmp4* mRNA is expressed within the nascent villi, but not in the mesenchyme underlying the proliferative cells in the intervillus regions. In mature villi, BMP4 protein expression was strong in the intervillus mesenchyme, while response to BMP signaling was predominantly in the differentiated villus epithelial cells. Transgenic mice in which BMP signaling was blocked were normal until about 3 weeks of age. At 4 weeks of age, ectopic crypts form within villi, suggesting that stem cells have migrated out of the crypts. These ectopic crypts generated Paneth, goblet, enteroendocrine, and absorptive cells. The resulting aberrant structures appear similar to those observed in familial juvenile polyposis syndrome, indicating a role for disrupted BMP signaling in this disease (45). Aberrant crypt formation following BMP disruption has also been reported by He et al., who suggest that Wnt signaling is necessary, but not sufficient, to regulate stem cell proliferation. Their data indicate that Wnt and BMP signals are integrated through phosphoinositide-3 (PI3) and Akt kinases to maintain the stem cell compartment (115).

The stem cells have been thought to reside in a relatively fixed position in the crypts, constrained by the factors that constitute their niche. If the stem cells can move in the epithelium when BMP signaling is blocked, this suggests that their location depends on a response to the signal, or probably a gradient of the signal. Since both BMP and response were observed primarily in the villus, these data also raise questions about how the signal could affect cells in the crypt. Finally, the morphological changes were observed in the fourth postnatal week, after the establishment of the mature intestinal villus and crypt architecture, suggesting that unknown, developmentally regulated factors are also involved.

LINEAGE DETERMINATION

The four cell lineages of the small intestine arise from the stem cell. A number of different approaches have identified Notch signaling as a key step in lineage specification. Constitutively active Notch1 eliminates goblet, enteroendocrine, and Paneth lineages, while increasing the proliferating cell population. This Notch activation upregulated Hes-1 and repressed Math1 and ngn3, confirming the role of Notch in lineage allocation (116). Elimination of Notch1 signaling by deletion of a key intermediate causes hyperplasia of the goblet cells at the expense of proliferating progenitor cells (117). Similarly, the use of soluble inhibitors of γ-secretase, which blocks the activation of Notch signaling, increases the number of goblet cells in the small intestine (118, 119). It has also been reported that in the developing intestine, Notch signals cause a reversible arrest of morphogenesis, with a depletion of progenitor cells, while in the adult Notch affects cell fate decisions, without altering morphogenesis (120). Key roles for Math1, Hes1, and Ngn3, all known targets of Notch signaling, have been established. Knockout of Math1, a transcription factor important in lineage determination in neural cells, eliminates Paneth cells, goblet cells, and enteroendocrine cells, leaving only the absorptive cells (121). Thus Math1 is critical for establishing the secretory lineage. Math1 is thought to be repressed by the expression of another transcription factor, Hes1, that is extinguished in the secretory lineage, but continues to be expressed in the early stages of the absorptive cell lineage. In Hes1 null mice, elevated levels of endocrine cells are found in both the intestine and pancreas, indicating that Hes1 functions as an inhibitor of the endocrine lineage (122). Secretory precursor cells first express both Math1 and the transcription factor Gfi1, then the lineage separates into an enteroendocrine lineage expressing Gfi1 and Ngn3 and a lineage that gives rise to Paneth cells and goblet cells expressing Math1, in which expression of Gfi1 is extinguished. Thus, the current model is that Notch signaling between adjacent cells increases expression

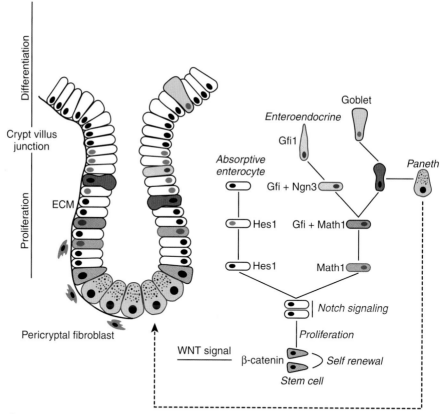

Figure 1-1 Diagram of the events in small intestinal stem cell differentiation and lineage allocation, showing the key genes expressed.

of Hes. Elevated Hes inhibits Math1 expression and these cells become absorptive cells. In cells with low Hes expression, Math1 is upregulated and these cells enter the secretory lineage, enteroendocrine cells expressing Gfi1, while Gfi1 is extinguished in the lineage giving rise to goblet and Paneth cells (Fig. 1-1). Hes1 is also required for enteroendocrine cell formation in the stomach and pancreas, as well as in the small intestine. Although required for goblet cell formation in the colon, KLF4 is not required for goblet cells in the small intestine (123). In contrast to the effects of lineage ablation in the stomach, ablation of the Paneth cell lineage in small intestine did not affect the other cell lineages (124). An interesting recent report describes a patient with severe enterocolitis and the apparent absence of Paneth, goblet, and enteroendocrine cells. There is a striking similarity to the transgenic mouse model with a Math1 deletion in which the same three lineages are abrogated, although the molecular basis of the patient's defect was not identified (125).

Evidence for the unitarian hypothesis of epithelial cell origin suggested that the crypts encompassed intermediate cells that were not completely committed to one lineage. Neurogenin 3 (ngn3) is essential for the differentiation of intestinal endocrine cells; germline knockout mice fail to develop endocrine cells in the pancreas or intestine, although endocrine cells of the stomach do develop. These mice express Math1, indicating that it is upstream of ngn3 (126). In the mature intestine, ngn3 is expressed in a small number of cells near the base of the crypt, suggesting that it is expressed early during differentiation, possibly in stem cells or their immediate descendents. Lineage analysis revealed that these progenitor cells differentiate into both endocrine and non-endocrine cell types, suggesting that ngn3 is initially expressed in progenitor cells that are not irreversibly committed to endocrine differentiation (127).

Cell cycle arrest is closely coupled to terminal differentiation of intestinal epithelial cells, but the mechanism remains obscure. Expression of *c-myc* is regulated by Wnt signaling and implicated as a critical mediator at the transition from proliferation to differentiation (128). In addition, the c-myc pathway has been identified as upregulated in intestinal progenitor cells (129). However, deletion of c-myc only transiently decreased crypt formation, but appeared to be dispensable for continued development (130). Two candidate cell proliferation inhibitors, p21 and p27, have been implicated by in vitro studies, but targeted deletions do not display an intestinal phenotype in vivo (131, 132). It is likely that there is co-operation among multiple family members, but this area remains to be elucidated. Further complicating the picture, absorptive enterocyte and Paneth cell differentiation may be induced by Rac1 without blocking proliferation (133).

Using a mouse model in which the Paneth cells are eliminated to increase the number of putative stem cells, Gordon's laboratory has undertaken an analysis of gene expression in these progenitor cells isolated by laser capture dissection. A number of upregulated and downregulated genes have been identified in an attempt to identify the genes critical for stem cell function (129). Similar analysis of the gastric progenitor cells has been undertaken (134). Several pathways and gene expression patterns were found in both small intestinal and stomach epithelial progenitor cells. Comparison of these expression patterns with those from hematopoietic stem cells (135, 136) have failed to identify any common genes. This may reflect difficulties in comparing different analyses or indicate that stem cells from different tissues have their own unique characteristics. It remains unclear whether or not there is a set of common 'stemness' genes or there exist unique sets of gene expression patterns for each tissue-specific stem cell (137).

STEM CELL NICHE

The microenvironment in which stem cells reside has been termed their niche (138). This term is often used to mean the physical location of the stem cells. It may also include other cells surrounding and supporting the stem cells and the signals that emanate from them. In the bone marrow, the niche of the hematopoietic stem cells (HSC) has recently begun to be delineated. The quiescent HSC are physically attached to osteoblastic cells via N-cadherin. The number of these N-cadherin-positive cells controls the number of HSCs and these cells influence HSCs by signaling through the Notch receptors (138). Since intestinal stem cells appear to have a fixed location near the base of the crypt and are known to be regulated by Wnt and BMP signaling, this is an attractive model. The reduction in proliferation resulting from deletion of integrinβ4 is consistent with a key role for this anchoring protein in stem cell function (139). The effects of deletion of E2F4 (140), Foxl1 (23), Indian hedgehog (28), and Nkx2.3 (141) on small intestinal cell proliferation suggest that they may all regulate aspects of the signaling that make up the stem cell niche. However, the mechanism by which these and other components interact remains unknown. In the absence of a definitive marker, it is unclear how restricted the location of the stem cells actually is. Furthermore, block of both the BMP signaling (45) and hedgehog signaling (142) pathways reportedly led to the formation of ectopic crypts on the villi, calling into question the concept of a fixed physical location of the stem cell niche. These data suggest that location of the stem cell is determined by gradients of these regulatory factors.

Much remains to be done to identify and characterize the small intestinal stem cell (ISC). In the future, it may be possible to isolate and use ISCs for therapeutic purposes as is currently being done with hematopoietic stem cells (HSC). In this context, it is of interest that trials are under way to use transplants of HSC to treat Crohn's disease patients (143).

Colon

Morphogenesis and Differentiation

A striking characteristic of the developing fetal colon is its initial similarity to the small intestine. The development of the colon is marked by three important cyto-differentiative stages: the appearance (from about 8–10 weeks) of a primitive stratified epithelium, similar to that found in the early development of the small intestine; the conversion of this epithelium to a villus-like architecture with developing crypts (about 12–14 weeks); and the remodeling of the epithelium at around 30 weeks of gestation when villi disappear and the adult-type crypt epithelium is established. Immunostaining for smooth muscle α-actin was detectable in the muscularis propria at 8 weeks of gestation and in the muscularis mucosae at 15 weeks (144). The apical surface of columnar colonocytes displays enterocyte-like microvilli (145), and glycogen stores are abundant (146). The quantity of intracellular glycogen, as well as the number of glycogen-positive cells identified by PAS staining, decreases from 13 weeks onward. From 30 to 36 weeks, very few glycogen-positive cells are found in fetal colon (146). During malignant transformation, glycogen expression reappears, and is a prominent feature of cell lines derived from human colonic adenocarcinomas (147).

Arsenault and Menard studied the kinetics and topography of cell proliferation in explanted fetal colon from 8 to 18 weeks of gestation. Cell proliferation occurred abundantly throughout the stratified epithelium. As villi formed, labeled cells were found principally in the intervillus region. At later stages, proliferation was limited to the crypts (148). In vitro, EGF, but not hydrocortisone, altered colonic cell proliferation (149).

Concurrent with the presence of villus morphology, the colonic epithelial cells express differentiation markers similar to those in small intestinal enterocytes. For example, Lacroix et al. (145) showed that SI was detectable at 8 weeks in fetal colon, increased 10-fold as villus architecture emerged at 11–12 weeks, peaked at 20–28 weeks and then decreased rapidly to barely detectable levels at term.

Stem cells

Mature epithelial cells of the large intestine are continuously replaced by stem cells located near the base of the colonic crypts (150). As with other putative stem cells in the gastrointestinal tract, two key issues are identification of the stem cells and confirmation that isolated cells are in fact stem cells. Progress has recently been reported by Whitehead and co-workers, who have developed an isolation and culture method for human colonic stem cells (151). These investigators found that colonic cells in the lower crypt expressed higher levels of integrinβ1 and used this characteristic to isolate putative stem cells by flow cytometry. When the isolated cells were cultured under previously established conditions, they formed larger numbers of colonies than unsorted cells (152). So far, these putative colonic stem cells have not been further characterized. Many of the regulatory genes and soluble factors that regulate small intestinal stem cells probably function in the colon as well. For example, an in situ analysis of mRNA expression identified many of the same Wnt signaling components in the small intestine and colon (111). As suggested for the small intestine, Musashi may provide a marker for the stem cell or the progenitor cell compartment in the colon also (153).

Hirschsprung's Disease

The most intensively studied aspect of the development of the large intestine is the mechanism of Hirschsprung's disease (HSCR), which is characterized by the absence of parasympathetic intrinsic ganglion cells in both the submucosal (Meissner's) and myenteric (Auerbach's) plexus of the hindgut. The disorder is caused by failure of vagal neural crest cells to migrate into the distal end of the intestine and represents the most common form of congenital bowel obstruction.

Analysis of mutant mouse models has elucidated the causes of the disease. In the lethal spotted mutant mouse, the terminal segment of the gut is congenitally aganglionic. The aganglionic colon results from the failure of migrating neural crest cells to penetrate an abnormally thickened basal lamina and colonize the bowel normally. Laminin in this basal lamina interacts with a receptor on the neural crest cells and causes them to stop migration prematurely. In a different mouse model, the congenital megacolon of transgenic mice overexpressing *hoxa-4* appears to arise from a similar defective interaction between enteric neuron precursors and smooth muscle.

The genetic and molecular mechanisms underlying the disease are the subject of intense investigation and have generated an extensive and growing literature. Numerous mutations associated with Hirschsprung's disease have been identified so far. Mutations in the coding regions of the genes, including missense, nonsense, and deletions, have been found, suggesting loss of function in the gene products. The most extensively studied are mutations in the *ret* receptor tyrosine kinase gene and in the endothelin-B receptor gene. The *ret* proto-oncogene encodes a transmembrane receptor tyrosine kinase. Its ligand has been identified as glial cell-line-derived neurotrophic factor (GDNF), which is expressed in the developing gut. Current evidence indicates that GDNF binds to another receptor, GDNFRα, and together they form a signaling complex with Ret. Mice homozygous for a truncated Ret protein lacking the kinase domain failed to form enteric ganglia. Numerous mutations in the *ret* gene have been identified in patients with HSCR. Manie et al. present a detailed review of the structure and function of the Ret receptor (154). Similarly, a targeted disruption of the endothelin-B receptor gene produces mice with aganglionic megacolon, consistent with a critical role for this receptor as well in migration or differentiation of the neural crest cells which give rise to the enteric ganglia. In addition to Ret and endothelin B receptor defects, deficits in the ligands GDNF and endothelin 3, as well as in endothelin-converting enzyme, all result in Hirschsprung's-like phenotypes in mouse models. Unrelated to either of these receptor/ligand systems, a mutation in *sox-10*, a transcription factor expressed early in neural crest cell development, has also been identified in Hirschsprung's patients. In contrast to earlier models, a recent mouse model expressing a dominant negative Ret mutation phenocopies human Hirschsprung's disease (155). Currently, eleven different susceptibility genes have been identified in humans and several other genes are associated with Hirschsprung's-like syndromes in mice (156).

Mutations in the *ret* gene are a major factor in HSCR. Mutations in the *ret* gene have been found in up to 50% of familial cases, but in the sporadic form coding mutations are found in only about 20% of patients. Recent studies suggest that mutations in the regulatory region of the *ret* gene also contribute to disease susceptibility. Sequence analysis of the *ret* locus identified polymorphisms associated with the disease but located in transcription factor binding sites, which were in conserved regions probably involved in transcriptional regulation (157). A detailed discussion of the current status of genetic analysis of HSCR may be found in Mendelian Inheritance in Man (MIM) 142623.

Sorting out the relative importance of proliferation, migration, and survival of neural crest cells has been one of the challenges in understanding the mechanisms of HSCR. Studies of isolated neural crest stem cells (NCSC) in a mouse model have begun to elucidate some of these questions. Iwashita et al. isolated NCSCs from the intestines of fetal rats and analyzed gene expression by microarray (158). They found that previously identified genes associated with HSCR were upregulated in the stem cells, data confirmed by RT-PCR, flow cytometry, and functional analysis. In vitro experiments demonstrated that GDNF promoted cell migration, but not proliferation or survival. Their data suggest that the GDNF and endothelin signaling pathways interact to regulate the migration of the neural crest stem cells. The possibility of therapeutic intervention has been tested by the demonstration that NCSCs engraft efficiently into endothelin receptor-deficient (159) and Ret-deficient (160) mouse intestine.

CONCLUSIONS

Key regulators of gastrointestinal development have been identified. Some of the genes critical in epithelial/mesenchymal interaction, long known to be a fundamental developmental process, are now known. Analysis of the expression pattern of the *hox* genes suggests that they act to pattern the gastrointestinal tract. The hedgehog proteins mediate several aspects of early development. Targeted disruption of several genes that regulate intestinal growth indicates that BMP secretion has a key developmental role in cell proliferation, villus morphology, and crypt location. Further understanding of the genetic regulation of gastrointestinal development should yield insights into the pathogenesis and treatment of gastrointestinal disorders.

REFERENCES

1. Hooper LV, Wong MH, Thelin A, et al. Molecular analysis of commensal host-microbial relationships in the intestine. Science 2001; 291:881–884.
2. Caicedo RA, Schanler RJ, Li N, Neu J. The developing intestinal ecosystem: Implications for the neonate. Pediatr Res 2005; 58:625–628.
3. Montgomery RK, Mulberg AE, Grand RJ. Development of the human gastrointestinal tract: Twenty years of progress. Gastroenterology 1999; 116:702–731.
4. Kim SK, Hebrok M. Intercellular signals regulating pancreas development and function. Genes Dev 2001; 15:111–127.
5. Zaret KS. Regulatory phases of early liver development: Paradigms of organogenesis. Nat Rev Genet 2002; 3:499–512.
6. Grapin-Botton A, Majithia AR, Melton DA. Key events of pancreas formation are triggered in gut endoderm by ectopic expression of pancreatic regulatory genes. Genes Dev 2001; 15:444–454.
7. Roberts DJ. Molecular mechanisms of development of the gastrointestinal tract. Dev Dynamics 2000; 219:109–120.
8. Wells JM, Melton DA. Vertebrate endoderm development. Annu Rev Cell Dev Biol 1999; 15:393–410.
9. Shivdasani RA. Molecular regulation of vertebrate early endoderm development. Dev Biol 2002; 249:191–203.
10. de Santa Barbara P, van Den Brink GR, Roberts DJ. Molecular etiology of gut malformations and diseases. Am J Med Genet 2002; 115:221–230.
11. Matsushita S, Ishii Y, Scotting PJ, et al. Pre-gut endoderm of chick embryos is regionalized by 1.5 days of development. Dev Dynamics 2002; 223:33–47.
12. Kanai-Azuma M, Kanai Y, Gad JM, et al. Depletion of definitive gut endoderm in sox17-null mutant mice. Development 2002; 129:2367–2379.
13. Henry GL, Melton DA. Mixer, a homeobox gene required for endoderm development. Science 1998; 281:91–96.
14. Hart AH, Hartley L, Sourris K, et al. Mixl1 is required for axial mesendoderm morphogenesis and patterning in the murine embryo. Development 2002; 129:3597–3608.
15. David NB, Rosa FM. Cell autonomous commitment to an endodermal fate and behaviour by activation of nodal signalling. Development 2001; 128:3937–3947.
16. Tremblay K, Hoodless P, Bikoff E, Robertson E. Formation of the definitive endoderm in mouse is a smad2-dependent process. Development 2000; 127:3079–3090.
17. Liu Y, Festing M, Thompson JC, et al. Smad2 and smad3 coordinately regulate craniofacial and endodermal development. Dev Biol 2004; 270:411–426.
18. Kedinger M, Simon-Assmann P, Bouziges F, Haffen K. Epithelial-mesenchymal interactions in intestinal epithelial differentiation. Scand J Gastroenterol Suppl 1988; 151:62–69.
19. Wells J, Melton D. Early mouse endoderm is patterned by soluble factors from adjacent germ layers. Development 2000; 127:1563–1572.
20. Ng AY, Waring P, Ristevski S, et al. Inactivation of the transcription factor elf3 in mice results in dysmorphogenesis and altered differentiation of intestinal epithelium. Gastroenterology 2002; 122:1455–1466.
21. Ang SI, Wierda A, Wong D, et al. The formation and maintenance of the definitive endoderm lineage in the mouse: Involvement of hnf3/forkhead proteins. Development 1993; 119:1301–1315.

22. Dufort D, Schwartz L, Kendraprasad H, Rossant J. The transcription factor hnf3β is required in visceral endoderm for normal primitive streak morphogenesis. Development 1998; 125:3015–3025.

23. Kaestner KH, Silberg DG, Traber PG, Schutz G. The mesenchymal winged helix transcription factor fkh6 is required for the control of gastrointestinal proliferation and differentiation. Genes Dev 1997; 11:1583–1595.

24. Perreault N, Katz JP, Sackett SD, Kaestner KH. Foxl1 controls the wnt/β -catenin pathway by modulating the expression of proteoglycans in the gut. J Biol Chem 2001; 276:43328–43333.

25. Cirillo LA, Lin FR, Cuesta I, et al. Opening of compacted chromatin by early developmental transcription factors hnf3 (foxa) and gata-4. Mol Cell 2002; 9:189–279.

26. Suh E, Traber PG. An intestine-specific homeobox gene regulates proliferation and differentiation. Mol Cell Biol 1996; 16:619–625.

27. Silberg DG, Sullivan J, Kang E, et al. Cdx2 ectopic expression induces gastric intestinal metaplasia in transgenic mice. Gastroenterology 2002; 122:689–696.

28. Ramalho-Santos M, Melton DA, McMahon AP. Hedgehog signals regulate multiple aspects of gastrointestinal development. Development Suppl 2000; 127:2763–2772.

29. Roberts DJ, Johnson Rl, Burke AC, et al. Sonic hedgehog is an endodermal signal inducing bmp-4 and hox genes during induction and regionalization of the chick hindgut. Development 1995; 121:3163–3174.

30. Roberts DJ, Smith DM, Goff DJ, Tabin CJ. Epithelial-mesenchymal signaling during the regionalization of the chick gut. Development Suppl 1998; 125:2791–2801.

31. Motoyama J, Liu J, Mo R, et al. Essential function of gli2 and gli3 in the formation of lung, trachea and oesophagus. Nat Genet 1998; 20:54–57.

32. Litingtung Y, Lei L, Westphal H, Chiang C. Sonic hedgehog is essential to foregut development. Nat Genet 1998; 20:58–61.

33. Mo R, Kim JH, Zhang J, et al. Anorectal malformations caused by defects in sonic hedgehog signaling. Am J Pathol 2001; 159:765–774.

34. Wang LC, Nassir F, Liu ZY, et al. Disruption of hedgehog signaling reveals a novel role in intestinal morphogenesis and intestinal-specific lipid metabolism in mice. Gastroenterology 2002; 122:469–482.

35. Pitera JE, Smith VV, Thorogood P, Milla PJ. Coordinated expression of 3′ hox genes during murine embryonal gut development: An enteric hox code. Gastroenterology 1999; 117:1339–1351.

36. Boulet AM, Capecchi MR. Targeted disruption of hoxc-4 causes esophageal defects and vertebral transformations. Dev Biol 1996; 177:232–249.

37. Pollock RA, Jay G, Bieberich CJ. Altering the boundaries of hox3.1 expression: Evidence for antipodal gene regulation. Cell 1992; 71:911–923.

38. Aubin J, Dery U, Lemieux M, Chailler P, Jeannotte L. Stomach regional specification requires hoxa5-driven mesenchymal-epithelial signaling. Development 2002; 129:4075–4087.

39. Kondo T, Dolle P, Zakany J, Duboule D. Function of posterior hoxd genes in the morphogenesis of the anal sphincter. Development 1996; 122:2651–2659.

40. Zakany J, Duboule D. Hox genes and the making of sphincters. Nature 1999; 401:761–762.

41. Walters JR, Howard A, Rumble HE, et al. Differences in expression of homeobox transcription factors in proximal and distal human small intestine. Gastroenterology 1997; 113:472–477.

42. Kawazoe Y, Sekimoto T, Araki M, et al. Region-specific gastrointestinal hox code during murine embryonal gut development. Dev Growth Differ 2002; 44:77–84.

43. Smith DM, Tabin CJ. Bmp signalling specifies the pyloric sphincter. Nature 1999; 402:748–749.

44. Theodosiou NA, Tabin CJ. Sox9 and nkx2.5 determine the pyloric sphincter epithelium under the control of bmp signaling. Dev Biol 2005; 279:481–490.

45. Haramis A-PG, Begthel H, van den Born M, et al. De novo crypt formation and juvenile polyposis on bmp inhibition in mouse intestine. Science 2004; 303:1684–1686.

46. Grand RJ, Watkins JB, Torti FM. Development of the human gastrointestinal tract. A review. Gastroenterology 1976; 70:790–810.

47. Menard D, Arsenault P. Maturation of human fetal esophagus maintained in organ culture. Anat.Rec 1987; 217:348–354.

48. Hitchcock RJ, Pemble MJ, Bishop AE, et al. Quantitative study of the development and maturation of human oesophageal innervation. J Anat 1992; 180:175–183.

49. Seery JP. Stem cells of the oesophageal epithelium. J Cell Sci 2002; 115:1783–1789.

50. Daniely Y, Liao G, Dixon D, et al. Critical role of p63 in the development of a normal esophageal and tracheobronchial epithelium. Am J Physiol Cell Physiol 2004; 287:C171–181.

51. Minoo P, Su G, Drum H, et al. Defects in tracheoesophageal and lung morphogenesis innkx2.1(-/-) mouse embryos. Dev Biol 1999; 209:60–71.

52. Goldstein I, Reece EA, Yarkoni S, et al. Growth of the fetal stomach in normal pregnancies. Obstet Gynecol 1987; 70:641–644.

53. Vanderwinden J, Mailleux P, Schiffmann S, et al. Nitric oxide synthase activity in infantile hypertrophic pyloric stenosis. N Engl J Med 1992; 327:511–515.

54. Huang PL, Dawson TM, Bredt DS, et al. Targeted disruption of the neuronal nitric oxide synthase gene. Cell 1993; 75:1273–1286.

55. Saur D, Vanderwinden J-M, Seidler B, et al. Single-nucleotide promoter polymorphism alters transcription of neuronal nitric oxide synthase exon 1c in infantile hypertrophic pyloric stenosis. Proc Natl Acad Sci 2004; 101:1662–1667.

56. Kim B-M, Buchner G, Miletich I, et al. The stomach mesenchymal transcription factor barx1 specifies gastric epithelial identity through inhibition of transient wnt signaling. Dev Cell 2005; 8:611–622.

57. Jacobsen CM, Narita N, Bielinska M, et al. Genetic mosaic analysis reveals that gata-4 is required for proper differentiation of mouse gastric epithelium. Dev Biol 2002; 241:34–46.
58. Takamoto N, You L-R, Moses K, et al. Coup-tfii is essential for radial and anteroposterior patterning of the stomach. Development 2005; 132:2179–2189.
59. Karam SM, Leblond CP. Dynamics of epithelial cells in the corpus of the mouse stomach. I. Identification of proliferative cell types and pinpointing of the stem cell. Anat Rec 1993; 236:259–279.
60. Karam S, Leblond CP. Origin and migratory pathways of the eleven epithelial cell types present in the body of the mouse stomach. Microsc Res Technique 1995; 31:193–214.
61. Li Q, Karam SM, Gordon JI. Diphtheria toxin-mediated ablation of parietal cells in the stomach of transgenic mice. J Biol Chem 1996; 271:3671–3676.
62. Menard D, Arsenault P. Cell proliferation in developing human stomach. Anat Embryol 1990; 182:509–516.
63. Akasaka Y, Saikawa Y, Fujita K, et al. Expression of a candidate marker for progenitor cells, musashi-1, in the proliferative regions of human antrum and its decreased expression in intestinal metaplasia. Histopathology 2005; 47:348–356.
64. Jung J, Zheng M, Goldfarb M, Zaret KS. Initiation of mammalian liver development from endoderm by fibroblast growth factors. Science 1999; 284:1998–2003.
65. Lee CS, Friedman JR, Fulmer JT, Kaestner KH. The initiation of liver development is dependent on foxa transcription factors. Nature 2005; 435:944–947.
66. Schmidt C, Bladt F, Goedecke S, et al. Scatter factor/hepatocyte growth factor is essential for liver development. Nature 1995; 373:699–702.
67. Rossi JM, Dunn NR, Hogan BL, Zaret KS. Distinct mesodermal signals, including bmps from the septum transversum mesenchyme, are required in combination for hepatogenesis from the endoderm. Genes Dev 2001; 15:1998–2009.
68. Matsumoto K, Yoshitomi H, Rossant J, Zaret KS. Liver organogenesis promoted by endothelial cells prior to vascular function. Science 2001; 294:559–563.
69. Shiojiri N. Development and differentiation of bile ducts in the mammalian liver. Microsc Res Technique 1997; 39:328–335.
70. Terada T, Nakanuma Y. Detection of apoptosis and expression of apoptosis-related proteins during human intrahepatic bile duct development. Am J Pathol 1995; 146:67–74.
71. Coffinier C, Gresh L, Fiette L, et al. Bile system morphogenesis defects and liver dysfunction upon targeted deletion of hnf1β. Development 2002; 129:1829–1838.
72. Kalinichenko VV, Zhou Y, Bhattacharyya D, et al. Haploinsufficiency of the mouse forkhead box f1 gene causes defects in gall bladder development. J Biol Chem 2002; 277:12369–12374.
73. McCright B, Lozier J, Gridley T. A mouse model of alagille syndrome: Notch2 as a genetic modifier of jag1 haploinsufficiency. Development 2002; 129:1075–1082.
74. McClean P, Weaver LT. Ontogeny of human pancreatic exocrine function. Arch Dis Child 1993; 68:62–65.
75. Gittes GK, Galante PE, Hanahan D, et al. Lineage-specific morphogenesis in the developing pancreas: Role of mesenchymal factors. Development 1996; 122:439–447.
76. Hebrok M, Kim SK, Melton DA. Notochord repression of endodermal sonic hedgehog permits pancreas development. Genes Dev 1998; 12:1705–1713.
77. Wilson ME, Scheel D, German MS. Gene expression cascades in pancreatic development. Mech Dev 2003; 120:65–80.
78. Harrison KA, Thaler J, Pfaff SL, Gu H, Kehrl JH. Pancreas dorsal lobe agenesis and abnormal islets of langerhans in hlxb9-deficient mice. Nat Genet 1999; 23:71–75.
79. Edlund H. Pancreatic organogenesis – developmental mechanisms and implications for therapy. Nat Rev Genet 2002; 3:524–532.
80. Offield MF, Jetton Tl, Laboskyl PA, et al. Pdx-1 is required for pancreatic outgrowth and differentiation of the rostral duodenum. Development 1996; 122:983–995.
81. Stoffers DA, Zinkin NT, Stanojevic V, et al. Pancreatic agenesis attributable to a single nucleotide deletion in the human ipf1 gene coding sequence. Nat Genet 1997; 15:106–110.
82. Colony PC. Successive phases of human fetal intestinal development. Raven Press; 1983.
83. Moxey PC, Trier JS. Specialized cell types in the human fetal small intestine. Anat Rec 1978; 191:269–285.
84. Trier JS, Moxey PC. Morphogenesis of the small intestine during fetal development. Ciba Found Symp 1979; 70:3–29.
85. Karlsson L, Lindahl P, Heath JK, Betsholtz C. Abnormal gastrointestinal development in pdgf-a and pdgfr-(alpha) deficient mice implicates a novel mesenchymal structure with putative instructive properties in villus morphogenesis. Development Suppl 2000; 127:3457–3466.
86. Frid MG, Shekhonin BV, Koteliansky VE, Glukhova MA. Phenotypic changes of human smooth muscle cells during development: Late expression of heavy caldesmon and calponin. Dev Biol 1992; 153:185–193.
87. McHugh KM. Molecular analysis of gastrointestinal smooth muscle development. J Pediatr Gastroenterol Nutr 1996; 23:379–394.
88. Smith VV, Milla PJ. Histological phenotypes of enteric smooth muscle disease causing functional intestinal obstruction in childhood. Histopathology 1997; 31:112–122.
89. Tachibana K, Hirota S, Iizasa H, et al. The chemokine receptor cxcr4 is essential for vascularization of the gastrointestinal tract. Nature 1998; 393:591–594.
90. Bevins CL. Events at the host-microbial interface of the gastrointestinal tract v. Paneth cell {alpha}-defensins in intestinal host defense. Am J Physiol Gastrointest Liver Physiol 2005; 289:G173–G176.

91. Bye WA, Allan CH, Trier JS. Structure, distribution, and origin of m cells in peyer's patches of mouse ileum. Gastroenterology 1984; 86:789–801.

92. Cheng H, Leblond CP. Origin, differentiation and renewal of the four main epithelial cell types in the mouse small intestine. V. Unitarian theory of the origin of the four epithelial cell types. Am J Anat 1974; 141:537–561.

93. Booth C, Potten CS. Gut instincts: Thoughts on intestinal epithelial stem cells. J Clin Invest 2000; 105:1493–1499.

94. Brittan M, Wright NA. Gastrointestinal stem cells. J Pathol 2002; 197:492–509.

95. Potten CS, Loeffler M. Stem cells: Attributes, cycles, spirals, pitfalls and uncertainties. Lessons for and from the crypt. Development 1990; 110:1001–1020.

96. Marshman E, Booth C, Potten CS. The intestinal epithelial stem cell. Bioessays 2002; 24:91–98.

97. Bjerknes M, Cheng H. Clonal analysis of mouse intestinal epithelial progenitors. Gastroenterology 1999; 116:7–14.

98. Ponder BA, Schmidt GH, Wilkinson MM, Wood MJ, Monk M, Reid A. Derivation of mouse intestinal crypts from single progenitor cells. Nature 1985; 313:689–691.

99. Schmidt G, Winton D, Ponder B. Development of the pattern of cell renewal in the crypt-villus unit of chimaeric mouse small intestine. Development 1988; 103:785–790.

100. Krause DS, Theise ND, Collector MI, et al. Multi-organ, multi-lineage engraftment by a single bone marrow-derived stem cell. Cell 2001; 105:369–377.

101. Wagers AJ, Sherwood RI, Christensen JL, Weissman IL. Little evidence for developmental plasticity of adult hematopoietic stem cells. Science 2002; 297:2256–2259.

102. Brittan M, Hunt T, Jeffery R, et al. Bone marrow derivation of pericryptal myofibroblasts in the mouse and human small intestine and colon. Gut 2002; 50:752–757.

103. Logan CY, Nusse R. The wnt signaling pathway in development and disease. Annu Rev Cell Dev Biol 2004; 20:781–810.

104. Korinek V, Barker N, Moerer P, et al. Depletion of epithelial stem-cell compartments in the small intestine of mice lacking tcf-4. Nat Genet 1998; 19:379–383.

105. Pinto D, Gregorieff A, Begthel H, Clevers H. Canonical wnt signals are essential for homeostasis of the intestinal epithelium. Genes Dev 2003; 17:1709–1713.

106. Kuhnert F, Davis CR, Wang H-T, et al. Essential requirement for wnt signaling in proliferation of adult small intestine and colon revealed by adenoviral expression of dickkopf-1. Proc Natl Acad Sci USA 2004; 101:266–271.

107. Sansom OJ, Reed KR, Hayes AJ, et al. Loss of apc in vivo immediately perturbs wnt signaling, differentiation, and migration. Genes Dev 2004; 18:1385–1390.

108. Andreu P, Colnot S, Godard C, et al. Crypt-restricted proliferation and commitment to the paneth cell lineage following apc loss in the mouse intestine. Development 2005; 132:1443–1451.

109. van Es JH, Jay P, Gregorieff A, et al. Wnt signalling induces maturation of paneth cells in intestinal crypts. Nat Cell Biol 2005; 7:381–386.

110. Shroyer NF, Wallis D, Venken KJT, et al. Gfi1 functions downstream of math1 to control intestinal secretory cell subtype allocation and differentiation. Genes Dev 2005; 19:2412–2417.

111. Gregorieff A, Pinto D, Begthel H, et al. Expression pattern of wnt signaling components in the adult intestine. Gastroenterology 2005; 129:626–638.

112. Sancho E, Batlle E, Clevers H. Live and let die in the intestinal epithelium. Curr Opin Cell Biol 2003; 15:763–770.

113. Ireland H, Kemp R, Houghton C, et al. Inducible cre-mediated control of gene expression in the murine gastrointestinal tract: Effect of loss of β-catenin. Gastroenterology 2004; 126: 1236–1246.

114. Bitgood MJ, McMahon AP. Hedgehog and bmp genes are coexpressed at many diverse sites of cell-cell interaction in the mouse embryo. Dev Biol 1995; 172:126–138.

115. He XC, Zhang J, Tong WG, et al. Bmp signaling inhibits intestinal stem cell self-renewal through suppression of wnt-β-catenin signaling. Nat Genet 1117; 36:1117–1121.

116. Fre S, Huyghe M, Mourikis P, et al. Notch signals control the fate of immature progenitor cells in the intestine. Nature 2005; 435:964–968.

117. van Es JH, van Gijn ME, Riccio O, et al. Notch/γ-secretase inhibition turns proliferative cells in intestinal crypts and adenomas into goblet cells. Nature 2005; 435:959–963.

118. Milano J, McKay J, Dagenais C, et al. Modulation of notch processing by γ-secretase inhibitors causes intestinal goblet cell metaplasia and induction of genes known to specify gut secretory lineage differentiation. Toxicol Sci 2004; 82:341–358.

119. Wong GT, Manfra D, Poulet FM, et al. Chronic treatment with the γ-secretase inhibitor ly-411,575 inhibits β-amyloid peptide production and alters lymphopoiesis and intestinal cell differentiation. J Biol Chem 2004; 279:12876–12882.

120. Stanger BZ, Datar R, Murtaugh LC, Melton DA. Direct regulation of intestinal fate by notch. Proc Natl Acad Sci USA 2005; 102:12443–12448.

121. Yang Q, Bermingham NA, Finegold MJ, Zoghbi HY. Requirement of math1 for secretory cell lineage commitment in the mouse intestine. Science 2001; 294:2155–2158.

122. Jensen J, Pedersen EE, Galante P, et al. Control of endodermal endocrine development by hes-1. Nat Genet 2000; 24:36–44.

123. Katz JP, Perreault N, Goldstein BG, et al. The zinc-finger transcription factor klf4 is required for terminal differentiation of goblet cells in the colon. Development 2002; 129:2619–2628.

124. Garabedian EM, Roberts LJ, McNevin MS, Gordon JI. Examining the role of paneth cells in the small intestine by lineage ablation in transgenic mice. J Biol Chem 1997; 272:23729–23740.

125. Shaoul R, Hong D, Okada Y, et al. Lineage development in a patient without goblet, paneth, and enteroendocrine cells: A clue for intestinal epithelial differentiation. Pediatr Res 2005; 58:492–498.

126. Jenny M, Uhl C, Roche C, et al. Neurogenin3 is differentially required for endocrine cell fate specification in the intestinal and gastric epithelium. EMBO J 2002; 21:6338–6347.

127. Schonhoff SE, Giel-Moloney M, Leiter AB. Neurogenin 3-expressing progenitor cells in the gastrointestinal tract differentiate into both endocrine and non-endocrine cell types. Dev Biol 2004; 270:443–454.

128. van de Wetering M, Sancho E, Verweij C, et al. The β-catenin/tcf-4 complex imposes a crypt progenitor phenotype on colorectal cancer cells. Cell 2002; 111:241–250.

129. Stappenbeck TS, Mills JC, Gordon JI. Molecular features of adult mouse small intestinal epithelial progenitors. Proc Natl Acad Sci USA 2003; 100:1004–1009.

130. Bettess MD, Dubois N, Murphy MJ, et al. C-myc is required for the formation of intestinal crypts but dispensable for homeostasis of the adult intestinal epithelium. Mol Cell Biol 2005; 25:7868–7878.

131. Brugarolas J, Chandrasekaran C, Gordon J, et al. Radiation-induced cell cycle arrest compromised by p21 deficiency. Nature 1995; 377:552–557.

132. Deng C, Zhang P, Wade Harper J, et al. Mice lacking p21 cip1/waf1 undergo normal development, but are defective in g1 checkpoint control. Cell 1995; 82:675–684.

133. Stappenbeck T, Gordon J. Rac1 mutations produce aberrant epithelial differentiation in the developing and adult mouse small intestine. Development 2000; 127:2629–2642.

134. Mills JC, Andersson N, Hong CV, et al. Molecular characterization of mouse gastric epithelial progenitor cells. Proc Natl Acad Sci USA 2002; 99:14819–14824.

135. Ivanova NB, Dimos JT, Schaniel C, et al. A stem cell molecular signature. Science 2002; 298:601–604.

136. Ramalho-Santos M, Yoon S, Matsuzaki Y, et al. 'Stemness': Transcriptional profiling of embryonic and adult stem cells. Science 2002; 298:597–600.

137. Eckfeldt CE, Mendenhall EM, Verfaillie CM. The molecular reperoire of the 'almighty' stem cell. Nat Rev Mol Cell Biol 2005; 6:726–737.

138. Li L, Xie T. Stem cell niche: Structure and function. Annu Rev Cell Dev Biol 2005; 21:605–631.

139. Murgia C, Blaikie P, Kim N, et al. Cell cycle and adhesion defects in mice carrying a targeted deletion of the integrin β 4 cytoplasmic domain. EMBO J 1998; 17:3940–3951.

140. Rempel RE, Saenz-Robles MT, Storms R, et al. Loss of e2f4 activity leads to abnormal development of multiple cellular lineages. Mol Cell 2000; 6:293–306.

141. Pabst O, Schneider A, Brand T, Arnold HH. The mouse nkx2–3 homeodomain gene is expressed in gut mesenchyme during pre- and postnatal mouse development. Dev Dynamics 1997; 209:29–35.

142. Madison BB, Braunstein K, Kuizon E, et al. Epithelial hedgehog signals pattern the intestinal crypt-villus axis. Development 2005; 132:279–289.

143. Oyama Y, Craig RM, Traynor AE, et al. Autologous hematopoietic stem cell transplantation in patients with refractory crohn's disease. Gastroenterology 2005; 128:552–563.

144. Romanska HM, Bishop AE, Moscoso G, et al. Neural cell adhesion molecule (ncam) expression in nerves and muscle of developing human large bowel. J Pediatr Gastroenterol Nutr 1996; 22:351–358.

145. Lacroix B, Kedinger M, Simon-Assmann P, et al. Developmental pattern of brush border enzymes in the human fetal colon. Correlation with some morphogenetic events. Early Hum Dev 1984; 9:95–103.

146. Rousset M, Robine-Leon S, Dussaulx E, et al. Glycogen storage in foetal and malignant epithelial cells of the human colon. Front Gastrointest Res 1979; 4:80–85.

147. Rousset M, Chevalier G, Rousset JP, et al. Presence and cell growth-related variations of glycogen in human colorectal adenocarcinoma cell lines in culture. Cancer Res 1979; 39:531–534.

148. Arsenault P, Menard D. Cell proliferation during morphogenesis of the human colon. Biol. Neonate 1989; 55:137–142.

149. Menard D, Corriveau L, Arsenault P. Differential effects of epidermal growth factor and hydrocortisone in human fetal colon. J Pediatr Gastroenterol Nutr 1990; 10:13–20.

150. Potten CS. Stem cells in gastrointestinal epithelium: Numbers, characteristics and death. Phil Trans R Soc Lond B Biol Sci 1998; 353:821–830.

151. Fujimoto K, Beauchamp RD, Whitehead RH. Identification and isolation of candidate human colonic clonogenic cells based on cell surface integrin expression. Gastroenterology 2002; 123:1941–1948.

152. Whitehead RH, Demmler K, Rockman SP, Watson NK. Clonogenic growth of epithelial cells from normal colonic mucosa from both mice and humans. Gastroenterology 1999; 117:858–865.

153. Nishimura S, Wakabayashi N, Toyoda K, et al. Expression of musashi-1 in human normal colon crypt cells: A possible stem cell marker of human colon epithelium. Dig Dis Scis 2003; 48:1523–1529.

154. Manie S, Santoro M, Fusco A, Billaud M. The ret receptor: Function in development and dysfunction in congenital malformation. Trends Genet 2001; 17:580–589.

155. Jain S, Naughton CK, Yang M, et al. Mice expressing a dominant-negative ret mutation phenocopy human hirschsprung disease and delineate a direct role of ret in spermatogenesis. Development 2004; 131:5503–5513.

156. Kapur R. Multiple endocrine neoplasia typ. 2b and hirschsprung's disease. Clin Gastroenterol Hepatol 2005; 3:423–431.

157. Burzynski GM, Nolte IM, Bronda A, et al. Identifying candidate hirschsprung disease-associated ret variants. Am J Hum Genet 2005; 76:850–858.
158. Iwashita T, Kruger GM, Pardal R, et al. Hirschsprung disease is linked to defects in neural crest stem cell function. Science 2003; 301:972–976.
159. Kruger GM, Mosher JT, Tsai Y-H, et al. Temporally distinct requirements for endothelin receptor b in the generation and migration of gut neural crest stem cells. Neuron 2003; 40:917–929.
160. Bondurand N, Natarajan D, Thapar N, et al. Neuron and glia generating progenitors of the mammalian enteric nervous system isolated from foetal and postnatal gut cultures. Development 2003; 130:6387–6400.

Chapter 2

Dietary Regulation of Gene Expression

Ian R. Sanderson, MD, MSc, FRCP, FRCPCH

Genes Controlling the Nutritional Requirements of Skeletal Muscle Cells
Effect of Intestinal Contents on Genes in the Intestinal Epithelium
Breast Milk and Gene Expression
DNA Methylation and Imprinting
Conclusions

Infancy is a time of great change in nutrient intake. This review will examine how nutritional changes alter the expression of genes in skeletal muscle (as an example of an end point of human action) and in the intestine (the point of interaction between the infant and the nutritional environment). Unlike other organs the intestine is not shielded from the major environmental changes of infancy. In the fetus, the intestinal lumen is sterile and the fetal circulation provides nourishment, while after birth it interacts with an extremely complex environment containing nutrients in varying concentrations. At weaning, this level of complexity increases further.

Altering the expression of genes has become a rapidly developing area of research in medicine. The realization that gene expression is important in a wide range of diseases, and not just in inherited disease, has resulted in the whole field of gene expression being recognized as one which may bring new therapeutic options. Although most recent attention has focused on the benefits of altering gene expression by inserting new genetic material into cells by a variety of vectors, the expression of genes can also be altered by other means, most notably by changing the molecular environment that cells inhabit. Utilizing the natural responses of a cell to changes in its surroundings offers a new and amenable way to alter the expression of its genes. Many ways of altering these surroundings can be proposed, but no single act alters the environment of the cells of the body more than the ingestion of food. Thus, the future of nutrition as a therapeutic tool may lie in its potential for influencing gene regulation. This chapter will examine this emerging field and will lay down some concepts which may prove useful in establishing the scientific basis from which future treatments may develop.

The survival of an infant to reproductive age and beyond requires an ability to respond to external demands. Every organ in the body is attuned to this need. Many organ systems have two levels of response to external changes. There is a rapid response, often occurring within seconds of a new stimulus: the contraction of muscle fibers following a neuronal impulse, or the breakdown of glycogen by the liver during hypoglycemia are examples of how cells can quickly change. Such responses do not involve changes in gene expression. The cells maintain themselves in a state of readiness by synthesizing proteins whose activity can quickly alter in response to external stimuli. Behind this immediate response, there lie other slower, but more lasting, responses that require genetic control. For example, when exercise increases on a regular basis, muscle mass increases, as does the activity of the attendant enzymes that serve the increased metabolic needs. Similarly, regular exposure of the liver to drugs induces the expression of enzymes that catalyze their breakdown.

There are few external stimuli on a child more important than its nutritional environment. The metabolic processes underlying the rapid response of cells to nutritional variations have long been documented in humans and other mammals (1). However, the mechanisms whereby gene expression changes in response to nutritional stimuli are still poorly understood in humans or indeed in any multi-organ animal. This is, at first, surprising because in bacteria the study of nutritional changes led to our understanding of some of the most fundamental mechanisms of gene expression. The elucidation of the induction of proteins that transport and hydrolyze lactose (the lac operon) after adding lactose to bacterial culture media (2) was the first examination of any form of gene regulation. These observations spawned an explosion of research in other regulatory genes in bacteria and in unicellular, eukaryotic organisms such as yeast. The upregulation of the bacterial genes that handle tryptophan when this amino acid is scarce (the Trp operon) has become another well-understood example of nutrient-gene interaction (3).

Progress in the study of nutrient-gene interaction in eukaryotic cells has been slower for two main reasons. First, the molecular mechanisms controlling gene expression are more complex than in bacteria; and second, it is more difficult to identify the metabolites of nutrients that may be responsible for inducing such changes. This review will therefore cover some of the recent advances in the study of the role of nutrition in gene expression in the human and, where necessary, in other mammals. Nutritional changes ultimately impinge on most cells in the body; however, it is the epithelium of the gastrointestinal tract that first encounters any variation in nutrient intake. Much of this chapter will therefore concentrate on how nutritional factors can alter the expression of genes in intestinal epithelial cells. The relevance of nutrient-gene interactions to human physiology will also be stressed. Finally, because manipulating nutritional intake may be a way of treating disease in children, the review will discuss nutritional therapy in childhood in the light of its effects on gene expression.

The effect of nutrients on gene expression may have different implications in different individual situations (4) (Table 2-1). First, genes may be upregulated to better utilize the supply of a particular nutrient when it is scarce. Transporters of nutrients and the enzymes that metabolize them are examples of proteins that may be induced by nutrients. Second, the expression of genes required for the storage of a particular nutrient may be altered according to that nutrient's abundance. Third, nutrients regulate the secretion of hormones that control the homeostasis of metabolic processes. For example, insulin synthesis increases after increased carbohydrate intake to maintain glucose homeostasis. Finally, food is part of our external

---

Table 2-1 The Physiological Importance of Nutritional Regulation of Gene Expression

1. To satisfy the nutritional needs of an organ
2. Managing storage fuels required by other organs
3. Production of hormones essential to whole body metabolism
4. Direct interaction with the body's external environment along the gastrointestinal tract

Adapted from (4) with permission.

environment and as such represents a challenge to the cells that come into intimate contact with it. This challenge is met, in the main, by the epithelial cells lining the gastrointestinal tract (5). The ability of these cells to alter the expression of their genes with changes in food intake is one of the ways by which the intestinal epithelium can dominate the intestinal environment.

Certain fundamental characteristics are found in the mechanisms that underlie each of these different aspects of nutrient-gene interactions. They include a specific interaction between the cell and a particular nutrient (sensing) and a pathway by which such an interaction may translate into alterations in gene expression (signal transduction). We have very little understanding of these mechanisms at the present time. However, some aspects of the molecular biology of these two functions will be examined later in this review.

GENES CONTROLLING THE NUTRITIONAL REQUIREMENTS OF SKELETAL MUSCLE CELLS

Survival of cells depends on their ability to extract nutrients and other essential molecules from their surroundings, and they synthesize proteins specifically for this purpose. There are broadly speaking two categories of genes involved: those genes that express proteins that transport nutrients across cell membranes; and those genes that express enzymes that metabolize nutrients. In both cases, genes are regulated purely to satisfy the requirements of an organ system. This form of gene regulation is similar in concept to the regulatory genes of bacteria such as the Trp operon (3). The cells are changing their phenotype to their own advantage, rather than to suit the needs of the body as a whole.

A good model of how cells may respond to their nutritional environment for their own needs is the utilization of glutamine by skeletal muscle (6). Glutamine availability modulates muscle turnover and glutamine is an important source of amino-nitrogen for muscle cells (7). Glutamine also critically regulates rapidly dividing cells such as lymphocytes (8) and intestinal epithelial cells (9). Glutamine and glutamate are transported into cells by sodium-coupled transporters. For experimental purposes, rat skeletal muscle can be grown as primary cell cultures. These cells exhibit an upregulation of the inward transport of both glutamine and glutamate when they are deprived of an exogenous glutamine supply (10–12). In addition, the activity of glutamine synthetase simultaneously increases. This enzyme catalyzes the addition of an amino group to the carboxyl moiety of the glutamate molecule to form glutamine. Two different nutrients, glutamine and glutamate, can therefore ultimately satisfy the glutamine requirements of the muscle cell through separate pathways, each of which is under genetic control. This system exemplifies how different nutrients can cross-stimulate the expression of a related set of proteins: removal of glutamine or glutamate from the cell medium results in an enhancement of the transport of both amino acids. Not only does lack of glutamine and glutamate enhance the expression of their own transport proteins, but deprivation of either substrate will also upregulate the transporter of the other (11). A study of the kinetics of transport (12) demonstrated that withdrawal of glutamine (or glutamate) enhanced the maximum rate at which the amino acid is transported into the cell (the V_{max}), and did not alter the affinity of the transporter for its amino acid. This suggests that deprivation resulted in an increase in the production of the number of transporters available. The time required to double the V_{max} was around 4 hours. This fact, taken together with the observation that the induction of both glutamate and glutamine transporters was lost when glutamine was withdrawn in the presence of actinomycin D (which inhibits RNA synthesis), indicates that their regulation is mediated through initiation of transcription.

Although there is much we still do not understand about the glutamine and glutamate transport systems, their examination is relatively straightforward because each amino acid has only two transporters, a sodium-dependent and a sodium-independent one. It is only the sodium-dependent transporter that responds to nutrient deprivation. Glutamate and glutamine regulation, although important, constitute only a minor part of nutrient homeostasis for skeletal muscle cells in vivo, whose energy requirements are mainly met by glucose and free fatty acids (4).

It has been unclear to what extent the diet affects skeletal muscle's ability to adjust to fat intake. Cameron-Smith et al. (13) demonstrated that a short-term high-fat diet upregulates lipid metabolism and gene expression in human muscle. They studied 14 athletes and gave two groups high-fat or isoenergetic high-carbohydrate diets for 5 days with a 2-week washout period and subsequent crossover, while maintaining matched exercise levels. Muscle biopsies and blood samples were taken on day 1 and after completing each stage of the diet. A greater gene expression of fatty acid translocase (a putative fatty acid transporter) and beta-hydroxyacyl-CoA dehydrogenase (beta oxidation pathway enzyme) and greater abundance of fatty acid translocase was found after the high-fat than after the high-carbohydrate diet. This would imply upregulation of genes necessary for fatty acid transportation and oxidative metabolism in skeletal muscle. The authors concluded that fatty acid interaction with genetic components of skeletal muscle is important in contributing to the adaptive capacity of the oxidative profile of muscle to the predominant food source. However, the exact details still require elucidation.

EFFECT OF INTESTINAL CONTENTS ON GENES IN THE INTESTINAL EPITHELIUM

The gastrointestinal tract is the only part of the body that normally comes into contact with nutrients before they are absorbed. The GI tract is therefore exposed to a wider variety of nutrient molecules than any other organ of the body. The picture is further complicated because the lumen of the intestine is not a direct reflection of the food ingested. It also contains bacteria and their by-products and factors secreted into the lumen in response to the ingestion of food. The study of the effects of nutrients on the enterocyte therefore should consider how changes in diet may affect the area around the apical aspect of a particular epithelial cell. The dissociation between nutrients ingested and the changes observed in the bowel lumen becomes greater the further one proceeds down the GI tract. The contents of the distal colon are completely different from food, although even here they are affected to some extent by dietary intake. This relationship between ingested nutrients and the local environment of the lumen is a separate issue from the interaction of that local environment with genes in the enterocyte.

It has been traditional to assume that the expression of genes in the small intestinal epithelium is preprogrammed and that their expression is not influenced by events in the lumen of the intestine. However, this view may be incomplete. An alteration in epithelial cell phenotype secondary to nutritional factors would have three possible advantages (4) (Table 2-2). First, the intestine could adapt to absorb nutrients more effectively if specific digestive enzymes and transporters of the epithelium were upregulated by the repeated intake of a particular nutrient. Second, as all mammals are fed from mother's milk, the opportunity exists for breast milk to influence the development of the epithelium through actions of its own constituents. Third, if the genes affected in the epithelium were immunologically important, the intestinal epithelium could influence mucosal immune responses, by signaling information to the mucosal immune system and beyond through changes in the

Table 2-2   Relevance of Dietary Regulation of Enterocyte Gene Expression

1. Intestinal adaptation
2. Influence of maternal breast milk
3. Signaling from lumen to mucosal immune system

Adapted from (4) with permission.

expression of epithelial cell genes. Each of these areas is likely to represent important physiological mechanisms which have implications for child health.

Polarity of Epithelia

Skeletal muscle cells do not depend on a separation of functions to different cellular poles. For example, muscle cells receive signals from the entry of glucose at any point on the plasma membrane and, as far as we can judge, the changes in gene expression are not affected by the site of glucose entry. Cells that form epithelia are different in that they exhibit polarity. This separation between the apical side (bordering the lumen in the case of the intestinal epithelium) and the basolateral side is central to epithelial activity. This property is well recognized in the field of intestinal transport. Ions (14), small molecules (15) and macromolecules (16) are all transported differently across the apical membrane than across the basolateral membrane. It is the polarity of the epithelium that gives direction to the movement of these substances across the epithelium into or out of the body. But this property must also be considered when examining all aspects of intestinal epithelial cell function. Polarity is also of fundamental relevance in the study of nutrient-gene interactions in the intestinal epithelium. The polarity of the epithelial cells distinguishes the two major mechanisms by which nutrients (and other luminal factors) affect genes – that of a direct luminal effect on enterocytes from an indirect effect mediated through hormones, growth factor and cytokines.

Furthermore, the intestinal epithelium acts as a barrier to the external environment contained within the gut lumen (17). The barrier is not complete as the intestine allows macromolecules to be sampled (18) and actively absorbs nutrients. It has become increasingly realized that the enterocyte itself acts an immune cell. For example, it has receptors for bacterial products (19), as well as expressing a wide variety of molecules on its surface that contain immunoglobulin domains. The epithelial cell also expresses proteins that may interact with immunocytes within the intestine. These include surface molecules such as class II MHC and cytokines that are released from the epithelium such as chemokines or IL-6.

These signaling proteins enable the epithelial cell to orchestrate events in the intestine. In our research group we have hypothesized that changes in the intestinal lumen regulate the expression of signaling molecules by the epithelial cell. By this means, the dietary effects on the intestinal lumen act through the epithelium to alter indirectly events in the intestine, particularly those of the mucosal immune system (20). There are two components within the signaling pathway linking diet and luminal bacteria to the mucosal immune system. First, the afferent limb comprises the mechanisms whereby luminal changes alter gene expression within the epithelium; and, second, the efferent limb is the effect of proteins expressed by the epithelial cell acting on the immune system of the intestine. There is now good evidence for both these pathways.

It is possible to examine molecular events in the epithelium induced by changes in diet (the afferent limb). A useful model is the expression of class II MHC in the epithelium following weaning of mice (21). Class II MHC is responsible for presentation of antigen, and its expression on the intestinal epithelium of the mouse occurs after weaning. It is therefore possible to wean mice on to a normal diet (mouse chow) or defined liquid formula (enteral nutrition) to examine the difference between these types of nutrition. The epithelial cells can then be isolated from the mice at varying time points after weaning to study the expression of class II MHC and invariant chain which is co-expressed. The effects of the enteral feeding (vivonex) was dramatically different from normal mouse chow.

Normal mice chow induced an expression of these genes between 20 and 30 days of age, whereas during this period enteral feeding did not result in their expression in the intestinal epithelium (21). It is known that the class II transactivator (a regulatory nuclear protein) is, for all cell types so far examined, both necessary and sufficient for class II MHC expression. Experiments were therefore designed to examine whether the diet acted through the class II transactivator (CIITA). In the mouse there are three isoforms of CIITA. Interestingly, a normal complex diet increased the expression of class II MHC though CIITA IV (22). In addition to the dietary regulation of class II MHC there was a slow time-dependent regulation and this was found to be due to CIITA III. These experiments show, therefore, that alterations in the diet have recognizable molecular pathways between the intestinal lumen and the signal transduction machinery of the epithelial cell.

Bacterial fermentation of unabsorbed carbohydrate in the intestine results in short-chain fatty acid production (23). Butyrate levels therefore reflect changes in bacterial populations and in the substrates available for bacterial metabolism. Butyrate levels vary greatly in response to external changes. For example, newborn babies have very low butyrate levels in either the small or large intestine. However, with time butyrate levels rise to adult levels by 2 years (24). Interestingly, butyrate levels are much higher in bottle-fed babies than they are in breast-fed babies during the first 6 months of life (24).

Butyrate levels therefore reflect events in the intestinal lumen and we hypothesized that their concentrations may alter epithelial cell signaling. We therefore examined their effects on IL-8 and monocyte chemotactic protein-1 (MCP-1) expression (25). Increasing the concentration of sodium butyrate increased IL-8 secretion while simultaneously decreasing MCP-1 expression. These effects were seen in resting epithelial cell lines but were much more marked in cells that had been stimulated with a pro-inflammatory agent such as LPS or IL-1β.

It is known that sodium butyrate alters histone acetylation. The nucleosome consists of a solenoid of histones wrapped around by an integral of two turns of DNA (26) (Fig. 2-1). Butyrate increases histone acetylation and this reduces the compactness of the histone. The DNA cannot wrap around the large nucleosome in a integral number of turns. The nucleosome can no longer be packaged into tight bundles. This exposes the DNA and makes it more amenable to transcription factors. We hypothesized that butyrate altered the expression of chemokines by this process (25). To test this hypothesis we used a fungicide, trichostatin A (TSA), which is 700 times more potent in inducing histone acetylation than butyrate. If the effects of butyrate on chemokine secretion were due to increased histone acetylation, we would expect them to be reproduced by the TSA. Experiments with TSA (Fig. 2-2) showed that TSA increased IL-8 secretion and decreased MCP 1 secretion. Figure 2-2 (lower part) shows that both TSA and butyrate increased the acetylation of histone 4. Non-acetylated histones move rapidly through the gel and form a single band, whereas acetylated histones form a ladder depending on the degree of acetylation. The histone 4 has four lysine residues which are acetylated and thus acetylation of histones will result in a ladder of five bands. This can be seen in the cells given butyrate or TSA. The upper part of the figure shows that TSA has a similar effect to butyrate. It increases IL-8 secretion and decreases

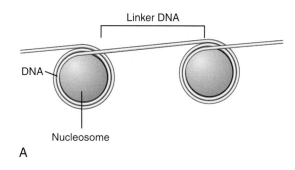

A

Figure 2-1 Relationship between nucleosomes and DNA. (A) DNA is wrapped two full turns around nucleosomes made up of unacetylated histones. (B) With butyrate-induced acetylation, the nucleosome expands, reducing the number of turns of DNA around the nucleosome to 1.8, with less linker DNA connecting each nucleosome. The result of this is that DNA cannot pass linearly from nucleosome to nucleosome but turns at an angle after every nucleosome, leading to disruption of nucleosome packaging. Reproduced from ref. 26 with permission from the Annual Review of Nutrition, Volume 20, ⓒ 2000 by Annual Reviews, www.annulreviews. com.

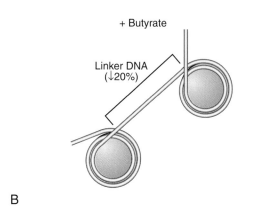

B

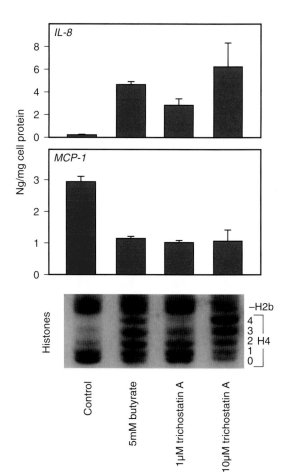

Figure 2-2 Effect of butyrate and trichostatin A in the induction of histone. Acetylation and chemokine secretion by Caco-2 cells. Both butyrate and trichostatin A increased the acetylation of histones. IL-8 secretion was simultaneously increased ($P < 0.0001$) and MCP-1 production decreased in Caco-2 cells stimulated with IL-1 ($P < 0.001$). Trichostatin A, a specific histone deacetylase inhibitor, acted in a manner similar to that of butyrate when given at concentrations that produced a comparable change in histone acetylation. Bars represent standard deviations of three different wells for each point. The data are representative of three experiments. Reproduced from ref. 25 with permission.

MCP 1 secretion. Furthermore, the degree of this increase in IL-8 varies with the degree of histone acetylation. Moreover, the effect of butyrate on histone acetylation was reversible (25). After removal of butyrate, histone acetylation returns to normal and the effects of IL-1b on IL-8 secretion and MCP 1 secretion return to those seen in the untreated cells. Different-length short-chain fatty acids have differing effects on histone acetylation. Butyrate is the most effective short-chain fatty acid in inducing histone acetylation while longer and shorter carbon lengths have lesser effects. This effect on histone acetylation is reflected by effects on the expression of IL-8 and MCP 1 (25). Butyrate causes the greatest increase in IL-8 secretion and the greatest decrease in MCP I secretion of the various short-chain fatty acids used.

In summary, these experiments show that sodium butyrate alters the expression of chemokines in the epithelial cell. In addition, short-chain fatty acids alter this expression through histone acetylation. These experiments, however, do not exclude the possibility that additional effects of sodium butyrate may occur through promoter systems. Indeed, recent studies have demonstrated that butyrate down-regulates insulin-like growth factor binding protein-3 (IGFBP-3) through acetylation of an inhibitory DNA binding protein (26). It is a challenge for future work to examine the interaction between chromosomal regulation, as is seen in these experiments, and promoter-based regulation with both butyrate and other luminal molecules.

Evidence for the effect of epithelial cell gene expression on the mucosal immune system (the efferent limb) has come from the ability to selectively alter the expression of genes in the intestinal epithelial cell by transgenic techniques (27). We have used chemokine expression by the epithelium as a model to show that the epithelium can orchestrate the mucosal immune system. The chemokine IL-8, which in the human results in recruitment of neutrophils, was the first identified chemotatic cytokine. However, IL-8 is not expressed in the mouse. To examine the effects of chemokines on the mucosal immune system, a system was developed whereby the chemokine macrophage inflammatory protein-2 (MIP-2), whose effects are very similar those of IL-8 in the human, was linked to an FABPI (fatty acid binding protein of the intestine) promoter (27). The promoter is only active in the epithelial cells of the small intestine and proximal colon. A construct was developed where the FABPI promoter and MIP-2 cDNA were linked to an intron and a polyadenylation site. This construct was injected into mouse oocytes. The epithelium from the first generation of the founder was shown to express MIP-2 mRNA (Fig. 2-3). Analysis showed effects both on neutrophil and on lymphocyte recruitment. The transgenic mice had an increased recruitment of neutrophils into the lamina propria, and into the epithelial cell fraction. The effects of the chemokine could be seen only in those tissues where the FABPI promoter was active. In the small intestine, where the FABPI promoter is active, the neutrophil recruitment, expressed as myloperoxidase activity (per unit weight of intestine), was significantly greater in the transgenic mice. In the proximal colon, where the FABPI promoter is also active, there was also an increase in neutrophil infiltration. However, in the distal colon, where the FABPI promoter is inactive, there was no effect. In addition, the liver and the spleen showed no increased infiltration in the transgenic mouse over the normal mouse. The FABPI promoter is not active in these organs. These data show for the first time that the epithelial cell can, through the release of chemokines, alter the mucosal immune function of the intestine in vivo.

Further analysis of the immune system demonstrated that the small intestine had increased lymphocyte infiltration, in addition to neutrophils (27). Lymphocyte numbers in the lamina propria were significantly increased, and there was also a doubling of the numbers of intraepithelial lymphocytes. Examination of the

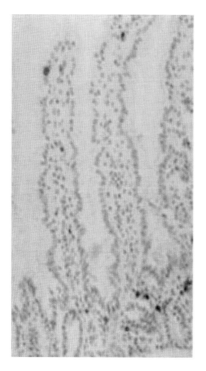
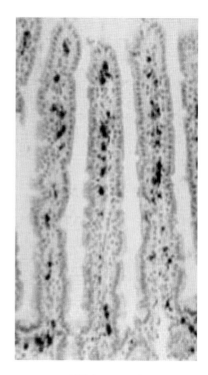

Wild-type   MIP-2 transgenic

Figure 2-3 Epithelial cell MIP-2 increases neutrophil recruitment. Transgenic mice express MIP-2 in the intestinal epithelium using an epithelial-specific promoter. Neutrophils were located by staining for myeloperoxidase. Reproduced from ref. 27 with permission from the BMJ Publishing Group.

receptors on the surface of the intraepithelial lymphocytes showed that they expressed the CXCR2 which is the receptor responsible for transducing MIP-2 activity. These experiments show therefore that altering the expression of only one chemokine in the epithelium has marked effects on both lymphocyte and neutrophil function. However, changes in the intestinal lumen may affect many chemokines as well as other cytokines which alter immune function. It is likely therefore that the changes in gene expression in the epithelium have far-reaching effects on the rest of the mucosal immune system.

We believe that these signaling processes are important not only in health but also in the treatment of disease. For example, the primary therapy of children with Crohn's disease in the United Kingdom is treatment with enteral feeds (28, 29). Although there are many mechanisms by which enteral feeds may have their activity, we think it possible that one of them is by radically altering the luminal environment to such an extent that it varies the signals from the intestinal epithelium to the mucosal immune element. This results in a downregulation of the inflammation of Crohn's disease. By this means there is a decrease in the inflammatory activity of Crohn's disease.

Glutamine and the Intestine

The earlier part of this chapter discussed the nutrient regulation of glutamine uptake into skeletal muscle cells. But glutamine also has profound effects on the infant intestine. A multicenter study (30) demonstrated that supplementation of premature infants on parenteral nutrition with glutamine significantly decreased the incidence of gastrointestinal problems, including bilious gastric acid aspirates and emesis, abdominal distension and blood in the stools. Neu and his laboratory have examined how glutamine may affect the expression of genes in the intestinal epithelial cell as a central point in the infant's pathophysiology. They studied two characteristics of the enterocyte in detail: (i) the ability of the epithelium to act as a barrier to the inappropriate passage of macromolecules; and (ii) the expression of inflammatory chemokines such as IL-8. Glutamine reduced the permeability of an epithelial cell monolayer (31); and it also reduced the cells' production of IL-8 in response to bacterial stimuli (32).

The group studied the disposition of the proteins (occludin, claudin-1 and ZO-1) central to tight junctional activity within epithelial cells to understand the changes in permeability (31). They demonstrated that glutamine deprivation impaired the occludin and claudin-1 from localizing at the tight junction, while having little effect on ZO-1. Separate experiments described the molecular basis of glutamine regulation of IL-8 expression. Immature intestinal biopsies express greater amounts of IL-8 in response to IL-1 (32) than do mature intestine. Neu and his co-workers demonstrated that glutamine maintains the ability of IkappaB to interrupt the signal transduction pathway from LPS to IL-8. The effect of glutamine deprivation on IkappaB depletion was greater in enterocytes derived from the human fetus than it was in other model epithelial cells (32).

BREAST MILK AND GENE EXPRESSION

The nutrition and protection of the infant are the primary roles of breast-feeding, and the nutritional and immunological properties of breast milk are reviewed in other chapters of this book. Nevertheless, the cells of the gastrointestinal tract are the first cells of the child to encounter breast milk, and it is not fanciful to suppose that breast milk may influence the development of these cells. A number of factors in milk can affect the expression of genes in the intestinal epithelium, particularly those genes that are associated with enterocyte differentiation. Growth factors such as EGF, VEGF and IGFs are found in breast milk (33–37) and EGF enhances brush-border enzyme activity. Although the exact effect of EGF in breast milk on the development of the intestinal epithelium depends on the age of the subject, its effect on enterocyte growth and development is not surprising. Less expected, perhaps, is the demonstration that other breast milk components such as nucleotides also affect these same genes (38, 39). A list of how each constituent in breast milk may affect expression of genes in the intestinal epithelium would not present an illuminating picture of how breast milk affected enterocyte expression. Instead it is more valuable to describe one factor, lactoferrin, as an example. We will examine what is known about its interactions with the intestinal epithelium, and how this knowledge may be added to in the future.

Lactoferrin

Lactoferrin, a glycoprotein with molecular weight of approximately 80 000, is a human iron-binding protein structurally similar to transferrin (40). Lactoferrin is present in high concentrations in breast milk, especially in colostrum (41). Although neutrophil granules contain lactoferrin (42), its concentration in plasma, in contrast to transferrin, is relatively low (43).

Specific binding sites for lactoferrin have been observed in intestinal brush-border membrane vesicles prepared from the human fetus (44), rhesus monkey (45), rabbit (46), and mouse (47). Lactoferrin is relatively resistant to proteolytic enzymes (48, 49), and it may therefore have a direct biological effect on the intestinal epithelium. An understanding of the actions of lactoferrin is particularly relevant as some artificial milk formulas now contain added bovine lactoferrin. Its major role is thought to be to deliver iron to the intestinal epithelium (50).

The number of lactoferrin-binding sites increases in cultured epithelial cells when depleted of iron (51), resulting in a specific increase of iron transport into enterocytes. The actions of lactoferrin are therefore interconnected with the actions of iron. Iron has well-characterized effects on the translation of ferritin and transferrin mRNA (52), but its effect on gene expression in the enterocyte is less well understood.

Although lactoferrin increases the bioavailability of iron in the neonatal intestine, recent studies suggest that lactoferrin may also act as a proliferative factor in a variety of cell types, including human lymphocytes (53), mouse embryo fibroblasts (54), and rat myoblasts (55). Lactoferrin also affects the proliferation of HT-29 human colon adenocarcinoma cells (56), and adult rat crypt cells (57). The effect of lactoferrin on the expression of brush-border enzymes has also been examined. In tissue culture experiments, the effect of lactoferrin on sucrase and alkaline phosphatase specific activities depended on whether or not the protein was saturated with iron (58).

There is a school of thought that proposes that the main function of lactoferrin in vivo is not to transport iron into the epithelium, but to scavenge iron (and possibly other substances) in the intestinal lumen. This unbound iron might otherwise cause free-radical-mediated damage to sensitive tissues (59). Accordingly, lactoferrin would have no direct effect with the intestinal epithelium, and only indirectly interact with it through the sequestration of other substances in the lumen. These luminal factors may, of course, if left free in solution have an impact on enterocyte gene expression. An example of this is lactoferrin's binding to lipopolysaccharide (60), thereby modulating the effect of this moiety on the epithelium. A purely luminal role for lactoferrin is, however, difficult to reconcile with the identification of specific receptors for lactoferrin on the surface of the small intestinal brush-border membrane (46). Initially, the binding of lactoferrin to brush borders was explained on the assumption that lactoferrin was binding to transferrin receptors (61), but the use of rhesus monkeys has enabled an examination of the specificity of lactoferrin binding to its receptor to be undertaken (45): binding was time-dependent and saturable; competitive experiments with excess unlabelled lactoferrin showed that the binding was specific; and monkey and human lactoferrin effectively inhibited the binding of rhesus lactoferrin at 50-fold excess, while a similar excess of bovine lactoferrin or human transferrin had no effect on binding. These results taken together are good evidence for a specific lactoferrin receptor. The lactoferrin receptor has now been isolated from human fetal and infant small intestine (44). Any direct effect of lactoferrin on gene expression should be transmitted through this receptor and its analysis may therefore give clues as to how lactoferrin might do this. However, it has been difficult to isolate sufficient lactoferrin receptor for structural analysis (62), but the size and number of peptide chains has been determined for both human (61) and mouse (63, 64) lactoferrin receptors. Recently the human lactoferrin receptor has been cloned (62) and its sequence determined.

Lactoferrin has the intriguing ability to bind to DNA at specific points of the protein structure. Despite this it does not appear that lactoferrin has a direct role in gene expression within the enterocyte nucleus (65). Nevertheless it binds to the bacterial DNA that is recognized by Toll-like receptor-9 (TLR-9). By this means, it may vary the responses (particularly in intestinal B cells) to DNA shed by luminal bacteria. (65)

DNA METHYLATION AND IMPRINTING

The chapter has described examples of nutrient regulation of gene expression in specific organs. However, mechanisms exist within the genome for affecting gene expression throughout the body. Imprinting is an important example of this. Genomic imprinting is the silencing of one of a pair of alleles, allowing preferential expression of a particular gene from either father or mother (66). For example, the maternally inherited allele of the gene encoding IGF-II is silenced, resulting in expression that is derived almost entirely from the father's DNA. Elegant studies in the late 1990s demonstrated that the phenomenon was due to differences in DNA methylation between the two alleles. Around 10% of adults (67) exhibit some loss of imprinting (LOI). LOI of the IGF-II is often present in a condition familiar to neonatologists, the Beckwith-Weidman syndrome (68), where infants are born with abdominal wall defects in association with hypoglycemia and large organs, most noticeably the tongue. In addition, LOI of IGF-II is associated with certain tumors of childhood, particularly nephroblastoma (Wilms' tumor) and hepatoblastoma.

The variable yellow allele (A^{vy}) of the agouti mouse is an excellent tool in which to study DNA methylation (69, 70). Expression of A^{vy} depends on a specific long terminal repeat (LTR). DNA methylation changes the gene's expression (and yellow color) by different amounts in genetically identical mice. Although the level of agouti expression alters a number of downstream processes such as obesity and longevity, the relation between DNA methylation and the coat color has enabled researchers (69, 70) to show that diets rich in nutrients that increase donation of methyl groups cause changes in DNA methylation that are reflected in coat color. These experiments raise the possibly that there is a direct relationship between diet, DNA methylation and gene expression. More recently Waterland and colleagues (71) have varied the diet and altered the DNA methylation and imprinting of the IGF-II gene in the maternal line of non-agouti mice, thus confirming that diet can alter the expression of genes through LOI.

CONCLUSIONS

The possible number of interactions between nutrients and genes is very large, but this chapter has focused on specific examples where such phenomena may be important in infant health and disease. The contents of the gastrointestinal tract have a major influence on gastrointestinal disease. We believe that the luminal regulation of epithelial signaling affects the intestinal inflammatory process, especially because the intestine is an organ where the variations of nutrients are greatest. The implications for this in neonatal gastroenterology are now being unraveled.

REFERENCES

1. Newsholme EA, Start C. Regulation in metabolism. London: Wiley; 1973.
2. Dickson R, Abelson J, Barnes W, et al. Genetic regulation: the lac control region. Science 1975; 187:27–35.
3. Platt T. Regulation of gene expression in the tryptophan operon of *Escherichia coli*. In: Miller JH, Reznikoff WS, eds. The operon. Cold Spring Harbor Laboratory; 1978: 213–302.
4. Sanderson IR. Nutrition and gene expression. In: Walker WA, Watkins JB, eds. Nutrition in Pediatrics. Hamilton: BC Decker; 1996: 213–232.
5. Sanderson IR, Walker WA. Mucosal barrier. In: Ogra R, Mestecky J, McGhee J, et al, eds. Handbook of mucosal immunology. San Diego: Academic Press; 1994: 41–51.
6. Rennie MJ, MacLennan PA, Hundal HS, et al. Skeletal muscle glutamine transport, intramuscular glutamine concentration and muscle protein turnover. Metabolism 1989; 38:47–51.
7. Feng B, Shiber SK, Max SR. Glutamine regulates glutamine synthetase expression in skeletal muscle cells in culture. J Cell Physiol 1990; 145:376–380.
8. Newsholme EA, Calder PC. The proposed role of glutamine in some cells of the immune system and speculative consequences for the whole animal. Nutrition 1997; 13(7-8):728–730.
9. Caicedo RA, Schanler RJ, Li N, et al. The developing intestinal ecosystem: implications for the neonate. Pediatr Res 2005; 58:625–628.
10. Durschlag RP, Smith RL. Regulation of glutamine production by skeletal muscle cells in culture. Am J Physiol 1985; 248:C442–C448.

11. Tadros LB, Willhoft NM, Taylor PM, et al. Effects of glutamine deprivation on glutamine transport and synthesis in primary tissue culture of rat skeletal muscle. Am J Physiol 1993; 265:E935–E942.

12. Low SY, Rennie MJ, Taylor PM. Sodium dependent glutamate transport in cultured rat myotubes increases after glutamine deprivation. FASEB J 1994; 8:127–131.

13. Cameron-Smith D, Burke LM, Angus DJ, et al. A short term, high fat diet upregulates lipid metabolism and gene expression in human skeletal muscle. Am J Clin Nutr 2003; 77(2):313–318.

14. Chang EB, Rao MC. Intestinal water and electrolyte transport. In: Johnson LR, ed. Physiology of the gastrointestinal tract, 3rd edn. New York: Raven Press; 1994: 2027–2081.

15. Sanderson IR, Parsons DS. Influence of vascular flow on amino acid transport across the frog small intestine. J Physiol 1980; 309:447–460.

16. Sanderson IR, Walker WA. Uptake and transport of macromolecules by the intestine: Possible role in clinical disorders (An update). Gastroenterology 1993; 104:622.

17. Sanderson IR, Walker WA. Mucosal barrier. In: Ogra R, Mestecky J, McGhee J, et al., eds. Handbook of mucosal immunology, 2nd edn. Academic Press; 1999: 5–17.

18. Sanderson IR, Walker WA. Uptake and transport of macromolecules by the intestine: Possible roles in clinical disorders (an update). Gastroenterology 1993; 104:622–639.

19. Naik S, Kelly EJ, Meijer L, et al. Absence of Toll-like receptor 4 explains endotoxin hyporesponsiveness in human intestinal epithelium. J Pediatr Gastroenterol Nutr 2001; 32:449–453.

20. Sanderson IR. Nutritional factors and immune functions of gut epithelium. Proc Nutr Soc 2001; 60(4):443–447.

21. Sanderson IR, Ouellette AJ, Carter EA, et al. Ontogeny of Ia messenger RNA in the mouse intestinal epithelium is modulated by age of weaning and diet. Gastroenterology 1993; 105:974–980.

22. Sanderson IR, Bustin SA, Dzennis S, et al. Age and diet act through distinct isoforms of the class II transactivator gene in mouse intestinal epithelium. Gastroenterology 2004; 127:203–212.

23. Sanderson IR. Short chain fatty acid regulation of signaling genes expressed by the intestinal epithelium. J Nutr 2004; 134(9):2450S–2454S.

24. Midtvedt AC, Midvedt T. Production of short chain fatty acids by the intestinal microflora during the first 2 years of human life. J Pediatr Gastroenterol Nutr 1992; 15:395–403.

25. Fusunyan RD, Quinn JJ, Fujimoto M, et al. Butyrate switches the pattern of chemokine secretion by intestinal epithelial cells through histone acetylation. Mol Med 1999; 5:631–640.

26. Sanderson IR, Naik SK. Dietary regulation of intestinal gene expression. Annu Rev Nutr 2000; 20:311–338.

27. Ohtsuka Y, Lee J, Stamm DS, Sanderson IR. MIP-2 secreted by epithelial cells increases neutrophil and lymphocyte recruitment in the mouse intestine. Gut 2001; 49(4):526–533.

28. Sanderson IR, Udeen S, Davies PSW, et al. Remission induced by an elemental diet in small bowel Crohn's disease. Arch Dis Child 1987; 62:123–127.

29. Sanderson IR, Boulton P, Menzies I, et al. Improvement of abnormal lactulose/rhamnose permeability in active Crohn's disease of the small bowel by an elemental diet. Gut 1987; 28:1073–1076.

30. Vaughn P, Thomas P, Clark R, et al. Enteral glutamine supplementation and morbidity in low birth weight infants. J Pediatr 2003; 142(6):662–668.

31. Li N, Lewis P, Samuelson D, et al. Glutamine regulates Caco-2 cell tight junction proteins. Am J Physiol Gastrointest Liver Physiol 2004; 287(3):G726–G733.

32. Liboni KC, Li N, Scumpia PO, et al. Glutamine modulates LPS-induced IL-8 production through IkappaB/NF-kappaB in human fetal and adult intestinal epithelium. J Nutr 2005; 135(2):245–251.

33. Siafakas CG, Anatolitou F, Fusunyan RD, et al. Vascular endothelial growth factor (VEGF) is present in human breast milk and its receptor is present on intestinal epithelial cells. Pediatr Res 1999; 45:652–657.

34. Oguchi S, Walker WA, Sanderson IR. Profile of IGF-binding proteins secreted by intestinal epithelial cells changes with differentiation. Am J Physiol 1994; 267:G843–G850.

35. Weaver LT, Walker WA. Epidermal growth factor and the developing human gut. Gastroenterology 1988; 94:845–847.

36. Chu SW, Walker WA. Growth factor signal transduction in human intestinal cells. In: Mestecky J, ed. Immunology of Milk and the Neonate. New York: Plenum Press; 1991: 107–112.

37. Berseth CL. Enhancement of intestinal growth in neonatal rats by epidermal growth factor in milk. Am J Physiol 1987; 253:G662–G665.

38. He Y, Chu SH, Walker WA. Nucleotide supplements alter proliferation and differentiation of cultured human (Caco 2) and rat (IEC 6) intestinal epithelial cells. J Nutr 1993; 123:1017–1027.

39. Sanderson IR, He Y. Nucleotide uptake and metabolism by intestinal epithelial cells in tissue culture. J Nutr 1994; 124:131S–137S.

40. Metz Boutigue MH, Jolles J, Mazurier J, et al. Human lactotransferrin: amino acid sequence and structural comparisons with other transferrins. Eur J Biochem 1984; 145:659–676.

41. Masson PL, Heremans JF. Lactoferrin in milk from different species. Comp Biochem Physiol 1971; 39B:119–129.

42. Masson PL, Heremans JF, Schonne E. Lactoferrin, an iron binding protein in neutrophilic leukocytes. J Exp Med 1969; 130:643–658.

43. Hansen NE, Malmquist J, Thorell J. Plasma myeloperoxidase and lactoferrin measured by radioimmunoassay: relation to neutrophil kinetics. Acta Med Scand 1975; 198:437–443.

44. Kawakami H, Lonnerdal B. Isolation and function of a receptor for human lactoferrin in human fetal intestinal brush border membranes. Am J Physiol 1991; 261:G841–G846.

45. Davidson LA, Lonnerdal B. Specific binding of lactoferrin to brush border membrane: ontogeny and effect of glycan chain. Am J Physiol 1988; 254:G580–G585.

46. Mazurier J, Montreuil J, Spik G. Visualization of lactotransferrin brush border receptors by ligand blotting. Biochim Biophys Acta 1985; 821:453–460.

47. Hu WL, Mazurier J, Sawatzki G, et al. Lactotransferrin receptor of mouse small intestinal brush border. Binding characteristics of membrane bound and Triton X 100 solubilized forms. Biochem J 1988; 249:435–441.

48. Davidson LA, Lonnerdal B. Persistence of human milk proteins in the breast fed infant. Acta Paediatr Scand 1987; 76:733–740.

49. Britton JR, Koldovsky O. Gastric luminal digestion of lactoferrin and transferrin by preterm infants. Early Hum Dev 1989; 19:127.

50. Cox TM, Mazurier J, Spik G, et al. Iron binding proteins and influx of iron across the duodenal brush border. Evidence for specific lactotransferrin receptors in the human intestine. Biochim Biophys Acta 1979; 588:120–128.

51. Mikogami T, Marianne T, Spik G. Effect of intracellular iron depletion by picolinic acid on expression of the lactoferrin receptor in the human colon carcinoma cell subclone HT29-18-C1. Biochem J 1995; 308:391–397.

52. Klausner RD, Rouault TA, Harford JB. Regulating the fate of mRNA: the control of cellular iron metabolism. Cell 1993; 72:19–28.

53. Hashizume S, Kuroda K, Murakami H. Identification of lactoferrin as an essential factor for human lymphocytic cell lines in serum free medium. Biochim Biophys Acta 1983; 763:377–382.

54. Azuma N, Mori H, Kaminogawa S, et al. Stimulatory effect of human lactoferrin on DNA synthesis in BALB/c 3T3 cells. Agric Biol Chem 1989; 53:31–35.

55. Byatt JC, Schmuke JJ, Comens PG, et al. The effect of bovine lactoferrin on muscle growth in vivo and in vitro. Biochem Biophys Res Commun 1990; 173:548–553.

56. Amouric M, Marvaldi J, Pichon J, et al. Effect of lactoferrin on the growth of a human colon adenocarcinoma cell line-comparison with transferrin. In Vitro 1984; 20:543–548.

57. Nichols BL, McKee KS, Henry JF, et al. Human lactoferrin stimulates thymidine incorporation into DNA of rat crypt cells. Pediatr Res 1987; 21:563–567.

58. Oguchi S, Walker WA, Sanderson IR. Iron saturation alters the effect of lactoferrin on of the proliferation and differentiation of human enterocytes (Caco-2) cells. Biol Neonate 1995; 67:330–339.

59. Sanchez L, Calvo M, Brock J. Biological role of lactoferrin. Arch Dis Child 1992; 67:657–661.

60. Miyazawa K, Mantel C, Lu L, et al. Lactoferrin-lipopolysaccharide interactions. Effect on lactoferrin biding to monocyte/macrophage-differentiated HL-60 cells. J Immunol 1991; 146:723–729.

61. Kawakami H, Dosako S, Lonnerdal B. Iron uptake form transferrin in human fetal intestinal brush-border membrane vesicles. Am J Physiol 1990; 261:G535–G541.

62. Lonnerdal B. Lactoferrin receptors in intestinal brush border membranes. Adv Exp Med Biol 1994; 357:171–175.

63. Hu WL, Mazurier J, Montreuil J, et al. Isolation and partial characterization of a lactotransferrin receptor form mouse intestinal brush border. Biochemistry 1990; 29:535–541.

64. Hu WL, Mazurier J, Sawatzki G, et al. Lactotransferrin receptor of mouse small intestinal brush border. Biochem J 1988; 248:435–451.

65. Mulligan P, White NR, Monteleone G, et al. Breast milk lactoferrin regulates gene expression by binding bacterial DNA CpG motifs but not genomic DNA promoters in model intestinal cells. Pediatr Res 2006; 118:124–129.

66. Feinberg AP. Imprinting of a genomic domain of 11p15 and loss of imprinting in cancer: an introduction. Cancer Res 1999; 59(7 Suppl):1743s–1746s.

67. Cui H, Cruz-Correa M, Giardiello FM, et al. Loss of IGF2 imprinting: a potential marker of colorectal cancer risk. Science 2003; 299(5613):1753–1755.

68. Weksberg R, Smith AC, Squire J, et al. Beckwith-Wiedemann syndrome demonstrates a role for epigenetic control of normal development. Hum Mol Genet 2003; 12(SPI/1):R61–R68.

69. Cooney CA, Dave AA, Wolff GL. Maternal methyl supplements in mice affect epigenetic variation and DNA methylation of offspring. J Nutr 2002; 132(8 Suppl):2393S–2400S.

70. Waterland RA, Jirtle RL. Transposable elements: targets for early nutritional effects on epigenetic gene regulation. Mol Cell Biol 2003; 23(15):5293–5300.

71. Waterland RA, Lin JR, Smith CA, et al. Post-weaning diet affects genomic imprinting at the insulin-like growth factor 2 (Igf2) locus. Hum Mol Genet 2006; 15(5):705–716.

Chapter 3

The Exocrine Pancreas

Steven L. Werlin, MD • Alan Mayer, MD

Time Course for Human Pancreatic Development
Molecular Embryology of Pancreatic Development
Pancreatic Function at Birth
Measurement of Pancreatic Function
Syndromes Associated with Pancreatic Abnormalities

TIME COURSE FOR HUMAN PANCREATIC DEVELOPMENT

The mature pancreas synthesizes and secretes more than 25 proteins and enzymes, most of which are required for digestion (reviewed in ref. 1). Histological examination of the early pancreas reveals predominantly undifferentiated epithelial cells, which by 9–12 weeks form a lobular-tubular pattern; zymogen granules are absent but the Golgi apparatus is present (2, 3) Primitive acini containing rough endoplasmic reticulum and recognizable zymogen granules are present by 14–16 weeks. Golgi vesicles become prominent at this time. Activity of secretory enzymes is first detectable at this age. By 16–20 weeks, large numbers of zymogen granules are present. As the pancreas matures, the luminal volume decreases and acinar cell volume increases. By 20 weeks of gestation, the acinar cells contain mature-appearing zymogen granules, well-developed endoplasmic reticulum, and highly developed basolateral membranes. Stroma continues to decrease. Acinar cells have a mature appearance. Postnatally, the volume of the exocrine pancreas continues to grow, nearly tripling in size during the first year of life from 5.5 g to 14.5 g (4). The adult pancreas weighs 85 g. During the first 4 months the ratio of acinar cells to connective tissue increases fourfold.

Centroacinar and duct cells, which are responsible for water, electrolyte, and bicarbonate secretion, are also found by 20 weeks. The ductal system contains less than 5% of the volume of the exocrine pancreas. The actual volume of the ductal system is only 0.5% of total pancreatic volume. In the postnatal period, luminal volume increases, along with the increase in acinar cell volume.

Islets are first identifiable at 12–16 weeks, at which time immunoreactive insulin is present in B cells. Mixed cells, those with characteristics of both acinar and islet cells that are only rarely seen in the adult, may be found (5). Endocrine cells of the fetus, but not the adult, may contain more than one hormone, and more than one hormone may be found within a single granule. The histological appearance of the term pancreas is similar to that of the adult.

The signals controlling both cytodifferentiation, the process by which pancreatic cells differentiate into the various structural elements, and morphogenesis are being increasingly understood and are discussed below.

Although duodenal and stool protease activity has been clearly demonstrated by many investigators, the time of first appearance of digestive enzymes in the fetal pancreas has been variably described. Unfortunately, until recently much of the available data not only were derived from methods no longer considered scientifically acceptable but also were contradictory. Only studies using modern, acceptable techniques are reviewed here.

Lieberman found proteolytic activity, both in the pancreas of the 500-g fetus after activation of pancreatic homogenate with enterokinase and in the meconium from similarly aged fetuses (6). Track and colleagues found that trypsin, chymotrypsin, phospholipase A, and lipase were all present in the 14-cm (14-week) fetus in low concentrations, and these steadily increased with gestational age but amylase was not found (3). Jodl and colleagues found increasing chymotrypsin activity in the stools collected from 42 low birth weight infants ranging in size from 750 to 2570 g with gestational age (7). Chymotrypsin activity was low at birth, peaked at age 3 days, then declined slightly. Similarly, Mullinger and Palasi detected trypsin and chymotrypsin in the stool of neonates (8). Wide day-to-day variation of enzyme concentration is found.

Using immunohistochemical techniques, Carrere and colleagues demonstrated that trypsinogen and chymotrypsinogen are present in all acinar cells at week 16 of gestation and progressively increase in concentration until birth (9). In contrast, lipase-containing cells were scattered until week 21. Fukayama and co-workers found pancreatic secretory trypsin inhibitor in the fetal pancreas at 10 weeks of gestation (10).

Using electrophoresis and immunohistochemistry with monoclonal antibodies, Davis and colleagues demonstrated that pancreatic amylase is present in amniotic fluid at 14 weeks of gestation (11). Immunologic activity is present in the pancreas at 16 weeks of gestation. In contrast, Mally and colleagues were unable to detect amylase mRNA in the human fetal pancreas (12). Thus amylase, lipase, trypsinogen, and chymotrypsinogen are present in the fetal pancreas by 16 weeks of gestation, the time of rapid development of zymogen granules.

Human mucin gene expression (Muc 1) was evaluated in the fetal pancreas by Batra and colleagues, who found that Muc 1 mRNA, a marker for differentiation of pancreatic cells, was not detectable until 18 to 19 weeks of gestation (13). In adults Muc 1 expression correlates with the differentiation state of pancreatic tumors.

MOLECULAR EMBRYOLOGY OF PANCREATIC DEVELOPMENT

Although morphogenesis of the pancreas was described over a century ago, molecular mediators underlying this complex process have been identified only recently. A recurrent theme of the molecular underpinning of pancreatic development is that both instructive and permissive factors must work in concert for proper organ formation. Given the stringency of these requirements, organogenesis is surprisingly robust and reproducible from animal to animal. Thus, multiple safeguards and redundancies are probably operative, many of which have yet to be discovered.

Patterning of the Endoderm

The parenchymal cells of the pancreas – both endocrine and exocrine glands – originate from the endodermal epithelium of the primitive gut tube (14). For example, before the pancreatic primordia evaginate from the primitive gut tube, many molecular programs that specify a pancreatic fate have been set in motion by the inductive influences of neighboring tissues. During gastrulation, the endoderm is subdivided into anterior and posterior domains by signals from the adjacent mesectoderm. Retinoic acid (15), bone morphogenic proteins (BMPs) and fibroblast growth factors (FGFs) (16) play an important role during late gastrulation in localizing the prepancreatic domain which will respond to subsequent instructive signals that induce pancreatic tissue.

The prospective ventral and dorsal pancreas are exposed to different local contacts, and therefore rely on distinct sources for their induction. The endoderm fated to become the ventral pancreas begins to express pancreatic genes first, induced by activin and BMP-family molecules derived from the adjacent lateral plate mesoderm (17). The dorsal pancreas is induced by a different mechanism. Its endoderm is transiently in contact with the notochord and then the dorsal aorta. Contact with the notochord induces a localized exclusion of sonic hedgehog (shh) from the prepancreatic endoderm. This signaling event is necessary for dorsal pancreatic development, since ectopic expression of shh interferes with subsequent events (18). Contact between endoderm and notochord ends with the interposition of the dorsal aorta, which also provides essential signals to promote pancreatic fate (19), among them vascular endothelial growth factor (20).

Pancreas Specification

The events described above contribute to rendering the prepancreatic endoderm competent to form pancreatic tissue. The next step involves expression of transcription factors in the endoderm and surrounding mesenchyme to further specify these cells to adopt a pancreatic fate. One of the essential genes is Hlx9, encoding the homeobox protein HB9. Its genetic ablation results in selective absence of the dorsal pancreas (21).

The pancreatic-duodenal homeobox gene 1(Pdx-1) gene, one of the first pancreas-specific transcription factors discovered (22), is expressed in both dorsal and ventral pancreatic primordia, and its ablation results in arrest of pancreatic development shortly after formation of these structures (23). A mutation in the human Pdx-1 gene was found to cause congenital pancreatic agenesis in an infant (24). The function of Pdx-1 is instructive, as evidenced by the ability to transform liver into pancreas by hepatic expression of the *Xenopus* Pdx-1 homolog fused to the VP16 transactivator (25). Pdx-1 also has a later role in the maintenance of β-cell identity and the transcription of the insulin gene.

Highlighting the role of the surrounding mesenchyme, the LIM homeodomain protein Isl1 is expressed in the dorsal pancreatic mesenchyme, and is required for its elaboration. In the absence of Isl1, the dorsal pancreas does not form, but the ventral pancreas is unaffected (26).

Cell Fate Specification: the Exocrine-Endocrine Decision

After specification of pancreatic cell fate and initial budding of the pancreatic primordium, the endodermal precursor cells become diversified into exocrine and endocrine lines (Fig. 3-1). The molecular effectors that influence these events have been deciphered in recent years, revealing a striking conservation of mechanism for cell fate allocation between different organ systems. Taking a cue from earlier work in neuronal cell fate allocation (27), researchers examined Notch signaling pathway mutant mice and discovered that Notch signaling is a key participant in the exocrine-endocrine cell fate allocation decision. Specifically, it was previously known that the basic helix-loop-helix (bHLH) transcription factor Neurogenin3 (Ngn3) is required for all endocrine cell lineages (28). Ngn3 activates expression of Notch ligands Delta, Serrate and Jagged, which then activate Notch signaling on adjacent cells. This signal results in expression of Hes-1, which in turn represses Ngn and other target genes. Thus an undifferentiated pancreatic

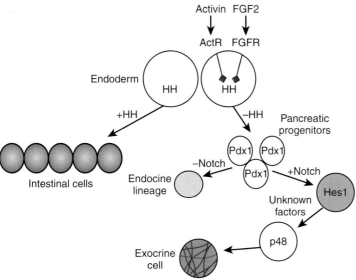

Figure 3-1 Molecular mediators of cell fate specification during pancreatic development. The endoderm is rendered competent to become pancreas by notochord-derived signals (Activin, FGF2) that act through their respective receptors (ActR, FGFR) and inhibit hedgehog (HH) expression in the pre-pancreatic endoderm. Ectopic hedgehog expression leads to intestinal cell fate. The HH-negative cells express Pdx1, which is essential for outgrowth of the pancreatic primordium. Exocrine-endocrine cells are partitioned by a "lateral inhibition" mechanism mediated by Notch signaling. Cells lacking Notch and its downstream mediators adopt endocrine fates, whereas Notch-expressing cells activate the transcriptional repressor Hes1, which represses neurogenin expression and other islet-specific genes. p48 is an exocrine-specific gene essential for the elaboration of the exocrine pancreas.(From Lowe ME, Pancreatic function and dysfunction. In: Walker WA, Goulet O, Kleinman R, Sherman P, Schneider B, Sanderson I, eds.Pediatric gastrointestinal disease: pathophysiology and management, 4th edition, p. 99. BC Decker, with permission.)

cell fated to become an islet cell will signal to its immediate neighbors to adopt an exocrine fate. By this mechanism, known as lateral inhibition, Notch signaling promotes the divergence of the pancreatic lineage into exocrine and endocrine fates (29).

Recent data have demonstrated a role for retinoic acid (RA) in the exocrine-endocrine cell fate decision, possibly upstream of Notch signaling (30). Interestingly, RA treatment seems to have divergent effects on the dorsal and ventral pancreas, promoting endocrine fate in the dorsal pancreas but exocrine fate in the ventral pancreas. These data stand as further evidence for distinct developmental programs in the dorsal and ventral primordia.

Endocrine Cells

Four endoderm-derived cell types are known to populate the islets: α-cells (glucagon-secreting), β-cells (insulin-secreting), δ-cells (somatostatin-secreting) and PP cells (pancreatic polypeptide). Each of these is derived from a common Ngn3-expressing precursor by a combinatorial hierarchy of transcription factors that promote a lineage-specific program. Beta2/NeuroD is a bHLH transcription factor activated by Ngn3 that is expressed in an alpha-beta cell progenitor, and subsequently regulates transcription of insulin and other β-cell specific genes (31). Pax4 is a paired-box homeodomain protein required for β- and δ-cells (32). Other transcription factors essential to proper islet differentiation include Pax6 (33), Nkx2.2, and Nkx6.1 (34, 35).

Maturity-onset diabetes of the young (MODY) is a group of dominantly inherited syndromes that predispose to the development of type 2 diabetes.

The loci have been mapped to six complementation groups and, of these, five result from mutations in transcription factors that are necessary for pancreatic development and insulin transcription. They include HNF4α (MODY1), HNF1α (MODY3), Pdx1 (MODY4), HNF1β (MODY5), and Beta2 (MODY6) (36). Mutations in Pax4, Isl1, and Ngn3 also predispose to late-onset diabetes (36).

Exocrine Pancreas

Compared to the islet cells, considerably less is known about the molecular determinants of exocrine pancreatic differentiation. As such, only two factors are known to be specifically required for exocrine differentiation: Ptf1a and Mist1. Ptf1 consists of a heterodimer comprising the ubiquitous transcriptional regulator E2A and a tissue-specific protein p48 (37). This complex binds to the promoter regions of exocrine-specific genes and activates their transcription. Genetic ablation of p48 in mice results in failure to form an exocrine pancreas, as well as morphological deformities of the islets (38). More recent studies utilizing Ptf1a-Cre knock-in mice have broadened our understanding of the role for p48 to include a much earlier function in specifying pancreatic identity from uncommitted endodermal precursors (39).

Mist1 is also a bHLH transcription factor expressed in the exocrine pancreas, but also in salivary gland and stomach (40). *Mist1* null mice exhibit lesions in the exocrine pancreas, possibly resulting from defective cell-cell adhesion, but still retain exocrine-specific gene expression (41). Mist1 has thus been proposed to function in cooperation with PTF1 to maintain a stable exocrine differentiated state.

PANCREATIC FUNCTION AT BIRTH

Pancreatic function is immature at birth, leading to physiological malabsorbtion for the first 6–12 months of life due to inadequate secretion of lipase and bile acids (42–46). Clinically significant fat malabsorbtion does not occur until pancreatic enzyme secretion is decreased to < 5–10% of normal, the range typically found in the newborn infant. Fortunately this is rarely a clinical problem. The relatively normal fat absorption found in premature and full-term infants is probably due to the presence of lingual and gastric lipase, neither of which are dependent on colipase or bile salts for activity.

Although amylase is present in the pancreas of the newborn, little is secreted (47). Adult levels of duodenal amylase are not reached until age 2–3 years. True isolated amylase deficiency has not been reported. Starch, in the form of corn syrup solids, which requires amylase for digestion, is a common carbohydrate source in infant formulas. Due to salivary amylase and glucoamylase, a brush-border enzyme, starch malabsorbtion leading to diarrhea is uncommon (48, 49). However, when an infant who is receiving a formula containing corn syrup solids or maltodextrins develops unexplained watery diarrhea, relative amylase deficiency should be suspected. The diagnosis of (relative) amylase insufficiency can be made by finding positive reducing substances in the stool following acid hydrolysis. The treatment is a formula change to one that does not contain starch.

MEASUREMENT OF PANCREATIC FUNCTION

The detection of pancreatic insufficiency has typically depended on screening tests as formal pancreatic function testing is invasive. A variety of markers have been used, each with a high incidence of false positives and negatives. For example, fat malabsorbtion, abnormal in pancreatic insufficiency, is also abnormal with mucosal diseases. Stool collections are distasteful and prone to error. Staining stool for fat globules is only 90–95% reliable. Since pancreatic enzymes are auto-digested as they pass through the intestines, stool levels of trypsin and chymotrypsin may be falsely low. However, pancreatic elastase, which is resistant to proteolytic digestion, passes through the intestinal tract undegraded. Fecal elastase has a high sensitivity and specificity for pancreatic insufficiency (50, 51). A normal fecal elastase has a 99% positive predictive value for excluding pancreatic insufficiency. However, fecal elastase may be low in normal premature infants. In older children decreased fecal elastase can also be found in small-bowel enteropathies. Measurement of fecal elastase by ELISA is commercially available.

Pancreatic Insufficiency

Except for cystic fibrosis (CF), disorders that may present with exocrine pancreatic insufficiency are uncommon. Newborns with CF may present with meconium ileus or ileal atresia but rarely with pancreatic insufficiency. Universal newborn screening for cystic fibrosis is recommended by the March of Dimes. CF has been added to the newborn screening panel in 16 states.

Definitive Morphogenesis: Rotation and Fusion of Dorsal and Ventral Buds

In mammals, the adult pancreas results from the fusion of the dorsal and ventral primordia, which occurs in concert with the rotation of the midgut. As the buds fuse, their respective ducts anastomose, with the ventral duct normally serving as the conduit for pancreatic secretions from both anlagen. In about 9% of people, the ducts fail to fuse completely and the two duct systems persist, causing the defect pancreas divisum, which may predispose to acute recurrent or chronic pancreatitis (52). Pancreas divisum has been observed in mice heterozygous for Indian hedgehog and sonic hedgehog null mutations, suggesting that hedgehog signaling may play a role in its pathogenesis (53). Mutation in these genes also causes overgrowth of the ventral pancreatic primordium, and can lead to annular pancreas, a congenital defect that often results in duodenal obstruction (53).

Complete and partial pancreatic agenesis due to a mutations in the IPF1 gene coding sequence and due to decreased half-life of insulin promoter factor 1 have both been described (22, 24). Dorsal pancreatic agenesis has been described in the retinoic-acid-deficient *Raldh2* mutant mouse (15). These conditions are often associated with diabetes and may be associated with sacral agenesis (54). Complete pancreatic agenesis is associated with exocrine pancreatic insufficiency as well as diabetes and is usually fatal (24).

Rare isolated deficiencies of enterokinase, required to activate trypsinogen to trypsin, trypsinogen, lipase and colipase have been reported. Patients with these deficiencies typically present with severe failure to thrive and malabsorbtion shortly after birth.

SYNDROMES ASSOCIATED WITH PANCREATIC ABNORMALITIES

A number of syndromes are associated with pancreatic insufficiency or abnormalities such as fibrosis. However, pancreatic insufficiency rarely presents in the newborn period.

The *Shwachman Diamond Syndrome* (*SBDS*) is an autosomal recessive disorder which includes fatty degeneration of the pancreas, bone marrow failure, hepatic, bony and other abnormalities. Pancreatic insufficiency is not typically apparent in the newborn (55, 56). The SDS gene has been identified and cloned and is located on chromosome 7 (57).

The *Johanson Blizzard Syndrome* is a rare autosomal recessive condition including exocrine pancreatic insufficiency due to absent pancreatic acini with intact ducts, aplasia or hypoplasia of the alae nasi and ectodermal scalp defects (58, 59). The *Johanson Blizzard Syndrome* is caused by a mutation in the UBR1 gene, located on chromosome 15q (58, 59). Variable features include deafness, hypothyroidism, and absent teeth. More variable features include developmental delay and cardiac and anorectal abnormalities. Endocrinopathies may include hypopituitarism, growth hormone deficiency and diabetes mellitus. While the syndrome is often recognized at birth due to the multitude of congenital abnormalities, unrecognized pancreatic insufficiency may be the cause of diarrhea, malabsorbtion and failure to thrive,

Jeune Syndrome, asphyxiating thoracic dystrophy, includes a complex of thoracic dystrophy, short-limbed dwarfism, and cystic dysplasia of the kidneys. Some reported cases have had exocrine pancreatic insufficiency (60). Histolological findings similar to Shwachman Diamond Syndrome have been found in some cases but not in others. Patients with Jeune syndrome should be screened for both pancreatic function and for the possibility of Shwachman Diamond Syndrome.

Pearson's Syndrome is a mitochondrial disorder characterized by bone marrow failure and exocrine pancreatic failure (60, 61). As in all mitochondrial disorders a variety of organ systems may be involved. Pancreatic insufficiency typically does not present in the newborn period.

The combination of renal, hepatic, and pancreatic abnormalities appears in several syndromes, including *Ivemark syndrome, trisomy 9, Meckel syndrome,* the *chondrodysplasias of Jeune* and of *Saldino and Noonan,* and *type II glutaric acidemia.* Bernstein et al. concluded that after exclusion of identifiable syndromes, the remaining cases of renal-hepatic-pancreatic dysplasia do not necessarily constitute a homogeneous group (62). Pancreatic dysfunction, although present in these patients, is not usually a major feature.

Hyperinsulinemic hypoglycemia (formerly called nesidioblastosis) caused by diffuse or focal beta cell hyperfunction is frequently treated with 95% or total pancreatectomy, which may then cause pancreatic exocrine insufficiency (63). Patients receiving major pancreatic resections should be assessed for exocrine pancreatic function.

REFERENCES

1. Werlin SL, Lee PC. Development of the exocrine pancreas. In: Polin RA, Fox WW, eds. Fetal and neonatal physiology, 3rd edition. Philadelphia, PA: WB Saunders; 2003: 1147–1151.
2. Lucia M, et al. The developing human fetal pancreas: an ultrastructural and histochemical study with special reference to exocrine cells. J Anat 1974; 117:619–634.
3. Track NS, et al. Enzymatic, functional and ultrastructural development of the exocrine pancreas II. The human pancreas. Comp Biochem Physiol 1975; 51A:95–100.
4. Schulz DM, et al. Weight of organs of fetuses and infants. Arch Pathol 1962; 74:244.
5. Lukinius A, et al. Ultrastructural studies of the ontogeny of fetal human and porcine endocrine pancreas, with special reference to colocalization of the four major islet hormones. Dev Biol 1992; 153:376–385.
6. Lieberman J. Proteolytic enzyme activity in fetal pancreas and meconium, demonstration of plasminogen and trypsinogen activators in pancreatic tissue. Gastroenterology 1966; 50:183–190.
7. Jodl J, et al. Chymotryptic activity in stool of low birth weight infants in the first week of life. Acta Pediatr Scand 1975; 64:619–623.
8. Mullinger M, Palasi M. Tryptic and chymotryptic activity of stools of newborn infants. Pediatrics 1966; 38:657–659.
9. Carrere J, et al. Immunohistochemical study of secretory proteins in the developing human exocrine pancreas. Differentiation 1992; 51:55–60.
10. Fukayama M, et al. Immunohistochemical localization of pancreatic secretory trypsin inhibitor in fetal and adult pancreatic and extra pancreatic tissues. J Histochem Cytochem 1986; 34:227–235.

11. Davis MM, et al. Pancreatic amylase expression in human pancreatic development. Hybridoma 1986; 5:137–145.

12. Mally MI, et al. Developmental gene expression in the human fetal pancreas. Pediatr Res 1994; 36:537–544.

13. Batra BK, et al. Human Muc 1 mucin gene expression in the fetal pancreas. Pancreas 1992; 7:391–393.

14. Slack JM. Developmental biology of the pancreas. Development 1995; 121:1569–1580.

15. Stafford D, Prince VE. Retinoic acid signaling is required for a critical early step in zebrafish pancreatic development. Curr Biol 2002; 12:1215–1220.

16. Wells JM, Melton DA. Early mouse endoderm is patterned by soluble factors from adjacent germ layers. Development 2000; 127:1563–1572.

17. Kumar M, et al. Signals from lateral plate mesoderm instruct endoderm toward a pancreatic fate. Dev Biol 2003; 259:109–122.

18. Hebrok M, Kim SK, Melton DA. Notochord repression of endodermal Sonic hedgehog permits pancreas development. Genes Dev. 1998; 12:1705–1713.

19. Lammert E, Cleaver O, Melton D. Induction of pancreatic differentiation by signals from blood vessels. Science 2001; 294:564–567.

20. Lammert E, et al. Role of VEGF-A in vascularization of pancreatic islets. Curr Biol 2003; 13:1070–1074.

21. Li H, et al. Selective agenesis of the dorsal pancreas in mice lacking homeobox gene Hlxb9. Nat Genet 1999; 23:67–70.

22. Ohlsson H, Karlsson K, Edlund T. IPF1, a homeodomain-containing transactivator of the insulin gene. Embo J 1993; 12:4251–4259.

23. Offield MF, et al. PDX-1 is required for pancreatic outgrowth and differentiation of the rostral duodenum. Development 1996; 122:983–995.

24. Stoffers DA, et al. Pancreatic agenesis attributable to a single nucleotide deletion in the human IPF1 gene coding sequence. Nat Genet 1997; 15:106–110.

25. Horb ME, et al. Experimental conversion of liver to pancreas. Curr Biol 2003; 13:105–115.

26. Ahlgren U, et al. Independent requirement for ISL1 in formation of pancreatic mesenchyme and islet cells. Nature 1997; 385:257–260.

27. Artavanis-Tsakonas S, Rand MD, Lake RJ. Notch signaling: cell fate control and signal integration in development. Science 1999; 284:770–776.

28. Gradwohl G, et al. Neurogenin3 is required for the development of the four endocrine cell lineages of the pancreas. Proc Natl Acad Sci USA 2000; 97:1607–1611.

29. Edlund H. Pancreas: how to get there from the gut?. Curr Opin Cell Biol 1999; 11:663–668.

30. Chen Y, et al. Retinoic acid signaling is essential for pancreas development and promotes endocrine at the expense of exocrine cell differentiation in Xenopus. Dev Biol 2004; 271:144–160.

31. Naya FJ, Stellrecht CM, Tsai MJ. Tissue-specific regulation of the insulin gene by a novel basic helix-loop-helix transcription factor. Genes Dev 1995; 9:1009–1019.

32. Sosa-Pineda B, et al. The Pax4 gene is essential for differentiation of insulin-producing beta cells in the mammalian pancreas. Nature 1997; 386:399–402.

33. St-Onge L, et al. Pax6 is required for differentiation of glucagon-producing alpha-cells in mouse pancreas. Nature 1997; 387:406–409.

34. Sander M, et al. Homeobox gene Nkx6.1 lies downstream of Nkx2.2 in the major pathway of beta-cell formation in the pancreas. Development 2000; 127:5533–5540.

35. Sussel L, et al. Mice lacking the homeodomain transcription factor Nkx2.2 have diabetes due to arrested differentiation of pancreatic beta cells. Development 1998; 125:2213–2221.

36. Habener JF, Kemp DM, Thomas MK. Minireview: transcriptional regulation in pancreatic development. Endocrinology 2005; 46:1025–1034.

37. Krapp A, et al. The p48 DNA-binding subunit of transcription factor PTF1 is a new exocrine pancreas-specific basic helix-loop-helix protein. Embo J 1996; 15:4317–4329.

38. Krapp A, et al. The bHLH protein PTF1-p48 is essential for the formation of the exocrine and the correct spatial organization of the endocrine pancreas. Genes Dev 1998; 12:3752–3763.

39. Kawaguchi Y, et al. The role of the transcriptional regulator Ptf1a in converting intestinal to pancreatic progenitors. Nat Genet 2002; 32:128–134.

40. Lemercier C, et al. Mist1: a novel basic helix-loop-helix transcription factor exhibits a developmentally regulated expression pattern. Dev Biol 1997; 182:101–113.

41. Pin CL, et al. The bHLH transcription factor Mist1 is required to maintain exocrine pancreas cell organization and acinar cell identity. J Cell Biol 2001; 155:519–530.

42. Hadorn B, et al. Quantitative assessment of exocrine pancreatic function in infants and children. J Pediatr 1968; 73:39–50.

43. Zoppi G, et al. Protein content and pancreatic enzyme activities of duodenal juice in normal children and in children with exocrine pancreatic insufficiency. Helv Paediatr Acta 1968; 23:577–590.

44. Zoppi G, et al. The electrolyte and protein contents and outputs in duodenal juice after pancreozymin and secretin stimulation in normal children and in patients with cystic fibrosis. Acta Paediatr Scand 1970; 59:692–696.

45. Zoppi G, et al. Exocrine pancreas function in premature and full term infants. Pediatr Res 1972; 6:880–886.

46. Norman A, et al. Bile acids and pancreatic enzymes during absorption in the newborn. Acta Paediatr Scand 1972; 61:571–576.

47. Lebenthal E, Lee PC. Development of functional response in human exocrine pancreas. Pediatrics 1990; 66:556–560.

48. Fisher SE, et al. Chronic protracted diarrhea: intolerance to dietary glucose polymers. Pediatrics 1981; 67:271–273.

49. Fagundes-Neto U, et al. Tolerance to glucose polymers in malnourished infants with diarrhea and disaccharide intolerance. Am J Clin Nutr 1985; 41:228–234.

50. Bebarry S, Ellis L, Corey M, et al. How useful is fecal pancreatic elastase 1as a marker of exocrine pancreatic disease? J Pediatr 2002; 141:84–90.

51. Cohen JR, Schall JI, Ittenbach RF, et al. Fecal elastase: pancreatic status verification and influence on nutritional status in children with cystic fibrosis. J Pediatr Gastroenterol Nutrit 2005; 40:438–444.

52. Klein SD, Affronti JP. Pancreas divisum, an evidence-based review: part pathophysiology. Gastrointest Endosc 2004; 60:419–425.

53. Hebrok M, et al. Regulation of pancreas development by hedgehog signaling. Development 2000; 127:4905–4913.

54. Wildling R, Schnedl WJ, Reisinger EC, et al. Agenesis of the dorsal pancreas in a woman with diabetes mellitus and in both her sons. Gastroenterology 1993; 104:1182–1186.

55. Ginzberg H, Shin J, Ellis L, et al. Shwachman syndrome: Phenotypic manifestations of sibling sets and isolated cases in a large patient cohort are similar. J Pediatr 1999; 135:81–88.

56. Ip WF, Dupuis A, Ellis L, et al. Serum pancreatic enzymes define the pancreatic phenotype in patients with Shwachman-Diamond syndrome. J Pediatr 2002; 141:259–265.

57. Boocock GRB, Morrison JA, Popovic M, et al. Mutations in SBDS are associated with Shwachman-Diamond syndrome. Nat Genetics 2002; 33:97–101.

58. Gershoni-Baruch R, Lerner A, Braun J, et al. Johanson-Blizzard syndrome: Clinical spectrum and further delineation of the syndrome. Am J Med Genet 1990; 35:546–551.

59. Zenker M, Mayerle J, Lerch MM. Deficiency of UBR1, a ubiquitin ligase of the N-end rule pathway, causes pancreatic dysfunction, malformations and mental retardation (Johanson-Blizzard Syndrome). Nat Genet 2005; 37:1345–1350.

60. Lacbawan F, Tifft CJ, Luban NL, et al. Clinical heterogeneity in mitochondrial DNA deletion disorders: a diagnostic challenge of Pearson syndrome. Am J Med Genet 2000; 95:266–268.

61. Gillis LA, Sokol RJ. Gastrointestinal manifestations of mitochondrial disease. Gastroenterol Clin North Am 2003; 32:789–817.

62. Bernstein J, Chandra M, Creswell J, et al. Renal-hepatic-pancreatic dysplasia: a syndrome reconsidered. Am J Med Genet 1987; 26:391–403.

63. Reinecke-Lüthge A, Koschoreck F, Klöppel G. The molecular basis of persistent hyperinsulinemic hypoglycemia of infancy and its pathologic substrates. Virchows Arch 2000; 436:1–5.

Chapter 4

Innate Immunity and Epithelial Biology: Special Considerations in the Neonatal Gut

Patricia W. Lin, MD • Andrew S. Neish, MD

Innate Intestinal Immunity Overview
Developmental Considerations in Intestinal Immunity
Clinical Considerations: Potential Clinical Strategies to Promote Intestinal Immunity

INNATE INTESTINAL IMMUNITY OVERVIEW

The mature intestine has remarkable physiological responsibilities. First and foremost, it functions as an organ of digestion and absorption, necessarily permeable to nutrients and fluids. However, the intestine is exposed to and must also protect itself from exposure to a vast bacterial flora, a wide array of food antigens, and physiochemical stresses caused by digestive processes and microbial metabolism. The intestine as a whole must be able to manage and even encourage microbial commensals, but also remain capable of responding to microbial threats in the form of enteric pathogens. The lumenal lining must remain quiescent in the face of high concentrations of non-endogenous chemical products and extremes of pH, yet be able to react to tissue injury caused by even more extreme stresses.

The neonatal gut faces even more daunting challenges; it must successfully negotiate the transition from a sterile lumen devoid of digestive and microbial metabolic products to the fully realized "bioreactor" of the adult gut. This chapter will describe how this dynamic tissue manages these challenges by focusing on the innate intestinal host defenses. Specifically, we will concentrate on the epithelial layer itself, the cells that form the actual interface. Each section will be organized along three components of innate immunity. First, we will describe the constitutive intrinsic structural barriers; second, the biochemical defenses; and finally the inducible inflammatory response.

The Epithelia

The mucosa of the large and small intestine allows bidirectional passage of liters of fluid and regulates the transport of nutrients and ions (1). Simultaneously, the lumenal surface of this tissue exists in physical contact with a diverse ecosystem of up to 10^{11} prokaryotic organisms/mL that comprises the normal flora. The eukaryotic-prokaryotic relationship in the GI tract can be described as symbiotic. The bacteria thrive in the nutrient-rich and temperature-controlled lumenal environment while serving a biochemical function to the host by metabolizing certain vitamins and degrading bile acids (2, 3). On the opposite side of the mucosa lie the host's interior and a biological system exquisitely sensitive to microbes and their products. A single-cell-layer columnar epithelium separates these compartments. This epithelial layer encompasses a surface area of approximately 200 m^2 organized into complex invaginations (crypts) and evaginations (villi). Stem cells located at the bases of these crypts proliferate, differentiate into enterocytes, and migrate to the villus tip where they eventually undergo a physiologic form of apoptosis (anokis) and slough into the lumen. The entire process, resulting in total reconstitution of the epithelium, occurs every 5 days (4). Thus, one form of defense against epithelial injury is the sheer proliferative and self-regenerating capacity of this interface.

In the embryological and topological sense, the intestinal lining forms a boundary with the external environment, as does the skin. And similar to the skin, the epithelial monolayer has physical adaptations to partially armor itself from exogenous stresses. Subapically located intercellular junctional complexes zipper together intestinal epithelial cells to form a barrier selective to even small molecules and ions (5). By selectively controlling the movement of small ions across this monolayer, enterocytes utilize Cl$^-$ and water secretion (secretory diarrhea) to flush unwanted pathogens or toxins from the intestinal lumen (6). Furthermore, specialized enterocytes (goblet cells) secrete gram quantities of mucins, a diverse mixture of complex glycoproteins, which form a thick protective layer over the intestinal mucosa. This mucus layer hampers direct microbial-epithelial binding, aggregates adherent bacteria, and enhances bacterial removal by reducing shear forces of the lumenal stream. Thus, the mature epithelia possess some degree of intrinsic adaptation to lumenal threats (6).

Antimicrobial Peptides

The gut also possesses chemical defenses. Paneth cells, specialized secretory enterocytes located at the base of small intestinal crypts, secrete lysozyme, phospholipase A2, and small cationic antimicrobial peptides (also secreted by absorptive enterocytes) which may regulate the composition and distribution of bacterial populations (7, 8). The two main families of intestinal-derived antimicrobial peptides are the defensins (α and β) and cathelicidins (7, 9). Both defensins and cathelicidins are present in epithelial, secretory and phagocytic cells throughout the body, each with a distinct conserved structure. Cathelicidins (LL-37/hCAP-18) are small linear peptides expressed near the top of large intestinal crypts. In humans, LL-37/hCAP-18 expression upregulates in response to *Salmonella* or *E. coli* infection (7). Defensins form a beta sheet through six disulfide-linked cysteine residues. In secretory or phagocytic cells, α-defensins are stored in granules in their proform and require subsequent post-translational cleavage by matrilysin (MMP-7 in mice) or Paneth cell trypsins (in humans) to become active (10, 11). These small cationic peptides were initially discovered in human neutrophils (human defensin neutrophil peptide or HNP1–4), where they play a key role in oxygen-independent killing of microbes (7). In the intestine Paneth cells secrete α-defensins (human defensin, HD5 and HD6) in response to microbial or cholinergic stimuli (9, 12). Intestinal epithelial cells primarily secrete β-defensins, with expression of hBD1 remaining relatively constant throughout the gastrointestinal tract. hBD3 and hBD2 are expressed primarily in the esophagus and stomach, respectively. Unlike hBD1, hBD2 exhibits NF-κB-dependent (see Section III) upregulation in response to enteroinvasive pathogens and other proinflammatory stimuli (7, 13, 14).

These antimicrobial peptides act by self-assembly into prokaryotic biomembranes to form anion-conductive channels, which depolarize cells and kill microbes

(9, 15–19). These peptides exhibit bioactivity against a wide range of microbes, including Gram-positive and Gram-negative bacteria, fungi, protozoa, spirochetes, and enveloped viruses (13, 20, 21). Interestingly, with the exception of hBD3, antimicrobial activity can be inhibited under high salt concentrations and may explain the propensity for pulmonary infections in cystic fibrosis patients (see "Clinical considerations" below) (9, 21). The strategic location of Paneth cells may allow concentrated secretion of α-defensins, thus creating the relatively sterile and protected environment within intestinal crypts (12).

In addition to direct antimicrobial action, recent studies have implicated antimicrobial peptides in other aspects of intestinal host defense. In vitro studies have demonstrated proinflammatory properties for cathelicidins, through direct chemotaxis for immune cells, induced immune cell differentiation, and activated secretion of chemokines (22). In vitro, certain murine Paneth cell α-defensins can form anion-conductive channels in eukaryotic (intestinal epithelial) cells, inducing Cl⁻ secretion, presumably protecting the crypt stem cell by flushing the crypt of unwanted pathogens and their toxins (23, 24). In addition, this channel formation can activate the intestinal epithelial inflammatory response through activation of NF-κB (see below) (25). Recent in vitro studies also demonstrate that murine β-defensins can induce chemotaxis for and maturation of certain immune cells (22). Future studies will be required to determine what role these additional defensin and cathelicidin-induced immune modulatory activities play in intestinal host defense in vivo.

The Inflammatory Response

An important and non-constitutive defense against potentially injurious threats is the inflammatory response. Inflammation is a programmed, tightly choreographed host response that serves to recruit leukocytes to aid in the defense against potential pathogens and in the initial response to damaged tissue. The inflammatory process begins when endogenous or exogenous signals of potential danger induce local release of soluble inflammatory mediators and chemotactic agents that serve to increase vascular permeability and attract inflammatory cells, initially neutrophils, and later monocytes and lymphocytes. Histopathologically, inflamed tissue exhibits edema and leukocyte infiltration. In the next section we will describe in detail the mechanisms by which the intestine responds to microbes and their products. We will first review how intestinal epithelia perceive microbes, then detail the signaling pathways activated by these sensors, and finally, describe the effector molecules induced by these signals and what role they play in host defense.

Epithelial Monitoring of Bacteria: MAMPs and PRRs

Enterocytes can perceive potential infection through a conserved, common circuitry for bacterial surveillance and response that has evolved in almost all forms of multicellular eukaryotic life, including lower invertebrates and plants (26, 27). Multiple receptors termed "pattern recognition receptors" (PRRs) specifically recognize and bind distinctive microbial ligands ("microbial associated molecule patterns" or MAMPs) and transmit signals into the cell. The term MAMP describes biochemical motifs that are restricted to, and definitive of, microbial organisms (28). MAMPs include complex macromolecules such as lipopolysaccharide (LPS), peptidoglycan (PGN), and lipoproteins; unmodified polypeptides (flagellin); and nucleic acids (CpG-rich DNA, dsRNA). Specific MAMPs may be characteristic of specific classes of microbes. For example, Gram-negative cell walls contain LPS, Gram-positive cell walls include PGN, and certain viral genomes encode dsRNA. Commensal intestinal organisms obviously contain MAMPs, and normal flora can be proinflammatory under abnormal host conditions (29).

From the viewpoint of host defense, MAMPs are optimally composed of patterns that are crucial to microbe viability, thus minimizing structural variation a prokaryote could evolve to avoid detection. Nevertheless, because of the efficiency of eukaryotic MAMP recognition, bacteria have developed significant ability to modify and conceal these structures. These strategies include encapsulation with complex carbohydrates, modifications in LPS structure, or genetically based phase-switching of flagellin genes. Perhaps the vertebrate adaptive immune system emerged in response to the escalating arms race between bacterial modification of existing MAMPs and additional duplication and modification of host cell PRRs.

The term PRR describes a eukaryotic receptor that specifically interacts with one or more MAMP(s). The most well-known PRRs in mammals are the now famous Toll-like receptors (TLRs). The human genome contains at least 10 known TLRs, and the corresponding MAMPs are known for some (Table 4-1), though some TLR ligands may not be MAMPs, but instead endogenous inflammatory mediators (30). This is an area of current intense research and revision (31). Structurally, TLRs are transmembrane receptors defined by the presence of two ancient, highly conserved structural motifs. The extracellular portion contains a leucine-rich repeat (LRR) domain and acts to recognize and bind MAMPs. The intracellular portion, known as the TIR (toll/IL-1R/plant resistance) domain, interacts with and activates cytoplasmic signal transducing proteins, which we will discuss in the next section (32).

Clearly, TLRs must not routinely be activated by commensal microflora and their products as to do so would result in a constant state of gut inflammation. The epithelial barrier and strategic localization of PRRs combine to prevent their activation. For example, TLR5 localizes along basolateral cell membranes, sheltered from the lumenal contents and poised to monitor breaches in cell-cell barriers (33). Other TLRs may be restricted to intracellular vacuolar membranes, positioned to monitor potentially threatening material sampled by cellular endocytosis or pinocytosis (34). Inappropriate TLR signaling may also be regulated by control of cytoplasmic signal transduction (35).

Epithelial cells can also detect soluble intracytoplasmic MAMPs to sense certain bacteria (*Shigella*, *Listeria*) and enteric viruses which have an intracellular stage of their lifecycle (36, 37). The NOD family of PRRs mediate cellular cytoplasmic monitoring for MAMPs, thus providing a means of detecting invading bacteria not perceived by surface receptors (36). Like TLRs, the NOD proteins exhibit a similar modular structure. The LRR ligand binding motifs interact with specific MAMPs (muropeptide component of PGN) (see Table 4-1). The C-termini of NOD1 and 2 proteins feature a caspase-recruitment domain (CARD), which is functionally analogous to the TIR domain of the TLRs that mediate second-messenger activation for subsequent signaling pathways.

Table 4-1	**Pattern Recognition Receptors and their Ligands**
TLR1:	Lipopeptides
TLR2:	Lipoprotein, lipoteichoic acid, others
TLR3:	Double-stranded RNA
TLR4:	Lipopolysaccharide
TLR5:	Flagellin
TLR6:	Unknown
TLR7:	Unknown
TLR8:	Unknown
TLR9:	Unmethylated CpG-containing DNA
TLR10:	Unknown
TLR11:	Uropathogenic *E. coli*
Nod1:	Gram-negative peptidoglycan
Nod2:	Gram-positive and -negative peptidoglycan

In summary, eukaryotic cells have evolved specific mechanisms to detect the fingerprints of prokaryotic life. The mechanisms by which this information is put into action will be discussed next.

Epithelial Reaction to Bacteria: NF-κB, MAPK and IRF Pathways

The binding of PRRs with their cognate MAMPs results in the activation of cytoplasmic signaling circuits. These pathways include the classic Rel/NF-κB, the mitogen-activated protein (MAP) kinase and the interferon regulatory factor (IRF) pathways. All three utilize post-translational signaling relays conducted by the controlled regulated transfer of covalent modifications (phosphorylation and ubiquitination) along a series of cytoplasmic protein intermediates. Rel/NF-κB, MAPK and IRF pathway activation ultimately results in the nuclear transfer of the transcription factors of the Rel, bZip, and IRF families respectively, binding of specific promoter elements and activation of programs of gene transcription involved in host defense.

NF-κB/REL PATHWAYS

NF-κB refers collectively to members of the Rel family of DNA binding transcription factors that bind characteristic sequence motifs in gene promoters that regulate immune and inflammatory responses. In the intestine, NF-κB usually exists as a heterodimer of two related proteins, p65 and p50. NF-κB activation is tightly regulated, normally sequestered in the cytoplasm (rendering it inactive) by the inhibitor of κB (IκB). The complex sequence of events by which bacteria activate NF-κB via TLRs and NOD proteins is diagrammed in Figure 4–1 (32, 38, 39). As currently understood, an appropriate MAMP binds to a TLR/NOD, resulting in dimerization and formation of a TIR domain that can then bind to a class of adaptor proteins (40). This family of adaptor proteins consists of MyD88, MAL/TIRAP and TRIF/TICAM (41). Emerging evidence suggests that these adaptor proteins may preferentially interact with specific TLRs and presumably tailor the most appropriate signaling pathways for a given MAMP/TLR interaction (42). All the MyD88 family adaptors interact with a second adaptor molecule, IRAK, of which several family members are known. Parenthetically, the specific role that this protein plays in managing bacterial stresses is underscored by the observation that mutations in IRAK4 cause a human genetic disorder manifested by recurrent pyogenic infections in childhood (43). IRAK, a serine kinase, then activates the cytoplasmic signaling intermediate TRAF6, possibly by phosphorylation. Upon activation, TRAF6 becomes ubiquitinated, which in turn activates the kinase TAK1, in complex with TAB1 and TAB2 (44–46). The TAK1/TAB1/TAB2 complex functions as an IkappaB kinase kinase (IκKK), which activates IkappaB kinase complexes (IκKs) (45).

The IκKs apparently function as a signaling nexus, receiving and integrating signals from multiple proinflammatory signal transduction pathways (47). In addition to TLR-mediated signals, many stimuli activate the IκK complex, including the proinflammatory cytokines TNF and IL-1, which both have dedicated receptors and IκK proximal signaling intermediates (48). After an appropriate MAMP binds to a NOD receptor, dimerization of the CARD domain induces interaction with the second messenger serine/threonine kinase RICK, which in turn activates IκK and may also directly activate apoptotic pathways (49, 50). Ca^{2+} mobilization can also activate these pathways (51). In each case, signaling converges on the IκK complex. The main catalytic subunits of the complex, IκK-α and IκK-β, phosphorylate two serine residues within IκB (48).

Phosphorylated IκB rapidly becomes polyubiquitinated by the ubiquitin ligase complex, β-TrCP-SCF (52, 53). The ubiquitin ligase complex consists of β-TrCP, which physically interacts with phospho-IκB, the ubiquitin ligase enzyme (E2),

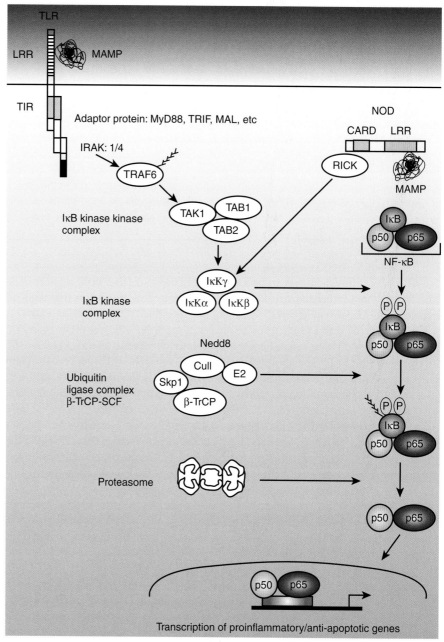

Figure 4-1 Diagram of the NF-κB activation pathway. See text. Transmembrane TLRs or intracytoplasmic NOD proteins bind PAMPs and transmit signals via cytoplasmic signaling intermediates to activate IkappaB kinase. This complex phosphorylates IκB that is subsequently ubiquitinated and degraded. Phosphorylation is indicated with a P and ubiquitination is depicted as a brush.

a linker subunit termed Skp-1, and a regulatory subunit, Cul-1, which itself is regulated by covalent modification of the ubiquitin-like molecule Nedd8 (54). IκB polyubiquitination targets it to the proteasome, resulting in proteolytic digestion of the IκB molecule (55–57). Following IκB degradation, the NF-κB translocates across the nuclear membrane, with subsequent DNA binding to relevant promoters, transcriptional activation and new mRNA synthesis.

Previously, we demonstrated that interaction of non-pathogenic bacteria with model epithelia in vitro inhibited NF-κB activation at the level of IκB ubiquitination (58). We have subsequently shown that this inhibition is due to bacterial-mediated loss of the Nedd8 modification of the Cul-1 regulatory subunit and consequent loss of IκB ubiquitin ligase complex enzymatic activity (59). These findings suggest mechanisms by which normal bacterial colonization in the gut could affect inflammatory (and as we shall see, survival) pathways.

While NF-κB is probably the key pathway activated by microbial signals (60), two other pathways can be rapidly activated by TLRs and probably act as modifiers to provide specific patterns of expression adapted for optimal responses to distinct classes of microbes (Fig. 4-2).

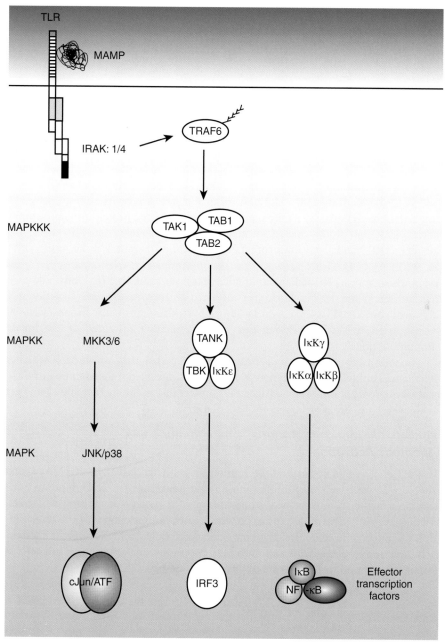

Figure 4-2 Schematic of NF-κB, MAPK and IRF pathways. Pathways of interacting proteins are indicated with arrows. The functional classes of enzymes are indicated on the left.

MAP KINASE PATHWAYS

The MAP kinase (MAPK) family of signaling molecules plays a role in many cellular functions, including control of proliferation and stress responses (61). Like the NF-κB pathway, the MAPK pathways integrate signals from various stimuli via regulated and sequential transfer of covalent modifications (phosphorylation) of signaling intermediates. MAPK pathways consist of a three-kinase relay, with the final kinase activating the target transcription factor (32). MAMP/TLR interaction causes TRAF6 activation, which in turn activates a MAP kinase kinase kinase (MAPKKK) such as the TAK complex. MAPKKK subsequently phosphorylates and activates a MAP kinase kinase (MAPKK), such as MKK3 or MKK6. The MAPKK in turn phosphorylates and activates the terminal MAPK. In bacterial responses, relevant MAPKs include JNK or p38 (58). These in turn phosphorylate the activation domain of the target transcription factors, cJun and CREB/ATF, respectively, leading to target gene mRNA synthesis. Cells contain multiple MAPK pathways, which can interact with each other through cross-activation.

INTERFERON REGULATORY FACTORS

The IRFs are a family of DNA binding transcription factors involved in anti-viral responses. IRF binding sites (ISREs) are found in chronic or lymphocytic inflammatory mediators, such as iNOS, IP-10, RANTES, VCAM-1, and several interferons (62). Many IRF family members are newly synthesized in response to dsRNA and other proinflammatory signals in order to mediate the secondary, chronic phase of inflammatory and adaptive responses. Specific family members, IRF3 and 7, can be activated by TLR3 and 4 signaling via a post-transcriptional pathway (63). Like NF-κB, IRF3 exists quietly as a cytoplasmic protein in the unstimulated cell. Recent studies have identified a pathway involving the TIR interacting adapter TRIF and activation of the IκK family members IκKe and TBK1 (a MAPKK) (64, 65). This activated kinase complex phosphorylates IRF3, an event which appears to mediate rapid nuclear translocation by a currently unknown mechanism. While IRF3 is classically considered an antiviral mediator, it is potently activated by LPS/TLR4, suggesting a role of these proteins in antibacterial responses (63). Much work remains in characterizing this arm of the innate immune response.

In summary, eukaryotic cells possess interrelated signal transduction schemes for the transmittal of alarm signals to the nucleus. Detailed understanding of these pathways provides important insight for clinicians as many therapeutic agents act at this level and are also targets for bacterial inhibition.

Epithelial Response to Bacteria: Innate Immune and Apoptotic Activation

In the initial events of bacterial perception by epithelial cells, NF-κB, MAPK and IRF3 are activated within minutes and nuclear appearance of DNA binding transcription factors results in new transcription of a battery of effector molecules. Studies utilizing large-scale expression profiling techniques demonstrate transcription of antibacterial peptides, cytokines, adhesion molecules, chemotactic messengers, anti-apoptotic proteins and metabolic enzymes (which play a role in bacterial killing and wound healing) (66–68).

Almost all promoters of inflammatory effector genes possess an NF-κB binding site required for activation (69). Additionally, effectors involved in early phases of inflammation often possess promoter-binding sites for MAPK-activated transcription factors (cJun, CREB/ATF). Initially, these transcription factors upregulate neutrophil-specific chemokines and leukocyte adhesion molecules. Neutrophil infiltration results in the classic histological changes of acute inflammation.

Secondary or chronic phase effectors often exhibit IRF binding sites in their promoters. Secondary effectors induce appearance of chemokines, growth factors and adhesion molecules (ICAM-1, MCP-1) necessary for recruitment of monocytic cells and leading to the histological appearance of lymphocytic infiltration and granuloma formation. In each case, the cJun, CREB/ATF and IRF proteins are thought to act in combination with NF-κB on the appropriate promoter to yield the optimal transcriptional output. Ultimately, the appearance of phagocytic neutrophils, sometimes followed by immunoregulatory (and phagocytic) macrophages and immunocompetent lymphocytes, mediate the removal of the offending microbe and initiate adaptive immunity (70).

We are beginning to recognize specificity of responses (41). Transcriptional profiling studies suggest that bacterial ligands (LPS and PGN) mediate responses optimal for antibacterial activity (71). Viral signals (dsRNA) transduced via TLRs 3 and 7 elicit genes with antiviral activity (63). The tailoring of specific transcriptional responses from specific TLR signals may be accomplished by the adaptor molecules that interact with the TIR domain of distinct TLR subsets (41). We must also keep in mind that in real-world infections, a given microbe offers several MAMPs to a host cell. Enteric floras contain both Gram-negative (LPS-TLR4) and Gram-positive (PGN-TLR2) representatives. Many are flagellated (TLR5) and all presumably possess CpG DNA (TLR9). These products are probably shed and/or released by dead organisms. Furthermore, upregulation of endogenous proinflammatory mediators, such as IL-1 and TNF, occurs during inflammatory processes, activating complex secondary patterns of gene expression.

While pathogens and other stressors elicit innate proinflammatory pathways (such as NF-κB) that culminate in cellular inflammation, they simultaneously stimulate pro-apoptotic pathways (mediated by caspases) that presumably lead to elimination of the infected or irreversibly injured cell. Apoptosis, or programmed cell death, is a morphologically distinct, genetically defined intrinsic mechanism by which individual cells can eliminate themselves while largely preserving the surrounding cells (72, 73). Apoptosis is mediated by an arsenal of effector cysteinyl aspartate-specific proteases (caspases) that in the active state carry out limited proteolysis on apparently dozens of cellular structural and regulatory proteins, thus effectively and harmlessly (for surrounding tissues) dismantling the cell and accounting for the morphologic changes characteristic of apoptosis (72). Understandably, this process is tightly regulated (Fig. 4-3). The *effector* caspases exist in inactive zymogen form until processed by an amplifying cascade of upstream *initiator* caspases. Caspase activation can occur by several mechanisms. In the **intrinsic** pathway, a variety of cellular stressors (metabolic stress, DNA damage, withdrawal of growth factors/hormones) results in the leakage of mitochondrial cytochrome-*c* into the cytosol, a process controlled by the balance of pro- and anti-apoptotic members of the Bcl-2 family. These proteins can heterodimerize with each other, and a relative excess of pro- over anti-apoptotic members is thought to permit formation of a mitochondrial "pore," allowing escape of cytochrome-*c* (74). The cytoplasmic presence of cytochrome-*c* nucleates the formation of a scaffold complex termed the apoptosome that serves to activate the initiator caspase 9 and the subsequent effector caspases. Alternatively, in the **extrinsic** pathway extracellular ligand binding events result in activation of death receptor complexes (classically, members of the TNF family of receptors (TNF-R, FAS, TRAIL, etc.)) mediating assembly of proteins bearing a "death domain" motif (DD). One example is TRADD (*T*NF *r*eceptor *a*ssociated *d*eath *d*omain protein). The death domain of TRADD interacts in a homotypical manner with secondary adaptor proteins also containing a death domain, such as FADD (*F*as *a*ssociated *d*eath *d*omain protein) (75). This protein contains a "death effector domain" (DED) that interacts in turn with proteins bearing the DED, such as procaspase 8.

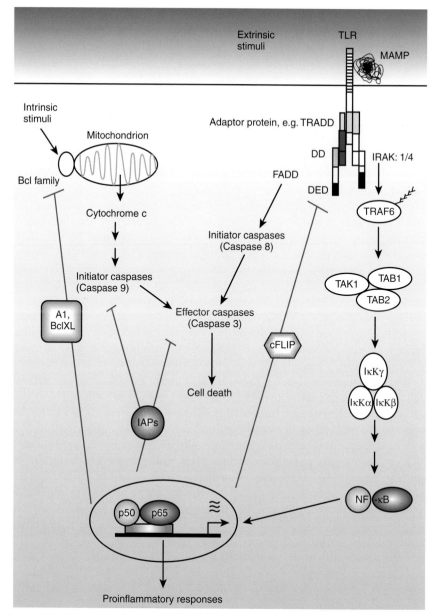

Figure 4-3 Apoptotic activation pathways. See text. Activating interactions are indicated with arrows, while inhibitory interactions are indicated with bars.

Assembly of procaspase 8 is thought to lead to autocatalytic activation of caspase 8 (according to the "induced proximity model") and subsequent cleavage of downstream effector caspases. Recently, it has become apparent that TLRs and NOD proteins can activate the extrinsic pathway of apoptosis and use much of the same signaling circuitry (76–78). Based on these findings, an emerging paradigm holds that when the cell is faced with a potentially damaging stimulus, whether microbial or physical (e.g. hypoxia), simultaneous activation of proinflammatory and pro-apoptotic pathways occurs as a default. Importantly, NF-κB (and MAPKK) activation is now well established as a cell survival pathway. Genetic mouse models have illustrated a crucial role of NF-κB as an anti-apoptotic control. Mice mutants lacking the p65 subunit of NF-κB die in utero due to massive apoptosis in the liver (79). A mouse strain harboring null alleles of IκK-β solely in intestinal enterocytes exhibited no abnormalities under normal conditions, but responded to a

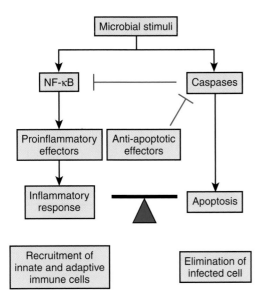

Figure 4-4 Summary of interrelationships of proinflammatory and pro-apoptotic pathways. Activating interactions are indicated with arrows, while inhibitory interactions are indicated with bars.

systemic stress (transient intestinal ischemia) with massive enterocyte apoptosis (80). Pharmacologic NF-κB inhibition, a potent pro-apoptotic stimulus, has been exploited as a chemotherapeutic agent (81). Why is NF-κB activation necessary for cell survival? In addition to inducing proinflammatory mediators, NF-κB activation also simultaneously induces anti-apoptotic effector proteins (e.g. A1, cFLIP, BCL family members and the IAP proteins), which serve to block apoptotic signaling at multiple control points and abort caspase activation (Fig. 4-3) (78). Under these conditions, apoptosis is arrested and cellular inflammation proceeds. On the other hand, if certain stressors result in reduced proinflammatory signaling, caspase activation may gain the upper hand; activated caspases can act as negative feedback to the survival pathways by degrading inflammatory signaling intermediates (Fig. 4-4). Under these circumstances, the stressed cell completes apoptosis and dismantles itself, by definition without lysis, thereby eliminating the invading bacteria without inducing secondary inflammation.

Numerous bacterial and viral pathogens have evolved protein effectors that inhibit activation of the NF-κB and MAPK pathways as a mechanism of immunosuppression and induction of apoptosis in regulatory cells (77). Collectively, these observations suggest caution when contemplating use of anti-inflammatory agents in contexts of cellular stress.

DEVELOPMENTAL CONSIDERATIONS IN INTESTINAL IMMUNITY

Now that we have completed our review of innate intestinal immunity in the normal adult host, we turn our attention to the immature host. Understanding how premature intestinal defenses potentially differ from mature defenses may provide insight into the pathogenesis of the most devastating intestinal disease neonatologists face, necrotizing enterocolitis (NEC). Furthermore, such knowledge can hopefully focus future research efforts and lead to better preventive and treatment strategies for premature infants who are at highest risk.

The Epithelia

Developmentally, the gastrointestinal epithelium forms largely during the first trimester of pregnancy (82). The initial enterocyte and goblet cell appears by 8 weeks

61

gestation and intestinal epithelia exhibit crypt-villus architecture by 12 weeks. Tight junctions form by 10 weeks and fetal intestines reportedly exhibit the ability to regulate tight junction organization (83). Therefore, the primitive intestinal epithelial barrier is formed early in fetal development. However, the machinery necessary to regulate secretion and absorption is only partially developed in the fetus, undergoing gradual maturation, under the influence of amniotic fluid, from 26 weeks to term (84). Mucus gene expression begins by 6.5 weeks gestation. However, developmental mucin gene expression changes throughout the intestine and appears to mimic adult pattern expression between 23 and 27 weeks (85). Paneth cells appear by week 12 and Paneth cell defensin production begins in the 13th week but lysozyme production is delayed until 20 weeks (82, 86). Gut length continues to increase especially rapidly during the second trimester and it continues to grow until 3–4 years of life (87).

As discussed earlier, this single-cell-layer epithelium reconstitutes itself every 5 days from the crypt stem cell pool. Maintenance of this intestinal epithelial lining requires tight regulation of cell proliferation and differentiation. The predominant signaling pathway responsible for this regulation is the canonical Wnt/β-catenin pathway (4, 88–90). Briefly, under quiescent conditions, a multiprotein complex sequesters and degrades cytoplasmic β-catenin. This degradation complex contains axin, adenomatous polyposis coli (APC), casein kinase I (CKI), and glycogen synthase kinase 3β (GSK3β). Reminiscent of NF-κB regulation, β-catenin becomes phosphorylated by the degradation complex, targeting it to ubiquitination by E3 ubiquitin ligase and subsequent proteasomal degradation. Receptor-mediated Wnt signaling blocks activity of the degradation complex, preventing phosphorylation, ubiquitination and degradation. The stabilized β-catenin accumulates, and translocates to the nucleus, where it can act as a transcription factor, binding promoters of target genes that presumably have a role in control of cell proliferation. Thus, appearance of nuclear β-catenin is the hallmark of canonical Wnt signal activation.

Studies confirm the importance of this pathway for maintenance of crypt-villus architecture. First, nuclear β-catenin accumulates in small and large intestinal crypts where stem cells reside. Secondly, genetically altered mice lacking components of Wnt/β-catenin signaling exhibited loss of crypt architecture, depleted intestinal secretory cells, and arrested intestinal epithelial proliferation and/or stem cell ablation. Finally, mutations in APC, the key inhibitor of Wnt signaling, are highly associated with adult colorectal cancer (4, 88–90). Perhaps not coincidentally, β-catenin degradation utilizes the same ubiquitin ligase complex as does IκB (52, 53). Furthermore, we have shown that commensal bacteria repress degradation of β-catenin and result in activation of this pathway (59). These biochemical events suggest another mechanism by which normal flora could influence epithelial signaling, in this case by controlling proliferation and differentiation.

Wnt/β-catenin signaling has not been studied in premature infants. However, it is tempting to speculate that disordered development of this pathway could result in immaturity of the constitutive barriers, predisposing neonates to perforations and/or NEC. Furthermore, a recent study reporting that dexamethasone suppresses Wnt signaling in human osteoblasts could provide another mechanism for steroid-associated spontaneous intestinal perforations in premature infants (91).

Antimicrobial Peptides

Antimicrobial peptides play a crucial role in intestinal host defense, which can obviously influence overall host health. Immaturity in defensin expression or regulation may play important roles in the clinical problems we face in the NICU. Developmental expression of intestinal β-defensins and cathelicidins has not been well studied. However, murine and human studies clearly demonstrate the developmental regulation of Paneth cell α-defensin expression (86, 92). Detection of human α-defensin expression correlates with the developmental appearance of Paneth cells. Human α-defensin transcript can be detected by 13.5 weeks gestation and becomes localized to the small intestine by 17 weeks gestation. However, Paneth cell number and α-defensin expression are markedly reduced in premature intestine (24 weeks) as compared to adult intestine. Furthermore, although pathological specimens demonstrate an increase in Paneth cell number and α-defensin transcript in infants undergoing surgery for NEC, actual amounts of α-defensin measured within the Paneth cell were much reduced compared to control (93). Plausibly, developmental disorders in α-defensin translation could account for the low peptide levels detected and/or the susceptibility to NEC in these patients.

Interestingly, human small intestines express the intracytoplasmic PRR NOD2 solely in Paneth cells, implying a role for NOD2 in regulating antimicrobial peptide expression (20). Indeed, recent studies in mice demonstrate that NOD2 influences α-defensin expression (94). NOD2 null mice exhibited increased susceptibility to gastrointestinal bacterial infections, plausibly due to decreased α-defensin. A recent clinical study in very low birth weight infants (VLBW) also demonstrated increased susceptibility to bacterial sepsis in infants with certain NOD2 mutations (95). While NOD2 mutations confer a predisposition to Crohn's disease (96), studies to date have not demonstrated a link to NEC (97). Future studies elucidating the ontogeny of β-defensin and cathelicidin expression, Paneth cell and NOD2 activity may shed some light on these problems and eventually allow us to better tailor our preventive and treatment strategies for maintaining premature intestinal health. In any event, in premature neonates, developmental immaturity of either the structural or biochemical barrier component of the epithelia may fail to keep bacteria at bay during the initial colonization period, again allowing bacterial invasion into deeper tissues and the inflammatory consequences described next.

The Inflammatory Response

When considering the defenses of the neonatal gut, one must bear in mind that the gut is totally naive to MAMPs while in utero, and is instantly challenged by their presence at birth with the introduction of the normal flora. Preliminary studies indicate that fetuses as early as 20 weeks exhibit basolateral TLR2 and TLR4 expression in intestinal crypts (98) though little is known regarding the functionality of innate immune signaling pathways during pre- and postnatal development in vivo. It is interesting to note that the NF-κB system apparently originally evolved as a developmental pathway in early fly embryos (38). What role NF-κB plays in mammalian gut development is unknown but is a tantalizing possibility.

Recent in vitro studies on cultured intestinal epithelial cells indicate that immature intestinal cells may exhibit a propensity for exaggerated inflammatory responses (as measured by IL-8 secretion) to pathogenic stimuli (99, 100). These authors hypothesize that developmentally deficient expression of the NF-κB inhibitor IκB may allow for enhanced NF-κB activity. In this model, an exaggerated inflammatory response would cause increased cellular inflammation and potentially uncontrolled tissue damage. Inflammation is a necessary and vital response for long-term survival in the microbe-rich environment of the intestine. However, the inflammatory response, like many immune reactions, is a classic two-edged sword. Inflammation results in collateral damage largely as a result of release of neutrophil-derived oxidants and proteases. This could lead to barrier damage and opportunistic access for microorganisms that would not normally be able to breach the epithelial barrier, thus allowing the noxious contents of the intestinal lumen to reach the subepithelial surface, perpetuating a vicious cycle of proinflammatory activation and tissue damage. Furthermore, anti-inflammatory strategies such as pharmacological intervention would be postulated to retard development of early NEC. More studies are needed to determine whether these findings can be confirmed in the ex vivo whole intestine or in vivo.

An alternative scenario could be envisioned in other pathophysiological situations. As we have discussed, activation of NF-κB and MAPK pathways by bacterial and other stimuli induces the transcriptional activation of a battery of proinflammatory effectors and resultant acute inflammation. Plausibly, an intrinsic failure in the ability to respond to bacterial challenges during the initial colonization of the gut, possibly due to developmental immaturity, inherited defects, or environmentally-mediated downregulation of signaling pathways, could lead to tissue damage. Clinically, adult patients who fail to generate an appropriate intestinal inflammatory response, such as those with inherited defects in innate immunity or acquired neutropenia, exhibit enhanced susceptibility to enteric bacterial infection, often resulting in systemic dissemination of disease (43, 101). Similarly, mice engineered with mutations in inflammatory regulators also show enhanced susceptibility to enteric infection (102, 103). Interestingly, Crohn's predisposing mutations in the NOD2 gene exhibit *loss of function*, showing defective rather than hyperactive NF-κB signaling (37). Additionally, in an experimental model of IBD, blockade of NF-κB via transgenic expression of a non-degradable version of IκB restricted to epithelial cells led to worse disease than control mice (104).

Reduced inflammatory signaling could allow for bacterial overgrowth, or may result in hypersensitivity to pro-apoptotic stimuli. Plausibly, a failure to activate inflammatory pathways may reduce induction of anti-apoptotic, cytoprotective factors. Thus, developmental immaturity of the inflammatory response would be expected to render a neonatal gut highly susceptible to apoptosis due to an environmental stress challenge whether due to microbial overgrowth or hypoxia. Clearly, host health depends upon a balance between too much proinflammatory activation (leading to tissue injury and clinical sequelae) and not enough (leaving mucosa undefended and/or poised to self-destruct) (Fig. 4-4). As described earlier, mice conditionally null for NF-κB activation in gut enterocytes responded to transient intestinal hypoxia with overwhelming epithelial apoptosis (80). Studies in a rat model of NEC report that early apoptosis plays a crucial role in the pathogenesis of NEC (105). Therefore, further studies are required to determine the relative in vivo role of hyperactive inflammatory processes leading to excessive inflammation, and/or hypoactive inflammation leading to uncontrolled bacterial growth and/or accelerated apoptotic responses. Both may play a role in different clinical scenarios or in distinct stages of pathogenesis and, once epithelial damage is initiated and propagated, may result in the syndrome of lesions recognized as NEC.

CLINICAL CONSIDERATIONS: POTENTIAL CLINICAL STRATEGIES TO PROMOTE INTESTINAL IMMUNITY

Now that we have reviewed the basic components of innate intestinal immunity and current knowledge of its developmental deficiencies, we will attempt to apply our knowledge to improve clinical practice. Understanding of basic physiology will allow better insight into the pathophysiology of neonatal intestinal disease. Hopefully, this will lead to better preventive and treatment strategies in promoting intestinal health.

The Epithelia

Many studies demonstrate the importance of diet in intestinal development. Dietary influences as early as the swallowing of amniotic fluid (week 16) play an important role in intestinal differentiation and growth. Non-nutritive dietary substances such as epidermal growth factor (EGF) and polyamines stimulate intestinal epithelial growth (82, 106). Clinically, this often places neonatologists in the difficult position of weighing the benefits of starting feeds against the risk of causing NEC. A reasonable compromise appears to be the practice of early trophic feeds. Indeed, in premature infants, trophic feeds have been shown to improve activity of some digestive enzymes and enhance digestive hormone release, intestinal blood flow, and motility. Infants fed early trophic feeds appear to have improved feeding tolerance and growth while exhibiting reduced hospital stay and sepsis incidence as compared to infants who are not. Furthermore, early trophic feeds do not increase the incidence of NEC (87, 107).

Clearly, commensal bacteria play a key role in intestinal development as well. Commensal bacteria induce genes responsible for barrier function, digestion, xenobiotic processing, angiogenesis, and immune function (3, 108, 109). Mice raised under germ-free (gnotobiotic) conditions exhibited villus hypoplasia, and recolonization with commensal bacteria normalized the intestinal epithelia. These studies suggest that normal flora plays a role in maintenance of cellular survival/ turnover and in stimulating normal epithelial proliferation (110). Since intestinal colonization develops postnatally as dietary changes occur, acquisition of flora may play an important role in the postnatal maturation of intestinal host defenses (111).

Another postulated role of the normal flora is competitive exclusion of frank pathogens. This is vividly illustrated in adults who can develop *Clostridial* pseudo-membranous colitis due to antibiotic-mediated suppression of normal colonic flora. Premature infants are particularly susceptible to pathologic intestinal bacterial colonization because of daily exposure to nosocomial flora and almost universal exposure to antibiotics upon admission to the NICU. In fact, studies have revealed abnormal duodenal colonization of *Enterobacteriaceae* in VLBW and shown that early abnormal stool colonization with *Clostridium perfringens* correlated with later development of NEC (112, 113). Thus, premature infants may be particularly susceptible to NEC due to pathologic bacterial infection secondary to suppression of normal flora. Therefore, as clinicians, we should continue to be wary of broad-spectrum antibiotic use in our patients.

Antimicrobial Peptides

Antimicrobial peptides play multiple roles in intestinal host defense. Indeed, genetically engineered mice lacking mature intestinal defensins (matrilysin knockout) exhibit increased susceptibility to certain oral bacterial infections (10). Current evidence indicates that premature infants demonstrate developmental deficiency in Paneth cell defensins. Broad-spectrum antibiotics may further inhibit defensin expression (114). Electrolyte homeostasis may also play an important role in preserving defensin function (20). In mice, Paneth cell secretion depends upon activity of a Ca^{2+}-dependent K^+ channel. Therefore, disruptions in Ca^{2+} and/or K^+ homeostasis could presumably have negative effects on innate intestinal defenses. Furthermore, mice lacking the cystic fibrosis transmembrane conductance regulator (CFTR, causing a defect in Cl^- transport) cannot release Paneth cell defensins, leading to intestinal bacterial overgrowth.

Recent advances in producing recombinant human defensins provide hope for developing the pharmaceutical potential of these antimicrobial peptides (21). These products could prove useful adjuncts to traditional antibiotic therapy and could potentially correct the intestinal defensin deficiency in our premature infants. Until then, clinicians should remember that maintaining normal electrolyte levels as well as limiting use of broad-spectrum antibiotics as much as possible could prove invaluable in preserving the limited intestinal defensin activity in our premature infants.

The Inflammatory Response

As previously mentioned, commensal bacteria can inhibit inflammatory pathways and perhaps plays a role in maintaining homeostasis (77). In vitro co-culture experiments with lactic acid bacteria show reduced inflammatory signaling; *Lactobacillus* can prevent colitis in spontaneous mouse models; and *Bacteroides thetaiotaomicron* can inhibit NF-κB by enhancing its nuclear export (115–117). We have previously shown that non-pathogenic bacteria are capable of inhibiting NF-κB proinflammatory pathways, via IκB ubiquitination blockade. Furthermore, we have also demonstrated mechanistically that a wide range of commensal bacterial can inhibit NF-κB via this mechanism, specifically by blockage of the Nedd8 modification necessary for enzymatic activation of the IκB ubiquitin ligase (58, 59). Conceivably, hyperactive inflammation in premature infants could be due to inadequate intestinal colonization and subsequent lack of bacterially mediated dampening of inflammatory pathways that occurs with the normal acquisition of flora.

Given the increasing awareness of the role that bacterial colonization plays in many intestinal diseases, probiotics are emerging as a promising therapy for intestinal diseases. Probiotics are defined as "living micro-organisms, which upon digestion in sufficient numbers, exert health benefits beyond basic nutrition" (118). Most commonly used microorganisms include *Lactobacilli*, *Bifidobacterium*, and *Saccharomyces*. They have been shown to reduce the severity of rotavirus- and antibiotic-associated diarrhea and improve outcomes in allergic diseases, such as cow-milk protein allergy and atopic dermatitis (118). Recently, a small randomized control trial demonstrated a significant reduction in NEC in VLBW infants fed breast milk with probiotics (containing *Lactobacillus* and *Bifidobacterium*) as compared with infants fed breast milk alone (119). Probiotics may prove an exciting preventive strategy for NEC, but further study is needed before universal use can be recommended. Clearly, larger follow-up studies are needed to confirm this beneficial effect while providing reassurance of no adverse effect. While not yet reported in VLBW infants, selective patient populations have reportedly suffered invasive disease from probiotic administration (120). How do probiotics mediate therapeutic effects? In neonates, probiotics can aid in the acquisition of normal flora. Numerous mechanisms have been postulated for the beneficial effects of probiotics, including enhancement of epithelial barrier function, competitive exclusion of pathogens, and direct anti-inflammatory effects on epithelial signaling pathways (121–123). Certain probiotic effects may require live organisms, presumably supplying beneficial effector proteins or small molecules. However, several recent observations have shown that purified TLR ligands themselves can have beneficial effects in the absence of viable organisms (124).

Another potential therapeutic strategy that carries less infectious risk is prebiotic therapy. Prebiotics are non-digestible dietary supplements, usually long-chain carbohydrates or mucins, which improve intestinal health by promoting proliferation of beneficial commensal bacteria, thus improving the ecological balance of the gut (125). Prebiotics have also been implicated in directly improving toxin removal, influencing immune responses, and promotion of commensal bacterial colonization. These bacteria in turn digest prebiotics and produce short-chain fatty acids, which can inihibit growth of intestinal pathogens, provide enterocyte nutrition (butyrate), promote mineral absorption, and relieve constipation. Preliminary studies demonstrate increased *Bifidobacterium* stool colonization and decreased pathogenic bacterial colonization in preterm infants fed special prebiotic-containing formula (90% short-chain galacto-oligosaccharide, 10% long-chain fructo-oligosaccharide) as compared to those fed control formula (126). Term infants exhibit decreased stool pH and increased stool short-chain fatty acids when fed this formula, reportedly comparable to that seen in breast-fed infants (127). Furthermore, preliminary evidence suggests a positive effect on overall host immune function (128). However, prebiotic administration is not without complications. Most commonly associated side-effects include flatulence, bloating, and diarrhea, which can be reversed by stopping treatment (125).

Finally, recent therapeutic strategies include the use of bacterial metabolites. Perhaps we can coin the term "post-biotics." Many members of the normal flora produce butyric acid, a 4-carbon short-chain fatty acid produced by the anaerobic catabolism of complex carbohydrates that reach the ascending colon largely undigested by the human gut. Butryate is a major energy source for the colonic enterocytes and has a widely recognized but poorly understood role in intestinal growth and differentiation (129, 130), inflammatory suppression (131–133), and apoptosis in vitro and/or in animal models (134, 135). It has been used with limited success in human inflammatory bowel disease (136). Perhaps this and other small-molecule products of the normal flora are at least partially responsible for the beneficial effects of the normal flora (and exogenous pro- and prebiotics), and could be employed as a more controllable therapeutic surrogate.

Interestingly, recent studies have discovered that the products of commensal bacteria can induce TLR-mediated protective responses that are crucial to maintaining intestinal health (124, 137, 138). It has been demonstrated that mice with intestines cleared of normal flora, and thus MAMPs, were markedly more sensitive to the chemical colitogen dextran sodium sulfate (DSS), and that the mucosal injury mediated by this compound could be ameliorated by oral administration of MAMPs such as LTA and LPS (124). Additionally, this study demonstrated that these protective effects were lost in TLR2 and 4 null mice, implicating TLR signaling as the protective mechanism. Beneficial effects of probiotic bacteria can be recapitulated by isolated MAMPs; for example, unmethylated probiotic CpG DNA has been shown to ameliorate DSS colitis in mice. Furthermore, the observed protective effects were lost in TLR9 null mice, directly implicating TLR signaling in intestinal cytoprotection (139). TLR signaling from MAMPs has also been shown to directly inhibit apoptotic processes in neutrophils (140). Other MAMP-inducible genes, such as stromal growth factors and angiogenic factors, have reparative functions, and may be protective in the sense of accelerating restitution. Taken together, these studies suggest that the mucosa (either epithelial cells, immunocompetent resident cells in the lamina propria, or both) can perceive the abundant MAMPs in the intestinal lumen and induce a transcriptional response that enhances cytodefenses. Potentially, oral administration of bioavailable TLR ligands could stimulate the upregulation of not yet fully defined survival genes or cytoprotective factors (e.g. heat-shock proteins, trefoil factors, anti-apoptotic effectors) and thus confer protective effects upon the epithelium. In this sense, MAMPs may induce an innate immune "trophic feed" effect. Of course, whether the neonatal epithelia respond to MAMPs from the normal flora in the same manner and intensity as the mature epithelium is unknown.

Probiotic use in premature infants could expose potentially hypersensitive epithelia with poor defenses to a microbial challenge too soon, with inflammatory or even septic complications. Perhaps the use of non-viable TLR ligands or bacterial metabolic products may be safer yet efficacious. More research is required to gain a clear picture of the development of the innate immune system, both intrinsic and inducible components. When does the proinflammatory response, with its anti-apoptotic component come "on-line": in utero or in neonatal life? Which processes are developmentally controlled and which are induced by diet or bacteria and their products? When are caspase cascades and PRRs expressed and functionally deployed? The answers to these questions are necessary before we can fully understand how probiotics or pharmacological modulators of inflammatory pathways can be employed clinically.

REFERENCES

1. Madara JL. Warner-Lambert/Parke-Davis Award lecture. Pathobiology of the intestinal epithelial barrier. Am J Pathol 1990; 137(6):1273–1281.
2. Xu J, Gordon JI. Inaugural Article: Honor thy symbionts. Proc Natl Acad Sci USA 2003; 100(18):10452–10459.
3. Hooper LV, Gordon JI. Commensal host-bacterial relationships in the gut. Science 2001; 292(5519):1115–1118.
4. Pinto D, Clevers H. Wnt control of stem cells and differentiation in the intestinal epithelium. Exp Cell Res 2005; 306(2):357–363.
5. Nusrat A, Turner JR, Madara JL. Molecular physiology and pathophysiology of tight junctions. IV. Regulation of tight junctions by extracellular stimuli: nutrients, cytokines, and immune cells. Am J Physiol Gastrointest Liver Physiol 2000; 279(5):G851–G857.
6. Hecht G. Innate mechanisms of epithelial host defense: spotlight on intestine. Am J Physiol 1999; 277(3 Pt 1):C351–C358.
7. Otte JM, Kiehne K, Herzig KH. Antimicrobial peptides in innate immunity of the human intestine. J Gastroenterol 2003; 38(8):717–726.
8. Scott MG, Hancock RE. Cationic antimicrobial peptides and their multifunctional role in the immune system. Crit Rev Immunol 2000; 20(5):407–431.
9. Ganz T. Defensins: antimicrobial peptides of innate immunity. Nat Rev Immunol 2003; 3(9):710–720.
10. Wilson CL, Ouellette AJ, Satchell DP, et al. Regulation of intestinal alpha-defensin activation by the metalloproteinase matrilysin in innate host defense. Science 1999; 286(5437):113–117.
11. Ghosh D, Porter E, Shen B, et al. Paneth cell trypsin is the processing enzyme for human defensin-5. Nat Immunol 2002; 3(6):583–590.
12. Ayabe T, Satchell DP, Wilson CL, et al. Secretion of microbicidal alpha-defensins by intestinal Paneth cells in response to bacteria. Nat Immunol 2000; 1(2):113–118.
13. Eckmann L. Innate immunity and mucosal bacterial interactions in the intestine. Curr Opin Gastroenterol 2004; 20(2):82–88.
14. O'Neil DA, Porter EM, Elewaut D, et al. Expression and regulation of the human beta-defensins hBD-1 and hBD-2 in intestinal epithelium. J Immunol 1999; 163(12):6718–6724.
15. Huttner KM, Bevins CL. Antimicrobial peptides as mediators of epithelial host defense. Pediatr Res 1999; 45(6):785–794.
16. Cociancich S, Ghazi A, Hetru C, et al. Insect defensin, an inducible antibacterial peptide, forms voltage-dependent channels in Micrococcus luteus. J Biol Chem 1993; 268(26): 19239–19245.
17. Kagan BL, Selsted ME, Ganz T, et al. Antimicrobial defensin peptides form voltage-dependent ion-permeable channels in planar lipid bilayer membranes. Proc Natl Acad Sci USA 1990; 87(1):210–214.
18. Lehrer RI, Ganz T, Selsted ME. Defensins: endogenous antibiotic peptides of animal cells. Cell 1991; 64(2):229–230.
19. Lehrer RI, Barton A, Daher KA, et al. Interaction of human defensins with Escherichia coli. Mechanism of bactericidal activity. J Clin Invest 1989; 84(2):553–561.
20. Ouellette AJ. Paneth cell alpha-defensins: peptide mediators of innate immunity in the small intestine. Springer Semin Immunopathol 2005; 27(2):133–146.
21. Chen H, Xu Z, Peng L, et al. Recent advances in the research and development of human defensins. Peptides 2006; 27(4):931–940.
22. Eckmann L. Defence molecules in intestinal innate immunity against bacterial infections. Curr Opin Gastroenterol 2005; 21(2):147–151.
23. Lencer WI, Cheung G, Strohmeier GR, et al. Induction of epithelial chloride secretion by channel-forming cryptdins 2 and 3. Proc Natl Acad Sci USA 1997; 94(16):8585–8589.
24. Merlin D, Yue G, Lencer WI, et al. Cryptdin-3 induces novel apical conductance(s) in Cl-secretory, including cystic fibrosis, epithelia. Am J Physiol Cell Physiol 2001; 280(2):C296–C302.
25. Lin PW, Simon PO Jr, Gewirtz AT, et al. Paneth cell cryptdins act in vitro as apical paracrine regulators of the innate inflammatory response. J Biol Chem 2004; 279(19):19902–19907.
26. Kim DH, Feinbaum R, Alloing G, et al. A conserved p38 MAP kinase pathway in Caenorhabditis elegans innate immunity. Science 2002; 297(5581):623–626.
27. Asai T, Tena G, Plotnikova J, et al. MAP kinase signalling cascade in Arabidopsis innate immunity. Nature 2002; 415(6875):977–983.
28. Barton GM, Medzhitov R. Toll-like receptors and their ligands. In: Beutler B, Wagner H, eds. Toll-like receptor family members and their ligands. New York: Springer; 2002: 81–92.
29. Cario E, Brown D, McKee M, et al. Commensal-associated molecular patterns induce selective toll-like receptor-trafficking from apical membrane to cytoplasmic compartments in polarized intestinal epithelium. Am J Pathol 2002; 160(1):165–173.

30. Gordon S. Pattern recognition receptors: doubling up for the innate immune response. Cell 2002; 111(7):927–930.
31. Takeda K, Kaisho T, Akira S. Toll-like receptors. Annu Rev Immunol 2003; 21:335–376.
32. O'Neill LAJ. Signal transduction pathways activated by the IL-1 receptor/Toll-like receptor super-family. In: Beutler B, Wagner H, eds. Toll-like receptor family members and their ligands. New York: Springer; 2002: 47–62.
33. Gewirtz AT, Navas TA, Lyons S, et al. Cutting edge: bacterial flagellin activates basolaterally expressed TLR5 to induce epithelial proinflammatory gene expression. J Immunol 2001; 167(4):1882–1885.
34. Hornef MW, Frisan T, Vandewalle A, et al. Toll-like receptor 4 resides in the Golgi apparatus and colocalizes with internalized lipopolysaccharide in intestinal epithelial cells. J Exp Med 2002; 195(5):559–570.
35. Liew FY, Xu D, Brint EK, et al. Negative regulation of toll-like receptor-mediated immune responses. Nat Rev Immunol 2005; 5(6):446–458.
36. Girardin SE, Tournebize R, Mavris M, et al. CARD4/Nod1 mediates NF-kappaB and JNK activation by invasive Shigella flexneri. EMBO Rep 2001; 2(8):736–742.
37. Inohara N, Nunez G. NODs: intracellular proteins involved in inflammation and apoptosis. Nat Rev Immunol 2003; 3(5):371–382.
38. Silverman N, Maniatis T. NF-kappaB signaling pathways in mammalian and insect innate immunity. Genes Dev 2001; 15(18):2321–2342.
39. Jobin C, Sartor RB. The I kappa B/NF-kappa B system: a key determinant of mucosal inflammation and protection. Am J Physiol Cell Physiol 2000; 278(3):C451–C462.
40. O'Neill LA, Fitzgerald KA, Bowie AG. The Toll-IL-1 receptor adaptor family grows to five members. Trends Immunol 2003; 24(6):286–290.
41. Kopp E, Medzhitov R. Recognition of microbial infection by Toll-like receptors. Curr Opin Immunol 2003; 15(4):396–401.
42. Hoebe K, Du X, Georgel P, et al. Identification of Lps2 as a key transducer of MyD88-independent TIR signalling. Nature 2003; 424(6950):743–748.
43. Picard C, Puel A, Bonnet M, et al. Pyogenic bacterial infections in humans with IRAK-4 deficiency. Science 2003; 299(5615):2076–2079.
44. Deng L, Wang C, Spencer E, et al. Activation of the IkappaB kinase complex by TRAF6 requires a dimeric ubiquitin-conjugating enzyme complex and a unique polyubiquitin chain. Cell 2000; 103(2):351–361.
45. Wang C, Deng L, Hong M, et al. TAK1 is a ubiquitin-dependent kinase of MKK and IKK. Nature 2001; 412(6844):346–351.
46. Ben-Neriah Y. Regulatory functions of ubiquitination in the immune system. Nat Immunol 2002; 3(1):20–26.
47. May MJ, Ghosh S. IkappaB kinases: kinsmen with different crafts. Science 1999; 284(5412):271–273.
48. Karin M, Ben-Neriah Y. Phosphorylation meets ubiquitination: the control of NF-[kappa]B activity. Annu Rev Immunol 2000; 18:621–663.
49. Inohara N, Koseki T, del Peso L, et al. Nod1, an Apaf-1-like activator of caspase-9 and nuclear factor-kappaB. J Biol Chem 1999; 274(21):14560–14567.
50. Kobayashi K, Inohara N, Hernandez LD, et al. RICK/Rip2/CARDIAK mediates signalling for receptors of the innate and adaptive immune systems. Nature 2002; 416(6877):194–199.
51. Gewirtz AT, Rao AS, Simon PO Jr, et al. Salmonella typhimurium induces epithelial IL-8 expression via Ca(2+)-mediated activation of the NF-kappaB pathway. J Clin Invest 2000; 105(1):79–92.
52. Winston JT, Strack P, Beer-Romero P, et al. The SCFbeta-TRCP-ubiquitin ligase complex associates specifically with phosphorylated destruction motifs in IkappaBalpha and beta-catenin and stimulates IkappaBalpha ubiquitination in vitro. Genes Dev 1999; 13(3):270–283.
53. Spencer E, Jiang J, Chen ZJ. Signal-induced ubiquitination of IkappaBalpha by the F-box protein Slimb/beta-TrCP. Genes Dev 1999; 13(3):284–294.
54. Read MA, Brownell JE, Gladysheva TB, et al. Nedd8 modification of cul-1 activates SCF(beta(TrCP))-dependent ubiquitination of IkappaBalpha. Mol Cell Biol 2000; 20(7):2326–2333.
55. Chen LW, Egan L, Li ZW, et al. The two faces of IKK and NF-kappaB inhibition: prevention of systemic inflammation but increased local injury following intestinal ischemia-reperfusion. Nat Med 2003; 9(5):575–581.
56. Read MA, Neish AS, Luscinskas FW, et al. The proteasome pathway is required for cytokine-induced endothelial-leukocyte adhesion molecule expression. Immunity 1995; 2(5):493–506.
57. Jobin C, Panja A, Hellerbrand C, et al. Inhibition of proinflammatory molecule production by adenovirus-mediated expression of a nuclear factor kappaB super-repressor in human intestinal epithelial cells. J Immunol 1998; 160(1):410–418.
58. Neish AS, Gewirtz AT, Zeng H, et al. Prokaryotic regulation of epithelial responses by inhibition of IkappaB-alpha ubiquitination. Science 2000; 289(5484):1560–1563.
59. Collier-Hyams LS, Sloane V, Batten BC, et al. Cutting edge: bacterial modulation of epithelial signaling via changes in neddylation of cullin-1. J Immunol 2005; 175(7):4194–4198.
60. Elewaut D, DiDonato JA, Kim JM, et al. NF-[kappa]B is a central regulator of the intestinal epithelial cell innate immune response induced by infection with enteroinvasive bacteria. Journal of Immunology 1999; 163(3):1457–1466.
61. Chang L, Karin M. Mammalian MAP kinase signalling cascades. Nature 2001; 410(6824):37–40.
62. Taniguchi T, Ogasawara K, Takaoka A, et al. IRF family of transcription factors as regulators of host defense. Annu Rev Immunol 2001; 19:623–655.

63. Doyle S, Vaidya S, O'Connell R, et al. IRF3 mediates a TLR3/TLR4-specific antiviral gene program. Immunity 2002; 17(3):251–263.

64. Fitzgerald KA, McWhirter SM, Faia KL, et al. IKKepsilon and TBK1 are essential components of the IRF3 signaling pathway. Nat Immunol 2003; 4(5):491–496.

65. Sharma S, tenOever BR, Grandvaux N, et al. Triggering the interferon antiviral response through an IKK-related pathway. Science 2003; 300(5622):1148–1151.

66. Boldrick JC, Alizadeh AA, Diehn M, et al. Stereotyped and specific gene expression programs in human innate immune responses to bacteria. Proc Natl Acad Sci USA 2002; 99(2): 972–977.

67. Eckmann L, Smith JR, Housley MP, et al. Analysis by high density cDNA arrays of altered gene expression in human intestinal epithelial cells in response to infection with the invasive enteric bacteria Salmonella. J Biol Chem 2000; 275(19):14084–14094.

68. Zeng H, Carlson AQ, Guo Y, et al. Flagellin is the major proinflammatory determinant of enteropathogenic Salmonella. J Immunol 2003; 171(7):3668–3674.

69. Collins T, Read MA, Neish AS, et al. Transcriptional regulation of endothelial cell adhesion molecules: NF-kappa B and cytokine-inducible enhancers. Faseb J 1995; 9(10):899–909.

70. Conlan JW. Critical roles of neutrophils in host defense against experimental systemic infections of mice by Listeria monocytogenes, Salmonella typhimurium, and Yersinia enterocolitica. Infect Immun 1997; 65(2):630–635.

71. Nau GJ, Richmond JF, Schlesinger A, et al. Human macrophage activation programs induced by bacterial pathogens. Proc Natl Acad Sci USA 2002; 99(3):1503–1508.

72. Adams JM. Ways of dying: multiple pathways to apoptosis. Genes Dev 2003; 17(20):2481–2495.

73. Meier P, Finch A, Evan G. Apoptosis in development. Nature 2000; 407(6805):796–801.

74. Green DR, Kroemer G. The pathophysiology of mitochondrial cell death. Science 2004; 305(5684):626–629.

75. Yeh WC, Pompa JL, McCurrach ME, et al. FADD: essential for embryo development and signaling from some, but not all, inducers of apoptosis. Science 1998; 279(5358):1954–1958.

76. Karin M, Lin A. NF-kappaB at the crossroads of life and death. Nat Immunol 2002; 3(3):221–227.

77. Collier-Hyams LS, Neish AS. Innate immune relationship between commensal flora and the mammalian intestinal epithelium. Cell Mol Life Sci 2005; 62(12):1339–1348.

78. Zeng H, Wu H, Sloane V, et al. Flagellin/TLR5 responses in epithelia reveal intertwined activation of inflammatory and apoptotic pathways. Am J Physiol Gastrointest Liver Physiol 2006; 290(1):G96–G108.

79. Beg AA, Baltimore D. An essential role for NF-kappaB in preventing TNF-alpha-induced cell death. Science 1996; 274(5288):782–784.

80. Chen Z, Hagler J, Palombella VJ, et al. Signal-induced site-specific phosphorylation targets I kappa B alpha to the ubiquitin-proteasome pathway. Genes Dev 1995; 9(13):1586–1597.

81. Dispenzieri A. Bortezomib for myeloma – much ado about something. N Engl J Med 2005; 352(24):2546–2548.

82. Rumbo M, Schiffrin EJ. Ontogeny of intestinal epithelium immune functions: developmental and environmental regulation. Cell Mol Life Sci 2005; 62(12):1288–1296.

83. Polak-Charcon S, Shoham J, Y Ben-Shaul. Tight junctions in epithelial cells of human fetal hindgut, normal colon, and colon adenocarcinoma. J Natl Cancer Inst 1980; 65(1):53–62.

84. Lebenthal A, Lebenthal E. The ontogeny of the small intestinal epithelium. JPEN J Parenter Enteral Nutr 1999; 23(5 Suppl):S3–S6.

85. Buisine MP, Devisme L, Savidge TC, et al. Mucin gene expression in human embryonic and fetal intestine. Gut 1998; 43(4):519–524.

86. Mallow EB, Harris A, Salzman N, et al. Human enteric defensins. Gene structure and developmental expression. J Biol Chem 1996; 271(8):4038–4045.

87. Newell SJ. Enteral feeding of the micropremie. Clin Perinatol 2000; 27(1):221–234viii.

88. Logan CY, Nusse R. The Wnt signaling pathway in development and disease. Annu Rev Cell Dev Biol 2004; 20:781–810.

89. Reya T, Clevers H. Wnt signalling in stem cells and cancer. Nature 2005; 434(7035):843–850.

90. Moon RT, Kohn AD, De Ferrari GV, et al. WNT and beta-catenin signalling: diseases and therapies. Nat Rev Genet 2004; 5(9):691–701.

91. Ohnaka K, Taniguchi H, Kawate H, et al. Glucocorticoid enhances the expression of dickkopf-1 in human osteoblasts: novel mechanism of glucocorticoid-induced osteoporosis. Biochem Biophys Res Commun 2004; 318(1):259–264.

92. Ouellette AJ, Greco RM, James M, et al. Developmental regulation of cryptdin, a corticostatin/ defensin precursor mRNA in mouse small intestinal crypt epithelium. J Cell Biol 1989; 108(5):1687–1695.

93. Salzman NH, Polin RA, Harris MC, et al. Enteric defensin expression in necrotizing enterocolitis. Pediatr Res 1998; 44(1):20–26.

94. Kobayashi KS, Chamaillard M, Ogura Y, et al. Nod2-dependent regulation of innate and adaptive immunity in the intestinal tract. Science 2005; 307(5710):731–734.

95. Ahrens P, Kattner E, Kohler B, et al. Mutations of genes involved in the innate immune system as predictors of sepsis in very low birth weight infants. Pediatr 2004; 55(4):652–656.

96. Hugot JP, Chamaillard M, Zouali H, et al. Association of NOD2 leucine-rich repeat variants with susceptibility to Crohn's disease. Nature 2001; 411(6837):599–603.

97. Habib Z, Arnaud B, de Pascal L, et al. CARD15/NOD2 is not a predisposing factor for necrotizing enterocolitis. Dig Dis Sci 2005; 50(9):1684–1687.

98. Fusunyan RD, Nanthakumar NN, Baldeon ME, et al. Evidence for an innate immune response in the immature human intestine: toll-like receptors on fetal enterocytes. Pediatr Res 2001; 49(4):589–593.

99. Nanthakumar NN, Fusunyan RD, Sanderson I. et al. Inflammation in the developing human intestine: A possible pathophysiologic contribution to necrotizing enterocolitis. Proc Natl Acad Sci USA 2000; 97(11):6043–6048.

100. Claud EC, Lu L, Anton PM, et al. Developmentally regulated IkappaB expression in intestinal epithelium and susceptibility to flagellin-induced inflammation. Proc Natl Acad Sci USA 2004; 101(19):7404–7408.

101. Sepkowitz KA. Gastrointestinal infections in neutropenic patients. In: Blaser MJ, et al., eds. Infections of the gastrointestinal tract. Philadelphia: Lippincott; 2002: 473–479.

102. Takeuchi O, Hoshino K, Akira S. Cutting edge: TLR2-deficient and MyD88-deficient mice are highly susceptible to Staphylococcus aureus infection. J Immunol 2000; 165(10): 5392–5396.

103. Sha WC, Liou H-C, Tuomanen EI, et al. Targeted disruption of the p50 subunit of NF-[kappa]B leads to multifocal defects in immune responses. Cell 1995; 80(2):321–330.

104. Russo MP, Boudreau F, Li F, et al. NF-kB blockade exacerbates experimental colitis in transgenic mice expression an intestinal epithelial cell specific IkB super-repressor (abst). Gastroenterology 2001; 120.

105. Jilling T, Lu J, Jackson M, et al. Intestinal epithelial apoptosis initiates gross bowel necrosis in an experimental rat model of neonatal necrotizing enterocolitis. Pediatr Res 2004; 55(4):622–629.

106. Pacha J. Development of intestinal transport function in mammals. Physiol Rev 2000; 80(4):1633–1667.

107. McClure RJ. Trophic feeding of the preterm infant. Acta Paediatr Suppl 2001; 90(436):19–21.

108. Hooper LV. Bacterial contributions to mammalian gut development. Trends Microbiol 2004; 12(3):129–134.

109. Hooper LV, Wong MH, Thelin A, et al. Molecular analysis of commensal host-microbial relationships in the intestine. Science 2001; 291(5505):881–884.

110. Falk PG, Hooper LV, Midtvedt T, et al. Creating and maintaining the gastrointestinal ecosystem: What we know and need to know from gnotobiology. Microbiol Mol Biol Rev 1998; 62(4):1157–1170.

111. McCracken VJ, Lorenz RG. The gastrointestinal ecosystem: a precarious alliance among epithelium, immunity and microbiota. Cell Microbiol 2001; 3(1):1–11.

112. Hoy CM, Wood CM, Hawkey PM, et al. Duodenal microflora in very-low-birth-weight neonates and relation to necrotizing enterocolitis. J Clin Microbiol 2000; 38(12):4539–4547.

113. de la Cochetiere MF, Piloquet H, des Robert C, et al. Early intestinal bacterial colonization and necrotizing enterocolitis in premature infants: the putative role of Clostridium. Pediatr Res 2004; 56(3):366–370.

114. Schumann A, Nutten S, Donnicola D, et al. Neonatal antibiotic treatment alters gastrointestinal tract developmental gene expression and intestinal barrier transcriptome. Physiol Genomics 2005; 23(2):235–245.

115. Wallace TD, Bradley S, Buckley ND, et al. Interactions of lactic acid bacteria with human intestinal epithelial cells: effects on cytokine production. J Food Prot 2003; 66(3):466–472.

116. Madsen KL, Doyle JS, Jewell LD, et al. Lactobacillus species prevents colitis in interleukin 10 gene-deficient mice. Gastroenterology 1999; 116(5):1107–1114.

117. Kelly D, Campbell JI, King TP, et al. Commensal anaerobic gut bacteria attenuate inflammation by regulating nuclear-cytoplasmic shuttling of PPAR-gamma and RelA. Nat Immunol 2004; 5(1):104–112.

118. Bourlioux P, Koletzko B, Guarner F, et al. The intestine and its microflora are partners for the protection of the host: report on the Danone Symposium 'The Intelligent Intestine', held in Paris, June 14 2002. Am J Clin Nutr 2003; 78(4):675–683.

119. Lin HC, BH Su, Chen AC, et al. Oral probiotics reduce the incidence and severity of necrotizing enterocolitis in very low birth weight infants. Pediatrics 2005; 115(1):1–4.

120. Kliegman RM, Willoughby RE. Prevention of necrotizing enterocolitis with probiotics. Pediatrics 2005; 115(1):171–172.

121. Teitelbaum JE, Walker WA. Nutritional impact of pre- and probiotics as protective gastrointestinal organisms. Annu Rev Nutr 2002; 22:107–138.

122. Mack DR, Lebel S. Role of probiotics in the modulation of intestinal infections and inflammation. Curr Opin Gastroenterol 2004; 20(1):22–26.

123. Sartor RB. Therapeutic manipulation of the enteric microflora in inflammatory bowel diseases: antibiotics, probiotics, and prebiotics. Gastroenterology 2004; 126(6):1620–1633.

124. Rakoff-Nahoum S, Paglino J, Eslami-Varzaneh F, et al. Recognition of commensal microflora by toll-like receptors is required for intestinal homeostasis. Cell 2004; 118(2):229–241.

125. Ouwehand AC, Derrien M, de Vos W, et al. Prebiotics and other microbial substrates for gut functionality. Curr Opin Biotechnol 2005; 16(2):212–217.

126. Knol J, Boehm G, Lidestri M, et al. Increase of faecal bifidobacteria due to dietary oligosaccharides induces a reduction of clinically relevant pathogen germs in the faeces of formula-fed preterm infants. Acta Paediatr Suppl 2005; 94(449):31–33.

127. Boehm G, Stahl B, Jelinek J, et al. Prebiotic carbohydrates in human milk and formulas. Acta Paediatr Suppl 2005; 94(449):18–21.

128. Fanaro S, Boehm G, Garssen J, et al. Galacto-oligosaccharides and long-chain fructo-oligosaccharides as prebiotics in infant formulas: a review. Acta Paediatr Suppl 2005; 94(449):22–26.

129. Tsukahara T, Iwasaki Y, Nakayama K, et al. Stimulation of butyrate production in the large intestine of weaning piglets by dietary fructooligosaccharides and its influence on the histological variables of the large intestinal mucosa. J Nutr Sci Vitaminol (Tokyo) 2003; 49(6):414–421.

130. Bartholome AL, Albin DM, Baker DH, et al. Supplementation of total parenteral nutrition with butyrate acutely increases structural aspects of intestinal adaptation after an 80% jejunoileal resection in neonatal piglets. JPEN J Parenter Enteral Nutr 2004; 28(4):210–22; discussion 222–223.

131. Kanauchi O, Andoh A, Iwanaga T, et al. Germinated barley foodstuffs attenuate colonic mucosal damage and mucosal nuclear factor kappa B activity in a spontaneous colitis model. J Gastroenterol Hepatol 1999; 14(12):1173–1179.

132. Yin L, Laevsky G, Giardina C. Butyrate suppression of colonocyte NF-kappa B activation and cellular proteasome activity. J Biol Chem 2001; 276(48):44641–44646.

133. Venkatraman A, Ramakrishna BS, Shaji RV, et al. Amelioration of dextran sulfate colitis by butyrate: role of heat shock protein 70 and NF-kappaB. Am J Physiol Gastrointest Liver Physiol 2003; 285(1):G177–G184.

134. Avivi-Green C, Polak-Charcon S, Madar Z, et al. Apoptosis cascade proteins are regulated in vivo by high intracolonic butyrate concentration: correlation with colon cancer inhibition. Oncol Res 2000; 12(2):83–95.

135. Mentschel J, Claus R. Increased butyrate formation in the pig colon by feeding raw potato starch leads to a reduction of colonocyte apoptosis and a shift to the stem cell compartment. Metabolism 2003; 52(11):1400–1405.

136. Scheppach W, Weiler F. The butyrate story: old wine in new bottles? Curr Opin Clin Nutr Metab Care 2004; 7(5):563–567.

137. Strober W. Epithelial cells pay a Toll for protection. Nat Med 2004; 10(9):898–900.

138. Abreu MT, Vora P, Faure E, et al. Decreased expression of Toll-like receptor-4 and MD-2 correlates with intestinal epithelial cell protection against dysregulated proinflammatory gene expression in response to bacterial lipopolysaccharide. J Immunol 2001; 167(3):1609–1616.

139. Rachmilewitz D, Katakura K, Karmeli F, et al. Toll-like receptor 9 signaling mediates the anti-inflammatory effects of probiotics in murine experimental colitis. Gastroenterology 2004; 126(2):520–528.

140. Francois S, El Benna J, Dang PM, et al. Inhibition of neutrophil apoptosis by TLR agonists in whole blood: involvement of the phosphoinositide 3-kinase/Akt and NF-kappaB signaling pathways, leading to increased levels of Mcl-1, A1, and phosphorylated Bad. J Immunol 2005; 174(6):3633–3642.

Chapter 5

The Intestinal Microbiota and the Microbiome

Erika C. Claud, MD • W. Allan Walker, MD

The preterm gut is essentially a fetal gut, expecting conditions of the intrauterine environment. This includes absence of bacteria, absence of food substrate, low oxygen consumption due to the role of the placenta as the primary organ of nutrition, and presence of amniotic fluid with proteins and hormones which may have a role in maturation. Rapid colonization of the intestine after birth with a variety of microbial species is a normal part of development. So begins a complex cross-talk between the gut and its microflora with implications for immune, inflammatory, and allergic responses. It is not merely the existence of bacteria but the balance of bacteria that affects a variety of signaling pathways and immune responses.

This chapter will review the effects of bacteria on the intestine and immune system as well as factors affecting colonization of the immature intestine. Implications for the disease necrotizing enterocolitis will be highlighted, including means by which bacteria in the form of probiotics may be beneficial in this disease.

INTESTINAL MICROBIAL FLORA IN THE HEALTHY HOST

The interaction between the intestine and bacterial microflora is a complex relationship with risk and benefit for the host. It is sobering to realize that of the estimated 10^{14} cells in the human body, only about 10% belong to the host and the remaining 90% represent the microbiota living in or on the host, containing a genome or "microbiome" collectively more extensive than our own (1). The human intestine is populated with more microorganisms than any other organ, and in fact

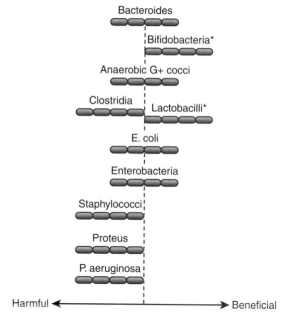

Bacteroides

Bifidobacteria*

Anaerobic G+ cocci

Clostridia   Lactobacilli*

E. coli

Enterobacteria

Staphylococci

Proteus

P. aeruginosa

Harmful ◄──────────────────────► Beneficial

* 95% of flora in breast fed infants in first month of life
  50% of flora in formula fed infants in first month of life (4,5)

Figure 5-1 Range of common organisms in gut micro-flora. The spectrum of gut microflora organisms can range from harmful to beneficial. Individual composition is affected by a variety of environmental and host defense influences. Adapted with permission from the American Journal of Clinical Nutrition. © Am J Clin Nutr. American Society for Clinical Nutrition (2).

some have considered the microflora itself equivalent to an ancillary body organ based on weight, genetic content, cellular content, and metabolic activity of these organisms. Many are difficult to grow in culture and are only now being identified via 16S ribosomal DNA polymerase chain reaction fingerprinting. In a healthy host, beyond merely colonizing the gut awaiting entry into the bloodstream, these microorganisms have a significant impact on intestinal health and gut function.

A variety of organisms, both beneficial and harmful, can colonize the gut. Some bacteria are almost always pathogenic, such as *Clostridia*, *Pseudomonas*, *Staphylococcus*, and *Proteus*. Others can be either pathogenic or beneficial such as *Bacteroides*, *Escherichia coli*, and *Enterobacteriae*. Still others are thought to be primarily beneficial, most commonly *Lactobacillus* and *Bifidobacterium* species (Fig. 5-1) (2).

Colonization begins at birth with bacteria that represent maternal vaginal and colonic flora in vaginally delivered infants. This flora contains many facultative anaerobic bacteria such as *Enterobacteriae*, *Enterococci*, and *Staphylococci*. As the number of aerobic and facultative anaerobic organisms increase, oxygen is consumed, allowing for colonization by anaerobic organisms (3). Thereafter colonization is affected by feeding, with bacteria introduced via either breast milk or formula feeds along with factors, particularly in breast milk, which influence colonization (4, 5). Weaning from breast milk, the introduction of solid foods, and the environment further affect colonization. This ultimately leads to complete adult colonization by 2 years of age with 400–1000 different species and a stable pattern that is unique for each individual. There is evidence that different organisms can affect different intestinal functions and it is likely that the synergy of the diversity of intestinal microbiota is important for the balance of intestinal health and appropriate control of pathogenic organisms.

Microbial flora is determined not only by the organisms to which the intestine is exposed, but also by intrinsic intestinal host defense mechanisms. The intestine has many physical barriers to bacteria including peristalsis, gastric acid, proteolytic enzymes, intestinal mucus, cell surface glycoconjugates, and tight

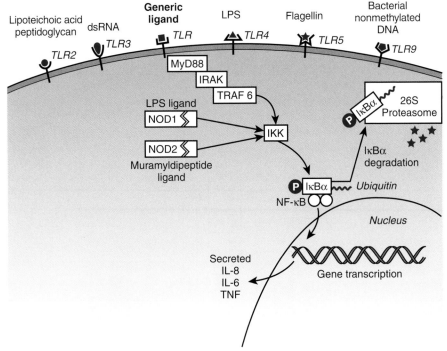

Figure 5-2 Schematic of TLR and NOD signaling leading to NF-κB activation. While different TLR and NOD receptors have specific ligands, post-receptor signaling events leading to NF-κB activation are the same. The signaling cascade begins with recruitment of the adaptor molecules MyD88, IRAK, and TRAF6, leading to IKK activation, which phosphorylates IκBα, targeting it for ubiquitination and degradation by the 26S proteasome. The NF-κB thus liberated translocates to the nucleus and binds to DNA, resulting in gene transcription. TLR, Toll-like receptor; LPS, lipopolysaccharide; IRAK, IL-1 receptor associated kinase; TRAF, tumor necrosis factor receptor associated factor; IKK, IkappaB kinase; IκB, inhibitor of kappaB; NF-κB, nuclear factor kappaB; P, phosphorylation; NOD, nucleotide-binding oligomerization domain.

junctions between intestinal epithelial cells. These are designed to limit bacteria to the gut lumen and prevent attachment and translocation across the intestinal epithelium. The intestine also has a complex system of immunologic host defense and biochemical factors designed to limit the growth of organisms that breach the physical barrier. This includes intestinal T and B lymphocytes, sIgA, human defensins secreted by Paneth cells, and intestinal trefoil factor secreted by the intestinal epithelium itself.

The intestine has developed multiple means of sampling and interacting with its microflora so that commensal bacteria can be recognized and tolerated while pathogenic organisms trigger inflammatory and immune responses. Three cell types can sample the microbial milieu: M cells, surface enterocytes, and dendritic cells (Fig. 5-3).

M cells are found throughout the digestive tract in the specialized follicle-associated epithelium of mucosal lymphoid follicles or Peyer's patches. They can transport antigens and bacteria to subepithelial dendritic cells via active vesicular transport across the epithelium using clathrin-mediated endocytosis, pinocytosis, or phagocytosis (6). This process is thought to be intended to regulate commensal flora and promote IgA antibody responses. However, while this mechanism can activate immune responses, it also allows a portal into the mucosa which can be exploited by pathogens.

Surface enterocytes can recognize bacterial products via a highly conserved family of pathogen-associated molecular pattern (PAMP) receptors called Toll-like

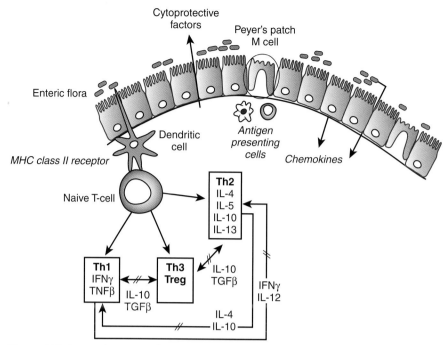

Figure 5-3 Host and gut microflora interaction. The intestinal epithelium can sample the microbial mileu via three cell types: dendritic cells, M cells in Peyer's patches, and intestinal epithelial cells. Interaction with bacteria can prime Th1 and Th2 immune responses, which are kept in balance by specific cytokines and T regulatory cells. In addition interaction with bacteria can result in the production of both chemokines and cytoprotective factors.

receptors (TLR) (Fig. 5-2). Each of these receptors recognizes a specific bacterial product. For example TLR-2 recognizes products of Gram-positive organisms such as peptidoglycan and lipoteichoic acid. TLR-4 recognizes lipopolysaccharide from Gram-negative organisms. TLR-5 recognizes flagellin, a proinflammatory subunit of bacteria flagella. TLR-9 recognizes nonmethylated bacterial DNA (7, 8). Binding of any of these receptors leads to activation of nuclear factor kappaB (NF-κB). In addition the intracellular receptors NOD1 and NOD2 (for nucleotide-binding oligomerization domain) also recognize bacterial motifs such as LPS and trigger activation of the NF-κB pathway (9, 10).

NF-κB represents a group of structurally related proteins that activate transcription of a wide variety of genes involved in inflammatory and immune responses. In its resting state NF-κB dimers are bound in the cytoplasm to the inhibitor of κB or (IκB) proteins (11–13). Cell stimulation can trigger signal transduction pathways leading to the activation of IκB kinase (IKK), which then phosphorylates IκB, targeting it for degradation by the proteasome. The NF-κB thus liberated moves to the nucleus, where it activates the transcription of genes including cytokines such as IL-6 and TNFα, chemokines such as IL-8, adhesion molecules, and regulators of apoptosis.

Dendritic cells are the antigen-presenting cells of the intestine (Fig. 5-3). They can extend between surface enterocytes, without disrupting tight junctions, and transmit live bacteria or bacterial antigens to mesenteric lymph nodes for immune responses (14). Antigens from either food or bacteria which come in contact with the intestinal epithelium are presented by dendritic cells in the context of MHC class II molecules to naive T lymphocytes in the Peyer's patches. Immune responses of the intestine to these bacterial signals are generally described in terms of two classes of CD4+ T cells, defined by their cytokine production (15, 16). T helper type 1 (Th1) cells produce interferon γ (IFNγ) and tumor necrosis factor β (TNFβ). These cytokines are important in the development of cell-mediated immunity. Inappropriate Th1 dominant responses are associated with autoimmune diseases. T helper type 2 (Th2) cells produce IL-4, IL-5, IL-10, and IL-13. These cytokines are associated with the development of IgE responses. Inappropriate Th2 responses result in allergy and atopy. CD4+ T lymphocytes are activated and differentiate based on the type and amount of antigen as well as by the cytokine balance. The presence of IL-12 primes for Th1 responses, while IL-4 primes for Th2 responses.

In the nondiseased mature state there is tight regulation of protective inflammatory and allergic host responses. Under baseline conditions the intestinal mucosa is in a constant "suppressed" state due to increased transforming growth factor beta (TGFβ) and IL-10 produced by regulatory T cells and Th3 cells (17, 18). If bacteria breech the mucosal barrier, allowing presentation of bacterial products in the context of TLR, Th1 responses are triggered, TH2 responses are suppressed, and appropriate inflammatory responses are induced to contain the bacterial insult. When no response is required, Th2 cells produce IL-4 and IL-10, which appropriately suppress Th1 responses, while Th1 cells produce IFNγ and IL-12, which appropriately suppress Th2 responses, returning the balance to its baseline state. Dysregulation can lead to conditions of inappropriate responses to bacteria such as inflammatory bowel disease, or to food antigens such as food allergies and celiac disease.

BENEFICIAL EFFECTS OF INTESTINAL FLORA

While the role of bacteria in pathogenesis is well understood, bacteria also provide many potential benefits to the host. Bacteria are responsible for provision of essential nutrients such as vitamin K, vitamin B12, and short-chain fatty acids such as butyrate. Bacteria are important in the metabolism of polysaccharides, so the host is not required to expend energy or develop pathways for these processes (19, 20). In addition, certain bacteria provide bacterial interference resulting in competitive colonization against pathogenic organisms. Commensal flora can interfere with infection by pathogenic organisms by competition for host binding sites, stimulation of host defense mechanisms, competition for nutrients and triggering cell-signaling events that limit the production of virulence factors.

Studies have also shown that certain bacteria promote cell viability. *E. coli*, *Streptococcus thermophilus*, *Lactobacillus*, and *Bifidobacterium* protect against cell death associated with pathogenic bacteria, while other studies have demonstrated that *Lactobacillus* alone protects against cytokine-mediated programmed cell death or apoptosis (21). Cell culture models indicate that *Lactobacillus GG* can specifically increase intestinal epithelial cell (IEC) survival by activating the cell protective anti-apoptotic pathway Akt, while simultaneously inhibiting the activation of the pro-apoptotic pathway p38/Map kinase by tumor necrosis factor (TNF), interleukin -1 (IL-1) alpha, or gamma interferon(22). In addition studies have shown an increased mitotic index of intestinal villi from germ-free animals mono-associated with LGG, suggesting cell growth and mucosal repair (23).

Next, bacteria regulate development of intestinal villus vascular architecture. These patterns are immature in adult germ-free mice with an arrested capillary network but can reach maturity and complexity with the addition of complete microbiota from conventional mice or again with the single organism *Bacteroides thetaiotaomicron*. This effect requires Paneth cells, further indicating the complexity of the relationship between organisms and specific aspects of the intestine (24).

Bacteria are also necessary for maturation of the intestine and appropriate containment of inflammatory responses. This is particularly relevant to the preterm infant with an immature gut. Many of the studies of the role of specific bacteria in the gut have been performed using gnotobiotic mice, with "known biota."

These mice can either be germ-free without any organisms, or mono-associated with specific organisms. These studies have demonstrated that compared to mice with conventional flora, germ-free mice have higher caloric intake, decreased epithelial cell turnover, disordered gut-associated lymphoid tissue (GALT), and abnormal gut motility (25). Microarray evaluation of the effect of just one commensal organism, *Bacteroides thetaiotaomicron*, on the intestine of germ-free mice revealed increased expression of genes involved in nutrient absorption, which may partially explain the higher caloric requirements of the germ-free animals. These included the Na^+/glucose transporter SGLT-1, genes involved in lipid absorption, and the copper transporter CRT1. This study also revealed an increase in small proline-rich protein 2 (sprr2a), which strengthens the barrier function of epithelium, and an increase in mRNA encoding a protein involved in neurotransmitter release and muscle systems which may have implications for the enteric nervous system and motility. Also noted were increased expression of polymeric immunoglobulin receptor, genes of the mucus layer (MUCLIN), and a receptor for trefoil peptides (26). Interestingly, when other commensal organisms such as *Bifidobacterium infantis* and *Escherichia coli* K12 were investigated in the same model, different patterns of gene expression were noted, indicating that different organisms have different roles.

Other studies have further evaluated the role of bacteria specifically in maturation of host defense. Studies have shown that cell-surface glycoconjugates which serve as adhesion sites for a variety of microbes have a different pattern of carbohydrate residues in the immature intestine compared to that of the adult intestine (27, 28). Examination of the maturation of these glycoconjugate patterns in germ-free and conventionalized mice demonstrates that conventional mice have increased fucosyl transferase activity over time and concomitant decreased sialyl transferase activity with maturity. In contrast, germ-free mice maintain the opposite immature pattern of low fucosyl transferase and high sialyl transferase activities. After 2 weeks of colonization with bacteria, however, the germ-free animals shifted the immature pattern to the normal mature pattern. This suggests that bacteria influence adherence patterns. Interestingly, other genetically programmed developmental brush-border enzyme patterns, such as increasing sucrase and decreasing lactase activities with maturation, were the same in the conventional and the germ-free animals (29).

Intestinal mucus is another barrier to infection that has been shown in animal studies to be developmentally mediated and potentially affected by bacterial colonization (30). Examination of the effect of intestinal colonization with a combination of the organisms *Streptococcus, Lactobacillus* and *Bifidobacterium* demonstrated induction of specific mucus genes MUC2, MUC3, and MUC5AC (21, 31).

Intestinal barrier function can also be influenced by bacterial colonization. The immature gut is "leaky" compared to mature IEC as demonstrated by permeability studies. One means of evaluating barrier function is measuring transepithelial resistance (TER). Studies have demonstrated that when intestinal cells are treated with commensal bacteria such as *E. coli, Streptococcus thermophilus, Lactobacillus*, and *Bifidobacterium*, TER increases, while treatment with pathogenic *Salmonella* decreases TER (21). Utilizing a model of directly measuring intestinal permeability to dextran or mannitol in the presence of different bacteria, it was similarly found that colonization with *E. coli, Klebsiella*, or *Streptococcus viridans* increased permeability while colonization with *Lactobacillus brevis* decreased permeability (32). This has clinical relevance, as a clinical study in infants demonstrated that when intestinal flora was manipulated to increase levels of anaerobic bacteria including *Bifidobacterium*, there were lower levels of serum endotoxin, suggesting decreased translocation of endotoxin-producing organisms (33).

BACTERIA AND MATURATION OF THE IMMUNE SYSTEM

Bacteria also influence responses to microflora. The gut-associated lymphoid tissue (GALT) is the largest mass of lymphoid tissue in the body. It consists of immune cells such as B and T lymphocytes, macrophages, antigen-presenting cells, including dendritic cells, and specific epithelial and intra-epithelial lymphocytes. A key unique feature of the intestine is its ability to process antigens from food or commensal bacteria and not mount an inflammatory response yet retain the ability to recognize and respond to pathogenic stimuli.

There is evidence that intestinal bacteria have an important role in maturation of the immune system. Studies of germ-free mice have noted several immunodeficiencies, including fewer splenic CD4+ T cells, structural splenic disorganization, fewer intraepithelial lymphocytes, decreased conversion of follicular associated epithelium to M cells, decreased secretory IgA, decreased ability to induce oral tolerance, and skewing towards a Th2 cytokine profile similar to the immature neonatal profile (34–36). Bacteria play an important role in the expansion of gut lymphoid tissues. When germ-free animals are colonized with intestinal flora GALT significantly expands. A recent study has demonstrated that *Bacteroides fragilis*, a common colonic Gram-negative organism, can accomplish this via a specific bacterial polysaccharide (PSA). Colonization with *B. fragilis* resulted in restoration of splenic CD4+ T cell numbers to normal levels, a response not seen with a *B. fragilis* PSA mutant. PSA itself, when cultured with primary T cells, induced production of IFNγ, suggesting induction of Th1 cytokines via Stat4 transcriptional regulation of IL-12 (34). Interestingly, *B. fragilis* has also been closely associated with maturation of IgA and IgM secretion, an important aspect of host defense which has been shown to be deficient in newborns and may not reach maturation until 6–8 years of age (37–39).

The immature immune system of neonatal mice and humans is known to have a Th2 bias, and bacteria from postnatal gut colonization are required to appropriately shift towards a Th1 response and thus balance the system. Failure to shift can result in an allergic bias (40, 41). Oral tolerance is a normal state of nonresponsiveness to antigens presented via the gut. An allergic reaction would be considered a failure to induce oral tolerance, resulting in an abnormally high IgE level. Recent data have shown an increase in asthma and allergy in the Western world. In general this represents an inappropriate Th2 bias. The hygiene hypothesis has been proposed, which states that "Over the past century declining family size, improved household amenities, and higher standards of personal cleanliness have reduced opportunities for cross-infection in young families. This may have resulted in more widespread clinical expression of atopic disease" (42, 43). A recent study found a relationship between high environmental levels of endotoxin, a cell wall component of Gram-negative bacteria, and decreased allergic sensitization in children from these environments compared to children from environments with low levels of endotoxin (44). At high doses endotoxin induces an inflammatory response; however, at low doses it can induce IL-12 and IFNγ, which stimulate Th1 responses while decreasing Th2 responses. Endotoxin can also stimulate defensins, which can enhance the host defense of a developing neonate (45).

The mechanism by which bacteria stimulate and maintain appropriate immune homeostasis is unclear. One means is via T regulatory cells, which via IL-10 decrease inflammation induced by colitis-inducing Th1 lymphocytes reactive with enteric bacterial antigens, by decreasing IL-12 secretion (35). It has been proposed that the decrease in childhood infections and overall antigenic stimulation has resulted in a decrease in IL-10 and possibly TGFβ – both produced by regulatory T cells to downregulate Th1 and Th2 responses. Tolerance is influenced by the development of the antigen-presenting cell, which in the gut is primarily dendritic cells (DC).

Regulatory T cells are antigen-specific suppressive T cells that turn off inflammatory immune responses. Immature DC which have not received an inflammatory stimulus induce differentiation of regulatory T cells, while mature DC which have seen an inflammatory stimulus induce maturation of Th1 or Th2 cells (46). *Lactobacillus* has been shown to influence dendritic cell maturation in mice and thus may influence whether a DC favors a Th1 or Th2 response (47).

More than the specific organisms or dose, however, timing appears to be critical. Protection against allergic disease can only be achieved by interventions in the neonatal period (45). Studies in germ-free mice have demonstrated that without bacteria Th2-mediated responses were intact, including elevated IgE and IgG1, but Th1 responses were decreased. Reconstitution of the flora of these germ-free animals with *Bifidobacterium infantis* allowed normalization of oral tolerance induction, but only when reconstitution was performed in neonates, not in older mice (36). Further studies looked prospectively at the flora from 76 infants at high risk for atopy at 3 weeks and 3 months of age. At 3 weeks those who developed atopy had relatively more *Clostridia* and less *Bifidobacterium*, but by 3 months there was no difference, suggesting that early colonization patterns are important for the maturation of human immunity to a nonatopic mode (48). In agreement with this, it has been shown that children who received antibiotics during infancy, which probably decreased intestinal flora, had a higher risk of allergy and atopy. Administration of *Enterococcus faecalis* or *Lactobacillus acidophilus* was able to prevent the Th2 shift induced by antibiotics (49).

Clinically allergic children are less often colonized with *Lactobacillus* and *Bifidobacterium* than are non-allergic children, and studies have noted decreased incidence of food allergy and atopic disease with lactobacillus administration (48, 50, 51). A further study looked at the effect of the administration of a probiotic *E. coli* and demonstrated that administration at birth decreased the risk of atopy compared to controls as far out as 10 and 20 years (52). Lastly, specific administration of probiotics to pregnant women and their subsequent newborns decreased the incidence of atopic dermatitis in the newborn (50).

The equilibrium between Th1 and Th2 immune responses is vital, with critical implications for host defense, auto-immune disease, atopy, and malignancies. Thus some bacterial contact is important to create an appropriate Th1/Th2 balance (41). T cells can travel beyond the gut, thus microbial flora may exert influence beyond the gut and beyond the newborn period by influencing immune responses. This may explain why enteral administration of bacteria such as lactobacillus can decrease asthma and arthritis (53). This raises the further intriguing possibility that colonization in the neonatal period can affect long-term health by imprinting immune patterns.

BACTERIA AND INFLAMMATION

In addition to maturation of immune responses, bacterial flora has a role in controlling intestinal inflammatory responses. The gut is in a constant controlled state of inflammation. Nonpathogenic organisms can decrease inflammatory signaling via NF-κB by inhibiting degradation of its inhibitor IκB. This is accomplished by interfering with the ubiquitin signal for its degradation (54). In addition *B. thetaiotaomicron* has specifically been shown to limit NF-κB signaling by inducing association of the transcriptionally active NF-κB subunit RelA and peroxisome proliferator activated receptor-γ (PPARγ). This subsequently enhances the nuclear export of NF-κB via a PPARγ-dependent pathway, limiting proinflammatory cytokine production (55).

It has recently been shown that commensal bacteria also have molecular patterns recognized by TLR. This leads to TLR activation critical for intestinal homeostasis.

If commensal organisms are unable to signal via TLR, as in MyD88 knockout animals or TLR2- or TLR4-deficient mice, there is increased morbidity associated with intestinal inflammation, possibly due to lack of ability to induce cytoprotective cytokines such as IL-6 and KC-1, as well as heat shock proteins (hsp) (56).

Another means of preventing immune responses to normal bacterial flora is via downregulation of Toll-like receptor responses. It has been shown for TLR4 and TLR2 that after multiple or prolonged exposure to ligand, there is decreased TLR signaling via decreased surface receptor expression and increased expression of Toll-interacting protein (57).

Lastly it has been shown that bacteria can upregulate cytoprotective pathways. Heat shock proteins (hsp) are highly conserved proteins that can be constitutively expressed and function to fold proteins into mature tertiary structures, or they can be induced and function to restore partially damaged proteins under conditions of stress. Heat is just one example of stress; others include bacterial infection or ischemia/reperfusion. Hsp are named by their molecular weight. Two of the induced forms of hsp are hsp 25, which stabilizes actin thus preserving cytoskeletal and tight junctions, and hsp 72, which binds and stabilizes critical cellular proteins preventing denaturation. Hsp are normally expressed by colonocytes, but not by small intestinal cells. It has been proposed that this can be explained by the constant exposure of colonocytes to bacteria. Consistent with this, studies using self-filling small intestinal loops resulting in chronic colonization, or self-emptying loops resulting in low levels of bacteria, have shown that continuous exposure to bacteria results in increased hsp 25 and 72 expression in the small intestine (58).

In summary, the healthy adult host is colonized with a wide variety of intestinal bacteria which play a significant role in intestinal health, maturation, immune regulation and control of inflammation.

PREMATURITY

In contrast to full-term infants or adults, the preterm infant has fewer organisms which tend to be more virulent. Colonization of the newborn intestine is affected by a variety of factors. Studies examining delivery method have shown that infants delivered vaginally have earlier colonization with *Bifidobacterium* and *Lactobacillus*, while infants delivered by cesarean section have colonization delayed up to 1 month for these species. In addition, infants delivered by cesarean section have very little *Bacteroides* and tend to have more *Clostridia* than vaginally delivered infants (59). Feeding is the next variable in the acquisition of intestinal flora. In breast-fed infants, *Bifidobacterium* is a primary organism, with *Lactobacillus* and *Streptococcus* as minor components. In formula-fed infants, similar amounts of *Bacteroides* and *Bifidobacterium* are found, with minor components of the more pathogenic species *Staphylococcus*, *Escherichia coli*, and *Clostridia* (60–64). This difference may be due to a variety of potentially antimicrobial factors found in breast milk such as antibodies, IgA, lysozyme, and lactoferrin which decrease the growth of pathogenic organisms. Concomitantly the growth of *Bifidobacterium* and *Lactobacillus* species is stimulated by the lower intestinal pH of breast-fed infants and the presence of specific oligosaccharides and glycoproteins in breast milk (65, 66) In addition, colonization is affected by gestational age. Although a wide range of aerobic and anaerobic flora colonizes normal infants by 10 days of age, infants in the neonatal intensive care unit undergo a delayed colonization with a limited number of bacterial species that tend to be virulent (5, 67). In particular it has been shown that in preterm infants, colonization with *Bifidobacterium* is delayed for several weeks (61, 68).

Many factors probably contribute to the altered intestinal microflora of preterm infants. Mothers in preterm labor and preterm infants themselves are often treated with antibiotics early in their hospital course. Human and animal models have demonstrated that antibiotic treatment in either mother or baby can result in long-term decreases in beneficial anaerobic organisms such as *Bifidobacterium*, *Lactobacillus* and *Bacteroides*, with concomitant increases in Gram-negative organisms, *Candida albicans* and *C. difficile* (46, 69). Admission to the neonatal intensive care unit itself, as a hospital environment, is likely to expose these infants to antibiotic-resistant organisms. Many preterm infants are unable to orally feed and thus require frequent instrumentation with nasogastric feeding tubes, which can alter colonization. Finally, the frequent use of acid-neutralizing medications and opioids which delay intestinal transit time removes important intestinal host defense mechanisms. Intestinal colonization patterns appear to be permanent and difficult to alter in adulthood. Thus the pattern of early colonization can be very important.

PREMATURITY AND NECROTIZING ENTEROCOLITIS (NEC)

Necrotizing enterocolitis is an inflammatory bowel necrosis that primarily affects preterm infants after the initiation of enteral feeds. While the exact pathophysiology is poorly understood, the primary risk factors are prematurity, bacterial colonization, enteral feeds and altered intestinal blood flow. It is known that the fetal intestine is exposed to amniotic fluid containing hormones and peptides that may have a role in intestinal maturation. At this stage, the fetal intestine is normally protected in its sterile environment and may not be prepared to respond to bacterial interaction. The preterm gut may not have completed maturation when colonized by bacteria and initially fed, potentially placing it at higher risk for NEC. One possible hypothesis is that intestinal injury in NEC may be the result of synergy in which enteral feeding results in colonization of the uniquely susceptible premature intestine with pathogenic bacteria, resulting in mucosal damage leading to an exaggerated inflammatory response (70).

WHY IS THE PRETERM INFANT UNIQUELY SUSCEPTIBLE?

A premature infant has an immature gut, and has potentially fewer organisms enhancing maturity and more pathogenic organisms, which collectively increases the risk of sepsis or NEC. Furthermore, data suggest that the immature preterm or fetal gut is unable to downregulate inflammatory responses.

Immature intestinal epithelial cells have an exaggerated response to endogenous inflammatory mediators such as tumor necrosis factor alpha (TNFα) or interleukin-1beta (IL-1β) and exogenous inflammatory mediators such as bacteria (71, 72). This exaggerated response is to either commensal or pathogenic bacteria (73). Studies comparing responses of fetal and adult human intestinal epithelial cells have found that there is no difference in receptor expression for these inflammatory mediators, but rather there is upregulation of NF-κB signaling secondary to decreased expression of its inhibitor IκB in immature enterocytes (73). In addition it has been shown that immune cells from the lamina propria or peripheral blood can limit proinflammatory gene expression despite induction of NF-κB signaling by bacteria (74). Thus a preterm infant with an immature immune system is at further risk for poorly regulated proinflammatory responses.

Increased NF-κB signaling leads to increased production of IL-8. IL-8 is a chemokine that stimulates migration of neutrophils from intravascular to interstitial sites and can directly activate neutrophils and regulate the expression of neutrophil adhesion molecules (75–77). Thus, by recruiting and activating immune cells, IL-8 may play an important role in inflammation. Previous studies have shown that serum IL-8 is significantly elevated in the first 24 h of severe cases of NEC (78). Surgical specimens of intestine from infants with acute NEC show up-regulation of IL-8 mRNA throughout the serosa, muscularis, and intestinal epithelium compared to those with other inflammatory conditions or those without disease (79).

Studies have also shown a differential response to bacterial toxins in immature enterocytes compared to adult enterocytes. Studies have demonstrated an increased receptor expression for cholera toxin and decreased receptor expression for shiga toxin and *C. difficile* toxin A (80–82).

In addition to differential expression, recent studies have demonstrated enhanced uptake of the toxin in immature enterocytes. Toxin is rapidly transported by endocytosis via a clathrin pathway in immature enterocytes, in contrast to decreased uptake in adult enterocytes via a caveolae/raft-mediated pathway (83). This may explain the more fulminant disease observed in young infants compared to older children. Increased endocytosis may increase capacity to uptake intact hormones and growth factors in the rapidly growing immature intestine, but if the immature intestine cannot distinguish between beneficial substances and harmful microorganisms, toxins, or antigens it is also at increased risk of harm (83)

WHAT IS THE ROLE OF BACTERIA?

Although clusters of cases of NEC have been reported, no specific organism has been linked to this disease. It is unclear whether bacteria are a primary effector of NEC or are passive participants, entering the bowel wall through a breech in the intestinal mucosal barrier. The presence of bacteria is a prerequisite for NEC, and indeed studies have shown that prophylactic antibiotics may decrease the incidence of NEC; thus antibiotics are a central aspect of NEC treatment (84). However, NEC is not believed to be an infection in the classical sense, but rather an exaggerated inflammatory response to the presence of bacteria with or without concomitant true sepsis, as only about 30% of infants with this disease have positive blood cultures.

Multiple studies have indicated that infants who develop NEC do not have unusual organisms in their GI tracts, but rather the "expected" flora (e.g. *E. Coli*, *Klebsiella, Enterococcus, Clostridium* species and coagulase-negative *Staphylococcus*) have been found in stool samples of affected infants (85–87). We know that the host has receptors that sense bacterial properties. In addition provocative studies suggest that the organisms themselves can sense the host environment and become more virulent for self-preservation in a stressed or undernourished host. Virulence in bacteria appears regulated by quorum sensing signals which regulate virulence gene expression based on bacterial number and growth. Studies in pseudomonas have indicated that the virulence-related attachment factor PA-1, which causes increased permeability of the intestinal epithelium to the cytotoxins of pseudomonas, is upregulated by surgical stress, intestinal epithelial hypoxia, and immune activation of the host. Moreover, it has been demonstrated that this virulence determinant can be induced by the apical cell supernatant of hypoxic intestinal epithelial cell monolayers, suggesting that bacteria sense a factor secreted into the milieu in contact with the bacteria that can trigger a transformation to a more virulent phenotype (88, 89). This suggests that potentially our sickest infants have the most virulent endogenous flora. This is particularly relevant because animal studies of a weanling rabbit ileal loop model demonstrated pathologic changes characteristic of NEC specifically be adherent *E. coli* strains, suggesting that patterns of adherence may influence the incidence of NEC (90).

Binding of pathogenic organisms is influenced by the underlying microbial ecology through competition for binding sites or nutrients, production of inhibiting agents, alteration in pH and synthesis of growth factors; thus the growth of competitive nonpathogenic strains of bacteria may protect the infant. Probiotics are living microorganisms in food and dietary supplements which have beneficial health effects beyond their inherent nutritive value. Ideally a probiotic should exert a beneficial effect without pathogenic or toxic side-effects, be capable of surviving and metabolizing in the gut, remain viable during storage and use, retain the ability to colonize the gut, and have well-understood properties including knowledge of its susceptibility to antibiotics. There are many commonly cited probiotics – primarily *Lactobacillus* and *Bifidobacterium*. These organisms are also components of commensal microflora. Probiotics have been shown to decrease the incidence and severity of diarrhea in children (91), and improve weight gain and feeding tolerance in preterm infants (92).

However, studies of probiotics in preterm infants have been small, and have used different organisms, in different populations, with different outcome measures. The outcome measurements have generally been clinical improvement in terms of weight gain, feeding tolerance, and incidence of infection including sepsis, urinary tract infection (UTI) and necrotizing enterocolitis. While some have documented colonization there has been little mechanistic study of effects on the intestine or inflammation that may account for the clinical effects seen. Studies have documented the ability of *Bifidobacterium breve* to colonize the intestine of preterm infants without side-effects, resulting in improved feeding tolerance and weight gain (93). This study found that early administration of this probiotic at < 24 h of birth resulted in a *Bifidobacterium*-predominant flora at an average of 2–4 weeks after birth, in contrast to the control group which did not receive the probiotic and in which the majority of the infants had no *Bifidobacterium* isolated during the entire observation period of 7 weeks (94). Similarly, studies of LGG administration have documented colonization and general safety, including no change in the amount of short chain fatty acids – acetic, propionic, and butyric acids – produced in the colon which are important in the nutrition of preterm infants (95).

Several probiotics, including *Bifidobacterium, Lactobacillus*, and *Saccharamyces boulardii*, have been studied in animal or human models of NEC (96, 97–99). Two studies, one prospective and one using historical controls, have suggested a decreased incidence of NEC with the combination of *Lactobacillus acidophilus* and *Bifidobacterium infantis* prophylactic administration (96, 98); however, with the small populations used and the low incidence of disease, it is unclear whether the conclusions are generalizable. However, an animal study using a well-accepted physiologic model of NEC in which preterm rat pups develop the disease after cold and hypoxia stress as well as formula feeding, demonstrated a significant decrease in the incidence of NEC associated with *Bifidobacterium infantis* colonization of the intestine and decreased plasma endotoxin levels (100). Studies of *Saccharamyces boulardii* in a hypoxia/deoxygenating model of NEC have also shown a decrease in the incidence of NEC (99). In contrast, a large placebo-controlled study of the effect of the administration of LGG to preterm infants did not document a significant change in the incidence of UTI, bacterial sepsis, or NEC, possibly because the incidence of each disease in both groups was low (97).

HOW CAN PROBIOTICS PROTECT AGAINST NEC?

Although the clinical studies have not been conclusive and mechanisms of action in infants are unknown, data in adult inflammatory bowel disease patients and models

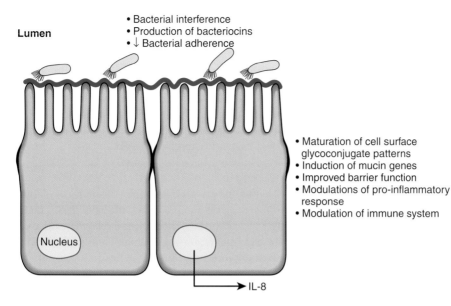

Lumen
- Bacterial interference
- Production of bacteriocins
- ↓ Bacterial adherence

- Maturation of cell surface glycoconjugate patterns
- Induction of mucin genes
- Improved barrier function
- Modulations of pro-inflammatory response
- Modulation of immune system

Nucleus

IL-8

Submucosa • Maturation of blood flow regulation

Figure 5-4 Potential beneficial effects of probiotics on the preterm intestine and NEC.

of adult colonic intestinal epithelial inflammation suggest means by which probiotics can influence the balance of inflammatory and anti-inflammatory processes in intestinal epithelial cells. Thus the benefit potential of probiotics extends beyond modulation of gut flora (Fig. 5-4).

As delineated above, specific bacteria play multiple roles in intestinal maturation, immune function, bacterial interference, and production of bacteriocins, which are substances produced by both Gram-negative and Gram-positive bacteria with a receptor-mediated antibiotic like bactericidal activity against similar organisms. Each of these factors may play a role. However, extrapolation of data from studies of inflammatory bowel disease suggests that there is evidence that probiotics may have the capacity to specifically influence aspects of the intestinal injury in NEC.

It has been hypothesized that the injury in NEC begins with a breach in the intestinal mucosal barrier leading to bacterial translocation across the epithelium, and exacerbation of the inflammatory cascade, resulting in the clinical signs of NEC. Predisposing features may be increased bacterial attachment, diminished intestinal barrier function, poor containment of pathogenic bacteria, ischemic injury to the gut mucosa, heightened inflammatory response, and lack of cytoprotective responses. Each of these features may be ameliorated by probiotics.

Adherence

While *E. coli* increases the incidence of NEC, *L. plantarum* has been shown to decrease the adherence specifically of enteropathogenic *E. coli* by increasing MUC2 and MUC3 mRNA expression (31). In addition, *L. acidophilus* has been shown to decrease cell attachment by pathogens such as enterotoxigenic *E. coli*, *Yersinia pseudotuberculosis*, *Salmonella typhimurium*, enteropathogenic *E. coli* (101).

Barrier Function and Bacterial Containment

Probiotics can improve intestinal barrier function. As previously noted, bacteria are normally involved in the maturation of the intestinal barrier; however,

Ussing chamber experiments of transport of intact proteins have demonstrated that LGG can specifically protect against increased intestinal permeability in suckling rats (102). *L. plantarum* has also been shown to protect against *E. coli*-induced intestinal permeability (103). In addition, as previously noted, bacteria have a role in the maturation of the intestinal immune system and preterm infants have an immature immune response. *E coli nissle* has been shown to induce specific and polyclonal immune responses, an important mechanism for containing bacteria which breach the intestinal mucosa (104).

Ischemic Injury

Probiotics may protect against ischemic injury. The newborn intestinal circulation must undergo changes as the neonate replaces the placenta with its GI tract as the means to obtain nutrition. During fetal life the fetal intestine is a relatively dormant organ engaged in minimal activity and thus requiring minimal blood flow and O_2 delivery. After birth, the intestine undergoes rapid growth necessitating dramatic increases in intestinal perfusion and O_2 delivery. The normal drop in vascular resistance leads to increased blood flow and oxygen delivery into the newborn intestine (105, 106).

Nitric oxide (NO) is produced by the endothelial cell isoforms of NO synthase (eNOS) during the enzymatic reduction of L-arginine. It then immediately diffuses to the vascular smooth muscle where it binds to the heme moiety of soluble guanylate cyclase, which then produces cGMP, which in turn reduces vascular smooth muscle Ca^{2+} and inactivates its contractile machinery, resulting in vasodilatation. The reduction of intestinal vascular resistance that occurs between postnatal days 1 and 3 is the consequence of increased endothelial production of the potent vasodilator NO.

Damaged endothelial cells can lead to the loss of the capacity of these cells to produce NO, leading to local intestinal ischemia and tissue damage and triggering an inflammatory response (72, 107, 108). LGG has been shown to induce NO production in intestinal epithelial cells primed by TNFα, IL-1β, and IFNγ by stimulating iNOS production by a mechanism involving NF-κB (109).

Exaggerated Inflammatory Response

As previously noted, preterm infants have an exaggerated inflammatory response associated with increased NF-κB activity. Studies in a rat model of NEC demonstrated increased NF-κB binding activity in the small intestine of the animals 0–3 h after the induction of NEC (110). This finding potentially suggests that NF-κB activation is an early step in the intestinal injury in NEC, and suggests a means by which bacteria can trigger an injury-inducing inflammatory response without causing traditional sepsis. It has been shown that the combination of probiotic organisms called VSL#3, containing a mixture of *Streptococcus*, *Lactobacillus* and *Bifidobacterium*, can decrease NF-κB activation by inhibition of the proteasome, preventing degradation of the inhibitor IκB (111). Preserving IκB may be specifically important as this is a point of developmental differentiation between immature and mature enterocytes, with immature enterocytes having less baseline expression of IκB (73). Furthermore, VSL#3 has been shown to decrease basal and LPS-stimulated TNFα secretion in the ileum of IL-10 knockout mice predisposed to inflammatory bowel disease (112). The ileum is the classic site of injury in NEC.

Cytoprotective Responses

Probiotics can increase cytoprotective mechanisms, specifically by inducing heat shock protein activation. It has been shown that VSL#3 can induce production of both hsp 25 and 72 specifically in intestinal epithelial cells, potentially leading to protection. Interestingly the same effects can be obtained using conditioned media obtained by growing the organisms in broth and then filtering the bacteria out – suggesting that the active component is a secreted factor.

Finally, probiotics have been taken beyond their role as just organisms to become tools to synthesize specific molecules. Proof of principal has been demonstrated by experiments in which *Lactococcus lactis* was designed to produce IL-10 within the gut, resulting in improvement in IBD (113). Perhaps other molecules could similarly be engineered, such as TGFβ, erythropoietin or platelet-activating factor acetylhydrolase, which have been shown to decrease inflammation in immature enterocytes and may decrease the incidence of NEC.

CONCERNS

Certainly there are concerns and issues of safety in using probiotics. First, do we really want to give live organisms to our relatively "immunocompromised" preterm patients? Cases of *Lactobacillus* sepsis have been documented and prompt caution (114). Two options for obtaining the beneficial effects of probiotics without the risks of administering live bacteria are the use of probiotic-conditioned media or the administration of prebiotics.

Interestingly some protective probiotic effects such as proteasome inhibition and hsp production can be obtained using bacteria-free probiotic-conditioned media (111). Broth containing the probiotic organisms is filtered to remove any live bacteria, leaving factors secreted by the bacteria in the resultant conditioned media. However, administering just a secreted factor may not confer all beneficial effects, such as effects on T regulatory cell function and colonization pattern imprinting.

Another option is the administration of prebiotics. Prebiotics are non-digestible food ingredients that benefit the host by selectively stimulating the growth or activity of a limited number of bacterial species already resident in the intestine. For example, lactulose is neither metabolized nor absorbed in the intestine and has been shown to decrease colonic pH by increasing production of organic acids, thus improving the environment for *Lactobacillus* and *Bifidobacteria* growth. It has been shown in IL-10 knockout animals at risk for colitis that increasing *Lactobacillus* species in the colon by prebiotics results in a concomitant decrease in levels of adherent and translocated bacteria, resulting in protection against colitis similar to results obtained by administering *Lactobacillus* directly (115). In addition, specific oligosaccharides such as fructooligosaccharide or galactooligosaccharide are thought to promote bifidobacterium (116, 117). Studies in adults have demonstrated that substitution of 15 g/day sucrose for 15 g/day oligofructose or inulin resulted in specific stimulation of *Bifidobacterium* (116). Furthermore, studies have demonstrated that feeding infants with a formula supplemented with a mixture of fructo and galactooligosaccharides as prebiotics resulted in a *Bifidobacterium* flora comparable to that of breast-fed infants (118). Lastly, a study of the effect of oligofructose supplementation in an animal model of NEC demonstrated an increase in *Bifidobacterium*, decrease in *Clostridia* species and a decrease in intestinal lesions, although not as effectively as the administration of *Bifidobacterium* itself as a probiotic agent (68). While the concept of prebiotics is intriguing as a means to support the growth of beneficial organisms in a probably cost-effective manner, without actually administering live bacteria, and thus with presumed minimal side-effects, clinical studies have not fully evaluated the efficacy of this intervention (66).

Another concern is efficacy and means of administration. In the clinical studies of the effect of probiotics on preterm infants numbers were small and populations used may or may not be generalizable. Further, no mechanism of action, dosage, or timing specifics are known. One problem is that different studies of probiotics have used different organisms. Multiple studies have shown that different organisms have different effects, and even different strains of the same organism may behave differently (47). The most specifically studied organism is *Lactobacillus GG*. One study in premature infants did show that orally administered LGG colonizes the gut of preterm infants; however, that study did not demonstrate evidence of clinical benefit (119). The previously cited study evaluating the effect of LGG on IEC apoptosis showed that other *Lactobacillus* strains (*L. acidophilus* and *L. casei*) stimulated Akt activity but did not affect TNF-stimulated p38, suggesting that different probiotic agents have different molecular effects (22). Microarray studies of intestinal epithelial cells from germ-free mice colonized with organisms including *Bacteroides thetaiotaomicron, Bifidobacterium infantis, E. coli,* or complete microflora, demonstrated bacteria-induced effects on gene expression affecting nutrient absorption, barrier function, intestinal mucus, gut motility, and toxin metabolism. However, not all bacteria affected all, or had the same effect, on all genes (26). Molecular techniques to evaluate mechanisms of action of specific probiotics and document survival and colonization of organisms after their administration will allow more specific application of probiotic therapy. Perhaps a combination of probiotics to produce a synergy of effects is best.

CONCLUSION

Appropriate colonization can lead to appropriate maturation of glycoconjugate pathways, improved barrier function, improved intestinal epithelial cell survival, competitive exclusion of pathogenic organisms, and appropriate maturation of the immune system. This may be of particular importance to the fundamentally immature preterm gut. Administration of probiotics is an intriguing option for influencing intestinal colonization. How well probiotics work, how to administer them, and safety are all issues of concern. However, there is a scientific basis to believe that influencing the microbial ecology of the preterm gut can have a significant impact on health, disease and gut development.

REFERENCES

1. Hooper LV, Bry L, Falk PG, et al. Host-microbial symbiosis in the mammalian intestine: exploring an internal ecosystem. Bioessays 1998; 20(4):336–343.
2. Bourlioux P, Koletzko B, Guarner F, et al. The intestine and its microflora are partners for the protection of the host: report on the Danone Symposium "The Intelligent Intestine", held in Paris, June 14, 2002. Am J Clin Nutr 2003; 78(4):675–683.
3. Karlsson H, Larsson P, Wold AE, et al. Pattern of cytokine responses to gram-positive and gram-negative commensal bacteria is profoundly changed when monocytes differentiate into dendritic cells. Infect Immun 2004; 72(5):2671–2678.
4. Benno Y, Sawada K, Mitsuoka T. The intestinal microflora of infants: composition of fecal flora in breast-fed and bottle-fed infants. Microbiol Immunol 1984; 28(9):975–986.
5. Orrhage K, Nord CE. Factors controlling the bacterial colonization of the intestine in breastfed infants. Acta Paediatr Suppl 1999; 88(430):47–57.
6. Neutra MR, Pringault E, Kraehenbuhl JP. Antigen sampling across epithelial barriers and induction of mucosal immune responses. Annu Rev Immunol 1996; 14:275–300.
7. Reichhart JM. TLR5 takes aim at bacterial propeller. Nat Immunol 2003; 4(12):1159–1160.
8. Medzhitov R. Toll-like receptors and innate immunity. Nat Rev Immunol 2001; 1(2):135–145.
9. Girardin SE, Tournebize R, Mavris M, et al. CARD4/Nod1 mediates NF-kappaB and JNK activation by invasive Shigella flexneri. EMBO Rep 2001; 2(8):736–742.
10. Kelsall B. Getting to the guts of NOD2. Nat Med 2005; 11(4):383–384.
11. Baeuerle PA, Henkel T. Function and activation of NF-kappa B in the immune system. Annu Rev Immunol 1994; 12:141–179.
12. Kopp EB, Ghosh S. NF-kappa B and rel proteins in innate immunity. Adv Immunol 1995; 58:1–27.
13. Ghosh S, Karin M. Missing pieces in the NF-kappaB puzzle. Cell 2002; 109:S81–S96.

14. Shanahan F. Physiological basis for novel drug therapies used to treat the inflammatory bowel diseases I. Pathophysiological basis and prospects for probiotic therapy in inflammatory bowel disease. Am J Physiol Gastrointest Liver Physiol 2005; 288(3):G417–G421.

15. Szabo SJ, Sullivan BM, Peng SL, et al. Molecular mechanisms regulating Th1 immune responses. Annu Rev Immunol 2003; 21:713–758.

16. Steinman RM, Hawiger D, Nussenzweig MC. Tolerogenic dendritic cells. Annu Rev Immunol 2003; 21:685–711.

17. Fehervari Z, Sakaguchi S. CD4+ Tregs and immune control. J Clin Invest 2004; 114(9):1209–1217.

18. Prioult G, Nagler-Anderson C. Mucosal immunity and allergic responses: lack of regulation and/or lack of microbial stimulation? Immunol Rev 2005; 206:204–218.

19. Salyers AA, West SE, Vercellotti JR, et al. Fermentation of mucins and plant polysaccharides by anaerobic bacteria from the human colon. Appl Environ Microbiol 1977; 34(5):529–533.

20. Vercellotti JR, Salyers AA, Bullard WS, et al. Breakdown of mucin and plant polysaccharides in the human colon. Can J Biochem 1977; 55(11):1190–1196.

21. Otte JM, Podolsky DK. Functional modulation of enterocytes by gram-positive and gram-negative microorganisms. Am J Physiol Gastrointest Liver Physiol 2004; 286(4):G613–G626.

22. Yan F, Polk DB. Probiotic bacterium prevents cytokine-induced apoptosis in intestinal epithelial cells. J Biol Chem 2002; 277(52):50959–50965.

23. Banasaz M, Norin E, Holma R, et al. Increased enterocyte production in gnotobiotic rats mono-associated with Lactobacillus rhamnosus GG. Appl Environ Microbiol 2002; 68(6):3031–3034.

24. Stappenbeck TS, Hooper LV, Gordon JI. Developmental regulation of intestinal angiogenesis by indigenous microbes via Paneth cells. Proc Natl Acad Sci USA 2002; 99(24):15451–15455.

25. Husebye E, Hellstrom PM, Midtvedt T. Intestinal microflora stimulates myoelectric activity of rat small intestine by promoting cyclic initiation and aboral propagation of migrating myoelectric complex. Dig Dis Sci 1994; 39(5):946–956.

26. Hooper LV, Wong MH, Thelin A, et al. Molecular analysis of commensal host-microbial relationships in the intestine. Science 2001; 291(5505):881–884.

27. Dai D, Nanthkumar NN, Newburg DS, Walker WA. Role of oligosaccharides and glycoconjugates in intestinal host defense. J Pediatr Gastroenterol Nutr 2000; 30(Supp. 2):S23–S33.

28. Chu SH, Walker WA. Developmental changes in the activities of sialyl- and fucosyltransferases in rat small intestine. Biochim Biophys Acta 1986; 883(3):496–500.

29. Nanthakumar NN, Dai D, Newburg DS, Walker WA. The role of indigenous microflora in the development of murine intestinal fucosyl- and sialyltransferases. Faseb J 2003; 17(1):44–46.

30. Snyder JD, Walker WA. Structure and function of intestinal mucin: developmental aspects. Int Arch Allergy Appl Immunol 1987; 82(3–4):351–356.

31. Mack DR, Michail S, Wei S, et al. Probiotics inhibit enteropathogenic E. coli adherence in vitro by inducing intestinal mucin gene expression. Am J Physiol 1999; 276(4 Pt 1):G941–G950.

32. Garcia-Lafuente A, Antolin M, Guarner F, et al. Modulation of colonic barrier function by the composition of the commensal flora in the rat. Gut 2001; 48(4):503–507.

33. Urao M, Fujimoto T, Lane GJ, et al. Does probiotics administration decrease serum endotoxin levels in infants? J Pediatr Surg 1999; 34(2):273–276.

34. Mazmanian SK, Liu CH, Tzianabos AO, et al. An immunomodulatory molecule of symbiotic bacteria directs maturation of the host immune system. Cell 2005; 122(1):107–118.

35. Cong Y, Weaver CT, Lazenby A, et al. Bacterial-reactive T regulatory cells inhibit pathogenic immune responses to the enteric flora. J Immunol 2002; 169(11):6112–6119.

36. Sudo N, Sawamura S, Tanaka K, et al. The requirement of intestinal bacterial flora for the development of an IgE production system fully susceptible to oral tolerance induction. J Immunol 1997; 159(4):1739–1745.

37. Gronlund MM, Arvilommi H, Kero P, et al. Importance of intestinal colonisation in the maturation of humoral immunity in early infancy: a prospective follow up study of healthy infants aged 0–6 months. Arch Dis Child Fetal Neonatal Ed 2000; 83(3):F186–F192.

38. Savilahti E. Immunoglobulin-containing cells in the intestinal mucosa and immunoglobulins in the intestinal juice in children. Clin Exp Immunol 1972; 11(3):415–425.

39. Burgio GR, Lanzavecchia A, Plebani A, et al. Ontogeny of secretory immunity: levels of secretory IgA and natural antibodies in saliva. Pediatr Res 1980; 14(10):1111–1114.

40. Wills-Karp M, Santeliz J, Karp CL. The germless theory of allergic disease: revisiting the hygiene hypothesis. Nat Rev Immunol 2001; 1(1):69–75.

41. Smits HH, van Beelen AJ, Hessle C, et al. Commensal Gram-negative bacteria prime human dendritic cells for enhanced IL-23 and IL-27 expression and enhanced Th1 development. Eur J Immunol 2004; 34(5):1371–1380.

42. Strachan DP. Family size, infection and atopy: the first decade of the "hygiene hypothesis." Thorax 2000; 55(Supp. 1):S2–S10.

43. Strachan DP. Hay fever, hygiene, and household size. BMJ 1989; 299(6710):1259–1260.

44. Braun-Fahrlander C, Riedler J, Herz U, et al. Environmental exposure to endotoxin and its relation to asthma in school-age children. N Engl J Med 2002; 347(12):869–877.

45. Bach JF. The effect of infections on susceptibility to autoimmune and allergic diseases. N Engl J Med 2002; 347(12):911–920.

46. Noverr MC, Huffnagle GB. Does the microbiota regulate immune responses outside the gut? Trends Microbiol 2004; 12(12):562–568.

47. Christensen HR, Frokiaer H, Pestka JJ. Lactobacilli differentially modulate expression of cytokines and maturation surface markers in murine dendritic cells. J Immunol 2002; 168(1):171–178.

48. Kalliomaki M, Kirjavainen P, Eerola E, et al. Distinct patterns of neonatal gut microflora in infants in whom atopy was and was not developing. J Allergy Clin Immunol 2001; 107(1):129–134.

49. Sudo N, Yu XN, Aiba Y, et al. An oral introduction of intestinal bacteria prevents the development of a long-term Th2-skewed immunological memory induced by neonatal antibiotic treatment in mice. Clin Exp Allergy 2002; 32(7):1112–1116.

50. Kalliomaki M, Salminen S, Arvilommi H, et al. Probiotics in primary prevention of atopic disease: a randomised placebo-controlled trial. Lancet 2001; 357(9262):1076–1079.

51. Majamaa H, Isolauri E. Probiotics: a novel approach in the management of food allergy. J Allergy Clin Immunol 1997; 99(2):179–185.

52. Lodinova-Zadnikova R, Cukrowska B, Tlaskalova-Hogenova H. Oral administration of probiotic Escherichia coli after birth reduces frequency of allergies and repeated infections later in life (after 10 and 20 years). Int Arch Allergy Immunol 2003; 131(3):209–211.

53. Rook GA, Brunet LR. Microbes, immunoregulation, and the gut. Gut 2005; 54(3):317–320.

54. Neish AS, Gewirtz AT, Zeng H, et al. Prokaryotic regulation of epithelial responses by inhibition of IkappaB-alpha ubiquitination. Science 2000; 289(5484):1560–1563.

55. Kelly D, Campbell JI, King TP, et al. Commensal anaerobic gut bacteria attenuate inflammation by regulating nuclear-cytoplasmic shuttling of PPAR-gamma and RelA. Nat Immunol 2004; 5(1):104–112.

56. Rakoff-Nahoum S, Paglino J, Eslami-Varzaneh F, et al. Recognition of commensal microflora by toll-like receptors is required for intestinal homeostasis. Cell 2004; 118(2):229–241.

57. Otte JM, Cario E, Podolsky DK. Mechanisms of cross hyporesponsiveness to Toll-like receptor bacterial ligands in intestinal epithelial cells. Gastroenterology 2004; 126(4):1054–1070.

58. Arvans DL, Vavricka SR, Ren H, et al. Luminal bacterial flora determines physiological expression of intestinal epithelial cytoprotective heat shock proteins 25 and 72. Am J Physiol Gastrointest Liver Physiol 2005; 288(4):G696–G704.

59. Gronlund MM, Lehtonen OP, Eerola E, et al. Fecal microflora in healthy infants born by different methods of delivery: permanent changes in intestinal flora after cesarean delivery. J Pediatr Gastroenterol Nutr 1999; 28(1):19–25.

60. Harmsen HJ, Wildeboer-Veloo AC, Raangs GC, et al. Analysis of intestinal flora development in breast-fed and formula-fed infants by using molecular identification and detection methods. J Pediatr Gastroenterol Nutr 2000; 30(1):61–67.

61. Gewolb IH, Schwalbe RS, Taciak VL, et al. Stool microflora in extremely low birthweight infants. Arch Dis Child Fetal Neonatal Ed 1999; 80(3):F167–F173.

62. Rubaltelli FF, Biadaioli R, Pecile P, et al. Intestinal flora in breast- and bottle-fed infants. J Perinat Med 1998; 26(3):186–191.

63. Tomkins AM, Bradley AK, Oswald S, et al. Diet and the faecal microflora of infants, children and adults in rural Nigeria and urban U.K. J Hyg (Lond) 1981; 86(3):285–293.

64. Wold AE, Adlerberth I. Breast feeding and the intestinal microflora of the infant—implications for protection against infectious diseases. Adv Exp Med Biol 2000; 478:77–93.

65. Ogawa K, Ben RA, Pons S, et al. Volatile fatty acids, lactic acid, and pH in the stools of breast-fed and bottle-fed infants. J Pediatr Gastroenterol Nutr 1992; 15(3):248–252.

66. Collins MD, Gibson GR. Probiotics, prebiotics, and synbiotics: approaches for modulating the microbial ecology of the gut. Am J Clin Nutr 1999; 69(5):1052S–1057S.

67. Kosloske AM. Epidemiology of necrotizing enterocolitis. Acta Paediatr Suppl 1994; 396:2–7.

68. Butel MJ, Waligora-Dupriet AJ, Szylit O. Oligofructose and experimental model of neonatal necrotising enterocolitis. Br J Nutr 2002; 87(Suppl. 2):S213–S219.

69. Bonnemaison E, Lanotte P, Cantagrel S, et al. Comparison of fecal flora following administration of two antibiotic protocols for suspected maternofetal infection. Biol Neonate 2003; 84(4):304–310.

70. Claud EC, Walker WA. Hypothesis: inappropriate colonization of the premature intestine can cause neonatal necrotizing enterocolitis. Faseb J 2001; 15(8):1398–1403.

71. Claud EC, Savidge T, Walker WA. Modulation of human intestinal epithelial cell IL-8 secretion by human milk factors. Pediatr Res 2003; 53(3):419–425.

72. Nanthakumar NN, Fusunyan RD, Sanderson I, Walker WA. Inflammation in the developing human intestine: A possible pathophysiologic contribution to necrotizing enterocolitis. Proc Natl Acad Sci USA 2000; 97(11):6043–6048.

73. Claud EC, Lu L, Anton PM, et al. Developmentally regulated IkappaB expression in intestinal epithelium and susceptibility to flagellin-induced inflammation. Proc Natl Acad Sci USA 2004; 101(19):7404–7408.

74. Haller D, Holt L, Parlesak A, et al. Differential effect of immune cells on non-pathogenic Gram-negative bacteria-induced nuclear factor-kappaB activation and pro-inflammatory gene expression in intestinal epithelial cells. Immunology 2004; 112(2):310–320.

75. Baggiolini M, Walz A, Kunkel SL. Neutrophil-activating peptide-1/interleukin 8, a novel cytokine that activates neutrophils. J Clin Invest 1989; 84(4):1045–1049.

76. Djeu JY, Matsushima K, Oppenheim JJ, et al. Functional activation of human neutrophils by recombinant monocyte-derived neutrophil chemotactic factor/IL-8. J Immunol 1990; 144(6):2205–2210.

77. Huber AR, Kunkel SL, Todd RF 3rd, et al. Regulation of transendothelial neutrophil migration by endogenous interleukin-8. Science 1991; 254(5028):99–102.

78. Edelson MB, Bagwell CE, Rozycki HJ. Circulating pro- and counterinflammatory cytokine levels and severity in necrotizing enterocolitis. Pediatrics 1999; 103(4 Pt 1):766–771.

79. Nadler EP, Stanford A, Zhang XR, et al. Intestinal cytokine gene expression in infants with acute necrotizing enterocolitis: interleukin-11 mRNA expression inversely correlates with extent of disease. J Pediatr Surg 2001; 36(8):1122–1129.

80. Mobassaleh M, Gross SK, McCluer RH, et al. Quantitation of the rabbit intestinal glycolipid receptor for Shiga toxin. Further evidence for the developmental regulation of globotriaosylceramide in microvillus membranes. Gastroenterology 1989; 97(2):384–391.

81. Isberg RR, Leong JM. Multiple beta 1 chain integrins are receptors for invasin, a protein that promotes bacterial penetration into mammalian cells. Cell 1990; 60(5):861–871.

82. Cohen MB, Guarino A, Shukla R, et al. Age-related differences in receptors for Escherichia coli heat-stable enterotoxin in the small and large intestine of children. Gastroenterology 1988; 94(2):367–373.

83. Lu L, Khan S, Lencer W, Walker WA. Endocytosis of cholera toxin by human enterocytes is developmentally regulated. Am J Physiol Gastrointest Liver Physiol 2005; 289(2):G332–G341.

84. Krediet TG, van Lelyveld N, Vijlbrief DC, et al. Microbiological factors associated with neonatal necrotizing enterocolitis: protective effect of early antibiotic treatment. Acta Paediatr 2003; 92(10):1180–1182.

85. Ballance WA, Dahms BB, Shenker N, et al. Pathology of neonatal necrotizing enterocolitis: a ten-year experience. J Pediatr 1990; 117(1 Pt 2):S6–S13.

86. Duffy LC, Zielezny MA, Carrion V, et al. Bacterial toxins and enteral feeding of premature infants at risk for necrotizing enterocolitis. Adv Exp Med Biol 2001; 501:519–527.

87. Hoy C, Millar MR, MacKay P, et al. Quantitative changes in faecal microflora preceding necrotising enterocolitis in premature neonates. Arch Dis Child 1990; 65(10 Spec No):1057–1059.

88. Kohler JE, Zaborina O, Wu L, et al. Components of intestinal epithelial hypoxia activate the virulence circuitry of Pseudomonas. Am J Physiol Gastrointest Liver Physiol 2005; 288(5):G1048–G1054.

89. Wu L, Estrada O, Zaborina O, et al. Recognition of host immune activation by Pseudomonas aeruginosa. Science 2005; 309(5735):774–777.

90. Panigrahi P, Gupta S, Gewolb IH, et al. Occurrence of necrotizing enterocolitis may be dependent on patterns of bacterial adherence and intestinal colonization: studies in Caco-2 tissue culture and weanling rabbit models. Pediatr Res 1994; 36(1 Pt 1):115–121.

91. Isolauri E, Juntunen M, Rautanen T, et al. A human Lactobacillus strain (Lactobacillus casei sp strain GG) promotes recovery from acute diarrhea in children. Pediatrics 1991; 88(1):90–97.

92. Robinson EL, Thompson WL. Effect on weight gain of the addition of Lactobacillus acidophilus to the formula of newborn infants. J Pediatr 1952; 41(4):395–398.

93. Kitajima H, Sumida Y, Tanaka R, et al. Early administration of Bifidobacterium breve to preterm infants: randomised controlled trial. Arch Dis Child Fetal Neonatal Ed 1997; 76(2):F101–F107.

94. Li Y, Shimizu T, Hosaka A, et al. Effects of bifidobacterium breve supplementation on intestinal flora of low birth weight infants. Pediatr Int 2004; 46(5):509–515.

95. Stansbridge EM, Walker V, Hall MA, et al. Effects of feeding premature infants with Lactobacillus GG on gut fermentation. Arch Dis Child 1993; 69(5 Spec No):488–492.

96. Hoyos AB. Reduced incidence of necrotizing enterocolitis associated with enteral administration of Lactobacillus acidophilus and Bifidobacterium infantis to neonates in an intensive care unit. Int J Infect Dis 1999; 3(4):197–202.

97. Dani C, Biadaioli R, Bertini G, et al. Probiotics feeding in prevention of urinary tract infection, bacterial sepsis and necrotizing enterocolitis in preterm infants. A prospective double-blind study. Biol Neonate 2002; 82(2):103–108.

98. Lin HC, Su BH, Chen AC, et al. Oral probiotics reduce the incidence and severity of necrotizing enterocolitis in very low birth weight infants. Pediatrics 2005; 115(1):1–4.

99. Akisu M, Baka M, Yalaz M, et al. Supplementation with Saccharomyces boulardii ameliorates hypoxia/reoxygenation-induced necrotizing enterocolitis in young mice. Eur J Pediatr Surg 2003; 13(5):319–323.

100. Caplan MS, Miller-Catchpole R, Kaup S, et al. Bifidobacterial supplementation reduces the incidence of necrotizing enterocolitis in a neonatal rat model. Gastroenterology 1999; 117(3):577–583.

101. Bernet MF, Brassart D, Neeser JR, et al. Lactobacillus acidophilus LA 1 binds to cultured human intestinal cell lines and inhibits cell attachment and cell invasion by enterovirulent bacteria. Gut 1994; 35(4):483–489.

102. Isolauri E, Majamaa H, Arvola T, et al. Lactobacillus casei strain GG reverses increased intestinal permeability induced by cow milk in suckling rats. Gastroenterology 1993; 105(6):1643–1650.

103. Mangell P, Nejdfors P, Wang M, et al. Lactobacillus plantarum 299v inhibits Escherichia coli-induced intestinal permeability. Dig Dis Sci 2002; 47(3):511–516.

104. Cukrowska B, LodInova-ZadnIkova R, Enders C, et al. Specific proliferative and antibody responses of premature infants to intestinal colonization with nonpathogenic probiotic E. coli strain Nissle 1917. Scand J Immunol 2002; 55(2):204–209.

105. Reber KM, Mager GM, Miller CE, et al. Relationship between flow rate and NO production in postnatal mesenteric arteries. Am J Physiol Gastrointest Liver Physiol 2001; 280(1):G43–G50.

106. Reber KM, Nankervis CA, Nowicki PT. Newborn intestinal circulation. Physiology and pathophysiology. Clin Perinatol 2002; 29(1):23–39.

107. Dvorak B, Halpern MD, Holubec H, et al. Epidermal growth factor reduces the development of necrotizing enterocolitis in a neonatal rat model. Am J Physiol Gastrointest Liver Physiol 2002; 282(1):G156–G164.

108. Caplan MS, Sun XM, Hseuh W, et al. Role of platelet activating factor and tumor necrosis factor-alpha in neonatal necrotizing enterocolitis. J Pediatr 1990; 116(6):960–964.

109. Korhonen R, Korpela R, Saxelin M, et al. Induction of nitric oxide synthesis by probiotic Lactobacillus rhamnosus GG in J774 macrophages and human T84 intestinal epithelial cells. Inflammation 2001; 25(4):223–232.

110. Chung DH, Ethridge RT, Kim S, et al. Molecular mechanisms contributing to necrotizing entero-colitis. Ann Surg 2001; 233(6):835–842.

111. Petrof EO, Kojima K, Ropeleski MJ, et al. Probiotics inhibit nuclear factor-kappaB and induce heat shock proteins in colonic epithelial cells through proteasome inhibition. Gastroenterology 2004; 127(5):1474–1487.

112. Madsen K, Cornish A, Soper P, et al. Probiotic bacteria enhance murine and human intestinal epithelial barrier function. Gastroenterology 2001; 121(3):580–591.

113. Steidler L, Hans W, Schotte L, et al. Treatment of murine colitis by Lactococcus lactis secreting interleukin-10. Science 2000; 289(5483):1352–1355.

114. Land MH, Rouster-Stevens K, Woods CR, et al. Lactobacillus sepsis associated with probiotic therapy. Pediatrics 2005; 115(1):178–181.

115. Madsen KL, Doyle JS, Jewell LD, et al. Lactobacillus species prevents colitis in interleukin 10 gene-deficient mice. Gastroenterology 1999; 116(5):1107–1114.

116. Gibson GR, Beatty ER, Wang X, Cummings JH. Selective stimulation of bifidobacteria in the human colon by oligofructose and inulin. Gastroenterology 1995; 108(4):975–982.

117. Rowland IR, Tanaka R. The effects of transgalactosylated oligosaccharides on gut flora metabolism in rats associated with a human faecal microflora. J Appl Bacteriol 1993; 74(6):667–674.

118. Rinne MM, Gueimonde M, Kalliomaki M, et al. Similar bifidogenic effects of prebiotic-supplemented partially hydrolyzed infant formula and breastfeeding on infant gut microbiota. FEMS Immunol Med Microbiol 2005; 43(1):59–65.

119. Millar MR, Bacon C, Smith SL, et al. Enteral feeding of premature infants with Lactobacillus GG. Arch Dis Child 1993; 69(5 Spec No):483–487.

Chapter 6

Intestinal Barrier Function: Implications for the Neonate and Beyond

Ricardo A. Caicedo, MD • Martha Douglas-Escobar, MD
• Nan Li, MD • Josef Neu, MD

The intestine serves a barrier function that is a critical component of the innate immune system (1, 2). A single layer of epithelial cells separates the luminal contents containing a myriad of microorganisms and food antigens from effector immune cells in the lamina propria and the internal milieu of the body. Breaching this single layer of cells can lead to pathologic stimulation of the mucosal immune system. Breakdown of the barrier is implicated in the pathogenesis of acute illnesses such as bacterial translocation leading to sepsis and multiple organ system failure (33). It also has been implicated in several diseases having their origins during infancy that manifest in later life. These include inflammatory bowel disease and celiac disease, as well as extraintestinal disorders such as type 1 diabetes and atopy. This chapter will provide an overview of the structure and function of one important component of the intestinal barrier, the intestinal epithelial tight junction (TJ), and how breakdown of this structure (leading to the so-called "leaky gut") may play a role in the pathogenesis of neonatal as well as pediatric diseases. We also point to areas wherein a better basic understanding of this structure might lead to prevention or treatment of neonatal pathology related to the "leaky gut" using nutritional or other means.

TIGHT JUNCTION STRUCTURE AND COMPOSITION

The gastrointestinal epithelium forms a barrier that separates the inner milieu of the body from the potentially harsh environment of the intestinal lumen. The plasma membrane of the intestinal epithelial cell serves as barrier to most hydrophilic solutes, but the interepithelial paracellular space is partially sealed and forms an intact epithelial barrier. Intestinal epithelial cells adhere to each other through junctional complexes, which are located at the lateral membranes. The interepithelial junction comprises three major components that have occlusive properties: tight junctions (TJ), adherens junctions (AJ) and desmosomes (Fig. 6-1).

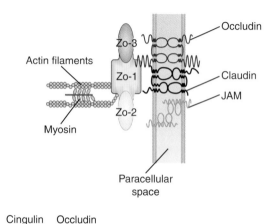

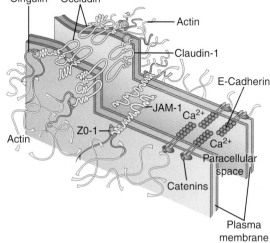

Figure 6-1 Tight junction proteins.

The TJ, sometimes also referred to as the zonula occludens (ZO), represent the major barrier within the paracellular pathway between intestinal epithelial cells (4). TJ appear as close cell-to-cell contacts by electron microphotograph (Fig. 6-2) and the contacts correspond to continuous rows of transmembrane protein particles by freeze fracture electronic microphotograph. TJ complex consists of integral proteins or "gatekeepers", plaque proteins that anchor the complex to actin cytoskeleton, and cytosolic and nuclear proteins that regulate transcription (and therefore paracellular solute permeability, cell proliferation, cell polarity and tumor suppression: see Table 6-1). This degree of complexity of the TJ complex correlates with its barrier function (5).

Multiple TJ integral proteins have been identified (Fig. 6-1): occludin and members of the claudins family, a group of at least 20 tissue-specific proteins, are the major sealing proteins (5). The claudins, a family of integral TJ proteins, form ion-selective pores within the TJ strands, whereas occludin and junctional adhesion molecule (JAM) may have an adhesive and/or signal transducing function as they interact with various cytosolic complexes (6). A third, junctional adhesion molecule (JAM) also appears to play a role, but is not as well delineated (4). Occludin was once thought to be the major protein contributing to TJ function. However, studies of occludin gene deletion mice demonstrated that they do not lose their intercellular structural morphology, and the barrier function of the intestine is not affected when examined electrophysiologically, despite growth failure and other phenotypic abnormalities (7). In the intestinal epithelium claudin-1 may directly associate with occludin laterally in the membrane within the same cell but not intercellularly (4). The combination of these two proteins functioning together

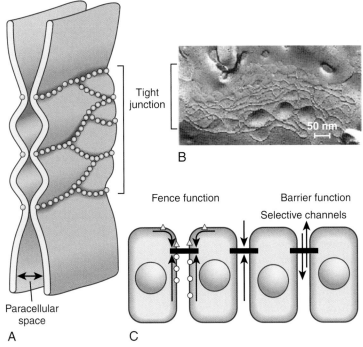

Figure 6-2 Schematic of TJ function, with freeze-fracture replica. From Sawada N, et al. Med Electron Microsc 2003; 36:147–156.

performs the major "gatekeeper" or barrier function of the tight junction. These sealing proteins, both transmembrane proteins, interact with cytoplasmic plaques that consist of different types of cytosolic proteins that function as adaptors between the TJ proteins and actin and myosin contractile elements within the cell. Acting together, they open and close the paracellular junctions (8).

TJ FUNCTION

The transcellular and the paracellular are two pathways through which substances cross epithelial membranes. The transcellular pathway allows molecules to enter from the luminal side of the enterocytes by endocytosis and exit on the serosal side. Here we will focus on the paracellular pathway, which is controlled primarily by the TJ, dynamic structures that readily adapt to a variety of developmental, physiological, and pathological circumstances. At the molecular level, TJ assume several major functions, two of which will be briefly mentioned here: the "barrier" and "fence" functions (Fig. 6-2).

Table 6-1 **Tight Junction Complex**		
TJ components	**Function**	**Examples**
Integral proteins	Modulate permeability	Occludin, claudins, JAM-1
Plaque proteins	Anchor the complex	Zonula occludens proteins (ZO-1, ZO-2, ZO-3), transmembrane associated guanylyl kinase inverted proteins (MAGI-1, MAGI-2, MAGI-3), multi PDZ domain proteins, etc.
Cytosolic and nuclear proteins	Coordinate paracellular solute permeability, cell proliferation, cell polarity and tumor suppression	Regulatory proteins, tumor suppressors, transcriptional and posttranscriptional factors

Barrier function refers primarily to the ability to selectively allow particles and solutes to pass through the intercellular space. This can be measured using transepithelial electric resistance (TER) of a monolayer of cells in culture or placing particles of different size and/or electrical charge on one side of the membrane and measuring the appearance on the other side. The latter measurements can be done in vitro or in vivo. The relationship between the number of TJ strands and TER is not a linear but a logarithmic one (9).

The *fence* function of the TJ maintains polarity of the cell. Heteropolymers of transmembrane proteins (primarily occludin, claudins and JAM) make up TJ strands, which encircle the top of epithelium to delineate the border between the apical and basolateral membrane. There are major differences in the composition of lipids and proteins that constitute the apical and basolateral surface of intestinal epithelial cells, and TJ impede the lateral diffusion of lipids and proteins between the apical and basolateral membrane (10), thus maintaining cell polarity. In other words, TJ prevent intermixing of molecules in the apical membrane with those in the lateral membrane.

TJ can adjust their integrity in response to physiological demands by adjusting their degree of phosphorylation. Sodium-glucose co-transport induces phosphorylation of myosin light chains in actin-myosin microfilaments surrounding the TJ, which contract and open the junctions, leading to increased permeability (11).

FACTORS AFFECTING TJ THAT ARE RELEVANT TO NEONATOLOGY

Intestinal Maturity

Pathology of the immature intestine, particularly necrotizing enterocolitis (NEC; discussed at length below), has been linked with barrier dysfunction. The levels of enteropathogen overgrowth reported in preterm neonates with NEC suggest an increased transmucosal passage of bacteria (12). In an early study, infants born before 34 weeks gestation had greater intestinal permeability to lactulose than more mature babies, while those of 34–37 weeks achieved a "mature" intestinal permeability to lactulose within 4 days of starting oral feeds (13). In neonates < 28 weeks, intestinal permeability at day 7 was higher and carrier-mediated monosaccharide absorption at day 14 was lower as compared with neonates of 28 weeks. The barrier function of the intestinal epithelium transiently decreases during the first week after birth in preterm neonates who are not enterally fed (14). However, a recent study concluded that in infants of 26–36 weeks, gut permeability is not related to gestational age or birth weight but is higher during the first 2 days of life than 3–6 days later.

Nutrition

In malnourished hospitalized patients, a significant increase in intestinal permeability is seen in association with phenotypic and molecular evidence of activation of lamina propria mononuclear cells and enterocytes (15). Undernutrition leads to villous atrophy, with rapid recovery of mucosal barrier function when the intestine is re-nourished. This is also the case when there is a lack of enteral nutrition. Despite being a beneficial therapy in many clinical settings, particularly the NICU, total parenteral nutrition (TPN) is the deprivation of enteral nutrition and is associated with intestinal changes in structure and function. Animal studies have demonstrated TPN-induced increases in bacterial translocation and intestinal permeability. In rats receiving TPN, loss of mucosal barrier function to both *E. coli* and the permeability marker phenol red was greater than in enterally fed rats (16).

TPN administration in newborn piglets led to mucosal atrophy and increased paracellular permeability and decreased intraepithelial lymphocytes (IELs), but bacterial translocation was not different between the two groups (17). Intestinal permeability was significantly reduced in TPN-dependent rats receiving an enteral low-residue diet (18).

In critically ill adult patients, TPN failed to improve urinary lactulose:mannitol ratios, markers of paracellular permeability, while enteral nutrition led to recovery of barrier function (19). In a study of preterm infants, early enteral feeding was associated with a reduction in gut permeability at 10 days of age, while feeding of human milk (vs. formula) was associated with decreased permeability at 28 days, and continuous vs. bolus feeding did not affect permeability (20). Because of feeding intolerance and the fear of NEC, very low birth weight (VLBW) neonates typically undergo a period of "luminal starvation", during which time they receive very little food via the gastrointestinal tract. The parenteral route supplies most of their nutrition. Long-term TPN has been associated with breakdown of the mucosal barrier and places VLBW infants at very high risk for mucosal atrophy-related pathology (21).

Individual Nutrients

VLBW infants and other highly stressed patients are frequently deprived of glutamine, a conditionally essential amino acid that has been demonstrated to improve intestinal barrier function (22). Glutamine plays a central role in numerous metabolic processes. In Caco-2 cells, a cell culture line widely used as a model of mature enterocytes, glutamine helps recovery from stress-induced increased permeability (23). Animal models and human patients have been shown to benefit from enteral or parenteral glutamine supplementation, which attenuates mucosal atrophy and decreases bacterial translocation, sepsis, and even mortality (24).

Both the ω-3 fatty acids eicosapentaenoic acid (EPA, C20) and gamma linolenic acid (C18) are known to be anti-inflammatory, and both have been show to up-regulate TJ function by increasing occludin in human vascular endothelial cell lines (25). However, EPA enhanced fluorescein sulfonic acid permeability and lowered transepithelial electrical resistance (TER) in Caco-2 cells (26). The reasons for differences in permeability depending on cell type are not understood.

Butyrate, a short-chain fatty acid, also is able to enhance restoration of mucosal barrier function after thermal and detergent injury to the rat distal colon in vitro (27). In Caco-2 cells, butyrate increases TER in a concentration-dependent manner. The mechanism may be through promotion of TJ protein synthesis, or through activation of lipooxygenase by histone acetylation of DNA (28). In HT29 colonocytes, butyrate significantly reduces paracellular permeability, probably through activation of peroxisome proliferator-activated receptor gamma (29).

Physiologic Stress

In severely stressed, critically ill patients, intestinal permeability is closely related to the presence of mucosal ischemia (30). Intestinal leakiness is triggered by a set of changes such as oxidative stress with increased production of nitric oxide and other reactive oxygen species, release of proinflammatory cytokines, reduction of intramucosal pH, and hypoxia. Potent oxidants damage cellular DNA and promote the peroxidation of lipid membranes and the down-regulation of the expression of several key TJ proteins of the ileum and colon (31). Critically ill neonates are subject to multiple physiologic stressors, including feeding restriction, ischemic injury of the intestinal mucosa, hemorrhagic shock, and systemic inflammatory response syndrome (SIRS, discussed below). All of these conditions are linked to excess production of oxidative free radicals.

Enteric Microbes

Interaction between intestinal epithelia and enteric microorganisms involves a complex and dynamic "cross talk". Commensal microbes maintain appropriate mucosal immune responses to both injury and pathogenic microbes. Enteric pathogens can disrupt the TJ of epithelial cells through a number of different virulence factors. Enteropathogenic *Escherichia coli* (EPEC) dissociates occludin from the TJ and promotes phosphorylation of the 20-kDa myosin light chain (MLC20), inducing cytoskeletal contraction and a large permeability increase (32). In a mouse model, EPEC significantly decreases barrier function in the ileum and colon through redistribution of occluding (33). The protozoan *Giardia lamblia* similarly uses myosin light chain kinase (MLCK) to disrupt TJ function (34). *Clostridium difficile* toxins cause disorganization of apical and basal filamentous (F-) actin and dissociation of occludin, ZO-1 and ZO-2 from the lateral TJ membrane in cultured intestinal epithelial cells (35). Rotavirus, the most common cause of infantile gastroenteritis worldwide, and the opportunistic protozoan *Cryptosporidium parvum* have both been shown to induce a rapid increase in gut permeability in the acute phase, with recovery of barrier function within 20 days (36). In polarized epithelial cells, rotavirus results in a paracellular leak and F-actin alteration (37). The NSP4 protein of rotavirus induces decreased TER, redistributes F-actin, and prevents lateral targeting of the TJ-associated ZO-1 protein (38). *Vibrio cholerae*, a diarrheagenic microbe, elaborates zonula occludens toxin (ZOT), which induces a redistribution of the F-actin cytoskeleton, correlating with increased mucosal permeability (39).

Cytokines

Cytokines and chemokines are soluble factors that mediate the inflammatory response by stimulating or activating lymphocytes and other immune cells. Interferon-gamma and tumor necrosis factor alpha are found in high concentrations in intestinal mucosa affected with inflammatory bowel disease (discussed below). These cytokines increase permeability of enterocyte culture monolayers (decrease the TER), also through activation of MLCK (40).

Pharmacologic Stress

One of the most commonly used drugs in the neonatal intensive care unit is the nonsteroidal anti-inflammatory agent indomethacin, primarily used for medical closure of the ductus arteriosus, but several studies associated its use with gastrointestinal perforations. Furthermore, the prostaglandin pathway, which is inhibited by indomethacin, has been linked with a major mechanism (the PI3 kinase pathway) related to control of TJ proteins. Prostaglandins stimulate recovery of decreased paracellular resistance caused by calcium depletion via a mechanism involving transepithelial osmotic gradients and PI3 kinase-dependent restoration of tight junction protein distribution (36). The short- and long-term effects of indomethacin on intestinal barrier function are yet to be determined.

ALTERED INTESTINAL PERMEABILITY IN NEONATAL AND PEDIATRIC DISEASES

In addition to neonatal necrotizing enterocolitis, the leaky gut phenomenon has been implicated in the pathogenesis of a variety of diseases that present later in childhood, many of them chronic. The association between barrier breakdown and disease was first recognized in the critical care setting, in patients with multi-organ dysfunction (41). A compromised intestinal epithelium, due to the combined effects of a genetic defect and stress or trauma, allows translocation of bacteria and antigens to the lamina propria, triggering an inappropriate or pathogenic immune response (1). The resultant disorder may be limited to the gastrointestinal tract, as with infectious enteritis, but often will have extraintestinal manifestations, as in celiac disease and atopic conditions. In many cases, barrier dysfunction is postulated as a cause of disease, but there is evidence suggesting that it may also, or even only, be a result of the disease process. Some of the more common pediatric conditions associated with altered intestinal permeability are discussed individually below.

Necrotizing Enterocolitis

Necrotizing enterocolitis (NEC), discussed in greater detail in another chapter of this volume, is one of the most feared diseases in the neonatal intensive care unit because it can progress rapidly from mild abdominal distension and feeding intolerance to fulminant septic shock, necrosis of the entire intestine and death. Its incidence is estimated to be 0.3–2.4 cases/1000 births, but it is 4–13% in neonates less than 1500 g of birth weight (42). Of 2500 annual cases reported in the USA, 20–60% would require surgery (43) and the mortality remains high (20–28%). The primary risk factor for NEC is prematurity, as the incidence varies inversely with gestational age. Approximately 90% of cases occur in premature infants and NEC is rarely seen in older infants and children. Some of the NEC-predisposing factors in premature infants include: incomplete innervation and poor motility of the premature gastrointestinal tract, stasis and bacterial overgrowth, low levels of protective mucus and secretory IgA, decreased regenerative mucosal capabilities, and increased intestinal permeability.

Animal models and clinical observations suggest that NEC requires at least three factors to develop: mucosal injury, formula feeding and the presence of bacteria (44). The common pathway leads to an inflammatory response and ischemia-necrosis.

Intestinal bacteria and/or their toxic products may translocate across a compromised epithelial barrier, activating mucosal immune responses. Gram-negative rods (E. coli, Klebsiella, Enterobacter and Pseudomonas) are common pathogens associated with NEC.

Figure 6-3 shows some of the measures that might be used to prevent NEC. The safest and most efficacious practices in the prevention of NEC include maternal breast-feeding, judicious advancement of enteral feedings and careful infection-control measures. Maternal breast milk may benefit the mucosal integrity by adding protective factors such as immunoglobulin, lysozyme, lactoferrin, macrophages, lymphocytes, neutrophils, gut maturation factors, glutamine, PAF acetylhydrolase and prostaglandin E1 (a splacnic vasodilator). Initiation of trophic feeds in very low weight infants and avoidance of high osmolar solutions reduced the incidence of NEC (45, 46).

To avoid unbalanced inflammatory responses in the GI, it is critical to maintain the commensal microbiota (avoiding the pathologic colonization). Use of probiotics may protect against NEC by different mechanisms (47): immune modulation, down-regulation of inflammatory responses, and regulation of intestinal permeability, increased mucin production, secretion of antimicrobial substances, inhibition of pathogens' mucosal adherence and stimulation of IgA production.

Systemic Inflammatory Response Syndrome (SIRS)

Severely stressed neonates with sepsis, trauma, and/or NEC are disposed to the development of systemic inflammatory response syndrome (SIRS), which may

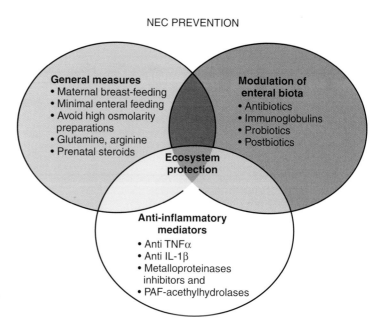

Figure 6-3 Measures for prevention of NEC.

lead to multi-organ dysfunction. SIRS may be regarded as the uncontrolled systemic expression of pro-inflammatory cytokines. A "leaky gut" can promote bacterial translocation, a phenomenon in which live bacteria and/or their products cross the intestinal barrier and can be retrieved in lymphoid tissues, liver, spleen and/or blood. Data in animal models clearly support its existence, and it is likely to also occur in humans, but this has been difficult to ascertain in well-designed studies (48). Gram-negative pathogens trigger SIRS through secretion of lipopolysaccharide, which in rats causes marked TJ morphological alteration, MLC phosphorylation, intestinal cytokine release and bacterial translocation (49).

Intensive care unit patients who developed SIRS had persistently abnormal intestinal permeability tests during their critical illness, and a significantly delayed improvement in permeability tests compared with the non-SIRS cohort (50). However, several clinical studies have demonstrated that bacteria isolated from patients with systemic infections are often of the same strain as bacteria predominant in the fecal flora. The Gram-negative bacteria present in the intestine often are the agents responsible for infectious complications in high-risk hospitalized patients, and the presumably translocated enteric bacteria are sometimes recovered from the mesenteric lymph nodes of these patients (51). The value of enteral feeding should not be underestimated in critically ill patients. Early enteral feeding can improve intestinal permeability and is associated with a decrease in multiple organ dysfunction syndrome (52).

Inflammatory Bowel Disease

Chronic inflammatory bowel disease (IBD) has a worldwide prevalence of over 1 million, and a rising incidence, estimated at 50 000 new cases yearly. The incidence of both Crohn's disease and ulcerative colitis is also increasing in the pediatric population. An estimated 25–30% of IBD patients have the onset of symptoms and/or are diagnosed before the age of 20 years (53). This early onset implies a higher lifetime morbidity burden; in the USA, the healthcare costs of IBD are estimated to exceed $1 billion annually (54). The pathogenetic mechanisms are as yet undefined, but are likely to involve a combination of genetic, environmental, and immunologic factors. One such innate immune factor, intestinal barrier function, has been associated with the development of IBD. Intestinal permeability is increased in humans with both ulcerative colitis (UC) (55) and Crohn's disease (56). Noninvasive permeability measurements such as urinary ^{51}Cr-labeled EDTA or lactulose:mannitol excretion ratio have been shown to correlate with disease activity (57). Abnormal sugar probe tests have predicted clinical relapse in Crohn's disease as much as 1 year in advance (58). Increased permeability has also been documented in asymptomatic first-degree relatives of IBD patients (59), suggesting a genetic predisposition. A very recent study in healthy first-degree relatives of Crohn's patients found a significant association between abnormal lactulose:mannitol excretion ratios and a NOD2/CARD15 mutation (60).

In both active and inactive IBD, interepithelial tight junction (TJ) structure is altered. Colonic mucosa from patients with UC and Crohn's revealed dramatic, global down-regulation of the key TJ transmembrane protein occludin in regions of active neutrophilic infiltration and in quiescent areas in the biopsy samples (61). Occludin and zonula occludens proteins are dislocated from the apical to basolateral surface of epithelia from inactively inflamed Crohn's mucosa (62). Translating these findings to barrier function, Soderholm et al. (63) demonstrated that in similar Crohn's mucosa luminal stimuli produce ultrastructural dilatations in TJ and induce a rapid increase in permeability to ^{51}Cr-EDTA. This impaired intestinal barrier function is believed to allow the passage of luminal antigens to the lamina propria, where they stimulate an immune response, which when dysregulated produces chronic inflammation. Activated macrophages secrete proinflammatory mediators, which act on the TJ to perpetuate the permeability defect. Two such cytokines, central to the cascade leading to IBD, are tumor necrosis factor alpha (TNF-α) and interferon-gamma (IFN-γ). TNF-α disrupts TJ assembly and increases endosomal uptake of luminal antigens in ileal Crohn's, while IFN-γ induces endocytosis of major TJ proteins claudin-1 and occludin (5). In synergy, they activate myosin light chain kinase (MLCK), leading to cytoskeletal changes that open the TJ, promoting a vicious cycle of increased leakiness and abnormal immune stimulation (64).

Clinical diagnosis of IBD relies primarily on histological and radiographic findings. Intestinal permeability markers have been proposed as screening tests for IBD, with utility in active small bowel Crohn's disease, but not in other phenotypes. In patients with Crohn's disease in clinical remission, an increased intestinal permeability can predict those at significant risk of relapse in the next few months, with less than 20% of those with normal barrier function relapsing over the ensuing 6 months (65).

Treatment of IBD is evolving beyond immunosuppression and surgery. Enteral nutrition therapy with elemental diets has been shown to produce remission of active Crohn's disease and restore intestinal permeability (66). Targeted molecular therapy of IBD with infliximab, a monoclonal antibody directed against TNF-α, has resulted in significant clinical improvement in both pediatric and adult patients. It curtails inflammation by inducing apoptosis of effector T lymphocytes, downregulating IFN-γ production, and restoring mucosal architecture (58). Crohn's patients treated with infliximab had significant decreases in permeability measured by ^{51}Cr-EDTA excretion, accompanied by decreased disease activity indices (67). Along the same lines, the barrier disruption may be corrected by inhibiting MLCK or using the anti-inflammatory cytokine IL-10 to counter IFN-γ (58), making these attractive targets for future therapies.

Celiac Disease

Also known as sprue or gluten-sensitive enteropathy, celiac disease (CD) is thought to be among the most common genetically determined conditions to affect humans, with a prevalence rate of 0.5–1% of the general population (68). Classically a disease of early childhood, it is now recognized as a common condition (up to 1:100 in some regions) with a wide spectrum of clinical manifestations that could be diagnosed at any age (69). The disease develops as a result of immune-mediated intestinal inflammation triggered by gluten, a protein component of certain grains, including wheat, barley, and rye. It occurs in individuals with a genetic predisposition, which is strongly linked to the human leukocyte antigen (HLA) DQ2 and DQ8 genotypes.

Intestinal barrier dysfunction is thought to be an early event in the pathogenesis of CD. Structural changes in small intestinal epithelial cell TJ associated with increased ionic permeability have been observed in biopsies from children with active CD (70). The proposed mechanism involves increased expression of zonulin, a reversible mediator of TJ disassembly (71). Enterocytes secrete higher levels of zonulin in response to gliadin peptides found in gluten, and zonulin subsequently induces actin polymerization, followed by cytoskeletal changes leading to "opening" of TJ (72). This permits the passage of gliadin into the lamina propria, where it is deamidated by tissue transglutaminase (tTG), producing antigenic epitopes. These bind to HLA receptors on the surface of antigen-presenting cells and are presented to specific T lymphocytes, leading to an abnormal adaptive immune response that involves the release of cytokines and zonulin, perpetuating the epithelial injury. Gliadin itself was found to have a direct effect on TJ in Caco-2 cell cultures, reorganizing actin filaments and altering expression of occludin, claudin-3 and claudin-4 (73).

CD is widely under-diagnosed, due to under-recognition of its protean manifestations, and, until recently, low yield and limited availability of screening tests. Improved methods have conferred sensitivity of 91%, specificity of 97%, and positive predictive value of 97% on measurement of IgA directed against tTG (74). The gold standard for diagnosis is small bowel biopsy demonstrating villous atrophy and intraepithelial lymphocytic infiltration. The utility of intestinal permeability tests for screening a general population for CD has been studied (75), but these tests are not being widely used. The only treatment for CD with documented efficacy is a strict gluten-free diet, and treatment is recommended because of associated long-term outcomes, including increased risk of intestinal malignancy, recalcitrant anemia, osteoporosis, liver injury, and neurological deficits. Within 2 months of starting a gluten-free diet, small intestinal barrier function, as measured by sugar probe permeability tests, recovers and this precedes histological and morphometric recovery (76). Furthermore, a gluten-free diet reverses gliadin-induced downregulation of the TJ component zonula occludens-1 (77). A recent prospective cohort study of CD patients treated with strict gluten avoidance demonstrated that permeability normalized in 87% after 1 year of treatment, and that permeability testing correlates better with trace gluten ingestion than serological testing (78). Adherence to a strict gluten-free diet is difficult; the searches for an alternative, more palatable treatment for CD, will probably target molecules involved in altered permeability.

Type 1 Diabetes

The defining features of type 1 diabetes (T1D), insulin deficiency and hyperglycemia, result from an immune-mediated destruction of insulin-secreting beta cells in the pancreatic islets (79). Autoimmune insulitis may result from dysregulated oral tolerance to dietary antigens combined with increased intestinal inflammation and permeability in genetically predisposed individuals (80). A permeability defect has been documented in animal models of T1D as well as in humans with the disease. The diabetes-prone BB (BBDP) rat has increased lactulose:mannitol excretion ratios prior to the onset of diabetes, with disease incidence reduced by feeding hydrolyzed casein (81). This abnormality of the rodent gut barrier is associated with low expression of the major TJ protein claudin-1 (82), so the correlation between structure and function applies to this condition as well. Oral administration of a zonulin inhibitor to BBDP rats blocks autoantibody formation and zonulin-mediated intestinal permeability increase, reducing the incidence of diabetes (83). Permeability to mannitol, which is normal in healthy children, young adult controls, and adult patients with type 2 diabetes, is increased in uncomplicated T1D (84). T1D patients without CD had structural alterations such as aberrant microvilli and thickened tight junctions in their intestinal epithelia, as seen by transmission electron microscopy, and these correlated with abnormal sugar probe tests (85).

As in CD and the BBDP rat, zonulin may play a central role in mediating this passage of non-self antigens through the gut epithelium. Sapone and colleagues (86) very recently reported a large subgroup of T1D patients in whom serum zonulin levels are elevated in correlation with increased lactulose:mannitol excretion ratios. This zonulin up-regulation was found in individuals at genetic risk for T1D and precedes the onset of overt T1D. Paralleling CD, the loss of intestinal barrier function preceding T1D may permit a switch from tolerance to immunity to non-self antigens that continuously cross the intestinal mucosa (87). The high prevalence (up to 10%) of CD in the T1D patient population and shared HLA haplotype associations between the two diseases (88) suggest a common mechanism of underlying intestinal barrier dysfunction. In addition to a role in T1D pathogenesis, increased intestinal permeability leads to higher variation in postprandial blood glucose levels, complicating metabolic control (89).

Atopic Disease

More than 50 million Americans suffer from atopic diseases, generally referred to as allergy. Allergies are the sixth leading cause of chronic disease in the USA, costing the healthcare system $18 billion annually. Environmental and genetic factors play a role in susceptibility to allergy. The hygiene hypothesis of atopic disease suggests that environmental changes in the industrialized world have led to reduced microbial contact at an early age and thus resulted in the growing epidemic of atopic eczema, allergic rhinoconjunctivitis, and asthma (90). Atopy involves a T lymphocyte-dependent generation of allergen-specific antibody.

The commensal microflora in the gut is essential for antigenic stimulation that leads to the Th1-type response of the gut-associated lymphoid tissue (GALT) and protects against the development of intestinal inflammation. The absence of commensal bacteria in animal models (e.g. germ-free mouse model) produces Th2-type hyperresponsiveness and lack of tolerance to orally administered antigens (Fig. 6-4) (91).

Murine models implicate signaling via Toll-like receptor 4 (TLR4) as a mechanism by which the luminal flora can influence the response to food antigens. Antibiotic administration during the neonatal period reduced and altered gut wild-type microflora and TLR4-deficient, inducing an allergic phenotype. When commensal flora is allowed to repopulate (during the newborn period) the allergen-specific IgE and Th2 cytokine responses are reduced in antibiotic-treated mice (92).

Gastrointestinal disorders have been reported in children with atopic eczema in several studies. Caffarelli et al. (93) showed that gastrointestinal symptoms (such as diarrhea, vomiting and regurgitation) are more common among patients with eczema than in healthy controls. The frequency of symptoms correlated with extent of the disease.

Some microbial products have been shown to be efficacious for the treatment and/or prevention of allergy in both experimental models and clinical trials. New research on probiotics suggests that certain types of bacteria, especially lactobacilli,

SCIENTIFIC OVERVIEW AND DEVELOPMENTAL PERSPECTIVES

I

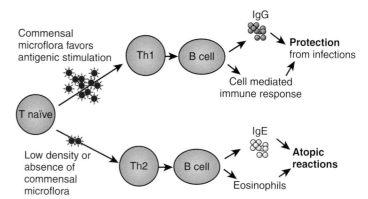

Figure 6-4 Diagram of the Th1-Th2 paradigm. Th, T-helper cell; Ig, immunoglobulin; Tnaïve, naïve T cell.

can ameliorate allergic inflammation. A prospective study (94) of 159 children with a family history of atopy showed that increased intakes of retinol, calcium, zinc and perinatal administration of probiotics reduced the risk of developing eczema.

In a double-blinded, placebo-controlled study (95) of 62 mother-infant pairs, administration of probiotics to the pregnant and lactating mother increased the anti-inflammatory transforming growth factor β-2 in the breast milk. The risk of developing atopic eczema during the first 2 years of life in infants whose mothers received probiotics was significantly reduced in comparison with that in infants whose mothers received placebo (15% and 47%, respectively; relative risk, 0.32 [95% CI, 0.12–0.85]; $P < 0.01$). The infants most likely to benefit from maternal probiotic supplementation were those with an elevated cord blood IgE concentration. Administering probiotics during pregnancy and breast-feeding may enhance the immunoprotective potential of breast-feeding and provide protection against atopic dermatitis during the first 2 years of life.

Mucosal permeability modulation and timing of antigen exposure are promising research areas in prevention of atopic diseases.

Autism

Autistic spectrum disorder (ASD) is a pervasive developmental disorder, with a complex clinical diagnosis as defined by the American Psychiatric Association (96), and without known biomarkers or clear etiology. There have been many anecdotal reports of increased nonspecific gastrointestinal symptoms (such as abdominal pain, diarrhea, bloating, food aversion) in ASD patients. Figure 6-5 illustrates how GI dysfunction may predispose to autism. Mucosal inflammatory responses to dietary proteins could be an explanation for a subset of ASD patients with gastrointestinal complaints. Non-allergic food hypersensitivity (adverse reaction) to dietary proteins is mostly mediated by cellular immunity and in small proportion by immunoglobulin E. A recent study (97) showed that peripheral blood monocytes in patients with ASD and gastrointestinal symptoms have elevated production of TNF-α and IL-12 in response to cow's milk protein.

There is growing evidence that children with ASD have an immune dysregulation with pro-inflammatory imbalance. Wakefield et al. (98) performed endoscopies and biopsies in 12 autistic children with gastrointestinal complaints and found ileal lymphoid nodular hyperplasia (LNH) in 10/12 and nonspecific colitis in 8/12. The same group investigated 60 ASD patients versus a control group of 37 non-ASD children with gastrointestinal symptoms (99). They found that a greater proportion of the ASD patients had nonspecific inflammatory bowel changes (93% LNH vs.

HYPOTHESIS OF GASTROINTESTINAL
ROLE IN AUTISTIC SPECTRUM DISORDER

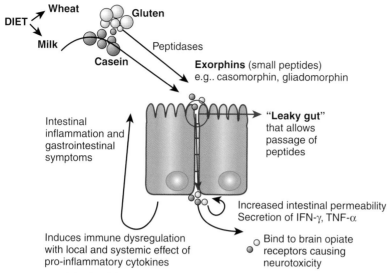

Figure 6-5 Potential role of the GI tract in autism.

14% control, 88% chronic colitis, and 8% active ileitis). Ileo-colonoscopy was performed in a prospective study (100) involving a cohort of 148 children with ASD and gastrointestinal symptoms and the findings were compared with 30 developmentally normal children with abdominal symptoms ("controls"). The prevalence of ileal LNH was 90% in children with ASD vs. 30% in the controls. The prevalence of LNH in colon was 59% in ASD children vs. 23% in controls. The same cohort was subjected to immune profiling and showed evidence of a significant systemic and intestinal mucosal immune dysregulation (101). In peripheral blood and mucosa, pro-inflammatory cytokine-producing lymphocytes were increased, and anti-inflammatory cytokine-producing lymphocytes were low compared with controls.

Jyonouchi et al. (102) found that children with ASD have exaggerated innate immune responses most evident in TNF-α production (dominant T_H2 pattern). Cytokines have widespread systemic effects including the central nervous system and may be factors contributing to changes in mood and sleep patterns in ASD patients. Between 30 and 70% of ASD patients have circulating anti-brain auto-antibodies such as antibodies to neuron-axon filament proteins (103), cerebellar neurofillaments, myelin basic protein, caudate nucleus (104), serotonin receptor, brain endothelial cells (105) and brain tissue. This evidence suggests autoimmunity as an important factor in ASD but it does not clarify whether this is an etiologic factor or a secondary phenomenon (106).

Abnormal intestinal permeability has been reported in 43% of ASD children without clinical or laboratory findings consistent with a known intestinal disorder (107).

Dietary proteins such as gluten and casein are digested by intestinal peptidases in the lumen of the small intestine. The resulting shor-chain peptides (e.g. gliadomorphin and casomorphin) are very similar to endorphins and are called "exorphins" (108). These exorphins are neuroactive and may interfere directly with the function of the CNS if they enter the body (109–110). Exorphins have a high and physiologically significant affinity with the binding sites of endogenous opioid receptors (111). Intravenous infusion of the exorphin B casomorphin-7 (exorphin) activates rat brain cells (112). The neonate is more likely to experience this effect of exorphins because of the more permeable gastrointestinal tract and immature nervous system.

There are reports that gluten-free and casein-free diets improve behavior in ASD patients (113). The improvement but not elimination of the neurobehavioral symptoms raises the possibility that elevated exorphins cause permanent damage to the infant brain. There is evidence of a strong association between gut, immune dysregulation, and ASD patients, but the present data are insufficient to prove causality.

A good understanding of the GI mucosal permeability may provide future answers about the pathology and treatment of the ASD.

Other Diseases

A role for or an association with gut barrier breakdown and dysfunction has been reported in a wide variety of clinical conditions, some of which affect infants and children. A reversible impairment in gut permeability, associated with local immune cell and enterocyte activation, occurs in patients with obstructive cholestasis, paralleling observations in a rat model (114). Other examples of diseases in which gut leakiness has been observed include juvenile rheumatoid arthritis, systemic lupus erythematosus, acute pancreatitis, and chronic renal failure (115).

SUMMARY

Barrier function, especially the role of interepithelial tight junctions, is integral to overall gastrointestinal function. Barrier dysfunction, or increased intestinal permeability, may be a pathogenetic mechanism underlying diseases such as NEC and SIRS affecting the neonate, as well as autoimmune and inflammatory conditions that present later in infancy or childhood. More studies are needed to further elucidate the mechanisms by which the intestinal barrier integrity is breached. Multiple factors early in life can affect tight junctions and barrier function, potentially leading to lifelong consequences.

REFERENCES

1. Fasano A, Shea-Donohue T. Mechanisms of disease: the role of intestinal barrier function in the pathogenesis of gastrointestinal autoimmune diseases. Nat Clin Pract Gastroenterol Hepatol. 2005; 2:416–422.
2. Medzhitov R, Janeway C. Innate immune recognition: mechanisms and pathways. Immunol Rev 2000; 173:89–97.
3. Lichtman S. Bacterial translocation in humans. J Pediatr Gastroenterol Nutr 2001; 33:1–10.
4. González-Mariscal L, Betanzos A, Nava P, Jaramillo BE. Tight junction proteins. Prog Biophys Mol Biol 2003; 81:1–44.
5. Tsukita S, Furuse M. The structure and function of claudins, cell adhesion molecules at tight junctions. Ann N Y Acad Sci 2000; 915:129–135.
6. Schneeberger EE, Lynch RD. The tight junction: a multifunctional complex. Am J Physiol Cell Physiol 2004; 286:C1213–C1228.
7. Saitou M, Furuse M, Sasaki H, et al. Complex phenotype of mice lacking occludin, a component of tight junction strands. Mol Biol Cell 2000; 11:4131–4412.
8. Matter K, Balda MS. Signalling to and from tight junctions. Nat Rev Mol Cell Biol 2003; 4:225–236.
9. Claude P. Morphological factors influencing transepithelial permeability: a model for the resistance of the zonula occludens. J Membr Biol 1978; 39:219–232.
10. Sawada N, Murata M, Kikuchi K, et al. Tight junctions and human diseases. Med Electron Microsc 2003; 36:147–156.
11. Turner JR, Rill BK, Carlson SL, et al. Physiological regulation of epithelial tight junctions is associated with myosin light-chain phosphorylation. Am J Physiol 1997; 273:C1378–C1385.
12. Duffy LC, Zielezny MA, Carrion V, et al. Concordance of bacterial cultures with endotoxin and interleukin-6 in necrotizing enterocolitis. Dig Dis Sci 1997; 42:359–365.
13. Weaver LT, Laker MF, Nelson R. Intestinal permeability in the newborn. Arch Dis Child 1984; 59:236–241.

14. Rouwet EV, Heineman E, Buurman WA, et al. Intestinal permeability and carrier-mediated mono-saccharide absorption in preterm neonates during the early postnatal period. Pediatr Res 2002; 51:64–70.

15. Welsh FKS, Farmery SM, MacLennan K, et al. Gut barrier function in malnourished patients. Gut 1998; 42:396.

16. Deitch EA, Xu D, Naruhn MB, et al. Elemental diet and IV-TPN-induced bacterial translocation is associated with loss of intestinal mucosal barrier function against bacteria. Ann Surg 1995; 221:299–307.

17. Kansagra K, Stoll B, Rognerud C, et al. Total parenteral nutrition adversely affects gut barrier function in neonatal piglets. Am J Physiol Gastrointest Liver Physiol 2003; 285:G1162–G1170.

18. Ohta K, Omura K, Hirano K, et al. The effects of an additive small amount of a low residual diet against total parenteral nutrition-induced gut mucosal barrier. Am J Surg 2003; 185:79–85.

19. Hadfield RJ, Sinclair DG, Houldsworth PE, Evans TW. Effects of enteral and parenteral nutrition on gut mucosal permeability in the critically ill. Am J Respir Crit Care Med 1995; 152:1545–1548.

20. Schulman RJ, Schanler R, Lau JC, et al. Early feeding, antenatal glucocorticoids, and human milk decrease intestinal permeability in preterm infants. Pediatr Res 1998; 44:519–523.

21. Kudsk KA. Current aspects of mucosal immunology and its influence by nutrition. Am J Surg 2002; 183:390–398.

22. Van Der Hulst RR, Von Meyenfeldt MF, Van Kreel BK, et al. Gut permeability, intestinal morphology, and nutritional depletion. Nutrition 1998; 14:1–6.

23. Li N, DeMarco VG, West CM, Neu J. Glutamine supports recovery from loss of transepithelial resistance and increase of permeability induced by media change in Caco-2 cells. J. Nutr Biochem 2003; 14:401–408.

24. Duggan C, Gannon J, Walker WA. Protective nutrients and functional foods for the gastrointestinal tract. Am J Clin Nutr 2002; 75:789–808.

25. Jiang WG, Bryce RP, Horrobin DF, Mansel RE. Regulation of tight junction permeability and occludin expression by polyunsaturated fatty acids. Biochem Biophys Res Commun 1998; 244:414–420.

26. Usami M, Muraki K, Iwamoto M, et al. Effect of eicosapentaenoic acid (EPA) on tight junction permeability in intestinal monolayer cells. Clin Nutr 2001; 20:351–359.

27. Venkatraman A, Ramakrishna BS, Pulimood AB. Butyrate hastens restoration of barrier function after thermal and detergent injury to rat distal colon in vitro. Scand J Gastroenterol 1999; 34:1087–1092.

28. Ohata A, Usami M, Miyoshi M. Short-chain fatty acids alter tight junction permeability in intestinal monolayer cells via lipoxygenase activation. Nutrition 2005; 21:838–847.

29. Kinoshita M, Suzuki Y, Saito Y. Butyrate reduces colonic paracellular permeability by enhancing PPARgamma activation. Biochem Biophys Res Commun 2002; 293:27–31.

30. Pastores SM, Katz DP, Kvetan V. Splanchnic ischemia and gut mucosal injury in sepsis and the multiple organ dysfunction syndrome. Am J Gastroenterol 1996; 91:1697–1710.

31. Banan A, Fields JZ, Decker H, et al. Nitric oxide and its metabolites mediate ethanol-induced microtubule disruption and intestinal barrier dysfunction. J Pharmacol Exp Ther 2000; 294:997–1008.

32. Simonovic I, Rosenberg J, Koutsouris A, Hecht G. Enteropathogenic Escherichia coli dephosphorylates and dissociates occludin from intestinal epithelial tight junctions. Cell Microbiol 2000; 2:305–315.

33. Schiflett DE, Clayburgh DR, Koutsouris A, et al. Enteropathogenic E. coli disrupts tight junction barrier function and structure in vivo. Lab Invest 2005; 85:1308–1324.

34. Scott KG, Meddings JB, Kirik DR, et al. Intestinal infection with Giardia spp. reduces epithelial barrier function in a myosin light chain kinase-dependent fashion. Gastroenterol 2002; 123:1179–1190.

35. Walsh SV, Hopkins AM, Chen J, et al. Rho kinase regulates tight junction function and is necessary for tight junction assembly in polarized intestinal epithelia. Gastroenterol 2001; 121:566–579.

36. Zhang Y, Lee B, Thompson M, et al. Lactulose-mannitol intestinal permeability test in children with diarrhea caused by rotavirus and cryptosporidium. J Pediatr Gastroenterol Nutr 2000; 31:16–21.

37. Dickman KG, Hempson SJ, Anderson J, et al. Rotavirus alters paracellular permeability and energy metabolism in Caco-2 cells. Am J Physiol Gastrointest Liver Physiol 2000; 279:G757–G766.

38. Tafazoli F, Zeng CQ, Estes MK, et al. NSP4 enterotoxin of rotavirus induces paracellular leakage in polarized epithelial cells. J Virol 2001; 75:1540–1546.

39. Fasano A, Fiorentini C, Donelli G, et al. Zonula occludens toxin modulates tight junctions through protein kinase C-dependent actin reorganization, in vitro. J Clin Invest 1995; 96:710–720.

40. Zolotarevsky Y, Hecht G, Koutsouris A, et al. A membrane-permeant peptide that inhibits MLC kinase restores barrier function in in vitro models of intestinal disease. Gastroenterol 2002; 123:163–172.

41. DeMeo MT, Mutlu EA, Keshavarzian A, Tobin MC. Intestinal permeation and gastrointestinal disease. J Clin Gastroenterol 2002; 34:385–396.

42. Lemons JA, Bauer CR, Oh W, et al. Very low birth weight outcomes of the National Institute of Child Health and Human Development Neonatal Research Network, January 1995 through December 1996. Available at: www.pediatrics.org/cgi/content/full/107/1/e1..

43. Hsueh W, Caplan MS, Qu XW, et al. Neonatal necrotizing enterocolitis: clinical considerations and pathogenic concepts. Ped Dev Path. 2002; 6:6–23.

44. Lee JS, Polin RA. Treatment and prevention of necrotizing enterocolitis. Semin Neonatol 2003; 8:449–459.

45. Berseth CL, Bisquera JA, Paje VU. Prolonging small feeding volumes early in life decreases the incidence of necrotizing Enterocolitis in VLBW infants. Pediatrics 2003; 111:529–534.

46. Book LS, Herbst JJ, Atherton SO, et al. NEC in low birth weight infants fed elemental formula. J Pediatr 1975; 87:602.

47. Isolauri E, Sutas Y, Kankaanpaa P, et al. Probiotics: effects on immunity. Am J Clin Nutr 2001; 73:444S–450S.

48. Lichtman SM. Bacterial translocation in humans. J Pediatr Gastroenterol Nutr 2001; 33:1–10.

49. Moriez R, Salvador-Cartier C, Theodorou V, et al. Myosin light chain kinase is involved in lipo-polysaccharide-induced disruption of colonic epithelial barrier and bacterial translocation in rats. Am J Pathol 2005; 167:1071–1079.

50. Doig CJ, Sutherland LR, Sandham JD, et al. Increased intestinal permeability is associated with the development of multiple organ dysfunction syndrome in critically ill ICU patients. Am J Respir Crit Care Med 1998; 158:444–451.

51. DeSouza DA, Greene LJ. Intestinal permeability and systemic infections in critically ill patients: effect of glutamine. Crit Care Med 2005; 33:1125–1135.

52. Kompan L, Kompan D. Importance of increased intestinal permeability after multiple injuries. Eur J Surg 2001; 167:570–574.

53. Mamula P, Markowitz JE, Baldassano RN. Inflammatory bowel disease in early childhood and adolescence: special considerations. Gastroenterol Clin North Am 2003; 32:967–995.

54. Sandler RS, Everhart JE, Donowitz M, et al. The burden of selected digestive diseases in the United States. Gastroenterology 2002; 122:1500–1511.

55. Nejdfors P, Wang Q, Ekelund M, et al. Increased colonic permeability in patients with ulcerative colitis: an in vitro study. Scand. J. Gastroenterol 1998; 33:749–753.

56. Jenkins RT, Jones DB, Goodacre RL, et al. Reversibility of increased intestinal permeability to 51Cr-EDTA in patients with gastrointestinal inflammatory diseases. Am J Gastroenterol 1987; 82:1159–1164.

57. Miki K, Moore DJ, Butler R, et al. The sugar permeability test reflects disease activity in children and adolescents with inflammatory bowel disease. J Pediatr 1998; 133:750–754.

58. D'Inca R, DiLeo V, Corrao G, et al. Intestinal permeability test as a predictor of clinical course in Crohn's disease. Am J Gastroenterol 1999; 94:2956–2960.

59. Munkholm P, Langholz E, Hollander D, et al. Intestinal permeability in patients with Crohn's disease and ulcerative colitis and their first degree relatives. Gut 1994; 35:68–72.

60. Buhner S, Buning C, Genschel J, et al. Genetic basis for increased intestinal permeability in families with Crohn's disease: role of CARD15 3020insC mutation? Gut 2006; 55(3):342–347.

61. Kucharzik T, Walsh SV, Chen J, et al. Neutrophil transmigration in inflammatory bowel disease is associated with differential expression of epithelial intercellular junction proteins. Am J Pathol 2001; 159:2001–2009.

62. Oshitani N, Watanabe K, Nakamura S, et al. Dislocation of tight junction proteins without F-actin disruption in inactive Crohn's disease. Int J Mol Med 2005; 15:407–410.

63. Soderholm JD, Olaison G, Peterson KH, et al. Augmented increase in tight junction permeability by luminal stimuli in the non-inflamed ileum of Crohn's disease. Gut 2002; 50:307–313.

64. Clayburgh DR, Shen L, Turner JR. A porous defense: the leaky epithelial barrier in intestinal disease. Lab Invest 2004; 84:282–291.

65. Tibble JA, Bjarnason I. Non-invasive investigation of inflammatory bowel disease. World J Gastroenterol 2001; 7:460–465.

66. Zoli G, Carè M, Parazza M, et al. A randomized controlled study comparing elemental diet and steroid treatment in Crohn's disease. Aliment Pharmacol Ther 1997; 11:735–740.

67. Suenaert P, Bulteel V, Lemmens L, et al. Anti-tumor necrosis factor treatment restores the gut barrier in Crohn's disease. Am J Gastroenterol 2002; 97:2000–2004.

68. Hill ID. Celiac disease – a never ending story. J. Pediatr 2003; 143:289–291.

69. Green PH, Jabri B. Coeliac disease. Lancet 2003; 362:383–391.

70. Schulzke JD, Bentzel C, Schulzke I, et al. Epithelial tight junction structure in the jejunum of children with acute and treated celiac sprue. Pediatr Res 1998; 43:435–441.

71. Fasano A, Not T, Wang W, et al. Zonulin, a newly discovered modulator of intestinal permeability, and its expression in coeliac disease. Lancet 2000; 355:1518–1519.

72. Clemente MG, DeVirgilis S, Kang JS, et al. Early effects of gliadin on enterocyte intracellular signalling involved in intestinal barrier function. Gut 2003; 52:218–223.

73. Sander GR, Cummins AG, Henshall T, et al. Rapid disruption of intestinal barrier function by gliadin involves altered expression of apical junctional proteins. FEBS Lett, 2005; 579:4851–4855.

74. Tesei N, Sugai E, Vazquez H, et al. Antibodies to human recombinant tissue transglutaminase may detect coeliac disease patients undiagnosed by endomysial antibodies. Aliment Pharmacol Ther 2003; 17:1415–1423.

75. Johnston SD, Smye M, Watson RG, et al. Lactulose-mannitol intestinal permeability test: a useful screening test for adult coeliac disease. Ann Clin Biochem 2000; 37:512–519.

76. Cummins AG, Thompson FM, Butler RN, et al. Improvement in intestinal permeability precedes morphometric recovery of the small intestine in celiac disease. Clin Sci 2001; 100:379–386.

77. Pizzuti D, Bortolami M, Mazzon E, et al. Transcriptional downregulation of tight junction protein ZO-1 in active coeliac disease is reversed after a gluten-free diet. Dig Liver Dis 2004; 36:337–341.

78. Duerksen DR, Wilhelm-Boyles C, Parry DM. Intestinal permeability in long-term follow-up of patients with celiac disease on a gluten-free diet. Dig Dis Sci 2005; 50:785–790.
79. Atkinson MA, Maclaren NK. The pathogenesis of insulin-dependent diabetes mellitus. N Engl J Med 1994; 331:1428–1436.
80. Vaarala O. The gut immune system and T1D. Ann NY Acad Sci 2002; 958:39–46.
81. Meddings JB, Jarand J, Urbanski J, et al. Increased gastrointestinal permeability is an early lesion in the spontaneously diabetic BB rat. Am J Physiol 1999; 276:G951–G957.
82. Neu J, Reverte CM, Mackey AD, et al. Changes in intestinal morphology and permeability in the BioBreeding rat before the onset of Type 1 diabetes. J Pediatr Gastroenterol Nutr 2005; 40:589–595.
83. Watts T, Berti I, Sapone A, et al. Role of intestinal tight junction modulator zonulin in the pathogenesis of type1 diabetes in BB diabetic prone rats. Proc Natl Acad Sci USA 2005; 102:2916–2921.
84. Carratù R, Secondulfo M, de Magistris L, et al. Altered intestinal permeability to mannitol in diabetes mellitus type I. J Pediatr Gastroenterol Nutr 1999; 28:264–269.
85. Secondulfo M, Iafusco D, Carratu R, et al. Ultrastructural mucosal alterations and increased intestinal permeability in non-celiac, type I diabetic patients. Dig Liver Dis 2004; 36:35–45.
86. Sapone A, de Magistris L, Pietzak M, et al. Zonulin upregulation is associated with increased gut permeability in subjects with type 1 diabetes and their relatives. Diabetes 2006; 55:1443–1450.
87. Westerholm-Ormio M, Vaarala O, Pihkala P, et al. Immunologic activity in the small intestinal mucosa of pediatric patients with type 1 diabetes. Diabetes 2003; 52:2287–2295.
88. Lazzarotto F, Basso D, Plebani M, et al. Celiac disease and type 1 diabetes. Diabetes Care 2003; 26:248–249.
89. Damci T, Nuhoglu I, Devranoglu G, et al. Increased intestinal permeability as a cause of fluctuating postprandial blood glucose levels in Type 1 diabetic patients. Eur J Clin Invest 2003; 33:397–401.
90. Schaub B, Lauener R, von Mutius E. The many faces of the hygiene hypothesis. J Allergy Clin Immunol 2006; 117:969–977.
91. Tanaka K, Ishikawa H. Role of intestinal bacterial flora in oral tolerance induction. Histol Histopathol 2004; 19:907–914.
92. Bashir ME, Louie S, Shi HN. Toll-like receptor 4 signaling by intestinal microbes influences susceptibility to food allergy. J Immunol 2004; 172:6978–6987.
93. Caffarelli C, Cavagni G, Deriu FM, et al. Gastrointestinal symptoms in atopic eczema. ArchDis Child 1998; 78:230–234.
94. Laitinen K, Kalliomaki M, Poussa T, et al. Evaluation of diet and growth in children with and without atopic eczema: follow-up study from birth to 4 years. Br J Nutr 2005; 94:565–574.
95. Rautava S, Kalliomaki M, Isolauri E. Probiotics during pregnancy and breast-feeding might confer immunomodulatory protection against atopic disease in the infant. J Allergy Clin Immunol 2002; 109:119–121.
96. American Psychiatric Association 1994, Diagnostic and statistical manual of mental disorders (DSM IV) 4th edition. Washington, DC: APA; 1994.
97. Jyonouchi H, Geng L, Ruby A, et al. Evaluation of an association between gastrointestinal symptoms and cytokine production against common dietary proteins in children with ASD. J Pediatr 2005; 146:605–610.
98. Wakefield AJ, Murch SH, Anthony A, et al. Ileal lymphoid-nodular hyperplasia, non-specific colitis, and pervasive developmental disorder in children. Lancet 1998; 35:637–641.
99. Wakefield AJ, Anthony A, Murch SH, et al. Enterocolitis in children with developmental disorders. Am J Gastroenterol 2000; 95:2285–2295.
100. Wakefield AJ, Ashwood P, Limb K, et al. The significance of ileo-colonic lymphoid nodular hyoperplasia in children with autistic spectrum disorder. Eur J Gastroenterol Hepatol 2005; 17:827–836.
101. Ashood P, Wakefield AJ. Immune activation of peripheral blood and mucosal CD3+ lymphocyte cytokine profiles in children with autism and gastrointestinal symptoms. J Neuroimmunol 2006; 173:126–134.
102. Jyonouchi H, Sun S, Le H. Proinflammatory and regulatory cytokine production associated with innate and adaptive immune responses in children with ASD and developmental regression. J Neuroimmunol 2001; 120:170–179.
103. Singh VK, Warren R, Averett R, Ghaziuddin M. Circulating autoantibodies to neuronal and glial filament proteins in autism. Pediatr Neurol 1997; 17:88–90.
104. Singh VK, Rivas WH. Prevalence of serum antibodies to caudate nucleus in autistic children. Neurosci Lett 2004; 355:253–256.
105. Connolly AM, Chez MG, Pestronk A, et al. Serum autoantibodies to brain in Landau-Kleffner variant, autism, and other neurologic disorders. J Pediatr 1999; 34:607–613.
106. Ashwood P, Van de Water J. Is autism an autoimmune disease?. Autoimmunity Rev 2004; 3:557–562.
107. D'Eufemia P, Celli M, Finocchiano R, et al. Abnormal intestinal permeability in children with autism. Acta Paediatr 1996; 85:1076–1079.
108. Zioudrou C, Streaty RA, Klee WA. Opioid peptides derived from food proteins. The exorphins. J Biol Chem 1979; 254:2446–2449.
109. Hemmings WA. The entry into the brain of large molecules derived from dietary protein. Proc Roy Soc London 1978; 200:175–192.
110. Sun Z, Cade JR. A peptide found in schizophrenia and autism causes behavioral changes in rats. Autism 1999; 3:85–95.

111. Meisel H, FitzGerald RJ. Opioid peptides encrypted in intact milk protein sequences. Br. J Nutr 2000; 84:S27–S31.

112. Sun Z, Cade JR, Fregly MJ, Privette RM. B-casomorphin induces Fos-like immunoreactivity in discrete brain regions relevant to schizophrenia and autism. Autism 1999; 3:67–83.

113. Reichelt KL, Ekrein J, Scott H. Gluten, mil proteins and autism: dietary intervention effects on behavior and peptide secretion. J Appl Nutr 1990; 42:1–11.

114. Welsh FK, Ramsden CW, McLennan K, et al. Increased intestinal permeability and altered mucosal immunity in cholestatic jaundice. Ann Surg 1998; 227:205–212.

115. Farhadi A, Banan A, Fields J, Keshavarzian A. Intestinal barrier: an interface between health and disease. J Gastroenterol Hepatol 2003; 18:479–497.

Chapter 7

The Intestine as a Neuro-endocrine Organ

Carol Lynn Berseth, MD

Gastrointestinal Hormones and Peptides
The Enteric Nervous System
The ENS and Host Defense

The focus of this chapter will be the enteric nervous system (ENS). Many gastro-intestinal peptides function as true hormones for the gastrointestinal tract proper as well as neuropeptides for the ENS. Conversely, the ENS triggers the release of gut peptides responsible for the digestion of ingested nutrients as well as immune responses. For this reason, this chapter will review physiology related to gut hormones and peptides as well as the ENS.

GASTROINTESTINAL HORMONES AND PEPTIDES

The gut is the largest hormone-producing organ in the body, in terms of both the number of cells and the number of hormones produced. The first hormone was identified over 100 years ago, and by 1970 only three hormones, secretin, gastrin, and cholecystokinen, had been recognized. Since then over 100 bioactive peptides have been identified, and enteroendocrine cells comprise 1% of all epithelial cells.

Because mature enteroendocrine cells have a short life-span, they are replenished continuously. Stem cells give rise to absorptive cells or secretory cells (goblet, enteroendocrine, and Paneth cells), depending on transcription factors and the Notch signaling system. A cell that expresses high levels of Notch, which induces the transcription factor Hes1 and represses Math 1, becomes an absorptive cell (1), while those with low levels of Notch become secretory cells. Other components of the signaling pathway (including Ngn3 and BETA2/NeruoD, bHLH transcription factors) are also important, in that Ngn3-deficient mice fail to generate any intestinal endocrine cells (2). Paired box genes (Pax), which are expressed throughout the intestine, also regulate enteroendocrine cell differentiation. Pax 4-deficient mice have a marked reduction in the number of somatostatin and serotonin cells but a normal number of gastrin cells, while Pax 6-deficient mice have a severe reduction in somatostatin and gastrin cells and normal numbers of serotonin cells (3, 4).

It is now clear that many gastrointestinal peptides fail to function as true hormones, as described below. Instead, many express paracrine or neurocrine function, and some function as growth factors. A true hormone must exhibit the following features, as detailed by Walsh (5). (i) It is released into the blood when a biologic stimulus is presented, and, in turn, triggers a physiologic response in a target organ. (ii) It binds to an identifiable receptor. (iii) Its chemical structure is known and synthetically producible. (iv) When a synthetic peptide is infused into the plasma, it reproduces an effect on the target organ. (v) The target organ's physiologic response can be blocked by removing the peptide from the blood or by blocking the target receptor. Gastrin is an example of a classic hormone that is released by the G cell when protein is ingested. When released, it triggers the parietal cell to produce acid.

Fewer than a dozen intestinal peptides are recognized to be true hormones. Others have paracrine or neurocrine function. Peptides that have paracrine function are released by the paracrine cells and diffuse to local target receptors. An example of a peptide that has paracrine function is vasoactive peptide (VIP). Peptides that have neurocrine function are released by nerve terminals. An example of a peptide that has neurocrine function is substance P, which is found in nerve terminals of enteric nerves. Growth factors are peptides that exert trophic effects. An example of a growth factor is epidermal growth factor, which promotes growth in the upper intestinal mucosa.

Although some hormones and peptides function solely in one capacity (e.g. hormone, growth factor), some peptides function in more than one capacity. An example is gastrin-releasing peptide, which functions as both a true hormone and as a neuropeptide. Others may function as hormones and exert trophic effects, as is the case for gastrin. Furthermore, a specific nerve terminal may produce several neuropeptides. Interestingly, some of these peptides are also found in tissue extracts outside the gastrointestinal tract (neurotensin and somatostatin). Obviously, this newly recognized complexity of intestinal peptide function has made classification of gastrointestinal hormones and peptides much more difficult in the current era of gastroenterology. The evolution of cell and molecular biology has forced scientists to revise their understanding of gastrointestinal peptides, as proposed by Rehfeld (6).

Until recently gut peptides were classified by their *structural homology*. When this classical method of classifying gut peptides is used, approximately half are classified to be members of eight families based on the presence of amino acid sequences, as shown in Table 7-1. All peptides in a family are thought to have evolved from a single ancestor and to have preserved their tissue-specific expression during evolution. Peptides in the secretin family, for example, include secretin, glucagon, and VIP – all of which are found in the intestinal tract – as well as growth-hormone-releasing hormone and pituitary adenylyl cyclase-activating peptide.

A limitation of using structural homology to classify hormones is that many of the recently identified hormones and peptides are not members of the eight families. In addition, it has been shown that hormone genes can express *multiple phenotypes*. While it was previously thought that one gene encoded one hormone, it is now known that one gene can express several different bioactive peptides. They may do this by several mechanisms, including: alternate splicing of transcripts (calcitonin gene transcription may generate RNAs that encode for calcitonin peptides or CGRPs), processing prohormones to multiple product peptides of differing lengths which are biologically active (the I cell which produces proCCK releases a heterogeneous mixture of CCK products), or by encoding propeptides that contain different but homologous hormones (proglucagon may be processed at the local level to produce true glucagons or in the pancreatic islet cells to glucagon-like peptides I and II). Examples of these latter two events are schematically shown in Figure 7-1.

Many gastrointestinal peptides are *widely expressed* outside the intestine. The gastrin gene, for example, is expressed in the antroduodenal G-cell, as well as in fetal and neonatal pancreas (7), pituitary corticotrophs and melanotrophs (8), and human spermatogenic cells (9). Finally, peptide production is dependent upon *cell-specific prohormone processing* and *cell-specific peptide release*. The description of these activities is beyond the scope of this chapter and the reader is referred to Rehfeld's review (6).

Table 7-1 Gastrointestinal Peptide Families

Gastrin
Gastrin
Cholecystokinin
Secretin

Secretin
Glucagon and glucagons-like peptides
Gastric inhibitory polypeptide
Vasoactive intestinal polypeptide
Peptide histidine isoleucine
Growth hormone releasing hormone
Pituitary adenylyl cyclase-activating peptide

Insulin
Insulin-like growth factor I
Insulin-like growth factor II
Relaxin

Somatostatin
Somatostatin
Corticostatin

PP-fold
Pancreatic polypeptide
Peptide YY
Neuropeptide

Tachykinin
Substance P
Neurokinin A
Neurokinin B

EGF
Epidermal growth factor
Transforming growth factor
Amphiregulin

Ghrelin
Ghrelin
Motilin

PREPROCHOLECYSTOKININ

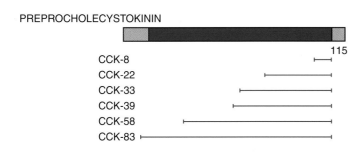

PREPROGLUCAGON

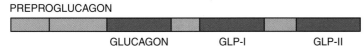

Figure 7-1 Multiple phenotypes of two gut hormones. The CCK gene encodes for a prepropeptide, which is processed to six CCK peptides varying in length from 83 to 8 amino acid residues through differentiated endoproteolytic cleavage. All six peptides have the same C-terminal bioactive octapeptide sequence. The glucagon gene encodes a prepropeptide that through cell-specific endoproteolytic cleavages is processed to either genuine pancreatic glucagons (in pancreatic islet cells) or to glucagon-like peptides I and II (GLP-I, GLP-II). Reproduced from Rehfeld JF. Gastrointestinal hormone, an overview. Horm Metab Res 2004; 36:735–741.

THE ENTERIC NERVOUS SYSTEM

The autonomic nervous system consists of the sympathetic, parasympathetic, and enteric nervous systems (ENS). The enteric nervous system is composed of nerves whose cell bodies lie within the gastrointestinal tract in numbers that are similar to those found in the spinal cord (10). Although considered to be similar to the sympathetic and parasympathetic nervous systems, the ENS is unique. Unlike the sympathetic and parasympathetic systems, which are directly under CNS control, the ENS functions independently of the central nervous system. The ultrastructure of the ENS differs from that of the sympathetic and parasympathetic systems, in that enteric neurons are supported by glia rather than Schwann cells and enteric neurons lack internal collagen (11). The vast network of the ENS is far more complex than those of the sympathetic or parasympathetic systems, as it is composed of numerous functional types of neurons with complex networks of connection, as will be detailed below. The ENS mediates motility as well as mucosal secretion and transport, and local blood flow. Investigation and physiology of the ENS has focused on two major areas: the migration and establishment of the major structures of the ENS and the function of the vast network at the level of the gut. Those two areas will be reviewed separately.

The ENS is formed when the gut is colonized by neural crest cells. The bulk of the cells migrate from the vagal region of the neural crest to colonize the entire gut in a rostral to caudal progression, but smaller numbers migrate from the sacral crest to colonize the postumbilical bowel and from the truncal crest to colonize the esophagus and stomach. These cells represent a heterogeneous population, and they evolve to their final form both during active migration and after arrival in the gut, depending upon their interactions with signaling factors in the surrounding matrix. Basic molecular and cellular science has recently permitted further understanding of this process, as will be detailed below in the discussion concerning clinical correlates. The final configuration consists of the myenteric (or Auerbach's) plexes, which are larger and more numerous, located between the circular and longitudinal muscle layers and the submucosal (or Meissner's) plexes which are located between the longitudinal and and submucosal layers.

At a local level, the ENS functions in subunits, each composed of intrinsic primary afferent sensory neurons (IPANs), interneurons, and motor neurons (Fig. 7-2) (12). The IPAN must be distinguished from the better-known primary afferent neuron, which has its cell body located in the nodose or dorsal root, and which mediates conscious sensation and pain. The intrinsic primary afferent neuron (whose cell body is located in the myenteric or submucosal plexuses) directs the minute-to-minute control of gastrointestinal function (see Bertrand and Thomas (13) for a more complete review). These neurons may respond to mechanical stimuli such as stretch or luminal chemical content such as pH. These neurons are multipolar and approximately half of them have three or more projections. Projections typically innervate the mucosal epithelium (where they come into contact with enteroendocrine cells), the submucosal or myenteric plexes, or other intrinsic neurons.

Motor neurons are classified as inhibitory, excitatory, or directed to the longitudinal muscle (the two former neuron types are largely directed to circular muscle). Interneurons are further classified as ascending, descending or interneurons. Muscle layers in the gut receive dual innervation by excitatory and inhibitory motor neurons. Acetylcholine is the primary neurotransmitter for excitatory motor neurons, while several substances may serve as cotransmitters for inhibitory motor neurons, including nitric oxide (NO), VIP, ATP, and pituitary adenylyl cyclase-activating peptide.

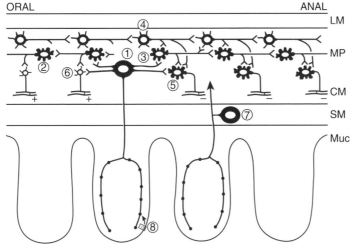

Figure 7-2 A schematic representation of the enteric neural circuitry for motility reflexes. Structures are identified as follows: 1, IPAN with cell body in the myenteric plexus; 2, ascending cholinergic interneuron; 3, descending interneuron in the local reflex pathway; 4, descending interneuron of the migrating motor complex pathway; 5, inhibitory-muscle motor neuron; 6, excitatory muscle motor neuron; 7, IPAN with cell body in the submucosal plexus; 8, enteroendocrine cell that releases excitant of the mucosal endings of IPANs; LM, longitudinal muscle; MP, myenteric plexus; CM, circular muscle; SM, submucosa; Muc, mucosa. Reproduced from Kunze WAA, Furness JB. The enteric nervous system and regulation of intestinal motility. Annu Rev Physiol 1999; 61:117–142.

Extensive mapping of ENS physiology has been performed in guinea pig (10). It is now believed that these structures function as micro-assemblies to form discrete reflex units that overlap one another along the length of the gut. It is estimated that each mm of length of gut contains 2500 nerve cells, 650 of which are IPANs, 400 are inhibitory motor units, 300 excitatory motor neurons, 500 provide input to the longitudinal muscle, 120 are ascending interneurons, and 120 are descending interneurons. Each villus tip is supplied by 65 IPANs. Because of the richness and complexity of this network of single reflex units, each supplying an approximately 2 mm circumferential band of intestine, localized reflex arcs are delivered via motor neurons while simultaneous information is transmitted along the length of the gut via interneurons in order to electrically couple muscle cells in groups.

IPANs and motor neurons interact reciprocally via excitatory ascending interneurons and descending inhibitory interneurons (14). Thus, when one activates IPANs in a small region of the gut, there is a contraction oral to the site of the activation, which is mediated via ascending cholinergic interneurons, and relaxation anally, which is mediated via descending neurons. When relaxation occurs at the anal site, it activates, which then triggers the muscle to contract, Hence, the "peristaltic reflex" perpetuates itself distally along the length of the intestine, pushing luminal contents anally (Fig. 7-3). This basic arrangement is made even more complex, as interneurons may mediate simultaneous transmission to release GI hormones and secretions, elicit vasodilatation (to alter blood flow patterns) and generate the motility patterns characteristic of various regions of the GI tract (Fig. 7-4).

THE ENS AND HOST DEFENSE

Just as the neural network that comprises the ENS contains as many neurons as the CNS, the digestive tract is recognized as the largest lymphoid organ in the body. When foreign antigens gain access to the intestinal mucosa, immunoneural signaling triggers the stereotypic behavior of power propulsion (15). This integrated activity results in copious secretion of water, electrolytes, and mucous as well as intense

PERISTALTIC REFLEX

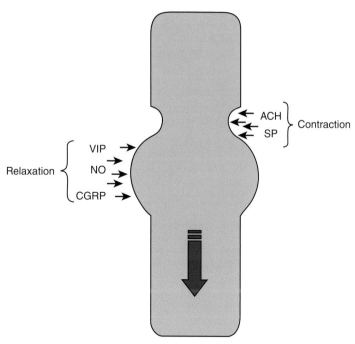

Figure 7-3 Schematic representation of the peristaltic reflex. When the intestinal mucosa is stimulated, it triggers a contractile response proximal to the site and a relaxation response distal to the site of stimulation. The occurrence of relaxation distends the luminal walls, and, in turn triggers another peristaltic reflex such that the area of relaxation will contract and the area distal to it will relax, thus propagating the reflex distally throughout the length of the intestine.

forward motor activity to culminate in the clinical expression of cramping abdominal pain, fecal urgency, and watery diarrhea. This activity literally "flushes" the offending material out of the intestinal tract. As described in the previous chapter, many immune cells are present throughout the length of the intestine. Each of these cells is anatomically associated with elements of the ENS, and the ENS works in concert with the immune system to provide one of the first lines of defense against foreign antigen. It is postulated that inflammatory mediators released by mast cells provide excitatory signals to the ENS, which, in turn, mediates the onset of power propulsion. Key mast cell–ENS mediators include histamine, 5-hydroxytryptamine, adenosine, interleukin-6, interleukin-1B, platelet-activating factor, leukotrienes, prostaglandins, NO, and mast cell proteases. The roles of all of these mediators have been explored extensively in animal models by inducing hypersensitivity to cow milk protein or intestinal parasites. Such work has provided better understanding about pharmacologic therapies for mast-cell-mediated illnesses than range from CNS-mediated anxiety and stress to irritable bowel disease (IBD).

Figure 7-4 Antroduodenal motor activity in a term infant. The upper line represents activity recorded from the antrum, and each successively lower line represents activity recorded from sites located 2.5 cm distally to the one above it. Phasic activity is present in the antrum (designated by the dagger) and it is temporally coordinated with migratory phasic activity in all three duodenal sites (designated by the double dagger). Three other duodenal clusters (designated by the asterisks) fail to migrate. Arrow indicates areas of the recording occupied by artifact caused by movement of the infant. Reproduced from Ittman PI, Amarnath R, Berseth CL. Maturation of antroduodenal motor activity in preterm and term infants. Dig Dis Sci 1992; 37:14–19.

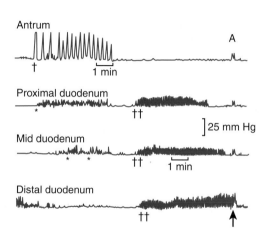

Table 7-2	Genetic Mutations Associated with Hirschsprung's Disease	
Mutation	Phenotype in mouse model	Human chromosome location
SOX10	Distal hind gut aganglionosis	22q13
RET/gdnf/gfrα1	Absence of ganglia in varying length of gut	10q25
RET/ntn/gfrα2	Decreased number of ganglia and decreased ganglia size	
Ednrb/edn3/ece1	Absence of ganglia in hind gut of varying length	1p36.1

Clinical Correlates

ENS Migration

Perhaps the best-studied neonatal intestinal neural abnormality is Hirschsprung's disease. Extensive molecular research of this pathologic condition has provided better understanding of regulation of normal maturation. Hirschsprung's disease is phenotypically characterized by the absence of ganglion cells in the submucosal and myenteric plexuses in the distal gut. It is a polygenic disorder characterized by mutations affecting a number of genes that control tyrosine kinase function and neurotropins that regulate neuronal differentiation, maturation and binding to the tyrosine kinase receptor. Mutations in seven genes may result in Hirschsprung's disease, including SOX10, ret, gdnf, ntn, ednrb, edn3, and ece1 (for more extensive reviews of this topic see Newgreen, DeGiorgio and co-workers: 16–18). Table 7-2 lists the gene mutations that are known to result in Hirschsprung's disease in humans. SOX10, a transcription factor, is expressed by neural crest cells before and during colonization of the gut. Neural crest cells deficient in SOX10 die during migration and the ENS fails to develop. If homozygotic, this mutation results in death in utero; however, heterozygotic mutation results in distal gut aganglionosis. Approximately half of infants with familial cases of Hirschsprung's disease and 20% of those with nonfamilial disease have mutations of RET-proto-oncogene or genes encoding for its ligands, glial-derived neurotrophic factor (GDNF) and neuroturin (NTN). The RET signaling pathway promotes survival, proliferation, and differentiation of neural crest cells. Other infants with Hirschsprung's disease have mutations in another signaling pathway with endothelin-3 (END3) and the endothelin-3 receptor (EDNRB) and endothelin-converting enzyme (ECE1).

Other intestinal neuronal dysplasias (INDB) are also considered to be phenotypic expressions of failure of normal migration and/or differentiation. While infants with Hirschsprung's disease are typically diagnosed during the neonatal period, infants with dysplasias typically present during infancy or early childhood with constipation and slowed intestinal transit time (16). Patients with type A, which is rare, display immaturity or hypoplasia of the ENS sympathetic nerves. Type B is associated with a variety of microscopic findings, including hyperganglionosis, enlarged ganglia, and ectopic ganglia (18). Patients with multiple endocrine neoplasia type 2B(MEN2B), a dominantly inherited neuroendocrine disorder, often have mutations of the RET oncogene.

Hirschsprung's disease was originally thought to be limited to the ENS. However, Hirschsprung's disease may also co-exist with autonomic dysfunction (19) or present as part of a syndrome such as MEN, Waardeberg Syndrome, or Haddad Syndrome (with central hypoventilation). As many as 28% of patients with Hirschsprung's disease also have neurological, genitourinary, skeletal, or cardiovascular anomalies (20). For this reason, Hirschsprung's disease is now considered to be included in the broader diagnostic category of neurocristopathies (21).

ENS Function

It is well known that stooling patterns of infants differ from those of toddlers, children, and adults. Breast-fed infants stool more frequently than formula-fed infants, and stooling occurs more frequently in all infants up to age 18–24 months. Khen et al. have shown that neurotransmitter function/expression matures throughout gestation and infancy, culminating in an adult-like expression by 2–3 years (22) This is particularly true for NO, one of the primary inhibitory mediators for the ENS. Interestingly, genetic defects that result in loss of NO, VIP, and somatostatin have been described in dysfunction of sphincteric regions, including achalasia and congential hypertrophic pyloric stenosis (23). Others have also demonstrated a paucity of Interstitial Cells of Cajal (ICC) in the tissues from these infants (24). Because ethical constraints have limited the study of tissues from age-matched control infants, it is not known whether these ENS patterns among infants with congenital hypertrophic pyloric stenosis reflect simply normal maturation or a delay in normal patterns.

Descriptive studies such as these have given neonatologists more insight into the use of prokinetics. Erythromycin, for example, which binds to motilin receptors, appears to trigger migrating motor complexes and increase the amplitude of motor contractions in stomach and intestine in infants whose gestational ages exceed 32 weeks, but this effect is not seen in infants who are more immature (25). Others have reported the efficacy of metoclopramide (26), a dopamine antagonist. Vagal modulation of gastric emptying is not fully present in some preterm infants (27) and drugs such as ophthalmics used for routine eye exams for retinopathy of prematurity may delay gastric emptying and cause transient feeding difficulties (28).

Feeding Intolerance

Although may neonatologists are now attempting to introduce enteral feedings within a few days after birth, approximately half of preterm infants are delayed in achieving full enteral feeding volumes beyond 2 weeks of life. The cause of this delay is rarely related to immaturity of digestion or absorption of nutrients, but rather is related to immaturity of motor function, expressed as delayed gastric emptying, prolonged intestinal transit, abdominal distension, and delayed passage of meconium. Ethical constraints limit the ability to perform full-thickness biopsies of gastrointestinal tissue, but studies using manometric and impedance techniques to assess motor function have shown that motor patterns are immature in the preterm antrum, upper small intestine, and colorectum. Moreover, evaluation of tissues from stillborn fetuses, preterm infants, and infants shows that acquisition of adult-like neurotransmission is delayed until 1–2 years after birth (22).

Although true gastrointestinal hormones may modulate gastrointestinal motor function in the adult, the plasma concentrations of many hormones in preterm infants are similar to those of term infants and older children. Thus, delay in the maturation of motor function in the preterm infant appears to largely reflect delay in maturation of neural regulation. Interestingly, local feedback of gastric emptying by hormone and/or local neural reflexes appears to be intact. For example, gastric emptying in the preterm infant is slowed when increased fat, acid, or osmotic density reaches the duodenum, just as is the case for adults. Similarly, nutrients that are hypo- or hyper-osmotic slow gastric emptying in the preterm infant, just as in adults. The maturation of regulation of motor function can be triggered precociously by giving small feedings to the preterm infant (29). However, there is no dose-response effect, in that larger feeding volumes do not enhance faster maturation than small feedings (30). Larger feedings cause the release of more gastrointestinal hormones, but motor function is not associated with higher plasma concentrations of hormones (30).

The practice of giving prokinetic drugs to preterm infants should be approached with caution for several reasons. First, depending upon the prokinetic drug, these agents bind to different receptor sites. It is not yet known which specific aspects of neurotransmission are abnormal in preterm infants, or if the specific site of immaturity varies among infants. Preterm infants who are less than 32 weeks gestation fail to respond to erythromycin (25); no other age-dependent studies have been performed in preterm infants. Secondly, it is not yet known whether the preterm gut benefits from these agents. Investigators have described the protective effect of the "ileal break" and the "duodenal brake," which slow the transit of intraluminal contents until more complete absorption of nutrients has occurred "downstream." One could speculate that prokinetic drugs would remove these protective braking mechanisms and permit the intraluminal contents to overwhelm the immature gastrointestinal tract. Thirdly, the side-effects of these agents are not fully understood. For example, in 25% of adults, chronic use of metoclopramide causes tardive dyskinesia. Although neonatologists give this drug to preterm infants who are attempting to achieve full oral feeding skills, it is not yet known whether this drug interferes with achievement of independent oral feeding skills.

A specific hormonal phenomenon that has been observed is the occurrence of hypergastrinemia in approximately 50% of infants who have short-bowel syndrome (31). Gastric hypersecretion results in hyperacidity which impairs micelle formation, decreases intraluminal digestion of proteins and complex carbohydrates, inactivates pancreatic lipase, and causes ulceration in the duodenum or upper small intestine. These limitations in digestion can result in increased intraluminal volume and osmotic load and promote diarrhea (31). These infants require treatment with H_2 blockers or proton pump inhibitors.

Gastroesophageal Reflux

Most neonatologists consider gastroesophageal reflux (GER) to consist of a constellation of symptoms that may include spitting, apnea, and/or behavioral activities such as facial grimacing and back arching. To the pediatric gastroenterologist, GER refers to the *physiologic* activity of permitting air to escape from the stomach with transient bathing of the distal esophagus with the acidic material that comprises the gastric bubble when it bursts in the distal esophagus. The pediatric gastroenterologist considers gastroesophageal reflux *disease* (GERD) to be a *pathologic* condition, wherein the presence of chronic prolonged acidic material in the distal esophagus causes erosion of the esophageal mucosa. Many neonatologists attempt to treat GER, while pediatric gastroenterologists prefer to limit treatment to infants who have GERD. Motor function in this region of the preterm GI tract is ubiquitously less mature than that of the term infant or older child, including esophageal peristalsis and gastric emptying (32). Interestingly, lower esophageal sphincter function is similar to that seen in an adult. As in the adult, the presence of transient lower esophageal sphincter relaxations (TLESRs) is associated with episodes of reflux of acidic material into the distal esophagus (33). No drug is currently approved for use by the FDA to reduce the occurrence of TLESRs. Thus, it should be no surprise that neonatologists, pediatric gastroenterologists, and adult gastroenterologists find few prokinetic drugs to be consistently, fully efficacious in treating symptoms of GER or GERD. However, these drugs may increase lower esophageal sphincter pressure and gastric emptying. Interestingly, H_2 blockers and proton pump inhibitors may relieve some – but not all – symptoms.

REFERENCES

1. Yang Q, Bermingham NA, Finegold MJ, Zogbi HY. Requirement of Math 1 for secretory cell lineage commitment in the mouse intestine. Science 2001; 294:2151–2155.

2. Jenny M, Uhl C, Roche C, et al. Neurogenin 3 is differentially required for endocrine cell fate specification in the intestinal and gastreic epithelium. EMBO J 2002; 21:6338–6347.

3. Sosa-Pineda B, Chowdhury K, Torres M, et al. The Pax4 gene is essential for differentiation of insulin-producing beta cells in the mammalian pancreas. Nature 1997; 386:399–401.

4. Larsson LI, St-Onge L, Hougaard DM, et al. Pax 4 and 6 regulate gastrointestinal endocrine cell development. Mechanism of Development 1998; 79:153–159.

5. Walsh JH. Gastrointestinal peptide hormones. In: Sleisenger MH, Fordtran JS, eds., Gastrointestinal Disease, 4th edn. Philadelphia: WB Saunders; 1989: 90–92.

6. Rehfeld JF. Gastrointestinal hormones, an overview. Horm Metab Res 2004; 92:735–741.

7. Larsson L-I, Rehfeld JF, Hakanson R, et al. Pancreatic gastrin in foetal and neonatal rats. Nature 1976; 262:609–610.

8. Larrson L-I, Rehfeld JF. Pituitary gastrins occur in corticotrophs and melanotrophs. Science 1981; 213:768–770.

9. Schalling M, Persson H, Pelto-Huikko M, et al. Expression and localization of gastrin mRNA and peptides in human spermatogenic cells. J Clin Invest 1990; 86:660–669.

10. Kunze WAA, Furness JB. The enteric nervous system and regulation of intestinal motility. Annu Rev Physiol 1999; 61:117–142.

11. Gershon MD, Kirchgessner AL, Wade PR. Functional anatomy of the enteric nervous system. In: Johnson LR, Alpers DH, Jacobson ED, Walsh JH, eds., Physiology of the gastrointestinal tract. New York: Raven Press; 1994: 381–422.

12. Costa M, Brookes SJH, Hennig GW. Anatomy and physiology of the enteric nervous system. Gut 2000; 47(Suppl IV):iv15–iv19.

13. Bertrand PP, Thomas EA. Multiple levels of sensory integration in the intrinsic sensory neurons of the enteric nervous system. Clin Exp Pharmacol Physiol 2004; 31:745–755.

14. Waterman SA, Tonini M, Costa M. The role of ascending excitatory and descending inhibitory pathways in peristalsis in the isolated guinea-pig small intestine. J Physiol 1994; 481:223–232.

15. Wood JD. Enteric neuroimmunophysiology and pathophysiology. Gastroenterology 2004; 127:635–657.

16. Newgreen D, Young HM. Enteric nervous system: development and developmental disturbances- Part 1. Pediatr Dev Pathol 2002; 5:224–247.

17. Newgreen D, Young HM. Enteric nervous system: development and developmental disturbances- Part 2. Pediatr Dev Pathol 2002; 5:329–349.

18. DeGeorgio R, Camilleri M. Human enteric neuropathies: morphology and molecular pathology. Neurogastroenterol Motil 2004; 16:515–531.

19. Staiano A, Santoro L, DeMarco R, et al. Autonomic dysfunction in children with Hirschsprung's disease. Dig Dis Sci 1999; 44:960–965.

20. Sarioglu A, Tanyel FC, Buyukpamukcu N, Hicsonmez A. Hirschsprung-associated congenital anomalies. Eur J Pediatr J Surg 1997; 7:331–337.

21. Shahar E, Shinawi M. Neurocristopathies presenting with neurologic abnormalities associated with Hirschsprung's disease. Pediatr Neurol 2003; 28:385–391.

22. Khen N, Jaubert F, Sauvat F, et al. Fetal intestinal obstruction induces alternation of enteric nervous system development in human intestinal atresia. Pediatr Res 0, 2004; 56:975–984.

23. Saur D, Seidler B, Paehge H, et al. Complex regulation of human neuronal nitric-oxide synthase exon 1c gene transcription. Essential role of Sp and ANF family members of transcription factors. J Biol Chem 2002; 277:25789–25814.

24. Vanderwinden JM, Liu H, De Laet MH, Vanderhaeghen JJ. Study of the interstitial cells of Cajal in infantile hypertrophic pyloric stenosis. Gastroenterology 1996; 111:279–288.

25. Jadcherla SR, Berseth CL. Effect of erythromycin on gastroduodenal contractile activity in developing neonates. J Pediatr Gastroenterol Nutr 2002; 34:16–22.

26. Sankaran K, Yeboah E, Bingham WT, Ninan A. Use of metoclopramide in preterm infants. Dev Pharmacol Ther 1982; 5:114–119.

27. AlTawil Y, Klee G, Berseth CL. Extrinsic neural regulation of antroduodenal motor activity in preterm infants. Dig Dis Sci 2002; 47:2657–2663.

28. Bonthala S, Musgrave V, Sparks J, Berseth CL. Mydriatics slow gastric emptying in preterm infants. J Pediatr 2000; 137:327–330.

29. Berseth CL. Early feedings induce functional maturation of preterm small intestine. J Pediatr 1992; 120:947–953.

30. Berseth CL, Bisquera JA, Paje VU. Prolonging small feeding volumes early in life decreases the incidence of NEC in very low birth weight infants. Pediatrics 2003; 111:529–534.

31. Ricketts RR. Surgical treatment of necrotizing enterocolitis and the short bowel syndrome. Clin Perinatol 1994; 21:356–387.

32. Omari TI, Miki K, Fraser R, et al. Esophageal body and lower esophageal sphincter function in healthy premature infants. Gastroenterol 1995; 109:1757–1764.

33. Omari TI, Barnett C, Snel A, et al. Mechanisms of gastroesophageal reflux in healthy premature infants. J Pediatr 1998; 33:650–654.

Chapter 8

Trophic Factors in the Neonatal Gastrointestinal Tract

Michael Janeczko, MD • Douglas G. Burrin, PhD

What is the Nature of Gut Growth?
Gut Adaptation in the Perinatal Period
How Soon and How Much to Feed Enterally?
What is the Trophic Role of Breast Milk vs. Formula?
Are there Key Nutrients to Provide Enterally?
What are the Key Gut Hormone and Growth Factors?

WHAT IS THE NATURE OF GUT GROWTH?

The neonatal period is a highly dynamic period of gastrointestinal growth and functional development. In the case of the intestine, this includes the development of swallowing and mature motility patterns (1), tissue vascular hemodynamics (2), and nutrient transporters (3). Together these physiological changes during the fetal-neonatal period facilitate the transition from placental nutrient assimilation to oral ingestion via the gastrointestinal tract. Intestinal epithelial growth at the tissue and cellular level is characterized by increased cell numbers, i.e. hyperplasia, and increased cellular size, i.e. hypertrophy. Intestinal growth also involves expansion of the number and size of crypt and villus units (4). An important aspect of growth in the gut is the continual proliferation, migration and loss of epithelial cells along the mucosal surface. In the intestine, this process involves four cell lineages (absorptive enterocyte, goblet, Paneth, endocrine) that differentiate from one pluripotent stem cell located in the crypt. Growth is also characterized by structural and functional changes in the innervation and vascularization within the gut. Gastrointestinal growth involves the proliferation, growth and development of cells and structures, including blood vessels, endothelial cells, smooth muscle cells, submucosal and myenteric nerves. The normal growth and development of the gastrointestinal tract is critical to normal development of the neonate, as the gut is not only a central organ for nutrient digestion and absorption, but also is a major environmental interface for innate immune function and nutrient sensing and neuroendocrine function between the gut and brain. The timing and characteristics of neonatal GI growth are exquisitely coordinated with the events of birth and weaning to ensure survival of the organism. The regulation of neonatal GI growth is complex and involves multiple and often redundant factors. Among these factors are intrinsic cell programs or signals arising from gene expression, as well as extracellular signals, such as peptide growth factors, hormones, nutrients, and microbes, which originate from surrounding cells, the circulation and the gut lumen.

GUT ADAPTATION IN THE PERINATAL PERIOD

Normal gastrointestinal growth and development during fetal life is critical to facilitate the successful adaptation from nutritional support via the umbilical circulation to that of oral ingestion of breast-milk. An increase in circulating fetal glucocorticoid concentration just prior to and during vaginal birth is an important trigger of gut functional development (5). In the neonatal period, growth of the GI tract is influenced by multiple physiological factors that serve to prepare the developing neonate for separation from maternal nutritional support (i.e. weaning). In addition, a number of important environmental cues signal adaptive changes in GI function to facilitate post-weaning survival. For example, the microbial colonization of the gut may serve to prime intestinal lymphoid cell development for normal innate immune function (6, 7). During these processes, extracellular signals, such as peptide growth factors, are often considered to be the major trophic factors that influence growth. However, the term trophic often pertains to nutrition and, in the case of the gut, nutrients present in amniotic fluid and breast milk are a major trophic influence. There are numerous extracellular trophic signals, including foods, nutrients, peptide growth factors, gut peptide hormones, steroid and thyroid hormones, microbes, neural inputs. The cells within fetal and neonatal GI tract are influenced by extracellular signals from multiple sources, including (i) blood-borne factors in the circulation such as hormones that act via endocrine mechanisms, (ii) luminal factors derived from amniotic fluid, mammary secretions or microbes, and (iii) local factors secreted via autocrine or paracrine mechanisms from surrounding cells.

The fact that many infants are born prematurely creates major problems for their adaptation to normal oral feeding and enteral nutrition. These problems are often manifested clinically as feeding intolerance, diarrhea, sepsis and necrotizing enterocolitis. These problems are linked with immature gastroduodenal motor function, hemodynamic regulation, nutrient malabsorption and mucosal immunity. Thus, the challenge for neonatologists and pediatric gastroenterologists is to provide the appropriate combination of clinical support, nutritional or otherwise, to stimulate the normal growth and development of these organs systems and physiological functions.

HOW SOON AND HOW MUCH TO FEED ENTERALLY?

Enteral nutrition is perhaps the most potent trophic stimulus of GI tract growth. The diet acts directly by supplying nutrients for growth and oxidative metabolism of the mucosal epithelial cells, but it also acts indirectly by triggering the release of local growth factors, gut hormones and activating neural pathways. Neonatal starvation causes reduced gut tissue mass, reduced mucosal surface area and generalized increased catabolism and decreased protein synthesis (8, 9). Evidence from numerous animal studies and some in humans shows that enteral nutrition is critical to maintain normal intestinal growth and development. The enteral nutrient stimulation of gut growth begins in the late-gestation fetus with the onset of amniotic fluid swallowing. Studies in fetal sheep and pigs have shown that preventing amniotic fluid swallowing by esophageal ligation suppresses intestinal growth (5, 10). In most infants, enteral feeding of breast milk or formula soon after birth continues to stimulate the growth and adaptive development of the gastrointestinal tract. However, premature infants normally receive a majority of their nutrition parenterally after birth due to poor feeding tolerance. Studies in neonatal pigs show that total parenteral nutrition (TPN) leads to significantly reduced growth and atrophy of the intestinal mucosa, marked by reduced cell proliferation, villus height and protein synthesis and increased apoptosis (11).

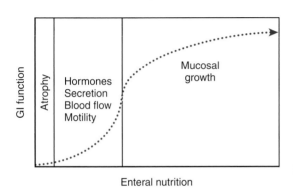

Figure 8-1 Illustration showing the relationship between enteral nutrition and GI function.

Additional studies with neonatal animals and human infants suggest that the lack of enteral nutrition is also associated with reduced secretion of many gut peptide hormones and growth factors and this may be linked to reduced gut functional development during TPN (12, 13).

Therefore, in premature infants the question is how soon and how much to feed enterally. A number of clinical studies have demonstrated that the practice of minimal enteral feeding or trophic feeding can enhance gastrointestinal motility and other functions (Fig. 8-1). The introduction of minimal enteral nutrition usually starts at birth at a daily intake of ~25 mL/kg, an amount that is insufficient for the total nutrient needs of the infant. Although meta-analysis shows that minimal enteral nutrition does reduce time to full feeding and length of hospital stay, the impact on the overall health and disease risk of premature infants is yet to be established (14). There is evidence that advancement of enteral feeding too rapid (by more than 20 mL/kg per day) can increase the risk of necrotizing enterocolitis (15). An underlying question in most of these clinical studies is how the enteral feeding level affects the growth, development and function of the gut. Recent clinical studies in premature infants indicated that the enteral feeding is positively linked to intestinal mucosal growth, but that lactose digestion is more closely correlated to lactase activity and gestational age (16, 17). Studies in piglets suggest that enteral nutrition is critical to maintain normal lactose digestion and glucose absorption (18). Studies in neonatal piglets suggest that an enteral intake of at least 40% of the total nutrient intake is necessary to maintain normal growth, which would imply that minimal enteral nutrition may not be trophic to gut mucosa (11). An additional consideration is whether to provide enteral nutrition orally, intragastrically, intraduodenally, as a bolus, or continuously. Evidence from clinical studies is equivocal as to the clinical outcome (19, 20). Studies in piglets suggest that, in comparison with continuous feeding, bolus feeding resulted in increased gut growth (21); however, this was not linked to secretion of trophic gut peptides (22).

WHAT IS THE TROPHIC ROLE OF BREAST MILK VS. FORMULA?

The relative significance of milk-borne trophic factors has been one of the most intensely studied areas of pediatric nutrition and gastroenterology (23–26). Several trophic peptide growth factors are present in breast milk, but not in infant formulas, and have been implicated in the beneficial outcomes of breast-fed infants, particularly reduced incidence of necrotizing enterocolitis and sepsis. Studies conducted in neonatal animals have confirmed the idea that breast milk has a greater trophic effect on the gastrointestinal tract than formula, as measured by typical indices of structural and cellular growth. However, the most significant advantage of breast milk on the neonatal intestine may not be related to growth, but rather mucosal barrier and immune function. There is considerable evidence suggesting that immunoprotective factors in breast milk (e.g. secretory IgA, lactoferrin, oligosaccharides) act to modulate mucosal immune function and bacterial colonization, thereby limiting the incidence of infection, sepsis, and necrotizing enterocolitis (27–30). Many of the trophic factors in milk are polypeptides that survive digestion, retain their biological activity, and interact with specific receptors present on the mucosal epithelium of neonates. A number of studies have shown that these milk-borne growth factors stimulate neonatal intestinal growth when given in purified and recombinant forms either orally or systemically. Moreover, in preterm neonates the presence of increased intestinal permeability could facilitate the intestinal absorption of milk-borne peptide growth factors; however, there are limited instances where this process has been found to be physiologically significant.

ARE THERE KEY NUTRIENTS TO PROVIDE ENTERALLY?

Despite the important functional effect of growth factors and immunological factors in human milk, the trophic stimulus on the neonatal intestine can be attributed to macronutrient content as much as to peptide growth factors. The chemical form and nutrient composition also influence the impact of enteral nutrition on GI growth and function (9, 12). Some studies indicate that enteral nutrition in a complex, polymeric form is more trophic to the small intestine than in a simpler, elemental form, yet a recent study in piglets refutes this idea (31). The dietary restriction of protein and energy generally suppresses gut growth and mucosal immune function. The enteral infusion of individual nutrients, by themselves, can have a trophic stimulus on the gut if administered in a sufficiently large amount. Cells within the gut are capable of responding to extracellular concentrations of nutrients directly via intracellular signaling pathways, including mammalian target of rapamycin (mTOR), that mediate downstream cellular functions, such as cell proliferation, protein synthesis and apoptosis (Fig. 8-2). However, there are a number of specific nutrients that have trophic actions when supplemented to a complete diet; among these are glutamine, arginine, nucleotides, and long-chain

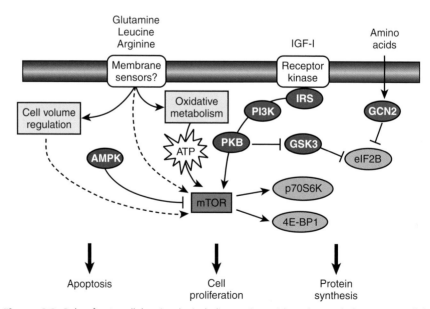

Figure 8-2 Role of extracellular signals, including amino acids and growth factors, on cellular signaling pathways that mediate cellular growth.

polyunsaturated fatty acids (LC-PUFA). In the past two decades, evidence of the metabolic and cellular effects of glutamine and arginine has prompted numerous studies aimed at evaluating the efficacy of their supplementation in clinical situations. This has spawned the concept of immunonutrition and the commercial introduction of immune-enhancing enteral diets that contain immune-enhancing nutrients, including arginine, glutamine, nucleotides, and n–3 long-chain fatty acids. Numerous clinical trials and meta-analysis of immune-enhancing diets with largely adult critical-care patients have shown reduced infectious complications, yet the relative role of specific immunonutrients remains to be established.

Glutamine

Glutamine is a key intestinal oxidative fuel that is extensively metabolized and oxidized to CO_2 by intestinal tissues when fed either enterally or parenterally (12, 32, 33) (Fig. 8-3). However, several studies have shown that enteral and parenteral glutamine also stimulates intestinal growth and enhances function in healthy and diseased conditions (34–36). Evidence from clinical studies with premature infants has also suggested that enteral glutamine may reduce infectious morbidity (37, 38). Further studies are warranted to determine whether enteral glutamine enhances gut immune function and whether this translates to reduced infectious morbidity. Studies in rodents indicate that enteral glutamine stimulates intestinal blood flow, yet a recent clinical study found no effect of glutamine on superior mesenteric arterial flow (39, 40). Studies in cultured intestinal epithelial cells indicate that glutamine, but not other non-essential amino acids, specifically stimulates cell proliferation, activates mitogenic intracellular signaling pathways, and may be a critical precursor for glucosamine, pyrimidine and arginine synthesis (41–45).

Arginine

Arginine is an essential amino acid for neonates and may be an especially important substrate for maintenance of intestinal nitric oxide synthesis, blood flow, and

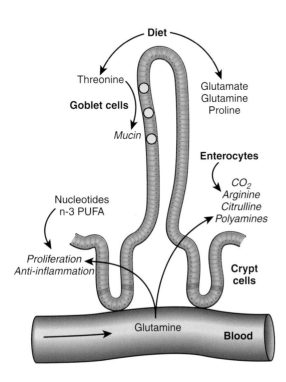

Figure 8-3 Functional roles of dietary nutrients in the intestinal mucosa.

immune function. L-Arginine is a precursor for the synthesis of nitric oxide, and nitric oxide plays a key role in regulating intestinal blood flow (46). A recent study in pigs demonstrates that arginine administered enterally or parenterally increases NO production in the GI tract (47). Arginine has also been shown to affect the molecular mechanisms of cell metabolism and growth. These include the downstream targets of mTOR, an amino-acid responsive serine/threonine kinase that affects cell growth. Specifically, arginine was shown to affect the phosphorylation of p70S6 kinase and 4E-BP-1, important components in the regulation of cell growth (48). Despite these findings, it is uncertain whether arginine can affect intestinal epithelial proliferation directly, but arginine has been shown to stimulate intestinal cell migration (49). Another study showed that arginine was able to re-epithelialize porcine ileal mucosa via iNOS, but only in the presence of serum (50).

A major cause of mortality and morbidity in preterm infants is necrotizing enterocolitis (NEC). The etiology of NEC has not been firmly established, but is associated with prematurity, enteral formula feeding, and small-bowel bacterial colonization. Additional, contributing factors thought to play a role in NEC are intestinal ischemia, proinflammatory stimulation, and an immature mucosal immune-barrier function. Arginine supplementation is a particularly attractive strategy to prevent the incidence of neonatal NEC because it is the immediate precursor for nitric oxide, which acts as a major vasodilator and participates in the inflammatory response, and because arginine also functions to augment B- and T-lymphocyte function. Some studies have shown that enteral arginine supplementation can reduce the incidence of NEC in neonatal infants and piglets (51, 52). A prospective study of 152 premature infants showed a significant reduction in the incidence of NEC in the group with arginine-supplemented enteral feeds. The study also showed that plasma arginine concentrations were lower in both groups at the time of diagnosis of NEC. Commercially available enteral formulas designed to enhance immune function in critically ill and surgical patients contain arginine, yet the safety and efficacy of these diets in infants are untested. Further studies are needed to characterize the impact of enteral arginine on intestinal blood flow, NO production, mucosal growth and immune function in neonatal infants and animal models.

Other nonessential amino acids, including glutamate, proline and citrulline, may have stimulatory actions on the gut, because they are precursors for glutamine and arginine synthesis (32, 53). This may be especially important in infants after small-bowel resection, since studies in rodents indicate that arginine is conditionally essential under these conditions due to the loss of intestinal citrulline production (54, 55). Threonine is also a key nutrient for the intestinal synthesis of threonine-rich mucins by goblet cells. Studies in piglets have shown that the gut extracts ~80% of the enteral threonine for intestinal mucosal protein synthesis (56). The sulfur-containing amino acids methionine and cysteine also may have important metabolic roles in maintaining antioxidant function in the neonatal intestine, which is exposed to increased oxidative stress. Methionine is metabolized via transsulfuration to cysteine, which is a precursor of glutathione, a critical antioxidant in the gut. Recent piglet studies indicate that intestinal metabolism accounts for ~30% of the daily methionine requirement (57).

Nucleotides

Nucleotides are ubiquitous, low-molecular-weight, intracellular compounds that are integral to numerous biochemical processes, and are especially important as precursors for nucleic acid synthesis in rapidly dividing cells, such as epithelial and lymphoid cells in the mucosa (58). Nucleotides consist of a purine or pyrimidine base, which can be synthesized within cells de novo from glutamine, aspartic acid, glycine, formate, and carbon dioxide as precursors. Human milk is an excellent source of dietary nucleotides for infants during the first months of life, and its nucleotide content is markedly higher than that of cow's milk and most infant formulas, although some commercial infant formulas contain added nucleotides. Numerous reports show that dietary supplementation with nucleosides, nucleotides, or nucleic acids supports small-intestinal mucosal function, growth and morphology. In an experimental short gut model, rats fed a diet containing supplemental orotate and uracil showed increased villus height when compared with rats fed a standard diet, demonstrating a possible role for nucleotides in adaptive gut growth (59). Clinical studies in term and preterm infants also showed that feeding nucleotide-supplemented formula increased superior mesenteric artery blood flow (60, 61).

n–3 PUFA

As with nucleotides, there is considerable interest in dietary long-chain fatty acids (LCFAs), because breast milk generally contains higher concentrations of n–3 LC-PUFAs than in formulas; many infant formulas are now formulated with these fatty acids. Interest in the n–3 LC-PUFAs or omega–3 fatty acids, particularly docosahexanoic acid (DHA), eicosapentaenoic acid (EPA) and arachidonic acid (AA), stems from studies showing that dietary supplementation can lower the incidence and inflammatory effects of NEC in neonatal infants and rats (62). There is limited information regarding the intestinal trophic effects of either n–3 LC-PUFA or other LCFA in developing animals. However, a series of studies have demonstrated that n–3 LC-PUFAs enhance intestinal adaptation after small-bowel resection, and their effects were greater than those of less-saturated oils; they also found that medium-chain triglycerides are less trophic than long-chain triglycerides (12). In contrast, studies with neonatal piglets indicated that the LCFA oleic acid can cause significant mucosal injury and increased permeability, and that this effect is more severe in newborn than in 1-month-old piglets (63).

WHAT ARE THE KEY GUT HORMONE AND GROWTH FACTORS?

Gut Hormones

The gut is one of the largest endocrine organs in the body and secretes numerous peptide hormones from specialized endocrine cells that act as chemical sensors that respond to the composition and amount of luminal nutrients (64) (Fig. 8-4). In many cases, these hormones function as neuroendocrine factors that activate extrinsic and intrinsic nerves, which mediate secretory and motor reflexes in the gastrointestinal tract. Some of the gut hormones that have been implicated in the stimulation of trophic functional response to minimal enteral nutrition include gastrin, cholecystokinin (CCK), and peptide YY (PYY) (13). Gastrin is secreted from the G-cells within the antrum of the stomach, and acts primarily to stimulate proliferation of parietal and enterochromaffin-like cells within the gastric mucosa (65). Cholecystokinin is expressed in endocrine cells of the gut and in neurons within the gut and brain, while its primary target tissues are the pancreas and gallbladder. CCK stimulates pancreatic growth and cell proliferation, and these trophic effects have been attributed exclusively to interaction via the CCK-A receptor. The neonate exhibits hypergastrinemia and comparatively high gastric pH, yet gastrin secretion is induced by feeding (13). The trophic effects of gastrin are most evident in the stomach and are mediated by increased ODC activity and cell proliferation (66). Peptide YY (PYY) is secreted from enteroendocrine L

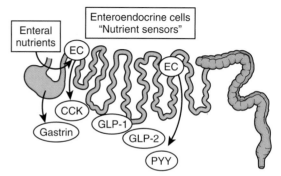

- Acid secretion
- Gastroduodenal motility
- Exocrine pancreas (enzymes)
- Endocrine pancreas (insulin)
- Mucosal blood flow
- Cell proliferation/survival

Enteral nutrients

Enteroendocrine cells "Nutrient sensors"

EC

EC

CCK

GLP-1

Gastrin

GLP-2

PYY

Figure 8-4 Role of enteroendocrine cells (EC) as nutrient sensors in the neonatal gastrointestinal tract.

cell and stimulates gut growth in developing rats (12). Apart from the effects on gastrointestinal tissue growth, CCK and PYY may be more important in the maturation and development of gastroduodenal motor and secretory function, which is critical for premature infants. CCK is a key hormone involved in pancreatic and biliary section and has been examined as a possible treatment for TPN-induced cholestasis; however, a recent clinical study suggested that CCK was ineffective (67, 68)

Glucagon-like peptide 2 (GLP-2) is a gut peptide that recently has gained considerable attention as an intestinal trophic factor (69). GLP-2, like PYY, is secreted by enteroendocrine L cells in response to enteral nutrition and secretion appears to be developmentally upregulated in late gestation (70). GLP-2 has significant trophic effects on the neonatal small intestine that are mediated by increased cell proliferation, protein synthesis, blood flow, and glucose transport (71, 72). Moreover, GLP-2 increased SMA blood flow without increasing systemic blood pressure or affecting brain blood flow in neonatal piglets, suggesting that its effects occur locally (73). GLP-2 treatment also has been shown to reduce proinflammatory cytokines and restore intestinal structure in animal models of GLP-2 inflammatory bowel disease and enteritis (69). GLP-2 may hold therapeutic potential, since it has been approved as an Orphan Drug and shown recently to improve gut function in adult patients with short-bowel syndrome (74, 75).

Tissue Growth Factors

Another class of molecules that may be key growth factors for the neonatal gut can be generally categorized as polypeptides that are secreted locally and act via a paracrine or autocrine mechanism to affect cellular growth and function (Table 8-1). Several of these growth factors are present in the blood, GI secretions and amniotic fluid and thus may act via endocrine mechanism, e.g. insulin-like growth factor I. More importantly, however, many of these growth factors are present in breast milk and thought to influence neonatal gut growth (12, 25, 76, 77). Among the most well-known of these is epidermal growth factor (EGF), a member of a family of peptides which includes transforming growth factor-α, heparin-binding EGF (HB-EGF), amphiregulin, epiregulin, betacellulin, neuregulin (78). Most of the EGF family peptides are trophic to the gut, stimulating cell proliferation and suppressing apoptosis; however, they also modulate a number of other physiological functions, including enhanced tooth eruption, decreased gastric acid secretion, increased mucus secretion and gastric blood flow, reduced gastric

Table 8-1	Tissue Growth Factors Present in Breast Milk and Produced Locally in Intestinal Mucosal Tissue

EGF
Intestinal cell growth
Stimulation of brush border enzymes
Stimulation of angiogenesis
Prevention of NEC

HB-EGF
Increased crypt cell proliferation
Inhibits epithelial cell apoptosis
Stimulation of brush border enzymes
Stimulation of angiogenesis
Prevention of NEC

IGF-I
Epithelial cell growth
Submucosal tissue growth
Intestinal smooth muscle growth
Increased lactase activity and glucose transport

VEGF
Vascular development and angiogenesis
Host defense/monocyte migration

KGF
Epithelial cell growth/proliferation
Inhibition epithelial cell apoptosis
Goblet cell hyperplasia
Increased glucose transport

emptying, and increased sodium and glucose transport (79–82). EGF also has been found to increase mucosal growth and functional adaptation following intestinal resection or TPN and to prevent the incidence of necrotizing enterocolitis (83–88). Recent reports in premature infants suggest that EGF concentrations in saliva, serum and urine are lower in infants who have NEC than in healthy infants (86, 89). Another EGF-family member, HB-EGF, has been shown to reduce the incidence of NEC in neonatal rats and intestinal injury resulting from ischemia/reperfusion injury in adult rats (77, 90). The mechanism whereby these two growth factors protect against NEC seems to involve their ability to induce cell proliferation and epithelial cell restitution and inhibit apoptosis. Enteral nutrition stimulates gastrointestinal secretion, resulting in the release of salivary and pancreatic EGF into the gut lumen, where it is postulated to play a protective role. Many neonatal animal studies have shown that oral EGF administration augments gut growth and functional development (12). These findings, combined with recent evidence from transgenic mice, support the idea that both local expression and milk-borne ingestion of EGF play a physiological role in neonatal gut growth and development.

The insulin-like growth factor (IGF) family of peptides includes insulin, IGF-I and IGF-II (12, 23, 91). Although insulin secretion is largely confined to the pancreas, both IGF-I and IGF-II are expressed throughout the body, including the gut. However, within the intestinal mucosa, expression of both IGF-I and II appears to be localized to subepithelial myofibroblast cells, although epithelial cells may also produce IGF-II. IGF-1 is also involved in growth of the submucosal and muscularis layers of the intestine. The expression of IGF-I and II in the gut is highest in the fetal and neonatal period and declines with age. The insulin and type I IGF receptors are present in epithelial cells; they are more abundant on the basolateral than apical membrane, and more abundant in proliferating crypt cells than in differentiated enterocytes. IGF-1 appears to stimulate intestinal smooth muscle cell growth and IGF-1 knockout mice exhibit thinning of the submucosa, identical to that in mice treated with dexamethasone (92). Diminishment of IGF-1 expression may play a role in spontaneous ileal perforation seen in LBW infants treated with dexamethasone (92). Numerous studies have shown that either administering IGF systemically or increasing its expression locally (as in transgenic mice) stimulates intestinal growth and function in normal animals and under conditions of TPN, gut resection, dexamethasone treatment, sepsis, and radiation therapy. Some studies with fetal and neonatal animals given pharmacological oral doses of insulin and IGF-I have demonstrated a stimulation of gut growth, disaccharidase activity and glucose transport (12). Yet others have shown only limited effects of oral IGF on the neonatal gut, suggesting that the IGFs may not have a physiological role in the neonate.

Vascular endothelial growth factor (VEGF), hepatocyte growth factor (HGF), and keratinocyte growth factor (KGF) are expressed in the gut tissues, and may play a role in mucosal angiogenesis, growth and repair (12). Vascular endothelial growth factor is expressed in the small intestine in the vascular endothelium and mast cells (12). The receptor (FLT-1) for the VEGF 165 amino acid isoform is present in intestinal epithelial cells; however, VEGF did not stimulate cell proliferation of these cells. VEGF receptor has also been found on human colonic vascular endothelial cells. VEGF can also be found in human milk, decreasing in concentration as lactation progresses (93, 94). The role of VEGF in the intestine remains uncertain, but unpublished work by Andersson, et al. showed that labeled VEGF was not absorbed by the intestine into systemic circulation, suggesting local action on the intestine. VEGF has also been shown to enhance monocyte migration, highlighting a possible role in intestinal host defense (95). A recent report in mice demonstrated that VEGF reduces the rate of crypt cell apoptosis following total body irradiation treatment. VEGF has been implicated in angiogenesis during intestinal repair (96).

Hepatocyte growth factor is expressed by mesenchymal, but not epithelial, cells, whereas the HGF receptor (c-met) is found in epithelial cells; the c-met receptor is localized on the basolateral membrane. Studies with cultured intestinal epithelial cells demonstrate that HGF stimulates cell proliferation and wound-closure proliferation, but decreases transepithelial resistance (97, 98). Hepatocyte growth factor is found in human milk mononuclear cells and partially accounts for the stimulatory effect of human milk on intestinal cell proliferation. Studies in rats have shown that HGF, given either systemically or orally, increased gut growth and nutrient transport after massive small-bowel resection. Increased local expression of KGF has been found in patients with inflammatory bowel disease, and administration of KGF enhanced mucosal healing in rats following induction of colitis (99). Studies in mice demonstrate that systemic KGF administration prevents intestinal apoptosis in TPN-fed mice and augments intestinal adaptation after massive small-bowel resection (100–104).

Acknowledgments

This work is a publication of the USDA/ARS Children's Nutrition Research Center, Department of Pediatrics, Baylor College of Medicine and Texas Children's Hospital, Houston, TX. The work was supported in part by federal funds from the U.S. Department of Agriculture Agricultural Research Service, Cooperative Agreement No. 58–6258–6001, and by the National Institutes of Health R01 HD33920. The contents of this publication do not necessarily reflect the views or policies of the U.S. Department of Agriculture, nor does the mention of trade names, commercial products, or organizations imply endorsement by the U.S. Government.

REFERENCES

1. Montgomery RK, Mulberg AE, Grand RJ. Development of the human gastrointestinal tract: twenty years of progress. Gastroenterology 1999; 116:702–731.
2. Nankervis CA, Reber KM, Nowicki PT. Age-dependent changes in the postnatal intestinal microcirculation. Microcirculation 2001; 8:377–387.
3. Buddington RK, Elnif J, Puchal-Gardiner AA, et al. Intestinal apical amino acid absorption during development of the pig. Am J Physiol Regul Integr Comp Physiol 2001; 280:R241–R247.
4. Cheng H, Bjerknes M. Whole population cell kinetics and postnatal development of the mouse intestinal epithelium. Anat Rec 1985; 211:420–426.
5. Sangild PT, Fowden AL, Trahair JF. How does the foetal gastrointestinal tract develop in preparation for enteral nutrition after birth?. Livestock Prod Sci 2000; 66:141–150.
6. Mackie RI, Sghir A, Gaskins HR. Developmental microbial ecology of the neonatal gastrointestinal tract. Am J Clin Nutr 1999; 69:1035S–1045S.
7. Brandtzaeg PE. Current understanding of gastrointestinal immunoregulation and its relation to food allergy. Ann NY Acad Sci 2002; 964:13–45.
8. Raul F, Schleiffer R. Intestinal adaptation to nutritional stress. Proc Nutr Soc 1996; 55:279–289.
9. Jenkins AP, Thompson RP. Mechanisms of small intestinal adaptation. Dig Dis 1994; 12:15–27.
10. Trahair JF, Sangild PT. Systemic and luminal influences on the perinatal development of the gut. Equine Vet J, 1997; Suppl 40–50.
11. Burrin DG, Stoll B, Jiang R, et al. Minimal enteral nutrient requirements for intestinal growth in neonatal piglets: how much is enough?. Am J Clin Nutr 2000; 71:1603–1610.
12. Burrin DG, Stoll B. Key nutrients and growth factors for the neonatal gastrointestinal tract. Clin Perinatol 2002; 29:65–96.
13. Berseth CL. Minimal enteral feedings. Clin Perinatol 1995; 22:195–205.
14. Tyson JE, Kennedy KA. Trophic feedings for parenterally fed infants. Cochrane Database Syst Rev 2005; CD000504.
15. Kennedy KA, Tyson JE, Chamnanvanakij S. Rapid versus slow rate of advancement of feedings for promoting growth and preventing necrotizing enterocolitis in parenterally fed low-birth-weight infants. Cochrane Database Syst Rev 2000; CD001241.
16. Shulman RJ, Wong WW, Smith EO. Influence of changes in lactase activity and small-intestinal mucosal growth on lactose digestion and absorption in preterm infants. Am J Clin Nutr 2005; 81:472–479.
17. Shulman RJ, Schanler RJ, Lau C, et al. Early feeding, feeding tolerance, and lactase activity in preterm infants. J Pediatr 1998; 133:645–649.
18. Burrin DG, Stoll B, Chang X, et al. Parenteral nutrition results in impaired lactose digestion and hexose absorption when enteral feeding is initiated in infant pigs. Am J Clin Nutr 2003; 78:461–470.
19. Schanler RJ, Shulman RJ, Lau C, et al. Feeding strategies for premature infants: randomized trial of gastrointestinal priming and tube-feeding method. Pediatrics 1999; 103:434–439.
20. Premji S, Chessell L. Continuous nasogastric milk feeding versus intermittent bolus milk feeding for premature infants less than 1500 grams. Cochrane Database Syst Rev 2003; CD001819.
21. Shulman RJ, Redel CA, Stathos TH. Bolus versus continuous feedings stimulate small-intestinal growth and development in the newborn pig. J Pediatr Gastroenterol Nutr 1994; 18:350–354.
22. van Goudoever JB, Stoll B, Hartmann B, et al. Secretion of trophic gut peptides is not different in bolus- and continuously fed piglets. J Nutr 2001; 131:729–732.
23. Donovan SM, Odle J. Growth factors in milk as mediators of infant development. Annu Rev Nutr 1994; 14:147–167.
24. Grosvenor CE, Picciano MF, Baumrucker CR. Hormones and growth factors in milk. Endocr Rev 1993; 14:710–728.
25. Koldovsky O. Hormonally active peptides in human milk. Acta Paediatr Suppl 1994; 402:89–93.
26. Hamosh M. Bioactive factors in human milk. Pediatr Clin North Am 2001; 48:69–86.
27. Bernt KM, Walker WA. Human milk as a carrier of biochemical messages. Acta Paediatr Suppl 1999; 88:27–41.
28. Claud EC, Walker WA. Hypothesis: inappropriate colonization of the premature intestine can cause neonatal necrotizing enterocolitis. FASEB J 2001; 15:1398–1403.
29. Walker WA. The dynamic effects of breastfeeding on intestinal development and host defense. Adv Exp Med Biol 2004; 554:155–170.
30. Forchielli ML, Walker WA. The role of gut-associated lymphoid tissues and mucosal defence. Br J Nutr 2005; 93(Suppl 1):S41–S48.
31. Stoll B, Price PT, Reeds PJ, et al. Feeding an elemental diet vs a milk-based formula does not decrease intestinal mucosal growth in infant pigs. J Parenter Enteral Nutr 2006; 30:32–39.
32. Stoll B, Burrin DG, Henry J, et al. Substrate oxidation by the portal drained viscera of fed piglets. Am J Physiol 1999; 277:E168–E175.
33. Reeds PJ, Burrin DG. Glutamine and the bowel. J Nutr 2001; 131:2505S–2508S.
34. Neu J. Glutamine in the fetus and critically ill low birth weight neonate: metabolism and mechanism of action. J Nutr 2001; 131:2585S–2589S.
35. Neu J, Demarco V, Li N. Glutamine: clinical applications and mechanisms of action. Curr Opin Clin Nutr Metab Care 2002; 5:69–75.
36. Ziegler TR, Bazargan N, Leader LM, et al. Glutamine and the gastrointestinal tract. Curr Opin Clin Nutr Metab Care 2000; 3:355–362.

37. Neu J, Roig JC, Meetze WH, et al. Enteral glutamine supplementation for very low birth weight infants decreases morbidity. J Pediatr 1997; 131:691–699.
38. Vaughn P, Thomas P, Clark R, et al. Enteral glutamine supplementation and morbidity in low birth weight infants. J Pediatr 2003; 142:662–668.
39. Houdijk AP, van Leeuwen PA, Boermeester MA, et al. Glutamine-enriched enteral diet increases splanchnic blood flow in the rat. Am J Physiol 1994; 267:G1035–G1040.
40. Mercier A, Eurin D, Poulet-Young V, et al. Effect of enteral supplementation with glutamine on mesenteric blood flow in premature neonates. Clin Nutr 2003; 22:133–137.
41. Rhoads M. Glutamine signaling in intestinal cells. J Parenter Enteral Nutr 1999; 23:S38–S40.
42. Wu G, Meininger CJ, Knabe DA, et al. Arginine nutrition in development, health and disease. Curr Opin Clin Nutr Metab Care 2000; 3:59–66.
43. Evans ME, Jones DP, Ziegler TR. Glutamine inhibits cytokine-induced apoptosis in human colonic epithelial cells via the pyrimidine pathway. Am J Physiol Gastrointest Liver Physiol 2005; 289:G388–G396.
44. Evans ME, Jones DP, Ziegler TR. Glutamine prevents cytokine-induced apoptosis in human colonic epithelial cells. J Nutr 2003; 133:3065–3071.
45. Nakajo T, Yamatsuji T, Ban H, et al. Glutamine is a key regulator for amino acid-controlled cell growth through the mTOR signaling pathway in rat intestinal epithelial cells. Biochem Biophys Res Commun 2005; 326:174–180.
46. Hansen MB, Dresner LS, Wait RB. Profile of neurohumoral agents on mesenteric and intestinal blood flow in health and disease. Physiol Res 1999; 47:307–327.
47. Bruins MJ, Luiking YC, Soeters PB, et al. Effects of long-term intravenous and intragastric L-arginine intervention on jejunal motility and visceral nitric oxide production in the hyperdynamic compensated endotoxaemic pig. Neurogastroenterol Motil 2004; 16:819–828.
48. Ban H, Shigemitsu K, Yamatsuji T, et al. Arginine and Leucine regulate p70 S6 kinase and 4E-BP1 in intestinal epithelial cells. Int J Mol Med 2004; 13:537–543.
49. Rhoads JM, Chen W, Gookin J, et al. Arginine stimulates intestinal cell migration through a focal adhesion kinase dependent mechanism. Gut 2004; 53:514–522.
50. Gookin JL, Rhoads JM, Argenzio RA. Inducible nitric oxide synthase mediates early epithelial repair of porcine ileum. Am J Physiol Gastrointest Liver Physiol 2002; 283:G157–G168.
51. Di Lorenzo M, Bass J, Krantis A. Use of L-arginine in the treatment of experimental necrotizing enterocolitis. J Pediatr Surg 1995; 30:235–240.
52. Amin HJ, Zamora SA, McMillan DD, et al. Arginine supplementation prevents necrotizing enterocolitis in the premature infant. J Pediatr 2002; 140:425–431.
53. Bertolo RF, Brunton JA, Pencharz PB, et al. Arginine, ornithine, and proline interconversion is dependent on small intestinal metabolism in neonatal pigs. Am J Physiol Endocrinol Metab 2003; 284:E915–E922.
54. Dumas F, De Bandt JP, Colomb V, et al. Enteral ornithine alpha-ketoglutarate enhances intestinal adaptation to massive resection in rats. Metabolism 1998; 47:1366–1371.
55. Wakabayashi Y, Yamada E, Yoshida T, et al. Arginine becomes an essential amino acid after massive resection of rat small intestine. J Biol Chem 1994; 269:32667–32671.
56. Schaart MW, Schierbeek H, Schoor SRD, et al. Threonine utilization is high in the intestine of piglets. J Nutr 2005; 135:765–770.
57. Shoveller AK, Stoll B, Ball RO, et al. Nutritional and functional importance of intestinal sulfur amino acid metabolism. J Nutr 2005; 135:1609–1612.
58. Carver JD. Advances in nutritional modifications of infant formulas. Am J Clin Nutr 2003; 77:1550S–1554S.
59. Evans ME, Tian J, Gu LH, et al. Dietary supplementation with orotate and uracil increases adaptive growth of jejunal mucosa after massive small bowel resection in rats. J Parenter Enteral Nutr 2005; 29:315–320.
60. Carver JD, Sosa R, Saste M, et al. Dietary nucleotides and intestinal blood flow velocity in term infants. J Pediatr Gastroenterol Nutr 2004; 39:38–42.
61. Carver JD, Saste M, Sosa R, et al. The effects of dietary nucleotides on intestinal blood flow in preterm infants. Pediatr Res 2002; 52:425–429.
62. Caplan MS, Jilling T. The role of polyunsaturated fatty acid supplementation in intestinal inflammation and neonatal necrotizing enterocolitis. Lipids 2001; 36:1053–1057.
63. Crissinger KD, Burney DL, Velasquez OR, et al. An animal model of necrotizing enterocolitis induced by infant formula and ischemia in developing piglets. Gastroenterology 1994; 106:1215–1222.
64. Raybould HE, Cooke HJ, Christofi FL. Sensory mechanisms: transmitters, modulators and reflexes. Neurogastroenterol Motil 2004; 16(Suppl 1):60–63.
65. Walsh JH. Gastrointestinal hormones. In: Johnson LR, et al, ed. Physiology of the gastrointestinal tract. Elsevier; 1994: 1–128.
66. Johnson LR. Regulation of gastrointestinal mucosal growth. In: Johnson LR, et al, ed. Physiology of the gastrointestinal tract. Elsevier; 1994: 611–641.
67. Teitelbaum DH, Tracy TF Jr, Aouthmany MM, et al. Use of cholecystokininoctapeptide for the prevention of parenteral nutrition-associated cholestasis. Pediatrics 2005; 115:1332–1340.
68. Tsai S, Strouse PJ, Drongowski RA, et al. Failure of cholecystokinin-octapeptide to prevent TPN-associated gallstone disease. J Pediatr Surg 2005; 40:263–267.
69. Estall JL, Drucker DJ. Glucagon-like peptide-2. Annu Rev Nutr 2006; 26:391–411.
70. Burrin D, Guan XF, Stoll B, et al. Glucagon-like peptide 2: a key link between nutrition and intestinal adaptation in neonates? J Nutr 2003; 133:3712–3716.

71. Cottrell JJ, Stoll B, Buddington RK, et al. Glucagon-like peptide-2 protects against TPN-induced intestinal hexose malabsorption in enterally refed piglets. Am J Physiol Gastrointest Liver Physiol 2006; 290:G293–G300.

72. Guan X, Karpen HE, Stephens J, et al. GLP-2 receptor localizes to enteric neurons and endocrine cells expressing vasoactive peptides and mediates increased blood flow. Gastroenterology 2006; 130:150–164.

73. Stephens J, Stoll B, Cottrell J, et al. Glucagon-like peptide-2 acutely increases proximal small intestinal blood flow in TPN-fed neonatal piglets. Am J Physiol Regul Integr Comp Physiol 2006; 290:R283–R289.

74. Jeppesen PB, Hartmann B, Thulesen J, et al. Glucagon-like peptide 2 improves nutrient absorption and nutritional status in short-bowel patients with no colon. Gastroenterology 2001; 120:806–815.

75. Jeppesen PB, Sanguinetti EL, Buchman A, et al. Teduglutide (ALX-0600), a dipeptidyl peptidase IV resistant glucagon-like peptide 2 analogue, improves intestinal function in short bowel syndrome patients. Gut 2005; 54:1224–1231.

76. Polk DB, Barnard JA. Hormones and growth factor in intestinal development. In: Sanderson I, Walker WA, eds. Development of the gastrointestinal tract; 37–56.

77. Feng J, El Assal ON, Besner GE. Heparin-binding EGF-like growth factor (HB-EGF) and necrotizing enterocolitis. Semin Pediatr Surg 2005; 14:167–174.

78. Barnard JA, Beauchamp RD, Russell WE, et al. Epidermal growth factor-related peptides and their relevance to gastrointestinal pathophysiology. Gastroenterology 1995; 108:564–580.

79. Seare NJ, Playford RJ. Growth factors and gut function. Proc Nutr Soc 1998; 57:403–408.

80. Thompson JS. Epidermal growth factor and the short bowel syndrome. J Parenter Enteral Nutr 1999; 23:S113–S116.

81. Uribe JM, Barrett KE. Nonmitogenic actions of growth factors: an integrated view of their role in intestinal physiology and pathophysiology. Gastroenterology 1997; 112:255–268.

82. Wong WM, Wright NA. Epidermal growth factor, epidermal growth factor receptors, intestinal growth, and adaptation. J Parenter Enteral Nutr 1999; 23:S83–S88.

83. Erwin CR, Helmrath MA, Shin CE, et al. Intestinal overexpression of EGF in transgenic mice enhances adaptation after small bowel resection. Am J Physiol 1999; 277:G533–G540.

84. Helmrath MA, Shin CE, Fox JW, et al. Adaptation after small bowel resection is attenuated by sialoadenectomy: the role for endogenous epidermal growth factor. Surgery 1998; 124:848–854.

85. Helmrath MA, Erwin CR, Warner BW. A defective EGF-receptor in waved-2 mice attenuates intestinal adaptation. J Surg Res 1997; 69:76–80.

86. Warner BW, Warner BB. Role of epidermal growth factor in the pathogenesis of neonatal necrotizing enterocolitis. Semin Pediatr Surg 2005; 14:175–180.

87. Clark JA, Lane RH, Maclennan NK, et al. Epidermal growth factor reduces intestinal apoptosis in an experimental model of necrotizing enterocolitis. Am J Physiol Gastrointest Liver Physiol 2005; 288:G755–G762.

88. Dvorak B, Halpern MD, Holubec H, et al. Epidermal growth factor reduces the development of necrotizing enterocolitis in a neonatal rat model. Am J Physiol Gastrointest Liver Physiol 2002; 282:G156–G164.

89. Shin CE, Falcone RA Jr., Stuart L, et al. Diminished epidermal growth factor levels in infants with necrotizing enterocolitis. J Pediatr Surg 2000; 35:173–176.

90. Pillai SB, Hinman CE, Luquette MH, et al. Heparin-binding epidermal growth factor-like growth factor protects rat intestine from ischemia/reperfusion injury. J Surg Res 1999; 87:225–231.

91. MacDonald RS. The role of insulin-like growth factors in small intestinal cell growth and development. Horm Metab Res 1999; 31:103–113.

92. Herman AC, Carlisle EM, Paxton JB, et al. Insulin-like growth factor-I governs submucosal growth and thickness in the newborn mouse ileum. Pediatr Res 2004; 55:507–513.

93. Sanderson IR. Vascular endothelial growth factor in human milk. NeoReviews 2003; 4:e125–e127.

94. Vuorela P, Andersson S, Carpen O, et al. Unbound vascular endothelial growth factor and its receptors in breast, human milk, and newborn intestine. Am J Clin Nutr 2000; 72:1196–1201.

95. Clauss M, Gerlach M, Gerlach H, et al. Vascular permeability factor: a tumor-derived polypeptide that induces endothelial cell and monocyte procoagulant activity, and promotes monocyte migration. J Exp Med 1990; 172:1535–1545.

96. Jones MK, Tomikawa M, Mohajer B, et al. Gastrointestinal mucosal regeneration: role of growth factors. Front Biosci 1999; 4:D303–D309.

97. Goke M, Kanai M, Podolsky DK. Intestinal fibroblasts regulate intestinal epithelial cell proliferation via hepatocyte growth factor. Am J Physiol 1998; 274:G809–G818.

98. Nusrat A, Parkos CA, Bacarra AE, et al. Hepatocyte growth factor/scatter factor effects on epithelia. Regulation of intercellular junctions in transformed and nontransformed cell lines, basolateral polarization of c-met receptor in transformed and natural intestinal epithelia, and induction of rapid wound repair in a transformed model epithelium. J Clin Invest 1994; 93:2056–2065.

99. Farrell CL, Rex KL, Chen JN, et al. The effects of keratinocyte growth factor in preclinical models of mucositis. Cell Prolif 2002; 35(Suppl 1):78–85.

100. Wildhaber BE, Yang H, Teitelbaum DH. Total parenteral nutrition-induced apoptosis in mouse intestinal epithelium: modulation by keratinocyte growth factor. J Surg Res 2003; 112:144–151.

101. Wildhaber BE, Yang H, Teitelbaum DH. Keratinocyte growth factor decreases total parenteral nutrition-induced apoptosis in mouse intestinal epithelium via Bcl-2. J Pediatr Surg 2003; 38:92–96.

102. Yang H, Antony PA, Wildhaber BE, et al. Intestinal intraepithelial lymphocyte gamma delta-T cell-derived keratinocyte growth factor modulates epithelial growth in the mouse. J Immunol 2004; 172:4151–4158.

103. Yang H, Wildhaber BE, Teitelbaum DH. 2003 Harry M. Vars Research Award. Keratinocyte growth factor improves epithelial function after massive small bowel resection. J Parenter Enteral Nutr 2003; 27:198–206.

104. Yang H, Wildhaber B, Tazuke Y, et al. 2002 Harry M. Vars Research Award. Keratinocyte growth factor stimulates the recovery of epithelial structure and function in a mouse model of total parenteral nutrition. J Parenter Enteral Nutr 2002; 26:333–340.

Chapter 9

Cholestasis in Neonates and Infants

Michael K. Davis, MD • Joel M. Andres, MD

Biliary Atresia, Biliary Hypoplasia and Choledochal Cyst
Hepatocellular Cholestasis
Non-Cholestatic Conjugated Hyperbilirubinemia
Perinatal Infections
Metabolic Cholestasis
Primary Mitochondrial Hepatopathies
Progressive Familial Intrahepatic Cholestasis (PFIC)
Treatment of Cholestasis

The most important cause of diminished bile flow and prolonged conjugated hyperbilirubinemia (neonatal cholestasis) in the first 2 months of life is biliary atresia. However, every effort must be made to diagnose non-surgical neonatal cholestatic disorders such as idiopathic "neonatal hepatitis"; various neonatal infections associated with cholestasis; neonatal metabolic disorders, including antitrypsin deficiency, cystic fibrosis, tyrosinemia, galactosemia, hereditary fructose intolerance, neonatal iron storage disease, and inborn errors of bile acid metabolism; in addition to the more rare problems of primary mitochondrial hepatopathy and familial intrahepatic cholestasis.

For the neonate with cholestasis, it is emphasized that the clinical features of most of the above liver diseases are similar. The neonatologist and hepatologist, however, need to establish a specific diagnosis, if possible; especially the differentiation of intrahepatic and extrahepatic cholestasis. It is the purpose of this chapter to review the differential diagnosis of cholestasis in neonates and infants and present an approach to these patients with cholestatic disorders (Table 9-1).

BILIARY ATRESIA, BILIARY HYPOPLASIA AND CHOLEDOCHAL CYST

Biliary Atresia

Biliary atresia is the end result of a destructive, inflammatory, idiopathic process involving the extrahepatic and intrahepatic bile ducts which leads to obliteration of the biliary tract and cirrhosis. Biliary atresia is the most common cause of chronic cholestasis in neonates and infants, and affects an estimated 1:8000 to 1:12 000 live births. Most infants with biliary atresia appear healthy at birth, developing progressive jaundice in the first weeks of life. Some infants have liver dysfunction at birth, possibly secondary to defective embryogenesis. These infants are described as having the syndromic, fetal or embryonic form of biliary atresia, perhaps 10–15%

Table 9-1 Cholestasis in Neonates and Infants

Biliary atresia, biliary hypoplasia and choledochal cyst
Biliary atresia
Biliary hypoplasia
Acute infections of the liver
Alagille's syndrome
Choledochal cyst

Hepatocellular cholestasis
"Neonatal hepatitis"
Galactosemia
Hereditary fructose intolerance
Inherited storage disease
Niemann-Pick
Gaucher's disease
Total parenteral nutrition (TPN)-associated hepatopathy

Non-cholestatic conjugated hyperbilirubinemia
Dubin-Johnson syndrome
Rotor syndrome

Perinatal infections
Bacterial infections
Congenital infections
Toxoplasmosis
Congenital Syphilis
Rubella
Cytomegalovirus
Herpes Simplex
Hepatitis B virus
Hepatitis A, C and D viruses
Human immunodeficiency virus
Echovirus, parvovirus, and adenovirus

Metabolic cholestasis
Antitrypsin deficiency
Cystic fibrosis
Tyrosinemia
Neonatal iron-storage disease
Inborn errors of bile acid metabolism

Primary mitochondrial hepatopathies

Progressive familial intrahepatic cholestasis
PFIC-1 (Byler's disease)
PFIC-2
PFIC-3

of the total. The fetal form is accompanied by other congenital anomalies in up to 20% of infants, including the polysplenia syndrome with cardiovascular defects, abdominal situs inversus, and positional anomalies of the portal vein and hepatic artery (1). The non-syndromic form of biliary atresia, also called the perinatal or postnatal form, occurs in approximately 90% of infants with biliary atresia. The apparent acquisition of biliary atresia after birth is not associated with anomalies and has led investigators to look for a causative environmental insult, such as a toxin or virus occurring in late gestation or after birth (2). Genetic predisposition, fetal-perinatal vascular compromise and altered or disordered immunologic response to injury are other etiologic possibilities. The etiopathogenesis of biliary atresia, however, remains elusive despite recent research initiatives. For example, messenger RNA expression using cDNA microarray analysis on RNA isolated from livers of patients with perinatal biliary atresia determined that gene profiles differentiated infants with end-stage biliary atresia from normal and diseased liver controls (3). The gene expression profiles were associated with cell signaling, transcription regulation and hepatic morpho-fibrogenesis. Genes with increased expression included collagen I, III, IV, VI and proteoglycan (implicated in development of hepatic fibrosis), in addition to osteonectin and metalloproteinases (involved in organization and destruction of the extracellular matrix). The results suggest that the pathogenesis of biliary atresia is orchestrated by a complex interplay of inflammation and morphologic and fibrogenic factors. For neonates with embryonic biliary atresia, another cRNA microarray study revealed a distinctive clinical phenotypic expression of regulatory genes, in addition to over-expression of some imprinted genes (4). The results of this small clinical study implied a failure to downregulate embryonic gene programs during maturation of the hepatobiliary system. These data may provide evidence for the transcriptional basis for pathogenesis of embryonic atresia, especially important because of the high incidence of laterality defects in this less-common form of biliary atresia.

Diagnostic algorithms for cholestasis are useful for excluding more frequent causes of direct hyperbilirubinemia (5). Histopathologic examination of liver biopsies may reveal the classic findings of biliary atresia: cholestasis, bile ductular proliferation, portal tract edema, and a neutrophilic inflammatory infiltrate (6). Screening hepatobiliary imaging studies include radionuclide scintigraphy (i.e., "IDA" scans using technetium99m iminodiacetic acid), magnetic resonance cholangiography, and ultrasonography (7). Endoscopic retrograde cholangiography has been suggested for diagnosis of biliary atresia, although few centers have the appropriate equipment or training to perform this more complex procedure in infants (8). Early diagnostic laparotomy with intraoperative cholangiography for suspected biliary atresia may prevent unnecessary delay in performing appropriate surgical intervention (9, 10)

Without surgery, biliary atresia produces progressive liver failure and death in the first years of life. In the past, the short-term prognosis for infants with biliary atresia correlated best for neonates and infants who had expert treatment performed by operating surgeons skilled in biliary microsurgery. However, overall survival in children with biliary atresia has improved because hepatic portoenterostomy (Kasai portoenterostomy) is complemented by liver transplantation. Successful portoenterostomy is usually defined by restoration in bile flow and subsequent normalization of serum bilirubin but not necessarily other liver function studies. Prediction of improved bile flow after operation is best correlated with time of surgery, extent of liver damage prior to surgery, and the surgeons' experience with the Kasai portoenterostomy (7). The short-term benefits for patients undergoing Kasai portoenterostomy are well-documented; however, 80–90% of these infants will eventually require liver transplantation (11). Predictors of a worse outcome after portoenterostomy include operative age greater than 2 months, although it can be argued that an attempt at reestablishing bile flow should still be considered in the infant with biliary atresia older than 60–90 days of age. Even though the Kasai procedure is not successful long-term, it may postpone the need for liver transplantation until the infant is older and larger, making the possibility of finding a suitable donor more likely (12). Other predictors of a poor outcome are presence of cirrhosis at initial biopsy, absence of bile ducts at transected liver hilus and subsequent development of varices or ascites. In general, it is clear that portoenterostomy, which is primarily palliative, has an initial complementary, but limited long-term, role in the treatment of most infants with biliary atresia. A knowledge of factors predictive of outcome allows for timely referral of biliary atresia patients for liver transplantation, which is usually a curative procedure.

The long-term outcome of liver transplantation for children with biliary atresia has been excellent. In 1976 pediatric patients undergoing primary orthotopic liver transplantation for biliary atresia in the USA from 1988 to 2003, the 5- and 10-year actuarial patient survival was greater than 87% and 85%, respectively (13). For children who received a live donor partial liver graft in lieu of a cadaveric partial/reduced liver graft, the 5-year actuarial survival rate improved to 98% (14). Other independent predictors of improved survival for children undergoing liver transplantation are age greater than 1 year and the absence of life support at the time of transplantion (13). Other factors that enhance survival include surgical technical precision, antimicrobial chemoproplylaxis and therapy, and judicious immunosuppression (15, 16)

Biliary Hypoplasia

Biliary hypoplasia is noted in infants with acute infections of the liver, various familial cholestasis syndromes such as arteriohepatic dysplasia syndrome (Alagille's syndrome) (17, 18) and the more common metabolic cholestasis syndrome, alpha-1-antitrypsin deficiency (19). The clinical course of infants with biliary hypoplasia is variable; overall survival is much longer than for infants with biliary atresia, but some patients require liver transplantation (20).

Choledochal Cyst

Clinical recognition of a jaundiced child with a choledochal cyst depends on cyst size and the presence of biliary obstruction (21). The classic triad of abdominal pain, jaundice and right epigastric mass is usually not present in infants. This cystic lesion may be detected at any age, with about 20% appearing before 1 year of age. Use of ultrasonography improves the preoperative diagnosis of this problem and should be the initial study in the evaluation of suspected choledochal cyst. Recommended treatment includes elimination of the entire cyst mucosal wall by complete excision of the cyst in order to avoid progressive biliary obstruction, cirrhosis and potential carcinoma in residual cystic tissue. Spontaneous perforation of a choledochal cyst in infancy has been reported (22). Ultrasound identification of the gallbladder, and change in size following oral feeding, also aids in the differential diagnosis of biliary obstruction versus a hepatocellular problem (23).

HEPATOCELLULAR CHOLESTASIS

Cholestasis may be secondary to immature or abnormal canalicular secretory mechanisms, damage to the hepatocyte canalicular membrane, or an anatomic abnormality of bile ducts. Cholestasis is always pathologic and usually associated with hepatocellular disease rather than biliary obstruction. A serum conjugated bilirubin level greater than 1.5 mg/dL should always be considered abnormal and secondary to hepatic injury. Hepatic excretion of organic anions such as bilirubin is dependent, in part, on the movement of bile acid and water across the canalicular membrane. Jaundice is usually closely associated with a reduction in bile flow or cholestasis; hence the term cholestatic jaundice.

Neonatal Hepatitis

Hepatocellular cholestasis syndromes (versus surgical or ductal cholestasis) include "neonatal hepatitis," which represents the diagnosis for the majority of neonates and infants with conjugated hyperbilirubinemia in the early months of life. Symptoms usually occur in the first 2 weeks after birth, and the typical presentation is that of an unwell, jaundiced infant with hepatomegaly. The main differential diagnostic consideration is ductal cholestasis, especially biliary atresia. The neonatologist should initiate an evaluation to determine the type of hyperbilirubinemia and establish an early diagnosis of a treatable disease. The basic studies include total and direct serum bilirubin; hemoglobin; Coombs test; blood glucose; serum amino acids; serum and urine for succinylacetone; serologic tests for toxoplasmosis, syphilis, hepatitis B virus, hepatitis C virus, and occasionally human immunodeficiency virus; urine for non-glucose-reducing substances and organic acids; blood cultures; and urine culture.

Galactosemia, Hereditary Fructose Intolerance

Infants with tyrosinemia, galactosemia, and hereditary fructose intolerance have similar clinical manifestations, usually within days to weeks after birth. Marked jaundice, hepatosplenomegaly, coagulation abnormalities, and failure-to-thrive are often prominent. However, infants with galactosemia may have less-apparent findings, after several months developing cataracts, cirrhosis, and psychomotor retardation. Similarly, the tyrosinemic infant may escape the acute phase of illness and be discovered months later to have cirrhosis, rickets, and renal disease. Infants with tyrosinemia will be discussed in more detail later; they have a high incidence of hepatoma. Cholestasis associated with a history of vomiting, distaste for sweet foods, and fructosuria would most likely result from fructose intolerance. Each of the above metabolic disorders may cause renal dysfunction manifested by aminoaciduria, glycosuria, and phosphaturia (Fanconi syndrome). Their definitive diagnosis depends on specific tolerance tests and the measurement of enzyme activity in red blood cells (galactosemia), enzyme activity in liver or kidney (fructose intolerance) and urine succinylacetone (tyrosinemia). Analyzing the urine for non-glucose-reducing sugars, organic acids, and amino acids is appropriate for initial screening. In addition, neonatal liver failure makes it mandatory to send urine and serum to special laboratories for analysis of primary bile acids and their metabolic intermediates. A family history of early neonatal death, oligohydramnios or hydrops fetalis suggests the possibility of iron-storage disease. Serum ferritin levels and analysis of iron in minor salivary glands (and liver iron quantitation, if biopsy is safe) helps the neonatologist rapidly establish the diagnosis of this rare metabolic problem.

Persistent jaundice is unusual in infants with cystic fibrosis, but it may occur when the disease is associated with meconium ileus, drug hypersensitivity, parenteral alimentation, or partial common duct obstruction secondary to inspissation of biliary secretions. Alpha-1-antitrypsin deficiency (24) is the most common metabolic disorder associated with liver disease in infants. The usual presentation is that of cholestasis with associated jaundice and hepatomegaly. Diagnosis is confirmed by a low serum alpha-1-antitrypsin level and Pi typing. No specific treatment is available yet, but the future of gene therapy is promising. It is essential to identify infants at risk and provide proper genetic counseling to the family. Liver transplantation is commonly performed in older infants and children with end-stage liver disease caused by alpha-1-antitrypsin deficiency (25). The prognosis is extremely variable. Despite persistence of mild hepatocellular dysfunction, clinical improvement may occur in infants a few months after birth. Biliary cirrhosis and portal hypertension eventually develop in some older children.

Inherited Storage Disease

Inherited storage diseases such as Niemann-Pick and Gaucher's disease usually cause hepatosplenomegaly in infants, but cholestasis is unusual. These storage diseases are rare and should not be considered in the initial evaluation of children with cholestatic jaundice.

Total Parenteral Nutrition (TPN)-Associated Hepatopathy

Total parenteral nutrition (TPN) is commonly associated with liver injury in neonates (26). TPN-associated hepatopathy typically manifests as cholestasis that resolves once intravenous alimentation is discontinued. In some infants, hepatic recovery may take several months, and others may develop permanent liver injury or liver failure requiring liver transplantation. Concomitant infection (e.g., sepsis), gastrointestinal surgery, and prematurity are often confounding factors in determining the precise cause of hepatic dysfunction. Because of these factors, the pathogenesis of TPN-associated hepatopathy is poorly understood. The primary treatment of these neonates and infants is the withdrawal of TPN with institution of judicious enteral feeds when practical.

NON-CHOLESTATIC CONJUGATED HYPERBILIRUBINEMIA

Dubin-Johnson Syndrome

Dubin-Johnson syndrome (27) is another type of familial jaundice that is considered a benign condition, but the child has a reduced capacity to secrete several organic anions, especially conjugated bilirubin and cholecystographic dye. This syndrome is caused by mutations in the *MDR2* gene (28). These patients, usually not infants, develop conjugated hyperbilirubinemia, not cholestasis. The syndrome is another example of a defect in hepatocyte canalicular transporter. Since the excretion of bile acids is normal, the term "noncholestatic jaundice" is more accurate and the extrahepatic and intrahepatic biliary trees are always patent. Recurrent episodes of jaundice, which can be precipitated by infection, may begin in infancy and can be misdiagnosed as acute hepatitis because of abrupt onset of illness. Routine tests of liver function are normal except for increased total bilirubin levels (usually less than 15 mg/dL) with predominance of conjugated bilirubin. Grossly, the liver has a black appearance due to accumulation of melanin-like pigment in lysosomes.

Rotor Syndrome

Rotor syndrome is similar to Dubin-Johnson syndrome except that pigmentation of hepatocytes has not been demonstrated and secretion of cholecystographic dye is normal. Also, the primary abnormality in infants with Rotor syndrome is a deficiency in the intracellular carrier proteins of the hepatocyte for binding anions (29). The carrier protein may be glutathione *S*-transferase. A deficiency of this intracellular storage protein results in movement of bilirubin conjugates back into the circulation rather than excretion through the canalicular membrane. There is also an increase in urinary coproporphyrin excretion in both of the above syndromes. Recognition of this benign noncholestatic jaundice syndrome and Dubin-Johnson syndrome may prevent unnecessary diagnostic evaluations.

Evaluation of Hepatocellular Cholestasis

The liver histology may suggest the cause of the infant's problem, but failure to make a specific diagnosis of hepatocellular cholestasis necessitates studies to determine patency of the biliary tree such as hepatobiliary scintigraphy. In general, infants with hepatocellular cholestasis who die have significantly more liver histologic abnormalities, including prominent periportal inflammation and fibrosis, and diffuse giant cell transformation (30). Approximately 30% of infants with hepatocellular cholestasis develop progressive liver failure, another 10% survive the early months of illness but have chronic disease including cirrhosis, and about 60% recover completely. Overall, the outlook for these patients is now markedly improved because of the success of liver transplantation.

PERINATAL INFECTIONS

Bacterial Infections

Jaundice and associated conjugated hyperbilirubinemia occur more frequently in neonates and infants with sepsis (31). The prompt diagnosis of sepsis is often difficult because jaundice may be the only clinical manifestation in an otherwise healthy-appearing neonate. For all age groups, jaundice may be the only sign of infection. However, disproportionate hyperbilirubinemia is probably less common in infants with bacteremia than in older children, except for neonates with hemolysis during the early phase of sepsis, when they experience elevated indirect bilirubin levels (31). Despite this, jaundice should not divert attention from other systemic problems such as urinary tract infection (32). Therapy always needs to be directed at the primary infection. In fact, the agent most commonly reported in neonates with sepsis is *Escherichia coli*, and the most common site of infection is the urinary tract. The routine evaluation of infants with jaundice, therefore, must always include a urinalysis and urine culture in addition to blood cultures. An abdominal ultrasound should be considered to exclude biliary obstruction. Liver histologic findings in neonates with sepsis include cholestasis and Kupffer cell hyperplasia.

Neonates have a greater susceptibility to Gram-negative bacterial infections. Bilirubin "overload" from brisk hemolysis and hepatocellular damage is more likely to occur in infancy. This may reflect immaturity of biliary excretory mechanisms with inhibition of membrane Na^+, K^+-ATPase by endotoxin, thereby interfering with the excretion of conjugated bilirubin into the bile canaliculi (33). Interestingly, bacteria are rarely isolated from the liver. In this regard, Kupffer cells, which can interact with other cellular components of the hepatic sinusoids and with hepatocytes, are capable of clearing bacteria from the blood. An inflammatory stimulus may lead to elaboration of secretory products from hepatic parenchymal macrophages, producing local hepatocyte damage. Endotoxin-exposed Kupffer cells can exert potentially harmful effects on hepatocyte function during sepsis (34). After interaction with macrophages, Kupffer cells are able to induce liver injury via leukotrienes (35).

Gram-positive infections are common in neonates, but associated liver abnormalities are distinctly uncommon. Infection with *Listeria monocytogenes* is an exception in that hepatic manifestations are always present (36). The modes of transmission include transplacental passage or inoculation of the neonate via passage through an infected cervix or vagina. These neonates are critically ill, most develop meningitis, but some have jaundice and hepatomegaly. The liver histology is always abnormal, revealing either diffuse hepatitis or, more commonly, demarcated areas of necrosis or microabscesses.

Congenital Infections

Neonatal infections caused by the "TORCH" organisms are well known, often clinically indistinguishable, and may be inapparent in both the neonate and mother. Unfortunately, serious sequelae commonly occur even in asymptomatic infants (37). Although other agents are reported to produce similar congenital problems, only *Toxoplasma gondii*, *Treponema pallidum*, rubella virus, cytomegalovirus, and *Herpes simplex* will be discussed. The incidence of these infections is high, occurring in 0.5–2.5% of births (37).

Toxoplasmosis

When acute *T. gondii* infection occurs during pregnancy, it can cross the placenta and infect the fetus; the earlier the transmission, the more severe are the congenital lesions (38). Maternal infection during the first two trimesters may be mild or asymptomatic but is a prerequisite for the development of congenital toxoplasmosis during gestation which leads to severe disease, whereas later acquisition usually results in subclinical or no fetal infections (39). Manifestations of infection with *T. gondii* may include microcephaly, chorioretinitis, intracranial calcifications, meningoencephalitis and psychomotor retardation. The parasite is widely distributed in the host, including in the liver, but isolation of *Toxoplasma* from the liver is rare. Most neonates have hepatosplenomegaly but jaundice is only occasionally noted. The hepatic histology is mainly periportal inflammation and marked extramedullary hematopoiesis (39). Hepatitis may be the only manifestation of the disease. Microcalcifications have been noted in the liver on plain films of the abdomen (40). Serologic diagnosis can be made by immunoglobulin M (IgM-ELISA), which is highly sensitive and specific for the diagnosis of congenital *Toxoplasma* infection (41). Persistent infection beyond 2 months of life relies on IgG anti-*Toxoplasma* antibody tests. Infants with documented infection are treated with sulfadiazine and pyrimethamine with folinic acid to prevent hematologic toxicity of therapy.

Strategies for prenatal diagnosis and prevention of congenital toxoplasmosis are under development. For mothers who develop a primary *Toxoplasma* infection during pregnancy, prenatal amniotic fluid polymerase chain reaction (PCR) testing is available (42). Amniotic PCR has a high positive predictive value for the diagnosis of congenital toxoplasmosis although sensitivity is low. Thus, a negative amniotic PCR test does not rule out disease. Vaccines against congenital toxoplasmosis have been successful in animal models (43, 44); further research is needed if a human vaccine is to be developed.

Congenital Syphilis

Transplacental transmission of *Treponema pallidum* spirochetes to the fetus may result in mild to severe symptoms. When rash, skin and mucosal lesions and bone lesions are associated with hepatosplenomegaly, the diagnosis is easy to make at birth. Milder presentations occur with anicteric hepatitis and poor weight gain, but the diagnosis of congenital syphilis should be entertained in any neonate with hepatitis. Jaundice is often present, appearing in the first 24 h after birth, or a delayed onset may be observed (45). The liver histologic findings are usually a characteristic centrilobular fibrosis with mononuclear infiltration or a more typical histology of neonatal cholestasis. The diagnosis of congenital syphilis is based on serologic testing. First, a nontreponemal test such as Venereal Disease Research Laboratory (VDRL) or rapid plasma reagin (RPR) should be performed. Confirmatory tests are for specific treponemal antibodies (e.g., the fluorescent treponemal antibody absorption (FTA-ABS) test) (37). Cases of treatment failure have been seen in infants given parenteral penicillin. Hence, the approach to active infection should be a regimen of 10–14 days of crystalline or procaine penicillin (46). The administration of penicillin, however, can precipitate or exacerbate liver dysfunction in patients with congenital syphilis, which may persist for more than 6 weeks after adequate treatment (47). It is speculated that the products of *Treponema* lysis cause a toxic reaction (e.g., a hepatic Jarisch-Herxheimer reaction (48)). After appropriate therapy, serology may remain positive for up to 2 years. Prognosis depends on the extent of hepatic damage prior to therapy.

Rubella

The transplacental origin of rubella infection has been well documented. Prenatal infection can occur during the first trimester and result in chronic multisystem disease. Widespread use of the rubella vaccine, however, has led to a progressive decline in the number of reported cases in the USA (49). Liver involvement is frequent in congenital rubella, and hepatomegaly is a constant feature. Histologically, mononuclear inflammatory infiltrates are prominent in the portal tracts, and intralobular fibrosis and persistence of extramedullary hematopoiesis are present. More characteristic findings of hepatitis also occur and persist well into the first year. Congenital rubella infection should be diagnosed by culture because all infected neonates shed the rubella virus. If this is not possible, serologic tests and a latex agglutination test are available (37,50).

Cytomegalovirus

Neonates are infected with cytomegalovirus (CMV) in utero, at the time of birth, or postnatally from infected secretions (saliva or breast milk). It is a significant problem throughout the world and may occur in up to 2% of all live births (51). Most congenitally infected infants remain asymptomatic. Maternal immunity to CMV, unlike immunity to rubella and toxoplasmosis, does not prevent virus reactivation, nor does it control the spread of virus that can produce congenital infection (52). In general, recurrent infections yield a much lower risk of vertical transmission. A well-described syndrome of microcephaly, periventricular cerebral calcifications, chorioretinitis, purpura, psychomotor retardation, deafness, and hepatosplenomegaly occurs in congenital CMV infection. The onset of hepatomegaly and jaundice usually is noted within the first days of life. The histopathology of the liver reveals giant cell transformation and a severe inflammatory reaction. Large intranuclear inclusion bodies in bile duct epithelium and intracytoplasmic inclusion bodies in hepatocytes are rarely detected but confirm the diagnosis (53). Biliary cirrhosis and noncirrhotic portal fibrosis have been rarely described in children (54). Radiographic evidence of liver calcifications has been noted in congenital CMV disease (54). Generally, there is no evidence of severe liver disease after prolonged follow-up evaluation, in contrast to the devastating effects on the central nervous system (55, 56). A recognized complication of acquired immune deficiency syndrome (AIDS), papillary stenosis with sclerosing cholangitis, has been associated with CMV (57). All CMV-infected neonates shed virus in their urine from the time of birth. Therefore, diagnosis is confirmed by demonstrating the presence of CMV in the urine. PCR is now available to amplify and detect CMV DNA directly from liver tissue (58), serum, and other body fluids; however the usefulness of these studies has not been well defined (59). Ganciclovir has demonstrated efficacy in immunocompromised patients with CMV infections (60), and appears to reduce the risk of sensorineural hearing loss in congenital CMV infection (61). Valganciclovir, the orally bioavailable prodrug of ganciclovir, is a possible alternative to ganciclovir. Strong consideration should be given to the use of ganciclovir therapy in infants who demonstrate evidence of CMV-related CNS disease.

Herpes Simplex

Maternal herpes (HSV) infection can result in congenital and perinatal infections in the neonate, even subsequent to a first episode of genital herpes, because of asymptomatic cervical shedding of the virus (62). There is a significant perinatal morbidity, especially in those who acquire infection in the third trimester of pregnancy, making preventive measures, including antiviral chemotherapy, extremely important (62). Neonates born to mothers with a recurrent HSV infection are likely to have HSV antibody at birth. Within the first hours of life, the neonate with HSV infection appears seriously ill with generalized acute disease, and there are usually signs of encephalitis. Ulcerative, vesicular, or purpuric skin lesions are diagnostic. HSV hepatitis may be part of acute disease with jaundice and coagulation abnormalities. Liver histology reveals multifocal necrosis of the hepatic parenchyma in addition to characteristic intranuclear inclusions in hepatocytes. Scrapings of a skin vesicle or ulceration have been examined for giant cells, which are diagnostic for HSV infection (37). This method, known as a "Tzanck smear," has been largely supplanted by the more sensitive PCR test performed on blood, cerebrospinal fluid, and other clinical specimens (63). Viral cultures are needed to confirm the diagnosis. Acyclovir is useful in pregnant women with disseminated HSV infections. Intravenous acyclovir therapy of neonates with HSV is valuable in that mortality can be decreased in infants with disseminated and central nervous system disease (63).

Hepatitis B Virus

Since the discovery of a serologic marker for hepatitis B virus (HBV), the virus has been recognized to be endemic throughout many parts of the world and is characterized by a virus-host interaction leading to HBV immune tolerance. It is a DNA virus with surface and inner core antigens. The surface antigen (HBsAg) is the earliest indicator of the presence of acute infection. The other antigens are core antigen (HBcAg) in addition to e antigen (HBeAg), DNA polymerase, and HBV DNA, which correlates with HBV replication. Cytotoxicity of lymphocytes for liver cell antigens may be the mechanism of tissue injury rather than a direct cytopathic effect of HBV.

In the USA, HBV is an uncommon cause of cholestasis in infancy. However, in certain parts of the world, perinatal transmission of HBV from a chronic carrier mother or mother with acute HBV disease during the third trimester of pregnancy is common. Vertical transmission of HBV is more likely to occur if the mother is positive for the hepatitis Be antigen (64, 65). These infants will become positive for HBsAg between 1 and 3 months of age and are usually asymptomatic carriers of HBV. It has been estimated that 70% of infants born under these latter conditions acquire HBV and become chronic carriers of the antigen. This also suggests that HBV transmission most likely occurs during birth. The modes of transmission include passage of contaminated maternal blood directly from mother to neonate during birth, oral inoculation of the neonate by ingestion of maternal blood on passage through the vagina or at the time of Cesarean (C)-section, and contact with the mother during early infancy via ingestion of contaminated breast milk.

After perinatal acquisition of HBV, most infants develop the chronic carrier state and remain chronically infected into adult life (66). In rare instances, fulminant hepatitis can occur (67, 68). Some children have mild abnormalities of liver function but, if infected in the perinatal period and not treated, will eventually develop chronic HBV disease, including chronic hepatitis and cirrhosis (69, 70). It is known, however, even in countries with a high frequency of perinatal HBV transmission, that chronic hepatitis and cirrhosis occur most often in adults, not in infancy and early childhood (70). The long-term consequences of asymptomatic HBV in neonates are a major problem, especially the high risk of hepatocellular carcinoma (71). The prevention of neonatal HBV hepatitis could eventually decrease the incidence of cirrhosis and hepatocellular carcinoma in many parts of the world (72).

All infants born to high-risk mothers should be tested after birth if prenatal screening was not completed. The diagnosis of HBV infection is confirmed by detection of HBsAg or anti-HBc-IgM in the newborn's serum. Treatment with hepatitis B immunoglobulin (HBIG) and vaccine is instituted immediately if the neonate is found to be serologically negative. Recombivax-HB and Engerix-B are yeast recombinant (DNA) vaccines with comparable immunogenicity (69, 73). Primary vaccination for perinatal postexposure prophylaxis consists of three intramuscular doses of HBV vaccine, with the first given within 12 h of birth and the second and third given 1 and 6 months after the initial dose. For the neonate, 0.5 mL of HBIG is given with HBV vaccine (concurrently, but at a separate site) within 12 h of birth. Conclusive evidence favors the combination of active and passive immunization for infants born to HBsAg-positive chronic carrier mothers (74, 75). The overall protective efficiency rate in neonates given HBV vaccine and HBIG exceeds 93%, which was a substantial improvement over administration of either HBV or HBIG prophylaxis alone (74). The American Academy of Pediatrics recommends a combined strategy of screening all mothers, vaccinating all neonates, and then vaccinating all adolescents (76). Antiviral treatment in perinatally acquired HBV is controversial. Two medications are licensed for use in children with chronic HBV: interferon alpha and nucleosides (e.g., Adefovir and Entecavir). These antivirals have been shown to be most useful in children, not neonates and infants, with elevated liver enzymes and low levels of HBV DNA replication. HBV-infected infants are most commonly chronic carriers without active immunologic responses to HBV and, thus, are unlikely to have a significant response to the above medications (77).

Hepatitis A, C and D Viruses

Hepatitis A (HAV), an RNA virus, is transmitted by the fecal-oral route (ingestion of contaminated food or water). Pregnant women with hepatitis A infection probably do not transmit HAV to their infants, and it is generally assumed that this virus does not pose a risk to the fetus (65). However, neonates may be at a small risk of HAV infection if acute hepatitis occurs less than 2 weeks before the termination of pregnancy (70). Under these circumstances, it is prudent to administer a single 0.02 mL/kg dose of immune serum globulin shortly after birth (78). The hepatitis A vaccine is reserved for children greater than 12 months of age. A chronic carrier state for HAV has never been demonstrated. Therefore, isolation of infants from mothers convalescing from HAV hepatitis is not necessary (70).

It is now recognized that hepatitis C virus (HCV), a single-stranded RNA virus, is responsible for the majority of cases of transfusion-related and community-acquired non-A, non-B (NANB) hepatitis (79). Detection of HCV infection is by ELISA and recombinant immunoblot (RIBA) assays, in addition to serum HCV RNA by the PCR assay for identification of replicative disease. In contrast to HBV, sexually active individuals have a low risk of developing HCV infection. The risk of vertical transmission of HCV is small and infected infants have a high rate of spontaneous viral clearance (80). A long-term prospective study of infants born to HCV RNA positive mothers showed that eight of 60 (13.3%) infants acquired HCV infection, but only 2 (3.3%) were still infected by 24 months of age. Moreover, the absence of viremia in the mother seems to predict an exceedingly low risk of HCV vertical transmission (81, 82). In another study, 56 out of 903 (6.2%) of infants born to HCV RNA PCR-positive mothers became infected, while no infants of HCV RNA PCR-negative mothers became infected. Coinfection with HIV is an independent risk factor for increased mother-to-infant transmission (81). Vertical transmission of HCV has been shown to occur in as many as 22% of HIV-positive mothers versus 4% of HIV-negative mothers. Female infants are twice as likely to become infected as males (83). The reason for this gender predilection is unknown but does not seem to be related to excessive deaths of infected males in utero. By contrast, mode of delivery and breast-feeding do not influence rates of mother-to-infant transmission significantly (83). No evidence for a protective effect of elective C-section delivery has been elicited. Although some investigators have detected HCV RNA in breast milk, no definite case of mother-to-infant transmission of HCV via breast milk has been reported (81). HCV-positive mothers should be allowed to breast-feed provided there is no nipple trauma or bleeding and no HIV coinfection (84). Universal screening for HCV in pregnant mothers is not recommended; however, selective HCV screening of high-risk mothers and their infants should be performed (84). Infants may retain maternal antibody for up to 18 months; thus testing for anti-HCV should be deferred until the infant reaches this age. Earlier diagnosis is possible with HCV RNA PCR testing between 1 and 2 months of age; however, there is no FDA-approved therapy available for treatment of HCV-infected infants. The clinical course of HCV infection in infancy is relatively benign, but the perinatal route of infection is a risk factor for HCV-related disease progression.

Transmission of the hepatitis D virus (delta agent) from mother to infant has been reported (85). This RNA virus requires HBV for replication; therefore, it is possible that the transmissions of delta agent and HBV to the infant, and prevention of disease for both, are similar. The delta agent is frequently responsible for more serious liver disease such as fulminant hepatitis. No therapy is available to treat this viral infection, which is currently uncommon in the USA. Because hepatitis D virus requires HBV co-infection for virulence, HBV immunization offers protection against both viruses.

Human Immunodeficiency Virus

In the last decade, strategies for reducing perinatal transmission of human immunodeficiency virus (HIV) (86, 87) have demonstrated remarkable success in resource-rich nations (88). In the developing world, however, perinatally acquired HIV continues to be a public health crisis. HIV is a retrovirus with a glycoprotein envelope and a characteristic core protein that surrounds genomic RNA. For infants, the most important route of transmission is maternal transfer of virus during pregnancy or the perinatal period. Approximately 80% of HIV infections in children are acquired via the perinatal route; most of these infants are born to mothers who have AIDS or are at risk of developing the disease (89, 90). A large percentage of mothers of congenitally infected children are asymptomatic at the time of birth, but they have immunologic evidence of HIV infection. For these children, the risk of perinatal acquisition of HIV and subsequent development of AIDS is estimated to be as high as 50% (91, 92). Breast milk has also been implicated in the transmission of HIV (93); it is recommended that HIV-infected mothers refrain from breast-feeding.

For perinatal HIV infection, clinical symptoms can develop as early as 1 month of age, but the median interval from birth to symptoms is 8 months (94). The most common early manifestations of disease in infants include the triad of poor growth, interstitial pneumonitis, and hepatosplenomegaly (89, 90, 91, 95–97). Acute hepatitis, however, can be the first manifestation of HIV infection in early infancy (98). Multiorgan involvement is common in all patients with HIV infection. A form of autoimmune hepatitis was discovered in four older infants (1.5–6 years of age) with clinical and immunologic characteristics of HIV infection (99). Liver histology was remarkable for prominent lymphocytic infiltration of the portal and lobular areas, interface hepatitis, and bridging fibrosis, but no obvious intranuclear viral inclusions. Marked lymphocytic infiltration and sinusoidal cell hyperplasia have been previously described in CMV (100) and EBV-induced hepatitis. Also, CMV may perturb bile ductular epithelium in the neonate (101), but a sclerosing cholangitis syndrome has not been described in infants with HIV infection.

Methods for diagnosing perinatally acquired HIV infection have shifted from antibody and antigen testing to the more accurate PCR-based techniques (88). HIV antibody testing in infants is unreliable due to the transplacental transmission of maternal immunoglobulin G (IgG) antibodies and the persistence of these antibodies in the child's serum for up to 12 months (102). The HIV DNA PCR assay on peripheral blood has yielded sensitivities and specificities as high as 87 and 99% respectively (103). For infants born to HIV-infected women, HIV DNA PCR testing is recommended at birth, 1–2 months of age and 2–4 months of age (104). Two separate blood samples must test positive for the diagnosis of HIV infection; thus any positive test should be repeated.

No curative therapy exists for HIV infection, but antiviral agents such as azido-3-deozythymidine (AZT) continue to be prescribed and investigated. Antepartum and intrapartum AZT treatment of mothers with HIV disease, combined with neonatal AZT therapy, reduces the risk of maternal-infant HIV transmission by approximately two-thirds (105). Also, development of an effective vaccine may become a reality in the future (106).

Echovirus, Parvovirus, and Adenovirus

Echovirus, an RNA enterovirus, can cause neonatal morbidity and mortality. Echovirus 11, the most commonly implicated serotype, is transmitted from mothers during the perinatal period, presumably by transplacental passage of virus prior to parturition. Four cases of fatal echovirus 11 disease occurred in premature infants during a community outbreak of enteroviral disease (107). Each infant developed jaundice in the first week of life and subsequent fulminant liver failure (108). One infant survived acute echovirus 11 hepatitis and subsequent hepatic failure but developed intractable ascites (109), and a neonate underwent successful treatment of fulminant liver failure by orthotopic liver transplantation (110). Because echovirus is a potentially treatable infection, the neonatologist should always consider this diagnosis as a cause of neonatal liver disease and order cultures for viral isolation, and appropriate serologic tests. Finally, it should be noted that there have been several cases of another enterovirus, Coxsackie B, causing fatal neonatal disease with neonatal hepatitis as a common feature (111, 112). Pleconaril, an anti-picornaviral drug (113), and intravenous immunoglobulin (IVIG) (114) have been used to treat severe neonatal enteroviral disease, although the efficacy of these therapies has not been established.

Parvovirus B-19, a DNA virus, may cause severe intrauterine infection responsible for leukoerythroblastic reaction in the liver and spleen, in addition to granular hemosiderin deposition in hepatocytes and Kupffer cells (115). This leads to profound anemia, nonimmune hydrops, and death. Infection by parvovirus is confirmed by maternal serology for parvovirus IgM and parvovirus DNA detection in fetal organs (116). The practical utility of PCR as a diagnostic method for discovery of intrauterine fetal parvovirus infection has also been examined (116, 117).

Adenovirus, a respiratory-tract pathogen, may cause hepatitis in the neonate. Acute adenoviral disease is usually fatal because of massive hepatic necrosis (118, 119). Prominent intranuclear inclusions are noted in hepatocytes. There is no known treatment for neonatal adenovirus infection.

METABOLIC CHOLESTASIS

Antitrypsin Deficiency

Alpha-1-antitrypsin (AAT) is a major plasma protease inhibitor which controls the proteolytic activity of neutrophil elastase that hydrolyzes structural proteins.

These serine protease inhibitors (Pi), known as serpins, play a role in regulating proteolysis in coagulation, fibrinolysis, and inflammation by inhibiting destructive neutrophil proteases and elastases (120). The AAT gene is a 12-kb single-copy gene on chromosome 14 and is known to have numerous variants, including the normal "M" type (121). About 2% of neonates have AAT alleles containing the deficiency "Z" type AAT gene, a variant associated with reduced serum antitrypsin. Other clinically relevant variants such as "S" type and the "null" type have been associated with low serum antitrypsin levels; however, only homozygotes for the Pi ZZ defect are subject to early-onset hepatocellular disease (122). Homozygous Pi ZZ is a relatively common autosomal recessive disorder affecting 1 in 2000 live births (123). Isoelectric focusing analysis has been used to detect varying degrees of AAT migration for type classification. The normal "M" variant migrates to the middle (M), while the abnormal variants A-L migrate faster and the N-Z variants migrate more slowly. The Z AAT gene differs from the normal M gene by a single base guanine-to-adenine change in the codon GAG of Glu (342) that modifies the residue to lysine (124). Abnormal Z-mutant AAT is then retained in the endoplasmic reticulum (ER) of hepatocytes with consequent intracellular accumulation and 80–85% decrease in serum AAT levels. Much of the retained AAT is degraded but the remainder aggregates to form insoluble intracellular inclusions of misfolded AAT proteins that are unable to traverse the secretory pathway (125). Although the precise mechanism is not known, these inclusions are associated with hepatocyte damage; only about 17% of neonates with homozygous ZZ antitrypsin develop clinically significant liver disease in infancy (126). This AAT deficiency, however, is the most frequent genetic cause of liver disease in children, and the most common genetic disease for which children undergo liver transplantation. It has been proposed that additional genetic traits may account for the net accumulation of mutant AAT and subsequent susceptibility to liver disease. In cellular transduction studies, it was determined that there was marked delay in degradation of mutant AAT after accumulation in fibroblasts from ZZ patients with liver disease compared to those without liver disease (127). More recent investigations have suggested the apparent involvement of cytoplasmic proteasome activity in this degradation process (128). It does not appear that immunoregulatory genes play a role in the pathogenesis of AAT liver damage (129).

At present, liver transplantation is the only therapy available to children with severe liver disease due to AAT deficiency. For older AAT-deficient patients with emphysema, a condition that does not affect children, future non-transplantation therapy potentially includes intravenous and aerosol AAT, inhibitors of neutrophil elastase and gene transfer by viral vectors. Replacement of AAT in the intravenous form has been problematic due to the risks and complications of infusing a product of human plasma and has only been studied in adults (130). Currently, recombinant forms of AAT are cleared too quickly from the human circulation to be practical therapies. There is active research in genetic approaches to mitigate or cure AAT deficiency. The normal human AAT gene has been successfully introduced into striated muscle cells using an adeno-associated virus vector in animal models and human studies are in development (131).

There is no precise method of predicting the severity of liver disease in an infant with AAT deficiency. Prolonged jaundice is often noticed in the first months of life as the initial sign of liver involvement. A small number of infants have hepatosplenomegaly with ascites and liver dysfunction. Some of these AAT-deficient patients develop fulminant liver failure in the neonatal period (132). Parents of affected children should receive genetic counseling regarding the potential risk for future PiZZ pregnancies. Up to 72% of PiZZ siblings of PiZZ probands will have liver disease and 29% will have concordantly severe liver disease (133). In this setting the perinatologist might want to consider chorion villus sampling for prenatal diagnosis of AAT deficiency. Primer designed, polymerase chain reaction methods are available for detection of the nucleotide base change in AAT deficiency at the Z mutation site (134).

Cystic Fibrosis

Cystic fibrosis (CF) is an epithelial electrolyte transport disorder identified, in part, by an elevated sweat chloride level. Since the elucidation of abnormal electrolyte transport across epithelial tissue as the basic physiologic disturbance in CF, there has been the identification and cloning of the gene on chromosome 7 encoding the CF transmembrane conductance regulator (CFTR). This CFTR proved to be not only the substrate for phosphorylation activation of the chloride channel, but also the actual cyclic-AMP-regulated chloride channel (135). It is now well established that CF is associated with nearly 1000 mutations in the CFTR gene, the most frequent being the delta F508, a three-base deletion removing phenylalanine 508 from the coding region. The delta F508 mutation is present in over 90% of patients with CF in the USA. The mechanisms by which CFTR mutations cause disease include a reduction (or absence) of CFTR synthesis, defective protein maturation, premature degradation, disordered regulation of CFTR function, defective chloride conductance, or accelerated CFTR turnover (135).

While CF is best known to disturb chloride secretion of sweat glands and the respiratory tract, defective forms of CFTR are also responsible for inspissation of pancreatic juice and hepatobiliary secretions. In fact, hepatobiliary disease is one of the commonest non-pulmonary causes of mortality in CF; neonates may present acutely with cholestatic jaundice, especially those with a history of meconium ileus (136). CFTR is normally distributed along the apical domain of biliary epithelial cell plasma membranes and is not expressed on hepatocytes (137). The apical location of CFTR in biliary cells assists in our understanding of how the CFTR-regulated chloride channel contributes to normal biliary secretion.

The classic presentation for CF is malabsorption in infancy with an increasing incidence of respiratory-tract infections during childhood and adolescence. Many neonates present with intestinal obstruction resulting from meconium ileus. Only some present with neonatal cholestasis suggestive of biliary atresia. Older children occasionally present with cirrhosis and portal hypertension prior to the diagnosis of CF. Many patients with severe liver disease secondary to inspissated bile flow and consequent biliary cirrhosis require liver transplantation. Treatment with ursodeoxycholic acid is the only available non-transplant therapeutic approach, although its effect on the progression of liver disease is unclear (138). With the discovery that CFTR is localized to both submucosal glands and surface epithelium, these sites may be important future targets for gene therapy. It is reasonable, therefore, to believe that the respiratory manifestations of CF could be prevented by transfer and expression of normal CFTR cDNA to airway epithelium. In like manner, the hepatobiliary manifestations of CF perhaps could be prevented by transfer of CFTR cDNA to the intrahepatic biliary epithelial cells (139). These biliary cells can be studied by adenovirus-mediated delivery and the defective CFTR complemented. This potential preventive therapy of CF liver disease by genetically reconstituting CFTR in the biliary tract (140) is also an opportunity to study and determine the mechanisms responsible for hepatobiliary disease in children with CF.

Tyrosinemia

Hereditary tyrosinemia (HT), an inborn error of amino acid metabolism, is caused by a deficiency of the last enzyme in the catabolic pathway of tyrosine (Fig. 9-1)

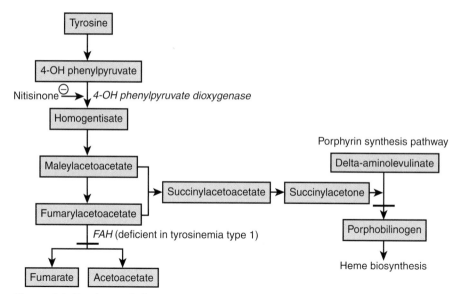

Figure 9-1 Tyrosine catabolism. Tyrosinemia type I is secondary to a deficiency of fumarylaceto-acetate hydrolase (FAH). Succinylacetone inhibits the synthesis of porphobilinogen. Nitisinone inhibits the enzyme 4-OH phenylpyruvate dioxygenase.

known as fumarylacetoacetate hydrolase (FAH). The disease is most commonly reported in neonates from French Canada (Saguenay, Quebec); in fact, 1 of 1846 newborns are affected in this region (141). Nucleotide changes were responsible for the decreased activity of FAH. A splice mutation was discovered in all of the neonates from the Saguenay area and in 28% of patients from other parts of the world (141). They were mostly homozygous for this prevalent mutation, a guanine-to-adenine change in the splice donor sequence of the gene. Other investigators have reported that the human FAH gene is 35kb long and is split into 14 exons, with nucleotide mutations from thymidine to guanine (142) and a change from trypto-phan to a stop codon at position 262 (143). Expression of FAH in livers of patients with HT has been analyzed at several molecular levels, including mRNA and enzy-matic activity, leading to differentiation of phenotypic variants. Many mutations in the FAH gene have been described in infants with tyrosinemia; there is heteroge-neity in the expression of FAH at the levels of mRNA, enzymatic and protein activity in the livers of these patients (144).

Until recently, there were no treatment options for infants with HT except for rapid institution of tyrosine-restricted diets and liver transplantation. The cloning of cDNA encoding FAH via retroviral and integrase-mediated gene transfer has led to the potential future consideration of gene therapy for this disorder (145, 146). It is already possible to restore FAH activity in fibroblasts from these deficient patients (147).

Use of a pesticide derivative, NTBC or nitisinone [2-(2-nitro-4-trifluoromethyl-benzoyl)-1,3-cyclohexanedione] is the first documented pharmacological therapy for HT (148). This chemical perturbs tyrosine metabolism via the inhibition of 4-hydroxyphenylpyruvate dioxygenase, preventing the formation and accumulation of succinylacetone and succinylacetoacetate (Fig. 9-1). In initial clinical trials, patients were given an oral dose of nitisinone (formerly known as NTBC) in the range 0.1–0.6 mg/kg/day (149). Serum succinylacetone decreased rapidly to almost undetectable levels and clinical symptoms generally improved. Also after treatment there was improvement in liver function and a decrease in serum fetoprotein. In response to the initial success of nitisinone in the treatment of HT, a multicenter study based in Gothenburg, Sweden, was established and has enrolled nearly

300 patients worldwide (150). Many of these patients have been treated for over 5 years with good clinical results. At present, it is not known to what degree this new pharmacological therapy will affect the possible development of hepatocellular carcinoma (HCC). While HCC is historically reported in up to 37% of tyrosinemic children, initial evidence from the Gothenburg study suggests a significantly lower incidence of HCC in those patients for whom nitisinone was started before 2 years of age (150). The current recommended dosage of nitisinone is 1mg/kg/day, to be combined with a phenylalanine- and tyrosine-restricted diet (148).

Liver transplantation is reserved for tyrosinemic children with acute liver failure, poor response to pharmacological management, and suspected HCC (148). When performed, liver transplant is curative for both hepatic tumor and the metabolic derangement of HT-1 (151, 152). Prior to the introduction of nitisinone, liver transplant was recommended for all infants with HT before the age of 12 months (153). Despite the dramatically improved metabolic control achieved with nitisinone therapy, HCC remains a significant risk for all patients with HT. Abnormal gene expression (154) and the development of hepatic dysplasia (155) are not corrected by nitisinone. The risk of HCC is increased when initiation of nitisinone therapy is delayed; thus nitisinone should be started as soon as feasible (148).

Classically, HT is divided into a chronic and an acute form. Patients with the chronic form have immunoreactive FAH at a level approximately 20% of normal enzymatic activity. No immunoreactive FAH was observed on immunoblots of liver, kidneys, and lymphocytes from patients presenting the acute form of this metabolic disease (156). Prior to the universal use of nitisinone therapy in HT, the probability of survival on dietary treatment alone was poor (157). The survival after the onset of symptoms varied with the age of onset – the earlier the symptoms, the poorer the outlook. The most common causes of death were liver failure and recurrent bleeding (67%), HCC (17%), and the porphyria-like syndrome with respiratory failure (10%). The 1-year survival probabilities after the onset of symptoms in children for whom the symptoms developed before 2 months, between 2 and 6 months, and after 6 months were 38%, 74%, and 96%, respectively. Based on these survival rates, a new classification was proposed: very early, early, and late presenting forms (> 6 months) of tyrosinemia (157). With the US FDA approval of nitisinone in January 2002, the true extent of improvement in morbidity and mortality of HT remains to be seen.

The acute form of HT can occur at any time, usually causes severe hepatocellular dysfunction, and is often associated with a marked increase in serum fetoprotein. Serum levels of tyrosine are usually elevated, and markedly increased urinary succinylacetone is diagnostic of this inborn error of tyrosine metabolism. Acute neurologic crises, while not emphasized as a significant complication, occurred in 42% of 48 children (158). This problem began at a mean age of 1 year and the episodes consisted of peripheral neuropathy with pain and extensor hypertonia, vomiting and paralytic ileus, muscle weakness, and self-mutilation. Between crises, most children regained normal function. A reliable biochemical marker for the neurologic crises was not found, including serum levels of tyrosine and urine succinylacetone. Urinary excretion of delta-aminolevulinic acid, a neurotoxic intermediate of porphyrin biosynthesis, was elevated during crises but also during asymptomatic periods. It has been suggested that succinylacetone might have neurotoxic effects. Interestingly, it has been noted in animal studies that brain tissue sequesters succinylacetone and that heme biosynthesis in the brain is adversely affected, possibly resulting in impaired oxidative metabolism (159). Succinylacetone, therefore, may be responsible for the central nervous system manifestations of tyrosinemia.

The chronic form of HT may occur with evidence of renal glomerular and tubular dysfunction in addition to involvement of the liver and neuromuscular system (160). Children with long-standing renal involvement may develop severe interstitial disease. In the nitisinone era, most patients regain normal renal tubular function after early institution of nitisinone therapy and few patients require renal transplantation (148).

Neonatal Iron-Storage Disease

Neonatal iron-storage disease (NISD) is a poorly understood, rare familial disorder of iron metabolism which is characterized by severe hepatic insufficiency of intra-uterine onset (161). This problem is often referred to as neonatal hemochromatosis because of its association with extrahepatic siderosis and sparing of the reticuloen-dothelial system. The precise cause of NISD and nature of the basic defect remain uncertain. It has been proposed that NISD may represent an unusual manifestation of adult-onset hereditary hemochromatosis because of a similar pattern of iron deposition; however, evolving genetic evidence suggests the two diseases are separate entities. While, mutations of the *HFE* gene are responsible for the vast majority of adult-onset hereditary hemochromatosis cases (162), this mutation is not found in NISD (163). Other genetic mutations described in adult-onset hereditary hemochromatosis are also notably absent in NISD (163). To further discount a possible link between NISD and adult-onset disease, a 30-year follow-up study for iron overload of a family in which 6 of 9 children died in utero or in the early neonatal period found no hereditary hemochromatosis or other iron-storage disease in the parents or surviving siblings (164). Patterns of familial occurrence of NISD and a higher-than-expected incidence of NISD in siblings of an index case (∼80%) make genetic inheritance difficult to explain. Some propose that NISD may be related to an acquired maternal factor such as a gestational alloimmune process. This would help explain the success of high-dose immunoglobulin during pregnancy for reducing morbidity of recurrent neonatal hemochromatosis in siblings of an index case (165).

Infants with NISD usually have normal serum iron and transferrin levels with markedly elevated serum ferritin. Although the physiology of iron entry into the fetal circulation and fetal cellular iron handling are not fully understood, placental transfer of iron is thought to be a carefully regulated process involving two key components, hepcidin and ferroportin (161). Hepcidin is a peptide released by the liver in response to high serum iron levels (166). The overexpression of hepcidin has been implicated in the anemia of inflammation and hepcidin deficiency has been associated with iron-overload syndromes. Hepcidin reduces the amount of ferroportin, a key regulator of cellular iron export in enterocytes, hepatocytes and macrophages. It is also noteworthy that excess iron deposition is observed in other disorders, e.g., tyrosinemia, which may result in significant antenatal liver injury. Therefore, NISD may be a secondary phenomenon and not a unique genetic disease involving perturbed iron metabolism.

If antenatal death does not occur, infants with NISD are usually severely ill at or near birth with hypoglycemia, coagulopathy, hyperbilirubinemia and early development of ascites. Neonatal iron-storage disease is one of the most common causes of perinatal cirrhosis. In a few cases, the diagnosis is associated with fetal nonimmune hydrops; therefore, there is the possibility of early diagnosis by the perinatologist (167). It is not known whether intrauterine liver disease secondary to infection can lead to NISD, but intra- and extrahepatic siderosis may accompany chronic fetal CMV liver disease (168) and more acute, neonatal echovirus 9 liver disease with associated exogenous iron overload (169). Inborn errors of metabolism are also associated with increased hepatic iron, especially tyrosinemia type I and disorders of bile acid synthesis (170). Neonatal liver disease secondary to iron overload may also be associated with maternal Sjogren's syndrome (171).

Table 9-2 **Inborn Errors of Bile Acid Metabolism Associated with Hepatocellular Cholestasis**

1. 3β-Hydroxy-C_{27}-steroid dehydrogenase/isomerase deficiency
2. Δ_4-3-Oxosteroid 5β-reductase deficiency
3. Oxysterol 7α-hydroxylase deficiency
4. 2-Methylacyl-CoA racemase deficiency
5. Sterol 27-hydroxylase deficiency
6. Bile acid-CoA:amino acid N-acyltransferase deficiency

The characteristic pathologic findings of NISD are marked siderosis of the liver, pancreas, kidneys, and adrenal glands with sparing of the reticuloendothelial system. Abnormal levels of iron are also detected in minor salivary glands, which are easily accessible via buccal mucosa biopsy. The hepatic hemosiderosis can be associated with prominent hepatocellular necrosis, regenerative nodules with true congenital cirrhosis, pseudoacinar changes, giant-cell transformation, and diffuse sinusoidal fibrosis (172). The iron-rich hepatic milieu may cause hepatocellular damage through iron-catalyzed lipid peroxidation, i.e., oxidative injury to cell membranes and organelle structures (173).

Deferoxamine has not proved to be effective in these infants with NISD (174), and liver transplantation as a definitive therapy is usually not possible because of delayed liver procurement in these very sick infants. When performed, however, liver transplant yields a 50% long-term survival and should be considered in those patients who do not respond to supportive medical care (175).

Infants with NISD have been treated with a combination of antioxidants, cryoprotective agents, and chelation. The potential efficacy of this antioxidant-chelation "cocktail" is controversial, with some reporting benefit in milder disease (176) and others reporting no change in outcomes (175, 177). To warrant this therapy, the infant should have at least a markedly elevated serum ferritin level; siderosis of minor salivary gland; and prominent siderosis involving liver, if the biopsy was not unsafe because of coagulopathy. Three antioxidants are used as follows: vitamin E, N-acetylcysteine, and selenium (176). Prostaglandin E1 and deferoxamine are used for the cryoprotective effect and iron chelation, respectively (176). The response to this therapy for a uniformly fatal NISD, while potentially beneficial, will need to be observed in larger group of patients.

Inborn Errors of Bile Acid Metabolism

It is now recognized that cholestasis and liver injury can result from failure to synthesize normal amounts of the primary bile acids, cholic and chenodeoxycholic acids (178). Several unique defects (Table 9-2) have been identified and together they represent approximately 2% of persistent cholestatic syndromes in infants. These neonates may present with liver failure and appear, at least initially, to have giant-cell hepatitis or even iron-storage disease (178, 179). It is essential for the neonatologist to make an early diagnosis of this problem because treatment improves the prognosis of an otherwise lethal inborn error of bile acid synthesis.

The bile acid synthetic pathway is a complex multi-step process in which the neutral sterol cholesterol is converted to cholic and chenodeoxycholic acids. Multiple enzymes are required as biosynthetic catalysts and, when deficient, can lead to the accumulation of toxic bile acid intermediates. Most of the known enzyme deficiencies cause varying degrees of liver disease, ranging from fulminant hepatitis to slowly progressive hepatic injury. The most commonly reported bile acid synthetic defect is 3β-hydroxy-$C27$-steroid dehydrogenase/isomerase deficiency

(3βHSD), which leads to the accumulation of di- and tri-hydroxy-δ-5-cholenoic acids (178, 180). While serum bile acid levels are normal in 3βHSD, the toxic bile acid precursors are qualitatively abnormal and poorly transported across canalicular membranes of cholangiocytes. The mechanism of hepatocyte toxicity is unknown. For most of the known defects of bile acid synthesis, clinical manifestations may appear in the neonatal period and often include a conjugated hyperbilirubinemia, elevated serum transaminases, and sequelae of malabsorption. Mass spectrometry for urinary bile acid analysis has provided a useful screening tool for rapid diagnosis of these disorders (181). While urinary bile acid excretion is minimal in normal individuals, those patients with increased accumulation of bile acid intermediates will have characteristic negative ion patterns on urine mass spectrometry.

While these inborn errors of bile acid metabolism are probably rare, their true incidence is not known. More importantly, bile acid therapy has been successful in many of these infants, with reversal of liver function abnormalities and normalization of liver histology. The administration of cholic acid repletes the bile acid pool and decreases the production of toxic bile acid intermediates. Combination therapy with cholic, chenodeoxycholic, and ursodeoxycholic acids has been given in the past; however, the efficacy of cholic acid is greatest when given as monotherapy (181). Bile acid synthesis defects which produce large quantities of unconjugated cholic acid, such as oxysterol 7α-hydroxylase deficiency and bile acid-CoA:amino acid N-acyltransferase deficiency, probably do not benefit from the administration of additional cholic acid (181).

PRIMARY MITOCHONDRIAL HEPATOPATHIES

The mitochondrial hepatopathies represent a group of rare disorders involving abnormalities of mitochondrial structure and function that have been associated with acute and chronic liver disease (182). The primary hepatopathies involving electron transport or fatty acid oxidation defects should be considered separately from secondary mitochondrial injury and dysfunction that may be acquired as a result of independent disease processes, such as the hepatic iron overload of NISD or Zellweger's syndrome, or conditions causing mitochondrial lipid peroxidation. Reduced activity of mitochondrial respiratory chain complexes, mitochondrial DNA depletion, and disruption of the oxidative phosphorylation pathway have been implicated in the pathogenesis of these complicated disorders (182). Hepatic dysfunction is commonly recognized in neonates who may even present with fulminant hepatic failure in the first few weeks of life. While the clinical manifestations of mitochondrial hepatopathies are protean, concomitant jaundice, lactic acidosis, ketotic hypoglycemia and neuromuscular involvement should raise suspicion for one of these disorders. Both microvesicular and macrovesicular steatosis are typical histologic findings (183). The degree of hepatocellular and canalicular cholestasis, bile ductular proliferation and periportal fibrosis depends on the stage of the disease. For a definitive diagnosis, liver biopsy specimens can be sent to a laboratory experienced in measurement of mitochondrial enzyme activity, determination of ultrastructural evidence of mitochondrial injury, histochemical evaluation, and mitochondrial DNA analysis (182). Antioxidants have been used to treat mitochondrial hepatopathies with limited success. Orthotopic liver transplantation may be a therapeutic option for those infants without extrahepatic manifestations of the mitochondrial defect (184).

PROGRESSIVE FAMILIAL INTRAHEPATIC CHOLESTASIS (PFIC)

Bile acids are actively transported across the hepatocyte canalicular membrane, the main determinant of bile secretion (185). Secretion across the canalicular membrane into bile occurs because of specific proteins such as P-type ATPases, bile salt export pump (BSEP) and multidrug resistance protein 3 (MDR3). The underlying progressive familial intrahepatic cholestasis (PFIC) abnormalities occur because of mutations in the above proteins.

PFIC-1 (Byler's Disease)

PFIC-1, or Byler's disease, is a rare complex disorder secondary to a mutation in the *FIC1* gene which encodes a P-type ATPase. The exact function of this protein is unknown, but appears to be related to ATP-dependent phospholipid transport (186). Hence, the physiologic defect is decreased canalicular bile acid transport with resultant formation of abnormal bile and consequent canalicular membrane damage leading to cholestasis. The histologic findings are dilatation of canalicular lumina, blebbing of canalicular membrane and loss of microvilli. Typically, the cholestasis is associated with a normal serum gamma-glutamyl transferase (GGT), suggestive of limited or no bile ductular injury.

PFIC-2

PFIC-2 is caused by a mutation in BSEP, with almost total absence of conjugated bile acids in bile (187). Cholestasis occurs as a result of the cytotoxic effect of bile acids which accumulate in the hepatocytes. Infants with this autosomal recessive disorder present with progressive cholestasis but, like Byler's disease, limited evidence of bile ductular injury with a normal serum GGT level.

PFIC-3

PFIC-3 is another rare syndrome secondary to a mutation of MDR3 with almost total absence of phosphatidylcholine in bile (188). The liver histology is characterized by bile duct proliferation and inflammatory infiltrates in portal tracts. Infants develop early jaundice and are noted to have an abnormal increase in serum GGT to suggest more significant bile ductular injury. Although long-term data are not available, empiric treatment with ursodeoxycholic acid has been used in patients with all of the above bile canalicular transport defects.

TREATMENT OF CHOLESTASIS

Therapy for neonates and infants with cholestasis is aimed at optimizing nutrition and controlling pruritus as one seeks to establish the underlying diagnosis. The use of a choleretic agent such as ursodeoxycholic acid (10–15 mg/kg/day) may effectively increase bile flow and improve cholestasis (189). Phenobarbital (5 mg/kg/day) is used in infants to increase the accuracy of hepatobiliary scintigraphy and improve bile acid independent bile flow. Rifampin (5–10 mg/kg/day), which inhibits hepatocyte uptake of bile acids, has been used to treat pruritus, especially refractory pruritus (190). Fat-soluble vitamins are also essential in these infants with cholestatic liver disease. Vitamin K is given in a starting dose of 2.5–5.0 mg every day or every other day. The dose is monitored by following the coagulation studies, especially INR and prothrombin time. Excessive vitamin K may cause hemolysis. Vitamin D is administered as the 25-hydroxy oral preparation (3–5 µg/kg/day). Serum levels of 25-hydroxy vitamin D are carefully monitored because vitamin D intoxication leads to hypercalcemia, which is responsible for central nervous system depression, ectopic calcification and nephrolithiasis. Vitamin A is usually effective as a water-miscible preparation (5000–25 000 IU/day). Deficiency of vitamin A can cause xerophthalmia, keratomalacia, and night blindness. Manifestations of vitamin

A toxicity are hepatotoxicity and pseudotumor cerebri. Vitamin E supplementation is indicated for all neonates and infants with cholestasis. Vitamin E-deficient patients develop hyporeflexia, occasionally areflexia, ptosis, mild truncal ataxia or hypotonia (191). Standard alpha-tocopherol acetate suspension or the vitamin E contents of gel capsules are sometimes administered (50 IU/kg/day). Tocopherol polyethylene glycol-1000 succinate (TPGS) is a water-soluble ester of vitamin E (Liqui-E) which is even more effective in maintaining vitamin E sufficiency (192). The dose of vitamin E is modified based on serum concentrations and the ratio of serum vitamin E to total serum lipid concentration (normal, above 0.8 mg/g).

REFERENCES

1. Silveira TR, Salzano FM, Howard ER, et al. Congenital structural abnormalities in biliary atresia: evidence for etiopathogenic heterogeneity and therapeutic implications. Acta Paediatr Scand 1991; 80(12):1192–1199.
2. Haber BA, Russo P. Biliary atresia. Gastroenterol Clin North Am 2003; 32(3):891–911.
3. Chen L, Goryachev A, Sun J, et al. Altered expression of genes involved in hepatic morphogenesis and fibrogenesis are identified by cDNA microarray analysis in biliary atresia. Hepatology 2003; 38(3):567–576.
4. Zhang DY, Sabla G, Shivakumar P, et al. Coordinate expression of regulatory genes differentiates embryonic and perinatal forms of biliary atresia. Hepatology 2004; 39(4):954–962.
5. Moyer V, Freese DK, Whitington PF, et al. Guideline for the evaluation of cholestatic jaundice in infants: recommendations of the North American Society for Pediatric Gastroenterology, Hepatology and Nutrition. J Pediatr Gastroenterol Nutr 2004; 39(2):115–128. Erratum in: J Pediatr Gastroenterol Nutr 2004; 39(3):306.
6. Li MK, Crawford JM. The pathology of cholestasis. Semin Liver Dis 2004; 24(1):21–42.
7. Kobayashi H, Stringer MD. Biliary atresia. Semin Neonatol 2003; 8(5):383–391.
8. Iinuma Y, Narisawa R, Iwafuchi M, et al. The role of endoscopic retrograde cholangiopancreatography in infants with cholestasis. J Pediatr Surg 2000; 35(4):545–549.
9. Senyuz OF, Yesildag E, Emir H, et al. Diagnostic laparoscopy in prolonged jaundice. J Pediatr Surg 2001; 36(3):463–465.
10. Okazaki T, Miyano G, Yamataka A, et al. Diagnostic laparoscopy-assisted cholangiography in infants with prolonged jaundice. Pediatr Surg Int 2006; 22(2):140–143. Epub 2005 Dec 8.
11. Lykavieris P, Chardot C, Sokhn M, et al. Outcome in adulthood of biliary atresia: a study of 63 patients who survived for over 20 years with their native liver. Hepatology 2005; 41(2):366–371.
12. Bielamowicz A, Weitzman JJ, Alshak NS, et al. Successful late Kasai portoenterostomy. J Pediatr Gastroenterol Nutr 1992; 14(2):232–236.
13. Barshes NR, Lee TC, Balkrishnan R, et al. Orthotopic liver transplantation for biliary atresia: the U.S. experience. Liver Transpl 2005; 11(10):1193–2000.
14. Chen CL, Concejero A, Wang CC, et al. Living donor liver transplantation for biliary atresia: a single-center experience with first 100 cases. Am J Transplant 2006; 6(11):2672–2679.
15. Tiao G, Ryckman FC. Pediatric liver transplantation. Clin Liver Dis 2006; 10(1):169–197, vii.
16. Bucuvalas JC, Ryckman FC. Long-term outcome after liver transplantation in children. Pediatr Transplant 2002; 6(1):30–36.
17. Alagille D, Odievre M, Gautier M, et al. Hepatic ductular hypoplasia associated with characteristic facies, vertebral malformations, retarded physical, mental, and sexual development, and cardiac murmur. J Pediatr 1975; 86(1):63–71.
18. Deprettere A, Portmann B, Mowat AP. Syndromic paucity of the intrahepatic bile ducts: diagnostic difficulty; severe morbidity throughout early childhood. J Pediatr Gastroenterol Nutr 1987 Nov-Dec; 6(6):865–871.
19. Sharp HL. The current status of alpha-1-antityrpsin, a protease inhibitor, in gastrointestinal disease. Gastroenterology 1976; 70(4):611–621.
20. Tzakis AG, Reyes J, Tepetes K, et al. Liver transplantation for Alagille's syndrome. Arch Surg 1993; 128(3):337–339.
21. Sherman P, Kolster E, Davies C, et al. Choledochal cysts: heterogeneity of clinical presentation. J Pediatr, Gastroenterol Nutr 1986; 5(6):867–872.
22. Ando K, Miyano T, Kohno S, et al. Spontaneous perforation of choledochal cyst: a study of 13 cases. Eur J Pediatr Surg 1998; 8(1):23–25.
23. Ikeda S, Sera Y, Akagi M. Serial ultrasonic examination to differentiate biliary atresia from neonatal hepatitis–special reference to changes in size of the gallbladder. Eur J Pediatr 1989; 148(5):396–400.
24. Sharp HL. The current status of alpha-1-antityrpsin, a protease inhibitor, in gastrointestinal disease. Gastroenterology 1976; 70(4):611–621.
25. Hood JM, Koep LJ, Peters RL, et al. Liver transplantation for advanced liver disease with alpha-1-antitrypsin deficiency. N Engl J Med 1980; 302(5):272–275.
26. Kaufman SS, Gondolesi GE, Fishbein TM. Parenteral nutrition associated liver disease. Semin Neonatol 2003; 8(5):375–381.

27. Arias IM. Inheritable and congenital hyperbilirubinemia. Models for the study of drug metabolism. N Engl J Med 1971; 285(25):1416–1421.
28. Kartenbeck J, Leuschner U, Mayer R, et al. Absence of the canalicular isoform of the MRP gene-encoded conjugate export pump from the hepatocytes in Dubin-Johnson syndrome. Hepatology 1996; 23(5):1061–1066.
29. Adachi Y, Yamamoto T. Partial defect in hepatic glutathione S-transferase activity in a case of Rotor's syndrome. Gastroenterol Jpn 1987; 22(1):34–38.
30. Suita S, Arima T, Ishii K, et al. Fate of infants with neonatal hepatitis: pediatric surgeons' dilemma. J Pediatr Surg 1992; 27(6):696–699.
31. Franson TR, Hierholzer WJ Jr, LaBrecque DR. Frequency and characteristics of hyperbilirubinemia associated with bacteremia. Rev Infect Dis 1985; 7(1):1–9.
32. Garcia FJ, Nager AL. Jaundice as an early diagnostic sign of urinary tract infection in infancy. Pediatrics 2002; 109(5):846–851.
33. Gamble JR, Vadas MA. Endothelial adhesiveness for blood neutrophils is inhibited by transforming growth factor-beta. Science 1988; 242(4875):97–99.
34. Keller GA, West MA, Harty JT, et al. Modulation of hepatocyte protein synthesis by endotoxin-activated Kupffer cells. Ann Surg 1985; 201(4):436–443.
35. Keppler D, Hagmann W, Rapp S, et al. The relation of leukotrienes to liver injury. Hepatology 1985; 5(5):883–891.
36. Becroft DM, Farmer K, Seddon RJ, et al. Epidemic listeriosis in the newborn. Br Med J 1971; 3(5777):747–751.
37. Alpert G, Plotkin SA. A practical guide to the diagnosis of congenital infections in the newborn infant. Pediatr Clin North Am 1986; 33(3):465–479.
38. Montoya JG, Liesenfeld O. Toxoplasmosis. Lancet 2004; 363(9425):1965–1976.
39. Watkins JB, Sunaryo FP, Berezin SH. Hepatic manifestations of congenital and perinatal disease. Clin Perinatol 1981; 8(3):467–480.
40. Remington JS, Desmonts G: Toxoplasmosis. In: Remington JS, Klein JO, eds., Infectious diseases of the fetus and newborn. Philadelphia: Elsevier Saunders; 2006: 984.
41. Naot Y, Desmonts G, Remington JS. IgM enzyme-linked immunosorbent assay test for the diagnosis of congenital Toxoplasma infection. J Pediatr 1981; 98(1):32–36.
42. Romand S, Wallon M, Franck J, et al. Prenatal diagnosis using polymerase chain reaction on amniotic fluid for congenital toxoplasmosis. Obstet Gynecol 2001; 97(2):296–300.
43. Buxton D, Thomson K, Maley S, et al. Vaccination of sheep with a live incomplete strain (S48) of Toxoplasma gondii and their immunity to challenge when pregnant. Vet Rec 1991; 129(5):89–93.
44. Ismael AB, Dimier-Poisson I, Lebrun M, et al. Mic1-3 Knockout of Toxoplasma gondii is a Successful Vaccine against Chronic and Congenital Toxoplasmosis in Mice. J Infect Dis 2006; 194(8):1176–1183.
45. Watkins JB, Sunaryo FP, Berezin SH. Hepatic manifestations of congenital and perinatal disease. Clin Perinatol 1981; 8(3):467–480.
46. Darville T. Syphilis. Pediatr Rev 1999; 20(5):160–164.
47. Long WA, Ulshen MH, Lawson EE. Clinical manifestations of congenital syphilitic hepatitis: implications for pathogenesis. J Pediatr Gastroenterol Nutr 1984; 3(4):551–555.
48. Pound MW, May DB. Proposed mechanisms and preventative options of Jarisch-Herxheimer reactions. J Clin Pharm Ther 2005; 30(3):291–295.
49. Banatvala JE, Brown DW. Rubella. Lancet 2004; 363(9415):1127–1137.
50. Meegan JM, Evans BK, Horstmann DM. Comparison of the latex agglutination test with the hemagglutination inhibition test, enzyme-linked immunosorbent assay, and neutralization test for detection of antibodies to rubella virus. J Clin Microbiol 1982; 16(4):644–649.
51. Griffiths PD. Cytomegalovirus and the liver. Semin Liver Dis 1984; 4(4):307–313.
52. Stagno S, Whitley RJ. Herpesvirus infections of pregnancy. Part I: Cytomegalovirus and Epstein-Barr virus infections. N Engl J Med 1985; 313(20):1270–1274.
53. Ahlfors K, Ivarsson SA, Harris S, et al. Congenital cytomegalovirus infection and disease in Sweden and the relative importance of primary and secondary maternal infections. Scand J Infect Dis 1984; 16(2):129–137.
54. Ghishan FK, Greene HL, Halter S, et al. Noncirrhotic portal hypertension in congenital cytomegalovirus infection. Hepatology 1984; 4(4):684–686.
55. Ahlfors K, Ivarsson SA, Harris S, et al. Congenital cytomegalovirus infection and disease in Sweden and the relative importance of primary and secondary maternal infections. Scand J Infect Dis 1984; 16(2):129–137.
56. Bale JF Jr, Blackman JA, Sato Y. Outcome in children with symptomatic congenital cytomegalovirus infection. J Child Neurol 1990; 5(2):131–136.
57. Jacobson MA, Cello JP, Sande MA. Cholestasis and disseminated cytomegalovirus disease in patients with the acquired immunodeficiency syndrome. Am J Med 1988; 84(2):218–224.
58. Wolff MA, Rand KH, Houck HJ, et al. Relationship of the polymerase chain reaction for cytomegalovirus to the development of hepatitis in liver transplant recipients. Transplantation 1993; 56(3):572–576.
59. Ross SA, Boppana SB. Congenital cytomegalovirus infection: outcome and diagnosis. Semin Pediatr Infect Dis 2005; 16(1):44–49.
60. Erice A, Jordan MC, Chace BA, et al. Ganciclovir treatment of cytomegalovirus disease in transplant recipients and other immunocompromised hosts. JAMA 1987; 257(22):3082–3087.

61. Schleiss MR. Antiviral therapy of congenital cytomegalovirus infection. Semin Pediatr Infect Dis 2005; 16(1):50–59.

62. Brown ZA, Vontver LA, Benedetti J, et al. Effects on infants of a first episode of genital herpes during pregnancy. N Engl J Med 1987; 317(20):1246–1251.

63. Kimberlin DW. Herpes simplex virus infections in neonates and early childhood. Semin Pediatr Infect Dis 2005; 16(4):271–281.

64. Wong VC, Lee AK, Ip HM. Transmission of hepatitis B antigens from symptom free carrier mothers to the fetus and the infant. Br J Obstet Gynaecol 1980; 87(11):958–965.

65. Tong MJ, Thursby M, Rakela J, et al. Studies on the maternal-infant transmission of the viruses which cause acute hepatitis. Gastroenterology 1981; 80(5 pt 1):999–1004.

66. Mulligan MJ, Stiehm ER. Neonatal hepatitis B infection: clinical and immunologic considerations. J Perinatol 1994; 14(1):2–9.

67. Delaplane D, Yogev R, Crussi F, et al. Fatal hepatitis B in early infancy: the importance of identifying HBsAg-positive pregnant women and providing immunoprophylaxis to their newborns. Pediatrics 1983; 72(2):176–180.

68. Watkins JB, Sunaryo FP, Berezin SH. Hepatic manifestations of congenital and perinatal disease. Clin Perinatol 1981; 8(3):467–480.

69. Stevens CE, Taylor PE, Tong MJ, et al. Yeast-recombinant hepatitis B vaccine. Efficacy with hepatitis B immune globulin in prevention of perinatal hepatitis B virus transmission. JAMA 1987; 257(19):2612–2616.

70. Stevens CE. Viral hepatitis in pregnancy: Problems for the physician dealing with the infant. Pediatr Rev 1980; 2:121.

71. Beasley RP, Hwang LY, Lin CC, et al. Hepatocellular carcinoma and hepatitis B virus. A prospective study of 22 707 men in Taiwan. Lancet 1981; 2(8256):1129–1133.

72. Snydman DR. Hepatitis in pregnancy. N Engl J Med 1985; 313(22):1398–1401.

73. West DJ, Calandra GB, Ellis RW. Vaccination of infants and children against hepatitis B. Pediatr Clin North Am 1990; 37(3):585–601.

74. Beasley RP, Hwang LY, Lee GC, et al. Prevention of perinatally transmitted hepatitis B virus infections with hepatitis B virus infections with hepatitis B immune globulin and hepatitis B vaccine. Lancet 1983; 2(8359):1099–1102.

75. Wong VC, Ip HM, Reesink HW, et al. Prevention of the HBsAg carrier state in newborn infants of mothers who are chronic carriers of HBsAg and HBeAg by administration of hepatitis-B vaccine and hepatitis-B immunoglobulin. Lancet 1984; 1(8383):921–926.

76. American Academy of Pediatrics. Childhood Immunization Support Program (CISP): 2006 Childhood Immunization Schedule and Catch-up Schedule. http://www.cispimmunize.org/. Accessed October 2006.

77. Slowik MK, Jhaveri R. Hepatitis B and C viruses in infants and young children. Semin Pediatr Infect Dis 2005; 16(4):296–305.

78. American Academy of Pediatrics. Hepatitis A. In: Pickering LK, Baker CJ, Long SS, McMillan JA, eds., Redbook: 2006 Report of the Committee on Infectious Diseases. 27th edn. Elk Grove Village, IL: American Academy of Pediatrics; 2006: 326–335.

79. Alter MJ, Hadler SC, Judson FN, et al. Risk factors for acute non-A, non-B hepatitis in the United States and association with hepatitis C virus infection. JAMA 1990; 264(17):2231–2235.

80. Ceci O, Margiotta M, Marello F, et al. Vertical transmission of HCV in a cohort of 2447 HIV-seronegative pregnant women: a 24-month prospective study. J Pediatr Gastroenterol Nutr 2001; 33:570–575.

81. Yeung LTF, King SM, Roberts EA. Mother-to-infant transmission of hepatitis C virus. Hepatology 2001; 34:223–229.

82. Dore GJ, Kaldor JM, McCaughan GW. Systematic review of role of polymerase chain reaction in defining infectiousness among people infected with hepatitis C virus. BMJ 1997; 315:333–337.

83. European Paediatric Hepatitis C. A significant sex-but not elective cesarean section-effect on mother-to-child transmission of hepatitis C virus infection. J Infect Dis 2005; 192:1872–1879.

84. American Academy of Pediatrics. Hepatitis C. In: Pickering LK, Baker CJ, Long SS, McMillan JA, eds., Redbook: 2006 Report of the Committee on Infectious Diseases, 27th edn. Elk Grove Village, IL: American Academy of Pediatrics; 2006: 355–359.

85. Zanetti AR, Ferroni P, Magliano EM, et al. Perinatal transmission of the hepatitis B virus and of the HBV-associated delta agent from mothers to offspring in northern Italy. J Med Virol 1982; 9(2):139–148.

86. Barre-Sinoussi F, Chermann JC, Rey F, et al. Isolation of a T-lymphotropic retrovirus from a patient at risk for acquired immune deficiency syndrome (AIDS). Science 1983; 220(4599):868–871.

87. Gallo RC, Salahuddin SZ, Popovic M, et al. Frequent detection and isolation of cytopathic retroviruses (HTLV-III) from patients with AIDS and at risk for AIDS. Science 1984; 224(4648):500–503.

88. Shetty AK. Perinatally acquired HIV-1 infection: prevention and evaluation of HIV-exposed infants. Semin Pediatr Infect Dis 2005; 16(4):282–295.

89. Rogers MF, Thomas PA, Starcher ET, et al. Acquired immunodeficiency syndrome in children: report of the Centers for Disease Control National Surveillance, 1982 to 1985. Pediatrics 1987; 79(6):1008–1014.

90. Shannon KM, Ammann AJ. Acquired immune deficiency syndrome in childhood. J Pediatr 1985; 106(2):332–342.

91. Pahwa S, Kaplan M, Fikrig S, et al. Spectrum of human T-cell lymphotropic virus type III infection in children. Recognition of symptomatic, asymptomatic, and seronegative patients. JAMA 1986; 255(17):2299–2305.

92. Rubinstein A, Bernstein L. The epidemiology of pediatric acquired immunodeficiency syndrome. Clin Immunol Immunopathol 1986; 40(1):115–121.

93. Ziegler JB, Cooper DA, Johnson RO, et al. Postnatal transmission of AIDS-associated retrovirus from mother to infant. Lancet 1985; 1(8434):896–898.

94. Rogers MF. AIDS in children: a review of the clinical, epidemiologic and public health aspects. Pediatr Infect Dis 1985; 4(3):230–236.

95. Oleske J, Minnefor A, Cooper R Jr, et al. Immune deficiency syndrome in children. JAMA 1983; 249(17):2345–2349.

96. Scott GB, Buck BE, Leterman JG, et al. Acquired immunodeficiency syndrome in infants. N Engl J Med 1984; 310(2):76–81.

97. Ammann AJ, Shannon KM. Recognition of acquired immune deficiency syndrome (AIDS) in children. Pediatr Rev 1985; 7:101.

98. Persaud D, Bangaru B, Greco MA, et al. Cholestatic hepatitis in children infected with the human immunodeficiency virus. Pediatr Infect Dis J 1993; 12(6):492–498.

99. Duffy LF, Daum F, Kahn E, et al. Hepatitis in children with acquired immune deficiency syndrome. Histopathologic and immunocytologic features. Gastroenterology 1986; 90(1):173–181.

100. Sacks SL, Freeman HJ. Cytomegalovirus hepatitis: evidence for direct hepatic viral infection using monoclonal antibodies. Gastroenterology 1984; 86(2):346–350.

101. Finegold MJ, Carpenter RJ. Obliterative cholangitis due to cytomegalovirus: a possible precursor of paucity of intrahepatic bile ducts. Hum Pathol 1982; 13(7):662–665.

102. Pyun KH, Ochs HD, Dufford MT, et al. Perinatal infection with human immunodeficiency virus. Specific antibody responses by the neonate. N Engl J Med 1987; 317(10):611–614.

103. Benjamin DK Jr, Miller WC. Rational testing of the HIV-exposed infant. Pediatrics 2001; 108(1):E3.

104. American Academy of Pediatrics. Human Immunodeficiency Virus Infection. In: Pickering LK, Baker CJ, Long SS, McMillan JA, Fiscas SA, et al., eds., Redbook: 2006 Report of the Committee on Infectious Diseases. 27th edn. Elk Grove Village, IL: American Academy of Pediatrics; 2006: 378–401.

105. Connor EM, Sperling RS, Gelber R, et al. Reduction of maternal-infant transmission of human immunodeficiency virus type 1 with zidovudine treatment. N Engl J Med 1994; 331(18): 1173–1180.

106. Lambert JS. HIV vaccines in infants and children. Paediatr Drugs 2005; 7(5):267–276.

107. Modlin JF. Fatal echovirus 11 disease in premature neonates. Pediatrics 1980; 66(5):775–780.

108. Mostoufizadeh M, Lack EE, Gang DL, et al. Postmortem manifestations of echovirus 11 sepsis in five newborn infants. Hum Pathol 1983; 14(9):818–823.

109. Gillam GL, Stokes KB, McLellan J, et al. Fulminant hepatic failure with intractable ascites due to an echovirus 11 infection successfully managed with a peritoneo-venous (LeVeen) shunt. J Pediatr Gastroenterol Nutr 1986; 5(3):476–480.

110. Chuang E, Maller ES, Hoffman MA, et al. Successful treatment of fulminant echovirus 11 infection in a neonate by orthotopic liver transplantation. J Pediatr Gastroenterol Nutr 1993; 17(2): 211–214.

111. Cheng LL, Ng PC, Chan PK, et al. Probable intrafamilial transmission of coxsackievirus b3 with vertical transmission, severe early-onset neonatal hepatitis, and prolonged viral RNA shedding. Pediatrics 2006; 118(3):e929–e933. Epub 2006 Aug 14.

112. Bryant PA, Tingay D, Dargaville PA, et al. Neonatal coxsackie B virus infection – a treatable disease? Eur J Pediatr 2004; 163(4–5):223–228. Epub 2004 Feb 18.

113. Aradottir E, Alonso EM, Shulman ST. Severe neonatal enteroviral hepatitis treated with pleconaril. Pediatr Infect Dis J 2001; 20(4):457–459.

114. Abzug MJ, Keyserling HL, Lee ML, et al. Neonatal enterovirus infection: virology, serology, and effects of intravenous immune globulin. Clin Infect Dis 1995; 20(5):1201–1206.

115. Maeda H, Shimokawa H, Satoh S, et al. Nonimmunologic hydrops fetalis resulting from intra-uterine human parvovirus B-19 infection: report of two cases. Obstet Gynecol 1988; 72(3 Pt 2):482–485.

116. de Jong EP, de Haan TR, Kroes AC, et al. Parvovirus B19 infection in pregnancy. J Clin Virol 2006; 36(1):1–7. Epub 2006 Feb 20.

117. Mark Y, Rogers BB, Oyer CE. Diagnosis and incidence of fetal parvovirus infection in an autopsy series: II. DNA amplification. Pediatr Pathol 1993; 13(3):381–386.

118. Abzug MJ, Levin MJ. Neonatal adenovirus infection: four patients and review of the literature. Pediatrics 1991; 87(6):890–896.

119. Krilov LR, Rubin LG, Frogel M, et al. Disseminated adenovirus infection with hepatic necrosis in patients with human immunodeficiency virus infection and other immunodeficiency states. Rev Infect Dis 1990; 12(2):303–307.

120. Law RH, Zhang Q, McGowan S, Buckle AM, et al. An overview of the serpin superfamily. Genome Biol 2006; 7(5):216.

121. Byth BC, Billingsley GD, Cox DW. Physical and genetic mapping of the serpin gene cluster at 14q32.1: allelic association and a unique haplotype associated with alpha 1-antitrypsin deficiency. Am J Hum Genet 1994; 55(1):126–133.

122. Crowther DC, Belorgey D, Miranda E, et al. Practical genetics: alpha-1-antitrypsin deficiency and the serpinopathies. Eur J Hum Genet 2004; 12(3):167–172.

123. Silverman EK, Miletich JP, Pierce JA, et al. Alpha-1-antitrypsin deficiency. High prevalence in the St. Louis area determined by direct population screening. Am Rev Respir Dis 1989; 140(4):961–966.

124. Brantly M, Courtney M, Crystal RG. Repair of the secretion defect in the Z form of alpha 1-antitrypsin by addition of a second mutation. Science 1988; 242(4886):1700–1702.

125. Carrell RW, Lomas DA. Alpha1-antitrypsin deficiency – a model for conformational diseases. N Engl J Med 2002; 346(1):45–53.

126. Sveger T. Liver disease in alpha1-antitrypsin deficiency detected by screening of 200,000 infants. N Engl J Med 1976; 294(24):1316–1321.

127. Wu Y, Whitman I, Molmenti E, et al. A lag in intracellular degradation of mutant alpha 1-antitrypsin correlates with the liver disease phenotype in homozygous PiZZ alpha 1-antitrypsin deficiency. Proc Natl Acad Sci USA 1994; 91(19):9014–9018.

128. Qu D, Teckman JH, Omura S, Perlmutter DH. Degradation of a mutant secretory protein, alpha1-antitrypsin Z, in the endoplasmic reticulum requires proteasome activity. J Biol Chem 1996; 271(37):22791–22795.

129. Doherty DG, Donaldson PT, Whitehouse DB, et al. HLA phenotypes and gene polymorphisms in juvenile liver disease associated with alpha 1-antitrypsin deficiency. Hepatology 1990; 12(2):218–223.

130. Juvelekian GS, Stoller JK. Augmentation therapy for alpha(1)-antitrypsin deficiency. Drugs 2004; 64(16):1743–1756.

131. Lu Y, Choi YK, Campbell-Thompson M, et al. Therapeutic level of functional human alpha 1 antitrypsin (hAAT) secreted from murine muscle transduced by adeno-associated virus (rAAV1) vector. J Gene Med 2006; 8(6):730–735.

132. Ghishan FK, Gray GF, Greene HL. Alpha 1-antitrypsin deficiency presenting with ascites and cirrhosis in the neonatal period. Gastroenterology 1983; 85(2):435–438.

133. Hinds R, Hadchouel A, Shanmugham NP, et al. Variable degree of liver involvement in siblings with PiZZ alpha-1-antitrypsin deficiency-related liver disease. J Pediatr Gastroenterol Nutr 2006; 43(1):136–138.

134. Dry PJ. Rapid detection of alpha-1-antitrypsin deficiency by analysis of a PCR-induced TaqI restriction site. Hum Genet 1991; 87(6):742–744.

135. Rowe SM, Miller S, Sorscher EJ. Cystic fibrosis. N Engl J Med 2005; 352(19):1992–2001.

136. Colombo C, Russo MC, Zazzeron L, Romano G. Liver disease in cystic fibrosis. J Pediatr Gastroenterol Nutr 2006; 43(Suppl 1):S49–S55.

137. Kinnman N, Lindblad A, Housset C, et al. Expression of cystic fibrosis transmembrane conductance regulator in liver tissue from patients with cystic fibrosis. Hepatology 2000; 32(2):334–340.

138. Paumgartner G, Beuers U. Ursodeoxycholic acid in cholestatic liver disease: mechanisms of action and therapeutic use revisited. Hepatology 2002; 36(3):525–531.

139. Grubman SA, Fang SL, Mulberg AE, et al. Correction of the cystic fibrosis defect by gene complementation in human intrahepatic biliary epithelial cell lines. Gastroenterology 1995; 108(2):584–592.

140. Yang Y, Raper SE, Cohn JA, et al. An approach for treating the hepatobiliary disease of cystic fibrosis by somatic gene transfer. Proc Natl Acad Sci USA 1993; 90(10):4601–4605.

141. Grompe M, St-Louis M, Demers SI, et al. A single mutation of the fumarylacetoacetate hydrolase gene in French Canadians with hereditary tyrosinemia type I. N Engl J Med 1994; 331:353.

142. Awata H, Endo F, Tanoue A, et al. Structural organization and analysis of the human fumaryl-acetoacetate hydrolase gene in tyrosinemia type I. Biochim Biophys Acta 1994; 1226(2):168–172.

143. St-Louis M, Leclerc B, Laine J, et al. Identification of a stop mutation in five Finnish patients suffering from hereditary tyrosinemia type I. Hum Mol Genet 1994; 3:69.

144. Phaneuf D, Lambert M, Laframboise R, et al. Type 1 hereditary tyrosinemia. Evidence for molecular heterogeneity and identification of a causal mutation in a French Canadian patient. J Clin Invest 1992; 90(4):1185–1192.

145. Held PK, Olivares EC, Aguilar CP, et al. In vivo correction of murine hereditary tyrosinemia type I by phiC31 integrase-mediated gene delivery. Mol Ther 2005; 11(3):399–408.

146. Montini E, Held PK, Noll M, et al. In vivo correction of murine tyrosinemia type I by DNA-mediated transposition. Mol Ther 2002; 6(6):759–769.

147. Phaneuf D, Hadchouel M, Tanguay RM, et al. Correction of fumarylacetoacetate hydrolase deficiency (type I tyrosinemia) in cultured human fibroblasts by retroviral-mediated gene transfer. Biochem Biophys Res Commun 1995; 208(3):957–963.

148. McKiernan PJ. Nitisinone in the treatment of hereditary tyrosinaemia type 1. Drugs 2006; 66(6):743–750.

149. Lindstedt S, Holme E, Lock EA, et al. Treatment of hereditary tyrosinaemia type I by inhibition of 4-hydroxyphenylpyruvate dioxygenase. Lancet 1992; 340(8823):813–817.

150. Holme E, Lindstedt S. Nontransplant treatment of tyrosinemia. Clin Liver Dis 2000; 4(4):805–814.

151. Mohan N, McKiernan P, Preece MA, et al. Indications and outcome of liver transplantation in tyrosinaemia type 1. Eur J Pediatr 1999; 158(Suppl 2):S49–S54.

152. Buyukpamukcu M, Varan A, Haberal M, et al. The efficacy of liver transplantation in malignant liver tumors associated with tyrosinemia: clinical and laboratory findings of five cases. Pediatr Transplant 2006; 10(4):517–520.

153. Freese DK, Tuchman M, Schwarzenberg SJ, et al. Early liver transplantation is indicated for tyrosinemia type I. J Pediatr Gastroenterol Nutr 1991; 13(1):10–15.

154. Luijerink MC, Jacobs SM, van Beurden EA, et al. Extensive changes in liver gene expression induced by hereditary tyrosinemia type I are not normalized by treatment with 2-(2-nitro-4-trifluoromethylbenzoyl)-1,3-cyclohexanedione (NTBC). J Hepatol 2003; 39(6):901–909.

155. Mohan N, McKiernan P, Preece MA, et al. Indications and outcome of liver transplantation in tyrosinaemia type 1. Eur J Pediatr 1999; 158(Suppl 2):S49–S54.

156. Tanguay RM, Valet JP, Lescault A, et al. Different molecular basis for fumarylacetoacetate hydrolase deficiency in the two clinical forms of hereditary tyrosinemia (type I). Am J Hum Genet 1990; 47(2):308–316.

157. van Spronsen FJ, Thomasse Y, Smit GP, et al. Hereditary tyrosinemia type I: a new clinical classification with difference in prognosis on dietary treatment. Hepatology 1994; 20(5):1187–1191.

158. Mitchell G, Larochelle J, Lambert M, et al. Neurologic crises in hereditary tyrosinemia. N Engl J Med 1990; 322(7):432–437.

159. Wyss PA, Boynton S, Chu J, et al. Tissue distribution of succinylacetone in the rat in vivo: a possible basis for neurotoxicity in hereditary infantile tyrosinemia. Biochim Biophys Acta 1993; 1182(3):323–328.

160. Russo PA, Mitchell GA, Tanguay RM. Tyrosinemia: a review. Pediatr Dev Pathol 2001; 4(3):212–221.

161. Whitington PF. Fetal and infantile hemochromatosis. Hepatology 2006; 43(4):654–660.

162. Feder JN, Gnirke A, Thomas W, et al. A novel MHC class I-like gene is mutated in patients with hereditary haemochromatosis. Nat Genet 1996; 13(4):399–408.

163. Kelly AL, Lunt PW, Rodrigues F, et al. Classification and genetic features of neonatal haemochromatosis: a study of 27 affected pedigrees and molecular analysis of genes implicated in iron metabolism. J Med Genet 2001; 38(9):599–610.

164. Dalhoj J, Kiaer H, Wiggers P, et al. Iron storage disease in parents and sibs of infants with neonatal hemochromatosis: 30-year follow-up. Am J Med Genet 1990; 37(3):342–345.

165. Whitington PF, Hibbard JU. High-dose immunoglobulin during pregnancy for recurrent neonatal haemochromatosis. Lancet 2004; 364(9446):1690–1698.

166. Papanikolaou G, Tzilianos M, Christakis JI, et al. Hepcidin in iron overload disorders. Blood 2005; 105(10):4103–4105.

167. Wisser J, Schreiner M, Diem H, et al. Neonatal hemochromatosis: a rare cause of nonimmune hydrops fetalis and fetal anemia. Fetal Diagn Ther 1993; 8(4):273–278.

168. Kershisnik MM, Knisely AS, Sun CC, et al. Cytomegalovirus infection, fetal liver disease, and neonatal hemochromatosis. Hum Pathol 1992; 23(9):1075–1080.

169. Bove KE, Wong R, Kagen H, et al. Exogenous iron overload in perinatal hemochromatosis: a case report. Pediatr Pathol 1991; 11(3):389–397.

170. Shneider BL, Setchell KD, Whitington PF, et al. Delta 4–3-oxosteroid 5 beta-reductase deficiency causing neonatal liver failure and hemochromatosis. J Pediatr 1994; 124(2):234–238.

171. Schoenlebe J, Buyon JP, Zitelli BJ, et al. Neonatal hemochromatosis associated with maternal autoantibodies against Ro/SS-A and La/SS-B ribonucleoproteins. Am J Dis Child 1993; 147(10):1072–1075.

172. Murray KF, Kowdley KV. Neonatal hemochromatosis. Pediatrics 2001; 108(4):960–964.

173. Ramm GA, Ruddell RG. Hepatotoxicity of iron overload: mechanisms of iron-induced hepatic fibrogenesis. Semin Liver Dis 2005; 25(4):433–449.

174. Jonas MM, Kaweblum YA, Fojaco R. Neonatal hemochromatosis: failure of deferoxamine therapy. J Pediatr Gastroenterol Nutr 1987; 6(6):984–988.

175. Rodrigues F, Kallas M, Nash R, et al. Neonatal hemochromatosis – medical treatment vs. transplantation: the king's experience. Liver Transpl 2005; 11(11):1417–1424.

176. Flynn DM, Mohan N, McKiernan P, et al. Progress in treatment and outcome for children with neonatal haemochromatosis. Arch Dis Child Fetal Neonatal Ed 2003; 88(2):F124–F127.

177. Sigurdsson L, Reyes J, Kocoshis SA, et al. Neonatal hemochromatosis: outcomes of pharmacologic and surgical therapies. J Pediatr Gastroenterol Nutr 1998; 26(1):85–9.

178. Bove KE, Heubi JE, Balistreri WF, et al. Bile acid synthetic defects and liver disease: a comprehensive review. Pediatr Dev Pathol 2004; 7(4):315–334.

179. Siafakas CG, Jonas MM, Perez-Atayde AR. Abnormal bile acid metabolism and neonatal hemochromatosis: a subset with poor prognosis. J Pediatr Gastroenterol Nutr 1997; 25(3):321–326.

180. Cheng JB, Jacquemin E, Gerhardt M, et al. Molecular genetics of 3beta-hydroxy-Delta5-C27-steroid oxidoreductase deficiency in 16 patients with loss of bile acid synthesis and liver disease. J Clin Endocrinol Metab 2003; 88(4):1833–1841.

181. Setchell KD, Heubi JE. Defects in bile acid biosynthesis–diagnosis and treatment. J Pediatr Gastroenterol Nutr 2006; 43(Supp. 1):S17–22.

182. Sokol RJ, Treem WR. Mitochondria and childhood liver diseases. J Pediatr Gastroenterol Nutr 1999; 28(1):14–16.

183. Bioulac-Sage P, Parrot-Roulaud F, Mazat JP, et al. Fatal neonatal liver failure and mitochondrial cytopathy (oxidative phosphorylation deficiency): a light and electron microscopic study of the liver. Hepatology 1993; 18(4):839–846.

184. Sokal EM, Sokol R, Cormier V, et al. Liver transplantation in mitochondrial respiratory chain disorders. Eur J Pediatr 1999; 158(Supp. 2):S81–84.

185. Trauner M, Meier PJ, Boyer JL. Molecular regulation of hepatocellular transport systems in cholestasis. J Hepatol 1999; 31(1):165–178.

186. Bull LN, van Eijk MJ, Pawlikowska L, et al. A gene encoding a P-type ATPase mutated in two forms of hereditary cholestasis. Nat Genet 1998; 18(3):219–224.

187. Shneider BL. Genetic cholestasis syndromes. J Pediatr Gastroenterol Nutr 1999; 28(2):124–131.

188. Elferink RP, Groen AK. The mechanism of biliary lipid secretion and its defects. Gastroenterol Clin North Am 1999; 28(1):59–74, vi.

189. Balistreri WF. Bile acid therapy in pediatric hepatobiliary disease: the role of ursodeoxycholic acid. J Pediatr Gastroenterol Nutr 1997; 24(5):573–589.

190. Yerushalmi B, Sokol RJ, Narkewicz MR, et al. Use of rifampin for severe pruritus in children with chronic cholestasis. J Pediatr Gastroenterol Nutr 1999; 29(4):442–447.

191. Sokol RJ, Guggenheim MA, Heubi JE, et al. Frequency and clinical progression of the vitamin E deficiency neurologic disorder in children with prolonged neonatal cholestasis. Am J Dis Child 1985; 139(12):1211–1215.

192. Sokol RJ, Heubi JE, Butler-Simon N, et al. Treatment of vitamin E deficiency during chronic childhood cholestasis with oral d-alpha-tocopheryl polyethylene glycol-1000 succinate. Gastroenterology 1987; 93(5):975–985.

Section II

Nutrition

Chapter 10

Regulation of Protein Synthesis and Proteolysis in the Neonate by Feeding

Tracy Gautsch Anthony, PhD • Susan Hazels Mitmesser, PhD

Basic Overview of Protein Metabolism
Mechanisms of Protein Synthesis
Mechanisms of Protein Degradation
Protein Nutrition in the Neonate

BASIC OVERVIEW OF PROTEIN METABOLISM

Introduction

There have been considerable efforts in the past decade toward understanding the regulation of protein metabolism in the neonate. This area of study is most appropriate in light of the fact that, during this same time, the rate of premature birth has risen substantially in the USA. In 2005, 12.5% of babies born in the USA were less than 37 weeks gestation, a 31% increase since 1981 (11). An increased incidence in premature birth and very low birth weight infants produces a larger population of neonates who require advanced nutritional support. Most neonatologists would agree that, although advances in perinatal care have improved survivability, current nutritional support standards are suboptimal for many premature and very low birth weight infants (2, 3). In general, there exists a great need to further explore how best to nutritionally support maximal growth of these fragile human beings.

Technological advances, using both isotopic amino acid tracers and basic molecular biology approaches, have begun to shed light on the mechanism and clinical impact of amino acids on catch-up growth and accretion of body proteins in the developing neonate. Data derived from these studies imply that current recommendations for protein and amino acid intake may be insufficient to maximize growth and protein accretion in the premature infant population (2, 3). Thus, the purpose of this chapter is twofold: first, to review our basic understanding of protein metabolism, synthesis and turnover, with an emphasis on neonatal growth needs. With this knowledge in hand, the second objective is to review the current recommended feeding practices in premature infants, with a focus on protein intake.

Interchange of Protein and Amino Acids

The process by which body protein is continually degraded and resynthesized is called protein turnover, a term that has been used collectively to include both protein synthesis and degradation. In addition to the exchange of amino acids into and out of protein, amino acids also are irreversibly lost through degradative pathways. For individuals in protein balance, the amount of amino acids degraded is equivalent to the amount ingested. Degradation involves the removal of nitrogen, primarily as urea and ammonia, and the breakdown of the remaining carbons, referred to as the carbon skeleton. The end result of the degradation of the carbon skeleton is the provision of energy, either directly or through the formation of simple compounds such as glucose and fatty acids, which can then be stored or metabolized to provide energy. The needs of the body regulate the directed flow rate, or flux, of amino acids through these possible pathways. Both energy balance and nitrogen balance influence whether amino acids and their carbon skeletons are used for the synthesis of amino acids and/or glucose versus oxidized for energy. It should be noted that if the breakdown of body proteins could be 100% reutilized to form the 20 classic amino acids, there would be little need to consume protein in the diet. However, certain amino acids cannot be synthesized by our bodies even in the face of ample nitrogen availability. These are called indispensable or essential amino acids.

Amino acids are also converted within the body to nonprotein end products. Nonprotein derivatives include compounds such as purine and pyrimidine bases, neurotransmitters (e.g., serotonin), and nonpeptide hormones (e.g., catecholamines). The quantities of amino acids involved in these nonprotein pathways are, in general, much smaller than the amounts of amino acids involved in protein synthesis and degradation. Because the amounts of amino acids irreversibly consumed in the synthesis of nonprotein compounds are normally much smaller than those consumed either by protein synthesis or by amino acid oxidation, these pathways often are ignored in the assessment of protein turnover and nitrogen balance. However, the amounts of some of these synthesized compounds can be substantial (e.g., heme, nucleic acids), and, for some amino acids, these pathways can become quantitatively significant during periods of insufficient protein intake.

Protein Turnover and Protein Balance

In the most simplified scheme, all the tissue and circulating proteins are considered together and, likewise, all the free amino acids are simplified to exist in a single, homogeneous "pool," rather than complex arrangements in blood, individual tissues, and subcellular compartments. This simplification has proved helpful in conceptualizing and developing methods for measuring the exchange of amino acids between the free and bound states. The exchange of free amino acids with body protein occurs through the processes of protein synthesis and protein degradation, and also through the entry and exit of amino acids by dietary intake and oxidation. Indispensible amino acids enter the body free pool from the digestion and absorption of dietary protein and from the degradation of body protein. Removal of amino acids from the free amino acid pool occurs either by the synthesis of protein or through excretion via oxidation to CO_2 and concomitant disposal of nitrogen, mainly as ammonia and urea. If the amount of free amino acid in the pool is constant, then the sum of the processes that remove amino acids (protein synthesis + oxidation) is equal to the sum of the processes by which amino acids enter the free pool (protein degradation + dietary amino acid intake). This can be easily expressed in the following equation:

$$S + E = D + I$$

In nitrogen equilibrium or protein balance, nitrogen intake (I) is equal to nitrogen excretion (E), and protein synthesis (S) is equal to protein degradation (D). For growth to occur, positive nitrogen balance must be obtained, and so for the neonate to be in positive nitrogen balance, there must be net protein synthesis or accretion $(S > D)$. The reverse is also true, for an individual to be in negative nitrogen balance there must be net protein degradation or loss $(S < D)$.

From the above-described relationships, it is clear that protein is retained in the body when synthesis exceeds degradation and that protein is lost from the body when degradation exceeds synthesis. Unlike the technique of nitrogen balance, which measures only net changes in body protein, estimates of protein synthesis and degradation indicate that changes in balance arise in a number of different ways. For example, loss of body protein can occur from a decrease in the synthesis of protein with no change in protein degradation, an increase in the degradation with no change in protein synthesis, or a change in both with one exceeding the other. In a number of pathological or stress conditions, body protein degradation exceeds synthesis, with both protein synthesis and degradation rates elevated over the rates in healthy individuals. Likewise, positive protein balance can be achieved by increases in protein synthesis, by decreases in protein degradation, or with changes in both protein synthesis and degradation, such that synthesis exceeds degradation. For example, in children recovering from malnutrition, the rates of both protein synthesis and degradation are increased, but the increase in synthesis is larger than the increase in protein degradation, producing a net positive protein balance. Thus, measurements of protein synthesis and degradation provide information about how the changes in balance are brought about. It is worth noting that, while the above explanation is presented in terms of whole-body protein, the concept of a balance between the processes of synthesis and degradation also occurs at the level of individual tissues or organs and for individual proteins (for more detail and further explanation on all of the above concepts, see McNurlan et al. (4)).

MECHANISMS OF PROTEIN SYNTHESIS

In its most general sense, the term protein synthesis describes the multiple processes required for a gene to be made into a functional protein. Each process comprises multiple steps, and regulation can occur at one or more of the steps within each process. Major advances in understanding the regulation of protein synthesis at the molecular level have been made in the last 30 years, and now with whole-genome sequences available for a growing number of different organisms, including rodents and humans, new information clarifying and extending our current understanding of the regulation of protein synthesis is accumulating at a faster rate than ever before.

The revelation that the human genome contains approximately 35 000 genes (5), one-third of original estimates and only about twice as many as found in invertebrates, has caused the scientific community to re-evaluate the influence of the genome in determining animal variety and complexity. It is now believed that the more global regulation of protein synthesis is the driver in determining cellular diversity.

Certainly, in terms of the preterm and full-term neonate, increases in protein synthesis drive growth and development. Major advances in our understanding of how feeding nutrients (amino acids and glucose, in particular) regulate protein synthesis in the preterm neonate have been achieved with the development of the neonatal piglet model (for recent reviews, see refs 6–8). The infusion of amino acid tracers in combination with established molecular biology methods has provided the scientific and medical community a deeper understanding of the factors that are controlling accretion of body protein. Furthermore, these technological advances have allowed examination of the effect of protein nutrition on individual tissues and organs in vivo.

In eukaryotic cells, the ability to express biologically active or functional proteins comes under major regulation at several points: deoxyribonucleic acid (DNA) transcription, ribonucleic acid (RNA) processing, messenger RNA (mRNA) stability, mRNA translation, and posttranslational protein modifications and folding. If cellular abundance of all proteins was determined at the level of transcription, the relationship between protein and mRNA levels would be linear. In fact, the correlation between mRNA levels and protein abundance in a single cell is poor, emphasizing the fact that posttranscriptional processes dominate in the regulation of cellular protein abundance. For this reason, the last two points of regulation (mRNA translation, and posttranslational protein modifications and folding) are of particular emphasis in this chapter.

Translation of mRNA

In the past few decades, the control of gene expression at the translational level has emerged as a means to regulate growth, proliferation, malignant transformation, and apoptosis (programmed cell death). Regulation of mRNA translation may alter the overall translational or ribosomal capacity of the cell (i.e., change in the number of ribosomes) or change the translational or ribosomal efficiency (i.e., amount of protein synthesized per ribosome). Furthermore, changes in ribosomal efficiency may be restricted to regulation of specific protein expression (e.g., ferritin mRNA) or affect the translation rate of specific proteins that are subsequently involved in mRNA translation and, thus, have global effects on the capacity and efficiency of mRNA translation (e.g., the TOP mRNAs, described below).

A change in ribosomal capacity implies alteration in the cellular abundance of the ribosomal proteins and rRNA. The time needed to modify these populations dictates that only chronic or sustained conditions, such as prolonged starvation or uncontrolled diabetes, can alter overall protein synthesis at the level of ribosomal capacity. There are also age-dependent differences at the level of RNA. Specifically, whole-body turnover rates for rRNA and tRNA in preterm infants are 3–4-times higher than in adults and mRNA turnover in neonates is 6-times higher than in adults (9, 10). This emphasizes the fact that the very high growth rates in neonates are made possible by the large capacity to make and utilize the translational machinery.

Each ribosome is composed of 80 different proteins and four RNA species (5S, 5.8S, 18S, and 28S). Three of the rRNA species (5.8S, 18S, and 28S) are transcribed from one gene (45S rDNA) by RNA polymerase I. Transcription of RNA polymerase I is enhanced by the transcription factor UBF (upstream binding factor). Conditions promoting anabolic growth may be accompanied by increased expression and/or activity of the UBF protein, resulting in increased 45S rDNA transcription. For example, hypertrophy of neonatal cardiomyocytes is promoted by increased activity of UBF (11).

Ribosomal capacity can also be influenced by ribosomal protein synthesis. Regulation of ribosomal protein synthesis occurs via the presence of a stretch of pyrimidines in the 5′-untranslated region of the gene. This terminal oligopyrimidine (TOP) motif is predominantly found in mRNAs that encode proteins that are involved in ribosome biogenesis and include the ribosomal proteins, mRNA translation factors such as elongation factors eEF1A and eEF2, and polyA-binding protein (12). Reduction in translation of TOP mRNAs reduces the overall protein-synthetic capacity of the cell because TOP mRNAs encode the translational machinery. A number of studies have implicated the phosphoinositide 3-kinase (PI3K) and mammalian target of rapamycin (mTOR) signaling pathways in the translational activation of TOP mRNAs (13, 14), but the precise role of each pathway in this process is not clearly defined at present. Feeding a protein-containing meal enhances TOP mRNA translation, whereas feeding an amino acid-deficient meal reduces translation of TOP mRNAs (15, 16). Although deprivation of amino acids can cause a decrease in the synthesis of essentially any protein, the synthesis of those proteins encoded by TOP mRNAs is repressed to a much greater extent than for most proteins. The exaggerated inhibition of TOP mRNAs by protein undernutrition is due to an "all or none" binary control mechanism that shifts the association of TOP mRNAs with polysomes (the translating population of ribosomes) into the sub-polysomes (the non-translating ribosome population) (12). In doing this, the translational machinery is effectively turned "off" or "on" in a non-permanent fashion.

A signaling pathway important in regulating TOP mRNA translation and thus ribosome biogenesis involves the mammalian target of rapamycin (mTOR) protein kinase. mTOR forms distinct signaling complexes with ancillary interacting proteins which then direct the translational machinery to respond appropriately to nutrients, insulin/growth factors, and energy state (17). In this way, the mTOR signal-transduction pathway is an important mechanism by which eukaryotic cells adjust their protein biosynthetic capacity in response to the cellular environment. The nutrient-sensitive mTOR complex 1 (mTORC1) responds to both hormones and amino acid status and activates the ribosomal protein S6 kinase (S6K1) pathway to control cell size (hypertrophy) and glucose homeostasis (18–20). A second mTOR complex (mTORC2) is identified as critical to modulating the actin cytoskeleton, an event important in tissue development and remodeling (21). Additional events controlled by mTOR activity include cell cycle progression, rRNA synthesis, processing of pre-rRNA, and autophagy (22). Thus, the mTOR signaling pathway controls a wide range of diverse events related to growth and development. To be sure, mTOR and its signaling complexes are centrally positioned in all matters of growth, and thus are absolutely essential for neonatal growth and anabolic response to nutrients (23).

The regulation of ribosomal capacity provides the organism with an ability to adapt to chronic or sustained conditions of change. In contrast, changes in ribosomal efficiency can be accomplished as needed without delay because all the protein-synthetic machinery is already present. Conditions that alter ribosomal efficiency include meal feeding, hypoxia, and hormone fluctuations. A change in ribosomal efficiency implies regulation at the level of mRNA translation.

Messenger RNA translation is a highly organized and multicomponent pathway that can be divided into three stages or steps: (1) initiation, (2) elongation, and (3) termination. During the initiation step, the small (40S) ribosomal subunit is recruited to a selected mRNA and joined with the large (60S) ribosomal subunit to form an 80S ribosome competent to identify the translation start codon and begin the process of elongation. The process of elongation involves the energy-expensive process of adding amino acids one after the other to the growing peptide chain. The termination step consists of recognition of the stop or termination codon and dissociation of the ribosomal subunits from the mRNA. Each of these steps is regulated by separate categories of protein factors called eukaryotic initiation factors (eIF), eukaryotic elongation factors (eEF), and eukaryotic release factors (eRF), respectively. Most of the protein factors regulating translation have multiple subunits and contain binding sites for interaction with other translation factors as well as for association with the ribosome. In addition, several are capable of catalytic activity that can be exploited to stimulate or inhibit translation.

Initiation

The majority of translational control lies at the initiation step (Fig. 10-1). This step can be further subdivided into three events that determine overall initiation activity (for detailed review see ref. 24). The first event involves the binding of the initiating tRNA (specifically, a methionyl-tRNA or Met-tRNAi) to the small ribosomal

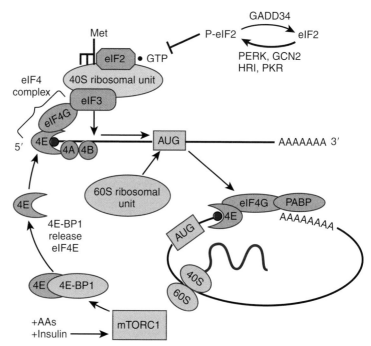

Figure 10-1 The pathway of eukaryotic mRNA translation initiation. Eukaryotic initiation factor (eIF) 2 bound to GTP is a necessary event that allows the binding of itself and the initiating tRNA (met-tRNAi) to the 40S ribosomal subunit. This event is regulated by the phosphorylation of eIF2 by a family of protein kinases which serve to inhibit pre-initiation complex formation under conditions of cell stress. Following this pre-initiation complex formation, the mRNA targeted for translation is selected by the eIF4 group of translation factors, which includes the mRNA cap binding protein, eIF4E and the scaffold protein, eIF4G. eIF4G is important for bringing the small ribosomal subunit in close proximity to the mRNA by interacting with eIF4E and eIF3 and has a role in mRNA circularization by binding the poly(A) binding protein (PABP). The mTOR complex regulates the activity of this step in part by modulating the association of eIF4G with eIF4E versus the translational repressor, 4E-BP1. Following successful formation of the eIF4 active complex and selection of mRNA, the 60S ribosomal subunit joins the 40S to form a competent 80S ribosome.

subunit. The Met-tRNAi is brought to the 40S ribosomal subunit by the protein factor eIF-2. The ability of eIF-2 and GTP (guanosine 5′- triphosphate) to associate with the initiating Met-tRNAi is regulated by the phosphorylation state of eIF-2. Increases in phosphorylated eIF-2 prevent association of Met-tRNAi with the small ribosomal subunit, resulting in global downregulation of mRNA translation. Under conditions of cellular stress, phosphorylation of eIF-2 also signals the need for increased expression of specific mRNAs that function to manage or alleviate cell stress. This paradoxical concept has been referred to as the Integrated Stress Response (25), and is initiated by a family of four eIF2 kinases. These family members are named: PERK (protein kinase R-like ER-resident kinase, also named pancreatic eIF2 kinase or PEK), which senses ER stress (26, 27), GCN2 (general control nonderepressible-2 kinase), which is activated by amino acid starvation and UV light (28), HRI (heme controlled inhibitor), which senses heme deprivation (29), and PKR (double-stranded RNA-dependent protein kinase), which is activated by viral infection (30). While these protein kinases primarily function to sense specific environmental stressors, they are also found to work cooperatively together, possessing auxiliary or secondary kinase activity when the primary responsive kinase is dysfunctional or nonfunctional.

The second event in translation initiation subject to regulation involves the binding of the small ribosomal subunit to the selected mRNA. This event requires a multicomponent complex, collectively called eIF-4 (or eIF-4F) (31). One of the proteins in this group, named eIF-4E, selects the mRNA to be translated by binding its 5′-cap structure. All eukaryotic mRNAs are "capped" with a 7-methylguanosine residue (m^{7}GTP). The covalently attached m^{7}GTP molecule serves to protect the mRNA from exonucleases but more importantly is recognized by the mRNA cap binding protein, eIF4E, for selection and binding to the small ribosomal subunit. A second member of the eIF4 group, called eIF-4G, functions to bring the small ribosomal subunit and the mRNA into proximity to each other. It accomplishes this task by serving as a scaffold, binding eIF-4E, eIF4A, and the 13-subunit protein complex, eIF-3, thereby facilitating their association with the 40S ribosome (32). A family of repressor proteins (4E-BPs and, specifically, 4E-BP1) can prevent eIF-4G from interacting with eIF-4E and thereby inhibit the 40S ribosome from binding mRNA (33).

A second function of eIF-4G is to associate with poly(A)-binding protein (PABP), a protein which binds a stretch of 20–250 adenosine residues at the 3′ end of the mRNA. These two binding events culminate in the 5′→3′ circularization of mRNA during translation. Circularization of mRNA is believed to be important for stabilizing recruited 40S ribosomal subunits and for efficient recycling of terminating ribosomes for another round of translation using the same mRNA (34). Thus, the eIF4G-PABP interaction is implicated in both enhancing the formation of 48S and 80S initiation complexes and ribosome recycling through mRNA circularization (35).

The final event in translation initiation involves the joining of the small ribosomal subunit (bound to mRNA) to the large ribosomal subunit. This event is catalyzed by several eIFs, including eIF-2, eIF-3, and eIF-5. Although the factors involved and their interactions have been explored, details surrounding potential regulation at this step are beyond the scope of this review.

With respect to feeding in the neonate, both insulin and amino acids are necessary to stimulate protein synthesis at the level of translation initiation (36–38). Amino acids, and in particular the branched-chain amino acid leucine, serve as signaling molecules to regulate the initiation step of mRNA translation by directing eIF4 complex formation and eIF2 phosphorylation (15, 16, 39). A physiological rise in leucine alone is all that is required to stimulate eIF4 formation and protein synthesis in the skeletal muscle of neonatal pigs (40). This finding is critically important for neonatal nutrition, as it indicates that amino acids have a very high priority in the cell to be used to promote growth of lean tissue. How exactly amino acids initiate a signal to turn on the translational machinery is still a mystery. What is known is that the mTOR kinase is one of the central players in sensing cellular availability of amino acids and that the stimulation in protein synthesis achieved from supplying leucine to neonates or young animals is promoted optimally when the amino acid signal occurs in combination with the activation of the insulin signal transduction pathway.

The signaling pathways elicited by insulin and amino acids converge at the level of mTOR, which then catalyzes the phosphorylation of 4E-BP1. Phosphorylation of 4E-BP1 causes its release of bound eIF4E, allowing eIF4G to bind eIF4E and eIF3, forming the eIF4F complex (33, 41). Both of these binding activities are blocked partially or fully by treatment with rapamycin, an mTOR inhibitor. Stimulation of mTOR activity also results in the activation of S6K1 phosphorylation. Phosphorylation of S6K1 activates ribosome biogenesis and other processes that serve to increase cell size (42). The S6K1 signaling pathway in response to amino acids or insulin is fully inhibited by rapamycin, whereas eIF4G binding activities are less so.

It is clear that the neonate is primed to respond to nutrients, with a very large capacity and efficiency of protein synthesis present at birth. However, the translational components and factors required to activate anabolic growth decline with age (43–45). This decline in translational capacity to respond to feeding occurs very rapidly, over the course of days in neonatal pigs. These data emphasize the point that early protein nutrition is critical in order to take advantage of the opportunity to maximally stimulate lean body growth in neonates. This may be why protein malnutrition early in life is hard to overcome later on, even with enhanced nutrition and hormone replacement not being able to reverse growth stunting (46). The capacity to respond to feeding is much reduced later in life.

Elongation

After initiation, the polypeptide is assembled with the amino acid sequence being specified by the mRNA sequence. This process requires a substantial amount of metabolic energy, cleaving two molecules of GTP for every added amino acid. The elongation step of mRNA translation involves fewer protein factors than the initiation step (just three eEFs versus more than a dozen eIFs), but the eEFs required are considered the workhorses of protein synthesis on the ribosome. At the start of elongation, the Met-tRNAi is base-paired with the mRNA start codon in a location named the peptidyl or "P" site within the ribosome. The protein factor eEF-1A (bound to GTP) then delivers the next correct aminoacyl-tRNA to the ribosome at the aminoacyl or "A" site. Upon correct codon-anticodon interaction, energy is released from eEF-1A in the form of GTP hydrolysis. A second factor, named eEF-1B, assists in regenerating active eEF-1A, ensuring continued deliverance of aminoacyl-tRNAs to the ribosome. A third and final factor, named eEF-2, mediates translocation of the peptidyl-tRNA from the P site to the A site, and facilitates movement of the ribosome along the mRNA. This ribosomal translocation also requires energy in the form of GTP hydrolysis. The level of eEF-2 in the cell reflects the level of protein synthesis activity. As such, mammary gland has 20-times more eEF-2 than liver, and is suggested to be the limiting factor for milk protein synthesis (47).

The activity of all three eEFs is subject to regulation by phosphorylation in mammalian cells. Phosphorylation of eEF-1A by insulin stimulates elongation activity (48), whereas phosphorylation of eEF-1B has no reported influence on elongation rates. On the other hand, insulin causes the dephosphorylation of eEF-2 to stimulate elongation activity (49). Phosphorylation of eEF-2 is the best-studied and perhaps the most important mechanism of reducing elongation rate. Phosphorylation of eEF-2 is catalyzed by a specific Ca^{2+}calmodulin-dependent eEF-2 kinase. Activity of the eEF-2 kinase is regulated by the mTOR kinase, but the manner in which mTOR causes its dephosphorylation is unclear (50).

Termination

The final step in translation, that of termination, occurs when the stop codon is positioned in the A site of the ribosome. This event is recognized by the protein eRF-1, which binds to the ribosome and, in a GTP-dependent fashion, catalyzes the cleavage of the bond between the nascent peptide and the tRNA, thereby releasing the protein. A second release factor called eRF-3 serves to stimulate eRF-1 activity in the presence of GTP.

Posttranslational Modifications and Folding of Proteins

Co- and posttranslational modifications are essential steps for the translocation, activation, regulation, and, ultimately, the degradation of proteins. In fact, there are probably only a small number of proteins that do not undergo some type of chemical change during or following synthesis. The N-terminal methionine residue is removed from many proteins, and other unnecessary regions of some proteins undergo cleavage. Other common modifications include, but are not limited to, glycosylation, acetylation, fatty acylation, and disulfide bond formation. Despite the omnipresence of protein modification in nature, much remains unknown about how these alterations affect the activity of each individual protein. This is mostly because a singular type of modification imparts different functions, depending on the target protein. For example, asparagine-linked glycosylation may stabilize the folding process of one polypeptide, whereas in a different protein it may play an important role in cellular recognition or function.

The mechanism for these and other protein modifications during and following translation is varied and complex. Nevertheless, it is important to point out that mutations in genes encoding proteins involved in protein modifications lead to various disorders, such as congenital disorders of glycosylation type I (GDG-I), a multisystem disorder that produces abnormal glycosylation of intestinal mucosa glycoproteins. CDG-I results in intestinal symptoms such as inflammation and abnormal enterocyte lipid transport or intestinal permeability. These human diseases emphasize the fact that co- and posttranslational modifications are germane events in regulating protein synthesis and also protein degradation, as will be detailed later in this chapter.

The majority of mRNA translation is initiated on cytosolic ribosomes. For distinct classes of proteins, the nascent polypeptide is targeted (via the signal recognition particle) to the endoplasmic reticulum (ER) for completion and for certain co- and posttranslational modifications to occur. These classes of proteins include ER and Golgi-resident proteins, membrane-associated proteins, proteins of the endosomal-lysosomal system, and proteins destined for secretion. Following translation and modification, nascent peptides located in the ER must be correctly folded and assembled prior to transit to intracellular organelles or the cell surface. A family of proteins referred to as molecular chaperones accomplishes this task, functioning as a quality-control system in nascent peptide synthesis. Unfolded or misfolded proteins in the ER lumen linger for a time, awaiting proper assembly. Proteins unable to be correctly assembled are eventually translocated from the ER and targeted for degradation in the cytosol by the proteasome (discussed in more detail below under "Mechanisms of protein degradation").

Unfolded Protein Response

ER homeostasis requires that the capacity of the protein-folding apparatus remains in balance with the demand. This balance can be disrupted by environmental stress (e.g., glucose starvation or disturbance of Ca^{2+} homeostasis during hypoxia), genetic mutations in proteins requiring ER assembly (e.g., cystic fibrosis transmembrane conductance regulator), or malfunctions in the folding machinery itself. When the balance becomes disrupted, unfolded or misfolded proteins accumulate in the lumen of the ER. This buildup of "cellular trash" initiates an adaptive mechanism, termed the unfolded protein response (UPR, or ER stress response) (Fig. 10-2; reviewed extensively in refs 51 and 52). The UPR encompasses three separate processes. First, the global rate of protein synthesis is slowed down to reduce the ER protein-folding load and directly inhibit cyclin D1 translation, thereby contributing to cell-cycle arrest. Second, ER-resident chaperones are transcriptionally induced to increase the folding capacity in these organelles. Third, a protein degrading system named endoplasmic reticulum-associated degradation (ERAD) is initiated to help clear the accumulating cellular waste. Activation of ERAD is important for the degradation of unfolded proteins through the ubiquitin-proteasomal pathway. If the ER stress cannot be alleviated by these three processes, then cellular pathways will be activated to induce programmed cell death.

Several ER-resident molecules detect the accumulation of unfolded proteins. One of these is the eIF2 kinase PERK, also named PEK. As mentioned above,

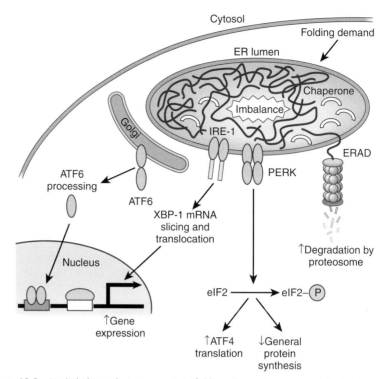

Figure 10-2 An imbalance between protein-folding demand versus protein-folding capacity imposes stress on the ER resulting in the tripartite mammalian unfolded protein response (endoplasmic reticulum stress response). A triad of stress sensors monitor environmental perturbations in the ER and elicit a temporal pattern of gene expression that collectively enhances processing, assembly and transport of secretory proteins while downregulating nascent protein synthesis. One stress sensor, ATF6, is a Golgi membrane-associated protein that, upon proteolytic cleavage, traffics into the nucleus to direct the transcription of genes subject to the UPR. The second sensor is IRE-1, a transmembrane ER protein kinase, whose associated RNase activity is important for splicing XBP-1 mRNA into a potent transcription factor that also serves to direct the transcription of UPR-target genes. The third UPR sensor is PERK, another ER transmembrane protein kinase that represses general protein synthesis via phosphorylation of eIF2. The resulting lowered protein synthesis would prevent further overload of the ER, and provide the cell sufficient time to reconfigure gene expression.

PERK/PEK induces phosphorylation of the translation factor eIF-2, resulting in a shutdown of translation at the initiation step (26). This response blocks new synthesis of proteins and prevents further accumulation of unfolded proteins that form toxic aggregates. At the same time, increases in the phosphorylation of eIF-2 allow the translation of a specific mRNA that encodes activating transcription factor-4 (ATF-4) (53). ATF-4 promotes the transcription of stress-remediation genes as well as genes that are linked to programmed cell death. The upregulation of specific mRNA translation in the face of global repression is a coordinated process (i.e., Integrated Stress Response) that highlights the capacity of the cell to sequester and channel multiple biologic processes in an organized fashion (25, 54). In addition, other ER-resident proteins, such as IRE-1 (a transmembrane protein with both kinase and endoribonuclease functions) and ATF-6 (a transmembrane transcription factor), respond to the accumulation of unfolded proteins by activating the transcription of other stress-response genes, all serving to increase folding capacity in the ER (55).

Although cellular stress is certainly a major activator of the UPR, it should be mentioned that not only harmful events trigger the UPR. To the contrary, recent studies show that cell differentiation associated with increased secretory-protein production is coupled with activation of these same signaling pathways. For example, terminal differentiation of a B lymphocyte into a mature antibody-secreting plasma cell requires the ER to assemble and ship out large quantities of antibodies with remarkable efficiency. This task requires enormous expansion of the ER protein-folding capacity during B-cell differentiation. The UPR mediates ER homeostasis as B cells transition into high-rate antibody secretion and serves to regulate events required for humoral immunity (56).

It is also clear that the UPR is required for normal cellular function. Patients with the rare autosomal-recessive disorder Wolcott-Rallison syndrome experience a severe form of neonatal or early infancy insulin-dependent diabetes, along with multiple defects in bone formation and growth retardation (57). The genetic mutation in these patients lies in the EIF2AK3 gene, which encodes the human form of the eIF-2 kinase, PERK. Mice with a functionally disrupted EIF2AK3/PERK gene demonstrate massive apoptosis of the exocrine pancreas a few weeks after birth, destroying the insulin-producing β-cells (58).

Finally, several studies indicate that signaling pathways related to the UPR have evolved to couple nutritional needs with some metabolic processes. A cellular stress response that is related to but distinct from the UPR involves the cellular response to amino acid deprivation. In response to limitation of essential amino acids, the eIF-2 kinase GCN2 phosphorylates the translation factor to reduce protein synthesis and initiate a cascade of events, not linked to protein folding, which results in the upregulation of genes involved in amino acid metabolism and transport (59). Animals lacking GCN2 are not able to cope with dietary essential amino acid deprivation and become moribund within days of feeding on a leucine-devoid diet (39). Thus, amino acid deprivation or starvation activates a cellular stress pathway that involves components of the UPR.

In addition to activating eIF2 phosphorylaion, amino acid deprivation causes signaling to mTOR to be less responsive to insulin and growth factors (60). The dominant proximal regulator of TORC1 signaling and kinase activity is the ras-like small GTPase Rheb (61). Amino acid depletion interferes with the ability of Rheb to activate mTOR. This effectually inhibits growth signals elicited upstream of Rheb, namely the insulin signal transduction pathway. The stimulation of mTOR signaling to promote anabolic growth via ribosome biogenesis, protein synthesis, nutrient import and cell-cycle progression requires dual input from both insulin/growth factors and amino acids. This is an important point for neonatal nutrition, that exogenous amino acids are critical for the most basic of human growth mechanisms to function properly in vitro and in vivo.

MECHANISMS OF PROTEIN DEGRADATION

In normal fasting newborns, the amino acid release from proteolysis is approximately 2–3-times greater than that of normal fasting adults (62). The reasons why higher rates of whole body turnover and muscle protein breakdown exist in preterm neonates are unclear, but a higher rate of proteolysis in immature neonates may contribute importantly to proper growth in order to provide amino acids for tissue remodeling, protein accretion and glucose homeostasis (63–65). Little is known regarding the molecular regulation of protein degradation in the neonate. Few studies in the premature infant exist concerning which of the major degradative systems are active and how. Thus, the following overview is provided in a general sense.

Once a protein is made, it is immediately a target for degradation. Some proteins, such as collagen and hemoglobin, are relatively resistant to degradation and therefore turn over slowly. Other proteins are readily degraded; especially those that have an important regulatory function or are damaged in some way or have errors in amino acid sequence due to errors in transcription. The details of the molecular basis of protein degradation, or proteolysis, have not been as fully described as for the system of protein synthesis. However, like synthesis, the regulation of protein degradation includes both a component that targets specific proteins and a component that regulates the overall rate of protein degradation in a tissue and facilitates changes in protein content. An example of how degradation of a single protein can cause disease is seen in cystic fibrosis. Deletion of phenylalanine at position 508 of the cystic fibrosis transmembrane regulator (CFTR) results in a temperature-sensitive folding defect and premature degradation in the cell, preventing its translocation to the cell surface (66, 67). The absence of CFTR at the airway epithelial cell surface disrupts luminal hydration and increases susceptibility to infection. An example of coordinated increases in the rate of degradation of all the proteins of a tissue, allowing the whole tissue to adapt to alterations in its environment, is the increased proteolysis of muscle tissue proteins that occurs in response to a number of stresses, including fasting, acidosis and thermal injury (68).

Protein degradation, or proteolysis, in eukaryotic cells is accomplished by a large number of specific and nonspecific proteases. Most of these degradative enzymes can be associated with one of three major systems of cellular protein breakdown: the ubiquitin-proteasome pathway (69), the autophagic-lysosomal system (70), and the calcium or calpain-dependent system (71, 72). The ubiquitin-proteasome system degrades mostly intracellular proteins, whereas the autophagy-lysosomal system degrades membrane and andocytosed proteins. The calcium-dependent thiol proteases, known as calpains, are widely expressed and have been implicated in a number of basic cellular processes, although their physiological function in human development is not well understood. Another proteolytic class not covered in detail in this chapter, but important to mention, is the caspase family of protein-degrading enzymes. The caspases are major players in the execution of apoptosis (i.e., programmed cell death), which serves to remove old, damaged or potentially dangerous cells (73). Investigations of the pathways directing protein degradation have proved that these processes are complicated and as exquisitely controlled as are the processes for protein synthesis.

Ubiquitin-Proteasome Pathway

The majority (up to 80–90%) of intracellular protein degradation is accomplished by the ubiquitin-proteasome pathway (Fig. 10-3). The ubiquitin-proteasome pathway is present in both the nucleus and cytoplasm of eukaryotic cells and plays a role in the degradation of both normal and abnormal proteins. This pathway is responsible for the regulated degradation of many critical proteins, including those required for the control of cell growth and proliferation, cell differentiation, immune and inflammatory responses, apoptosis, and metabolic adaptation. The ubiquitin-proteasome pathway also carries out housekeeping functions in basal protein turnover and the elimination of abnormal proteins that are miscoded, misfolded, mislocalized, damaged, or otherwise rendered inoperative. The ubiquitin-proteasome pathway plays a critical role in the control of muscle mass, and its activity is increased during muscle wasting (68). It also plays an important role in muscle recovery and remodeling (74).

The ubiquitin-proteasome pathway can be considered as made up of three sequential processes: (1) recognition of a protein substrate for degradation; (2) covalent addition of a polyubiquitin chain to mark the protein for degradation; and (3) proteolysis of the protein by a 2500 kDa complex called the 26S proteasome. The recognition of a protein for degradation typically takes advantage of certain structural changes in the protein, including the exposure of specific amino acid sequences that are normally buried, posttranslational modifications such as phosphorylation or hydroxylation, binding to or release from its ligand, interaction

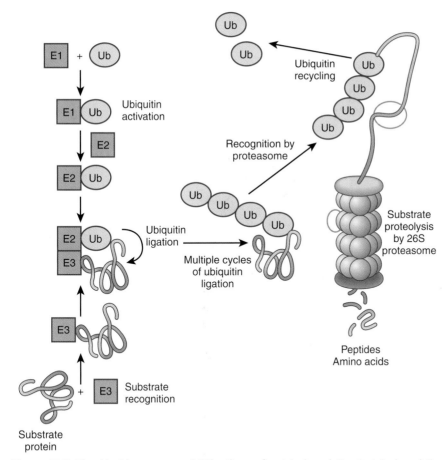

Figure 10-3 The ubiquitin-proteasome (UPS) pathway of protein degradation. Protein degradation through the UPS is a highly regulated, multistep process. The first step is ubiquitin activation by E1 (ubiquitin-activating enzyme), followed by ubiquitin delivery to E2 (ubiquitin-conjugating enzyme). The second step involves complex formation by E2, E3 (ubiquitin ligase) and the substrate. The third step comprises transfer of ubiquitins to the substrate lysine(s) to tag the substrate with a polyubiquitin chain. In the fourth step, a polyubiquitylated substrate is released from E3. Finally, the proteasome unfolds the substrate in ATP-dependent manner, removes the ubiquitin chain via proteasome-associated ubiquitin hydrolase activity, and feeds the unfolded protein into the proteasome chamber, where the protease active sites are located. The ubiquitin molecules are reused, whereas the peptides generated are degraded to amino acids and recycled for new protein synthesis.

with an adaptor protein or chaperone (e.g., the export of misfolded proteins via chaperones from the ER into the cytosol), or specific damage incurred to the protein such as oxidation or nitrosylation. Further, the presence of specific 'destabilizing' residues at the N-terminus (e.g., N-end rule pathway) targets a peptide for degradation (i.e., shorter half-life). It should also be mentioned, however, that not all proteins are tagged with ubiquitin before degradation. Alternatively, certain proteins undergo "default" degradation by the 20S core proteasomes. The purpose of this mode of breakdown is unclear, but it seems to happen to proteins with distinctly unstructured regions, imparting greater protein instability (75).

Once a protein has been identified as a substrate for degradation, it is covalently tagged with ubiquitin. Ubiquitin, a protein so-named because of its omnipresence in all cell types, is made up of 76 amino acid residues, including a C-terminal glycine and a lysine residue at position 48. Ubiquitin is covalently attached to the protein destined for degradation in a series of three reactions or steps catalyzed by enzymes known as E1 (ubiquitin-activating enzyme), E2 (ubiquitin-conjugating enzyme), and E3 (ubiquitin-ligating enzyme). There are two isoforms of E1, multiple isoforms of E2, and a very large number of E3 enzymes, allowing for much tissue- and substrate-specific regulation of this process (76).

In the first step, a molecule of ubiquitin is activated by binding to E1 in an ATP-dependent reaction, and the ubiquitin moiety is then transferred to an E2. Both E1s and E2s have active-site cysteinyl residues that form thioesters with the C-terminal glycine of ubiquitin. Finally, the ubiquitin attached to E2 is transferred, directly or via E3, to an internal lysyl residue on the substrate protein. E3 plays a critical function in recognition of a substrate protein for degradation and in mediating the formation of an E2-E3-substrate complex (76). Additional ubiquitins are similarly added to the monoubiquitinated substrate by forming isopeptide bonds between the C-terminal glycine of the ubiquitin molecule being added and lysine 48 of the ubiquitin molecule previously added. A chain of at least four ubiquitin molecules is required for polyubiquitinated proteins to be readily recognized and targeted to the 26S proteasome for destruction. The binding domains and activities of ubiquitin have been recently reviewed (77). It is important to note that the process of ubiquitination is reversible, with the deconjugation reaction accomplished by a class of cysteine proteases called the deubiquitinating enzymes. Deubiquitinating enzyme activites include reversal of ubiquitin conjugation, processing of ubiquitin precursors, editing of ubiquitin chains and recycling of ubiquitin. These activities are responsible for regulating several important pathways in development, including cell growth and differentiation (78).

The actual degradation of ubiquitinated proteins takes place within an inner chamber of the proteasome, but the ubiquitin molecules are first released so they can be reused. The 26S proteasome is a large, multisubunit complex that consists of a core 20S proteolytic complex with a regulatory 19S complex attached to one or both ends. The regulatory units are involved in recognition of tagged proteins, removal of the ubiquitin tag, and in the ATP-dependent unfolding and guiding of the client protein into the tunnel-shaped proteolytic core. The 20S core complex is composed of four stacked ring-like structures ($\alpha\beta\beta\alpha$) of seven subunits each, which together form a barrel-like structure. The central catalytic cavity of the structure contains a total of six proteolytic sites, contributed by the three separate catalytic subunits of each β-ring (79). These catalytic subunits are classified as N-terminal threonine hydrolases because the N-terminal threonine acts as the nucleophile catalyst. However, the three different subunits in each of the two rings differ in their preference for cleaving peptide bonds immediately after basic, hydrophobic, or acidic residues. The 20S core hydrolyzes incoming substrate into peptide fragments of approximately 3 to 30 amino acid residues. These peptide products are released from the proteasome and are further hydrolyzed by other proteases and aminopeptidases in the cell.

Regulation of proteolysis by the proteasome occurs on three levels. First, substrate recognition is regulated by features that uniquely specify the targeted protein for polyubiquitination. These are largely unidentified for most proteins and include phosphorylation, hydroxylation of a proline residue, or unmasking of a degradation signal contained in the primary sequence. Second, regulated degradation of specific classes of substrates may be achieved by association of E2-E3 complexes with different ancillary factors (80). For example, in some cases it is the E3 that must be modified or switched "on" by undergoing posttranslational modification to yield an active form that recognizes the substrate. In other cases, the stability of the protein substrate depends on its association with molecular chaperones that act as recognition elements and serve as a link to the appropriate ligase (81). For example, insulin decreases ubiquitin-mediated proteasomal activity by displacing an intracellular protease, the insulin-degrading enzyme, from 20S and 26S proteasomes (82). Finally, the ubiquitin-proteasome pathway can be regulated via interaction or altered expression of ubiquitin or proteasome subunits. An example of this can be seen following intravenous infusion or luminal provision of amino acids.

Increased supply of amino acids, but not glucose, reduces mRNA expression of ubiquitin, 14-kDa ubiquitin-conjugating enzyme (E2), and C9 subunit of the proteasome in the intestinal mucosa (83).

ER-Associated Degradation

The ER-associated degradation (ERAD) pathway functions in ER quality control, directing ubiquitin-mediated degradation of a variety of ER-associated misfolded and normal proteins. This is particularly important in professional secretory cells, where the capacity of ERAD critically determines the efficiency of protein secretion (84). Proteins located in the ER that are targeted for destruction are retrotranslocated (or dislocated) from the ER into the cytosol where the ubiquitin-conjugating enzymes and 26S proteosome are located. ERAD comprises three events: substrate selection, transport to the cytosol, and ubiquitin-mediated degradation (85). Substrate selection is mediated by the various molecular chaperones located in the ER, which facilitate gating and movement to the cytosol through a specific translocation. Dysfunctions in ERAD result in the build-up of cellular protein waste, leading to cell injury and death. Many diseases are linked to genetic mutations that lead to an overwhelmed ERAD, resulting in an accumulation of cytotoxic proteins in the cell (86).

Autophagy-Lysosomal System

Separate from the proteasome, cellular proteins are degraded within an intracellular compartment called the lysosome. Lysosomes are dispersed throughout the cytosol, where they form gradually from endosomes or phagosomes. Lysosomes contain a variety of hydrolytic enzymes that degrade proteins and other substances. The lysosomal system is less selective in targeting specific proteins for breakdown than is the ubiquitin-proteasome system.

Extracellular components, including plasma membrane components, enter the lysosomal system via endocytosis, whereas intracellular components (portions of the cytoplasm, including certain organelles) are sequestered by autophagy. In the process of autophagy, cytosolic components, including old organelles, destined for degradation by the lysosome are surrounded by a membrane to form an autophagic vesicle. This autophagic vesicle then fuses with a lysosome. On the other hand, in the process of endocytosis, vesicles are formed at the plasma membrane by pinching off and enclosing a portion of the extracellular matrix to form the early endosome. The early endosome, along with other vesicles carrying lysosomal membrane proteins, then fuses with the late endosome. The late endosome then matures to a multivesicular body before fusing with a lysosome. In both cases, within the lysosomes, the vesicular contents are broken down by degradative enzymes such as the cathepsins, and the degraded cellular components are then either recycled back into the cytosol or exported out of the cell via exocytosis. Recent studies have found that autophagy serves as an overflow pathway from the ER when ERAD is compromised, thus playing a more direct role in ER protein quality control than was previously thought (87).

Much of the information about the regulation of the lysosomal system is derived from studies in rats. Under conditions of nutrient starvation, autophagic proteolysis is induced to high levels and is referred to as macroautophagy (88). Although the lysosomal system is believed to be present in all tissues, e.g., the presence of autophagic cells is documented in the developing gut (89), macroautophagy is most actively expressed in the liver in response to nutrient deprivation (90). Macroautophagy is believed to be a major source of amino acids during starvation. It is also a major mechanism for establishing glucose homeostasis during periods of starvation in the neonate (91). Neonates initially adapt to the loss of nutrients derived from the placenta by inducing autophagy. The loss of auto-phagosome formation in mice deficient for the autophagy-related genes *Atg5* or *Atg7* results in the inability to manage short-term starvation and the pups die soon (~12 h) after birth (91). Thus, the release of amino acids from tissues allows for energy homeostasis during periods of neonatal starvation.

The rate of autophagy is physiologically controlled by amino acid concentrations, with activation of the system when amino acid supply is reduced and inhibition of the system when amino acid supply is increased (92). Protein kinase cascades including mTOR and eIF2 are involved in the regulation of autophagy, and amino acids appear to exert their effects through these pathways but separate from that of insulin (93). For example, an apparent cell surface receptor that is responsive to leucine in the suppression of macroautophagy has been reported in the literature, but this protein or factor has yet to be definitively identified (94).

Calpains

A third mechanism of cellular degradation is the calcium and/or calpain-dependent system. The calpain system consists of a widely-expressed family of at least 14 Ca^{2+}-activated proteolytic enzymes (95). The precise physiologic functions of the calpains remain to be determined, but so far they have been implicated in basic cellular processes, including cell proliferation, cell motility, and apoptosis (96). Calpain-generated degradation products also play important roles in neonatal brain development and synaptic activity (97). Mammalian calpains have a ubiquitous endogenous inhibitor protein, calpastatin, which is actually a group of at least eight polypeptide isoforms that are produced from a single gene by alternative splicing or use of alternate promoters (98). How calpastatin regulates calpain activity in living cells is not well understood. In the skeletal muscle and liver of animals, calpain and calpastatin activities decline markedly between birth and weaning (99, 100). Why this occurs is not well understood.

PROTEIN NUTRITION IN THE NEONATE

Nutrient Needs of the Preterm Infant

According to the neonatal community, infants born less than 37 completed weeks (< 259 days) of gestation are considered to be preterm (1, 101). Nearly term infants, defined as 35–37 completed weeks of gestational age, are many times placed in the term nursery and not monitored as preterm infants. The standard of practice for postnatal nutrition in premature neonates is one that mimics in utero fetal growth rates (102). However, when dealing with nearly term infants, many may fall through the guidelines as the healthcare professionals in the term nursery must be trained to be more observant and cautious of the nearly term neonate.

While healthy adults exist in a state of neutral nitrogen balance, infants need to be in a state of positive nitrogen balance in order to achieve normal growth and development. Infants are capable of retaining up to 80% of the metabolizable protein from both oral and intravenous diets (103, 104). However, the use and synthesis of amino acids by gut microflora influences the availability of amino acids to peripheral tissues, and so the amino acid requirement for growth is higher in neonates receiving enteral versus parenteral nutrition. The route of amino acid administration to neonates (enteral versus parenteral) is an important consideration well understood only recently.

Overall protein metabolism of the neonate is dependent upon both protein and energy intake. Higher energy intake alone improves nitrogen retention by enhancing amino acid reutilization for protein synthesis, whereas the addition of protein or amino acids to enteral or parenteral feedings further improves protein balance by limiting protein breakdown (105, 106). Recent studies show both an increase in whole body protein synthesis and leucine oxidation (107, 108), while other studies demonstrate that amino acids decrease in proteolysis and protein oxidation (109, 110) following infusion of glucose or insulin plus amino acids when given to preterm infants. The different results by these recent studies may be related to differences in study design, age/weight of study subjects, level of nonprotein energy provided, or methodological differences in the use of isotopic tracers to calculate nitrogen flux and utilization. Despite the differences in measured outcomes, it can be concluded that amino acids play a prominent and necessary role in improving net protein balance.

The influence of nonprotein energy composition on protein metabolism is more contentious. Early work showed that the addition of fat to the intravenous diet of postoperative neonates resulted in a reduction of protein oxidation, a decrease in the amount of protein contributed to energy expenditure, and an increase in protein retention (111). Other studies have demonstrated that a high-fat diet versus a high-carbohydrate diet had no effect with regard to protein synthesis, protein breakdown, protein oxidation/excretion, or total protein flux (112–114). On the other hand, more recent work suggests that in enterally fed, low birth weight infants, higher carbohydrate reduces protein oxidation more effectively (115). Yet higher carbohydrate intake in the first month of life results in premature neonates with greater fat mass and reduced insulin sensitivity (116, 117). More studies are needed to assess whether the macronutrient composition of nonprotein nutrition in preterm neonates is an important determinant of protein accretion and insulin sensitivity (118).

Current Practices

The current practice surrounding neonatal nutrition care is to "provide nutrients to approximate the rate of growth and composition of weight gain for a normal fetus of the same post conceptional age" (102). Unfortunately, even if recommended dietary intakes (RDIs) are met, they are rarely maintained throughout the infant's hospital stay (119, 120). Currently, RDIs are based on the needs required for normal growth and maintenance with no provision for "catch-up" growth in the preterm infant. Some have suggested that catch-up needs be added to those of normal growth and replaced in the neonate before hospital discharge (121, 122). Whether or not this practice is possible has yet to be confirmed.

Nonprotein substrate infusion is often used first in infants who are unable to receive enteral intake. At one time, carbohydrates were the only exogenous nutrient administered initially during the postnatal period of the premature infant. Amino acids were withheld due to previous mixtures resulting in metabolic acidosis and hyperammonemia (123, 124). Although improved approaches have since corrected this, it is not uncommon for neonatal intensive care units to limit amino acids in extremely low-birth-weight (ELBW) or sick neonates in the early neonatal period because of concerns about their ability to metabolize substrates. According to the recent article by Hay and Thureen (2), these are general misconceptions, for the most part, not supported by current reports. Indeed, in the absence of providing amino acids, the practice of intravenous glucose infusion does not suppress proteolysis, and the rate of proteolysis is not reduced from fasting values during either separate or combined glucose and lipid infusions (125).

There is wide variation among how healthcare professionals determine the appropriate rate of amino acid administration in the neonate. Currently, the common rate of parenteral amino acid administration ranges from 2.5 to 3.5 g/kg per day. While controversy remains as to where within the range is most appropriate, an upper limit of 6 g/kg per day has been determined and which toxicity has been observed. Due to more and more studies concluding the benefits of amino acid inclusion in early feedings, more practitioners are supporting more aggressive early strategies. For example, parenteral administration of amino acids (3 g/kg per day) to preterm infants in the first days of life leads to greater protein accretion as compared to a lower amino acid intake (1 g/kg per day) (108), and, in critically ill neonates on life support, insulin infusion limits the increase in protein breakdown and significantly improves net protein balance only when in combination with amino acids (at least 2 g/kg per day) (108). No toxicity appears to be associated with early protein administration up to 3.7 g/kg per day (106, 126–132).

In addition to nutrient composition, the route of nutrient administration influences whole body and tissue-specific measures of protein balance. Minimal enteral feeding (20 mL/kg per day) in the first week of life increases leucine uptake by the splanchnic tissues in preterm infants, implying greater splanchnic protein synthesis (133). Indeed, portal delivery of amino acids contributes to protein synthesis in the splanchnic tissues (intestines, stomach, pancreas, liver, spleen). This extensive "first-pass" metabolism of enteral amino acids can range from 20 to 96% of enteral intake, significantly influencing the composition of amino acids available to the periphery (reviewed in ref. 6). Thus, amino acid metabolism in the gut impacts whole-body amino acid requirements, resulting in significantly higher dietary requirements for the essential amino acids lysine, methionine, threonine, and the branched-chain amino acids (6). Enteral intake of amino acids is also utilized by the developing gut microflora, which recently were shown to also synthesize essential amino acids in addition to oxidizing significant quantities (134). The role of the intestinal microflora in influencing splanchnic protein balance requires further study.

Amino Acids

In addition to the amount, the composition of the amino acid mixture in total parenteral nutrition (TPN) solutions also influences measures of protein turnover, synthesis and breakdown (135). Glutamine is an important precursor for nucleotide synthesis and glutathione, and is the primary fuel for enterocytes, lymphocytes, and macrophages. Due to the short shelf-life when placed in solution, most commercial TPN solutions do not contain glutamine. Short-term studies in preterm babies have shown improvement in protein balance by adding glutamine to TPN. Glutamine supplementation elicits a protein-sparing effect via suppression of whole-body protein breakdown and oxidation (136, 137), resulting in reduced hospital costs due to fewer days on parental nutrition, less time on the ventilator, shorter length of time to full enteral feeds, and less incidence of necrotizing enterocolitis in the very low birth weight neonate (138, 139) (Fig. 10-4). On the other

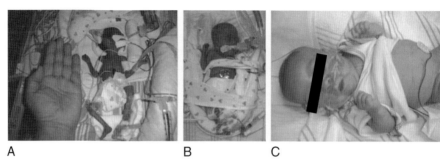

A   B   C

Figure 10-4 A preterm infant born with a birth weight of 434 g at 22 weeks gestation, (A) shortly after admission at birth, (B) at approximately 3 months, and (C) near hospital discharge at approximately 5 months. Photographs kindly provided by Dr. Gerardo A. Cabrera-Meza, Baylor College of Medicine.

hand, not all prolonged advantages such as reduction in mortality are consistently demonstrated (140, 141). It is possible that the addition of glutamine to intravenous nutrition may be of most benefit to certain populations of preterm infants. Additional studies are needed in this regard.

Arginine is indispensable for growth and nitrogen balance in neonates. The synthesis of arginine from its precursor proline occurs in the intestine, and the metabolism of proline to arginine in the gut provides about half of the whole-body arginine requirement (142). When enteral nutrition is not possible, recent studies in neonatal pigs demonstrate convincingly that it is necessary to provide arginine in TPN to prevent hyperammonemia (143). Supplementation of arginine in TPN can also provide the additional benefit of significantly reducing the development of all stages of necrotizing enterocolitis in premature infants (144, 145). This is important because necrotizing enterocolitis is a leading cause of mortality in preterm infants. The mechanism for this beneficial effect may be due to the fact that arginine serves as a precursor for the synthesis of nitric oxide which participates in the response to inflammation. Arginine also enhances immune cell responses, which serve to ward off bacterial infection.

Taurine is necessary for proper development of the brain and retina, and cysteine is required for the synthesis of all proteins, plus glutathione and taurine. Controversy still remains as to whether these two amino acids should be considered conditionally essential for neonates. Low plasma levels of cysteine and taurine in infants are corrected when added to the TPN or infant formula, indicating a need for supplementation (146). Very-low-birth-weight (VLBW) infants are at greater risk for taurine and cysteine deficiency than near-term or term infants because of immature tubular transport and impaired fat absorption, bile acid secretion, retinal function, and hepatic function (146). Recently, it was also reported that low neonatal taurine status adversely affects later neurodevelopment of preterm infants (147). Although retrospective in design, this study further supports the view that taurine is a conditionally essential nutrient for the preterm infant. Because supplementation of these amino acids has been a part of infant formula for over 25 years, is well tolerated and presents very low risk (148), maintaining a minimal requirement for cysteine and taurine in nutritional strategies implemented in premature infants is clinically relevant and appropriate (149).

Postnatal Malnutrition and Growth Retardation

A distinct relationship between nutrient intake and growth exists in all neonates. Poor growth postpartum is a direct result of inadequate protein intake (120). To optimize long-term growth and development, and prevent early growth retardation in neonates, adequate protein nutrition is essential. Furthermore, it is clear that if neonates are only fed intakes based on the RDIs, catch-up growth will not be achieved (122).

Growth retardation is observed in preterm infants as early as hospital discharge. Several studies suggest that a delay in nutrition can produce measurable growth failure upon hospital discharge (150–152). It has been noted that roughly 1% of stored protein is lost each day in a preterm infant who only receives supplemental glucose (153). Moreover, developmental outcomes and memory have been linked to early protein malnutrition. Research indicates that early protein intake is directly correlated to long-term developmental outcome of the preterm neonate and that consequences of inadequate early nutrition cannot be overcome even if adequate intake is eventually achieved (151). The practice of withholding amino acids needs to be reversed within the neonatal intensive care unit in order to reduce the incidence of poor weight gain upon hospital discharge and improve overall developmental outcomes.

Table 10-1	Protein Content of Commercially Available Human Milk Fortifiers	
Product name	Manufacturer	Protein content g per 100 cal
Enfamil Human Milk Fortifier (4 packet)	Mead Johnson Nutritionals, Evansville, IN	1.1 g
Similac Human Milk Fortifier (4 packet)	Ross Laboratories, Columbus, OH	1.0 g
Similac Natural Care Fortifier (liquid, 100 mL)*	Ross Laboratories, Columbus, OH	3.0 g

*To be diluted 1:1 with human milk.

Enteral Feeding Methods

Human Milk and Human Milk Fortifier

According to the American Academy of Pediatrics, the average value of protein in mature human milk (>28 days postpartum) is 1.0 g/100 mL (102, 154). Similarly, premature human milk (<32 weeks gestational age) typically contains protein levels ranging from 1.1 to 2.4 g/100 mL, depending on the number of weeks postpartum (155, 156). However, the protein needs of the preterm infant are much greater than those of the term infant. Once growth is established, specific nutritional needs of the premature neonate exceed the content readily available in human milk, such as protein, calcium, phosphorus, magnesium, sodium, copper, zinc, riboflavin, vitamins B6, C, D, E, K, and folic acid (157, 158). The higher protein concentration in milk from mothers of preterm infants within the first 2 weeks following delivery is sufficient to meet the growth requirements for nitrogen when consumed at a very high volume (180–200 mL/kg per day) (159). However, as the protein concentration decreases in the preterm milk over the first postpartum week, the protein content is inadequate to meet the needs of most preterm infants (160). In addition, researchers have documented many metabolic complications associated with a long-term use of unsupplemented human milk in preterm neonates, such as hyponatremia, hypoproteinemia, osteopenia, zinc deficiency, muscle weakness, and susceptibility to infection due to decreased immune function (106, 161–163).

While there does not appear to be a correlation between birth weight and the average protein concentration of preterm milk or the volume of milk produced, there is a correlation between protein content and lactational age. Specifically, a rapid decrease in protein content occurs during the first 4–5 days of lactation, followed by a more gradual linear decline over the next 28 days (160). This appears to be related to the increase in total milk volume output over time. Thus, the proportion of mothers able to meet the protein needs of their nursing preterm infant gradually declines with lactational age, even as early as the first week postpartum.

Human milk fortifiers are commercially designed to provide additional protein, minerals, and vitamins to preterm human milk (Table 10-1). While feeding tolerance has been an issue and concern with regard to fortified human milk, current research proves otherwise. In a recent meta-analysis, no differences in feeding tolerance were reported when comparing preterm infants fed fortified human milk or unfortified human milk (164). Feeding tolerance concerns should not deter clinicians from using human milk fortifiers, given the positive nutritional outcomes they can have on a preterm infant (Fig. 10-5). Preterm infants fed fortified human milk grow and develop similarly to infants fed preterm formula (165, 166). In addition to specialized human milk fortifiers packed with protein, the use of

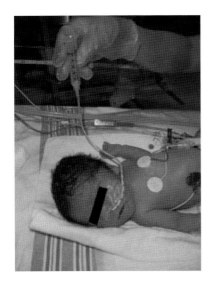

Figure 10-5 A preterm infant born at approximately 31 weeks gestation being given enteral feedings via nasogatric tube. Photograph kindly provided by Dr. Gerardo A. Cabrera-Meza, Baylor College of Medicine.

iron-fortified products can decrease the need for blood transfusions in VLBW infants (167). Researchers found preterm neonates fed an adjustable fortification regimen (2.3 g/100 mL) had improved growth compared to infants fed a standard human milk fortifier regimen (1.9 g/100 mL) (168). Thus, human milk fortifiers appear both safe and efficacious at improving health and weight gain in preterm infants fed breast milk.

Preterm Formula

While it is a rarity for a preterm infant to leave the hospital with a weight above the 10th percentile, it can be achieved and maintained with appropriate nutrition during the hospital stay and post-discharge. In the case of the formula-fed infant, the formula must contain adequate protein in order to sustain normal growth and development. Significant improvements in growth and cognitive development have been shown in preterm infants fed specially formulated preterm formulas when compared to standard formulas (169). However, not all preterm formulas are the same (Table 10-2). Recently, it has been documented that a formula containing 3.6 g/100 kcal of protein more appropriately meets the requirements of the preterm infant than 3.0 g/100 kcal of protein (170). And in another recent study, preterm infants fed a preterm formula ingested 24% more protein and experienced greater protein accretion as compared to premature infants fed fortified breast milk (171). It is clinically important to choose a formula designed to meet the individual needs of each neonate. Due to specific protein requirements, a particular preterm formula may be more desirable than another, based on the protein content of that formula.

Table 10-2	**Protein Content of Commercially Available Formulas for Low-Birth-Weight and Premature Infants**	
Product name	**Manufacturer**	**Protein content g per 100 kcal**
Similac® Special Care® 24	Ross Laboratories, Columbus, OH	3.0 g
Enfamil® Premature Lipil® 24	Mead Johnson Nutritionals, Evansville, IN	3.0 g
Neosure® Advance® 22 cal	Ross Laboratories, Columbus, OH	2.8 g
Enfacare®	Mead Johnson Nutritionals, Evansville, IN	2.8 g

Post-Discharge Nutrition

In the instance when a standard infant formula is fed to a preterm infant, the weight gain is the result of a higher percentage of fat when compared to a fetus of the same maturity (172). As compared to infants fed a standard formula for term infants or unfortified human milk, the preterm infant fed a specially formulated preterm formula and preterm human milk fortifier have a weight gain and bone mineralization more similar to that of the reference fetus. When and if intrauterine weight gain is achieved, catch-up growth is rarely reached and maintained until well after hospital discharge (173, 174). More attention to nutrition post-discharge is needed because, based on the work of Davis and colleagues (43, 44), there seems to be a finite period during which the protein-synthetic response to increased nutrient intake occurs maximally.

The AAP recommends the use of enriched formulas up to 9 months of age to promote greater linear growth and weight gain compared to the use of standard term formula (102, 175, 176). Preterm formulas, as well as human milk fortifiers, are commercially available and take into account the additional nutrient needs of the premature infant. Recently, a clinical study looked at the growth and efficacy of a commercially available preterm formula and found that preterm formula, supplemented with median worldwide human milk levels of DHA and ARA from single-cell algal and fungal oils, can enhance growth of premature infants to the extent that they achieve catch-up growth comparable to the breastfed infant (177).

Need for Earlier and More Aggressive Protein Nutrition

Large amounts of amino acids are available to the fetus in utero, which are utilized for protein synthesis and as a fuel source. Therefore, it seems logical to supply a neonate with adequate amounts of amino acids for energy, as well as a growth substrate to promote protein accretion for ongoing development. To prevent a loss of about 1% of total endogenous protein stores per day, an amino acid intake slightly greater than that of endogenous protein losses (e.g., 1–1.5 g/kg per day) is sufficient in most neonatal populations as long as a catabolic condition is not present. Recent studies have indicated that an amino acid intake of 2–2.5 g/kg per day and an energy intake of 35–50 kcal/kg per day result in a positive nitrogen retention without significant metabolic abnormalities (153, 178). Additionally, the AAP estimates the protein requirements of the preterm neonate to be 23–27 g/L (154).

Hay and Thureen (2) recommend administering amino acids via total parenteral nutrition (TPN) in the first hours after birth. It has been documented that high-dose amino acids (2.4 g/kg per day) introduced at birth are well tolerated and result in an anabolic state (108, 127). This is then combined with initially small, and then increasing, enteral feedings beginning on the first or second day of life. The role of the TPN is to provide rapid, maximal nutrition in order to prevent protein malnutrition. The purpose of the early enteral feedings is to stimulate normal gut development, which influences overall growth rate. The earlier the infant can engage in enteral nutrition and discontinue TPN, the better the chance of achieving a normal growth rate at discharge.

The early nutritional management of premature infants needs to be considered carefully. While preterm formulas and human milk fortifiers are commercially available, thoughtful consideration needs to be taken when choosing how to feed this vulnerable population. It is reasonable to presume that preterm infants who have less weight loss and are able to achieve and maintain catch-up growth sooner, are less likely to have inadequate nutrition-related ailments later in life. Importantly, although recent research has been helpful, the optimal amino acid requirements of premature infants remain undefined. Further studies are needed to establish optimal mixtures of amino acids for parenteral and enteral delivery.

Finally, studies to determine which and how much glucose and lipid are required to optimize protein accretion should be another major research thrust.

Considering the fact that preterm birth is the most frequent cause of infant death in the USA, currently representing at least one-third of infant deaths (179), this information cannot arrive too soon.

REFERENCES

1. Raju TN, Higgins RD, Stark AR, Leveno KJ. Optimizing care and outcome for late-preterm (near-term) infants: a summary of the workshop sponsored by the National Institute of Child Health and Human Development. Pediatrics 2006; 118:1207–1214.
2. Hay WW Jr, Thureen PJ. Early postnatal administration of intravenous amino acids to preterm, extremely low birth weight infants. J Pediatr 2006; 148:291–294.
3. Thureen PJ, Hay WW Jr. Early aggressive nutrition in preterm infants. Semin Neonatol 2001; 6:403–415.
4. McNurlan MA, Anthony TG. Protein synthesis and degradation. In: Stipanuk MH, ed. Biochemical, physiological, molecular aspects of human nutrition, Second edn. St. Louis: Saunders Elsevier; 2006: 319–359.
5. Ewing B, Green P. Analysis of expressed sequence tags indicates 35,000 human genes. Nat Genet 2000; 25:232–234.
6. Burrin DG, Davis TA. Proteins and amino acids in enteral nutrition. Curr Opin Clin Nutr Metab Care 2004; 7:79–87.
7. Pencharz PB, Ball RO. Amino acid needs for early growth and development. J Nutr 2004; 134:1566S–1568S.
8. van Goudoever JB, van der Schoor SR, Stoll B, et al. Intestinal amino acid metabolism in neonates. Nestle Nutr Workshop Ser Pediatr Program 2006; 95–102; discussion -8.
9. Sander G, Hulsemann J, Topp H, et al. Protein and RNA turnover in preterm infants and adults: a comparison based on urinary excretion of 3-methylhistidine and of modified one-way RNA catabolites. Ann Nutr Metab 1986; 30:137–142.
10. Schoch G, Topp H, Held A, et al. Interrelation between whole-body turnover rates of RNA and protein. Eur J Clin Nutr 1990; 44:647–658.
11. Hannan RD, Rothblum LI. Regulation of ribosomal DNA transcription during neonatal cardiomyocyte hypertrophy. Cardiovasc Res 1995; 30:501–510.
12. Hamilton TL, Stoneley M, Spriggs KA, Bushell M. TOPs and their regulation. Biochem Soc Trans 2006; 34:12–16.
13. Tang H, Hornstein E, Stolovich M, et al. Amino acid-induced translation of TOP mRNAs is fully dependent on phosphatidylinositol 3-kinase-mediated signaling, is partially inhibited by rapamycin, and is independent of S6K1 and rpS6 phosphorylation. Mol Cell Biol 2001; 21:8671–8683.
14. Reiter A, Anthony T, Anthony J, et al. The mTOR signaling pathway mediates control of ribosomal protein mRNA translation in rat liver. Int J Biochem Cell Biol 2004; 3 6:2169–2179.
15. Anthony T, Anthony J, Yoshizawa F, et al. Oral administration of leucine stimulates ribosomal protein mRNA translation but not global rates of protein synthesis in the liver of rats. J Nutr 2001; 131:1171–1176.
16. Anthony T, Reiter A, Anthony J, et al. Deficiency of dietary EAA preferentially inhibits mRNA translation of ribosomal proteins in liver of meal-fed rats. Am J Physiol Endocrinol Metab 2001; 281:E430–439.
17. Tokunaga C, Yoshino K, Yonezawa K. mTOR integrates amino acid- and energy-sensing pathways. Biochem Biophys Res Commun 2004; 313:443–446.
18. Proud C. Role of mTOR signalling in the control of translation initiation and elongation by nutrients. Curr Top Microbiol Immunol 2004; 279:215–244.
19. Ruvinsky I, Meyuhas O. Ribosomal protein S6 phosphorylation: from protein synthesis to cell size. Trends Biochem Sci 2006; 31:342–348.
20. Park IH, Erbay E, Nuzzi P, Chen J. Skeletal myocyte hypertrophy requires mTOR kinase activity and S6K1. Exp Cell Res 2005; 309:211–219.
21. Sarbassov DD, Ali SM, Kim DH, et al. Rictor, a novel binding partner of mTOR, defines a rapamycin-insensitive and raptor-independent pathway that regulates the cytoskeleton. Curr Biol 2004; 14:1296–1302.
22. Sarbassov DD, Ali SM, Sabatini DM. Growing roles for the mTOR pathway. Curr Opin Cell Biol 2005; 17:596–603.
23. Kimball SR, Jefferson LS, Nguyen HV, et al. Feeding stimulates protein synthesis in muscle and liver of neonatal pigs through an mTOR-dependent process. Am J Physiol Endocrinol Metab 2000; 279:E1080–1087.
24. Marintchev A, Wagner G. Translation initiation: structures, mechanisms and evolution. Q Rev Biophys 2004; 37:197–284.
25. Harding H, Zhang Y, Zeng H, et al. An integrated stress response regulates amino acid metabolism and resistance to oxidative stress. Mol Cell 2003; 11:619–633.
26. Harding HP, Zhang C, Bertolotti A, et al. *Perk* is essential for translational regulation and cell survival during the unfolded protein response. Mol Cell 2000; 5:897–904.

27. Sood R, Porter AC, Ma K, et al. Pancreatic eukaryotic initiation factor-2alpha kinase (PEK) homologues in humans, *Drosophila melanogaster* and *Caenorhabditis elegans* that mediate translational control in response to endoplasmic reticulum stress. Biochem J 2000; 346:281–293.

28. Kimball S, Anthony T, Cavener D, Jefferson L. Nutrient signaling through mammalian GCN2. In: Winderickx P, Taylor J, eds. Topics in current genetics: Nutrient-induced responses in eukaryotic cells. Berlin: Springer-Verlag; 2004: 113–130.

29. Chen J-J. Heme-regulated eIF2 kinase. In: Sonenberg N, Hershey J, Mathews M, eds. Translational control of gene expression. Cold Spring Harbor, NY: Cold Spring Harbor Laboratory Press; 2000: 529–546.

30. Kaufman RJ. Double-stranded RNA-activated Protein Kinase, PKR. In: Sonenberg N, Mathews MB, Hershey JWB, eds. Translational control of gene expression. Cold Spring Harbor, NY: Cold Spring Harbor Laboratory Press; 2000: 503–528.

31. Gingras A, Raught B, Sonenberg N. eIF4 Initiation Factors: Effectors of mRNA Recruitment to Ribosomes and Regulators of Translation. Annu Rev Biochem 1999; 68:913–963.

32. Hinton TM, Coldwell MJ, Carpenter GA, et al. Functional analysis of individual binding activities of the scaffold protein eIF4G. J Biol Chem 2006; 282:1695–1708.

33. Anthony J, Anthony T, Kimball S, Jefferson L. Signaling pathways involved in translational control of protein synthesis in skeletal muscle by leucine. J Nutr 2001; 131:856S–860S.

34. Mazumder B, Seshadri V, Fox PL. Translational control by the 3′-UTR: the ends specify the means. Trends Biochem Sci 2003; 28:91–98.

35. Gross J, Moerke N, van der Haar T, et al. Ribosome loading onto the mRNA cap is driven by conformational coupling between eIF4G and eIF4E. Cell 2003; 115:739–750.

36. Davis TA, Fiorotto ML, Burrin DG, et al. Stimulation of protein synthesis by both insulin and amino acids is unique to skeletal muscle in neonatal pigs. Am J Physiol Endocrinol Metab 2002; 282:E880–890.

37. O'Connor PM, Bush JA, Suryawan A, et al. Insulin and amino acids independently stimulate skeletal muscle protein synthesis in neonatal pigs. Am J Physiol Endocrinol Metab 2003; 284:E110–119.

38. O'Connor PM, Kimball SR, Suryawan A, et al. A Regulation of neonatal liver protein synthesis by insulin and amino acids in pigs. Am J Physiol Endocrinol Metab 2004; 286:E994–E1003.

39. Anthony T, McDaniel B, Byerley R, et al. Preservation of liver protein synthesis during dietary leucine deprivation occurs at the expense of skeletal muscle mass in mice deleted for eIF2 kinase GCN2. J Biol Chem 2004; 279:36553–36561.

40. Escobar J, Frank JW, Suryawan A, et al. Physiological rise in plasma leucine stimulates muscle protein synthesis in neonatal pigs by enhancing translation initiation factor activation. Am J Physiol Endocrinol Metab 2005; 288:E914–921.

41. Harris TE, Chi A, Shabanowitz J, et al. mTOR-dependent stimulation of the association of eIF4G and eIF3 by insulin. Embo J 2006; 25:1659–1668.

42. Ohanna M, Sobering AK, Lapointe T, et al. Atrophy of S6K1(-/-) skeletal muscle cells reveals distinct mTOR effectors for cell cycle and size control. Nat Cell Biol 2005; 7:286–294.

43. Davis TA, Nguyen HV, Suryawan A, et al. Developmental changes in the feeding-induced stimulation of translation initiation in muscle of neonatal pigs. Am J Physiol Endocrinol Metab 2000; 279:E1226–1234.

44. Suryawan A, Escobar J, Frank JW, et al. Developmental regulation of the activation of signaling components leading to translation initiation in skeletal muscle of neonatal pigs. Am J Physiol Endocrinol Metab 2006; 291:E849–859.

45. Suryawan A, Nguyen HV, Bush JA, Davis TA. Developmental changes in the feeding-induced activation of the insulin-signaling pathway in neonatal pigs. Am J Physiol Endocrinol Metab 2001; 281:E908–E915.

46. Gautsch TA, Kandl SM, Donovan SM, Layman DK. Growth hormone promotes somatic and skeletal muscle growth recovery in rats following chronic protein-energy malnutrition. J Nutr 1999; 129:828–837.

47. Christophersen CT, Karlsen J, Nielsen MO, Riis B. Eukaryotic elongation factor-2 (eEF-2) activity in bovine mammary tissue in relation to milk protein synthesis. J Dairy Res 2002; 69:205–212.

48. Chang YW, Traugh JA. Insulin stimulation of phosphorylation of elongation factor 1 (eEF-1) enhances elongation activity. Eur J Biochem 1998; 251:201–207.

49. Redpath NT, Foulstone EJ, Proud CG. Regulation of translation elongation factor-2 by insulin via a rapamycin-sensitive signalling pathway. Embo J 1996; 15:2291–2297.

50. Hait WN, Wu H, Jin S, Yang JM. Elongation factor-2 kinase: its role in protein synthesis and autophagy. Autophagy 2006; 2:294–296.

51. Kaufman R. Regulation of mRNA translation by protein folding in the endoplasmic reticulum. Trends Biochem Sci 2004; 29:152–158.

52. Marciniak SJ, Ron D. Endoplasmic reticulum stress signaling in disease. Physiol Rev 2006; 86:1133–1149.

53. Vattem KM, Wek RC. Reinitiation involving upstream ORFs regulates ATF4 mRNA translation in mammalian cells. Proc Natl Acad Sci USA 2004; 101:11269–11274.

54. Harding H, Novoa I, Zhang Y, et al. Regulated translation initiation controls stress-induced gene expression in mammalian cells. Mol Cell 2000; 6:1099–1108.

55. Calfon M, Zeng H, Urano F, et al. IRE1 couples endoplasmic reticulum load to secretory capacity by processing the XBP-1 mRNA. Nature 2002; 415:92–96.

56. Gass JN, Gunn KE, Sriburi R, Brewer JW. Stressed-out B cells? Plasma-cell differentiation and the unfolded protein response. Trends Immunol 2004; 25:17–24.

57. Delepine M, Nicolino M, Barrett T, et al. EIF2AK3, encoding translation initiation factor 2-alpha kinase 3, is mutated in patients with Wolcott-Rallison syndrome. Nat Genet 2000; 25:406–409.

58. Zhang P, McGrath B, Li S, et al. The PERK eukaryotic initiation factor 2a kinase is required for the development of the skeletal system, postnatal growth, and the function and viability of the pancreas. Mol Cell Biol 2002; 22:3864–3874.

59. Zhang P, McGrath B, Reinert J, et al. The GCN2 eIF2a kinase is required for adaptation to amino acid deprivation in mice. Molec Cell Biol 2002; 22:6681–6688.

60. Dann SG, Thomas G. The amino acid sensitive TOR pathway from yeast to mammals. FEBS Lett 2006; 580:2821–2829.

61. Avruch J, Hara K, Lin Y, et al. Insulin and amino-acid regulation of mTOR signaling and kinase activity through the Rheb GTPase. Oncogene 2006; 25:6361–6372.

62. Denne S, Kalhan S. Leucine metabolism in human newborns. Am J Physiol 1987; 253:E608–615.

63. Fryburg D, Louand R, Gerow K, et al. Growth hormone stimulates skeletal muscle protein synthesis and antagonizes insulin's antiproteolytic action in humans. Diabetes 1991; 41:424–429.

64. Scornik O. Protein synthesis and degradation during growth. In: Jones L, ed. Biochemical development of the fetus and neonate. New York: Elsevier; 1982: 866–894.

65. Ballard FJ, Haslam RR, Burgoyne JL, Tomas FM. Muscle protein breakdown in premature human infants. Revis Biol Celular 1989; 21:445–457.

66. Loo TW, Bartlett MC, Clarke DM. Rescue of folding defects in ABC transporters using pharmacological chaperones. J Bioenerg Biomembr 2005; 37:501–507.

67. Skach WR. CFTR: new members join the fold. Cell 2006; 127:673–675.

68. Jagoe RT, Goldberg AL. What do we really know about the ubiquitin-proteasome pathway in muscle atrophy? Curr Opin Clin Nutr Metab Care 2001; 4:183–190.

69. Lecker SH, Goldberg AL, Mitch WE. Protein degradation by the ubiquitin-proteasome pathway in normal and disease states. J Am Soc Nephrol 2006; 17:1807–1819.

70. Cuervo AM. Autophagy: in sickness and in health. Trends Cell Biol 2004; 14:70–77.

71. Farkas A, Tompa P, Friedrich P. Revisiting ubiquity and tissue specificity of human calpains. Biol Chem 2003; 384:945–949.

72. Friedrich P, Tompa P, Farkas A. The calpain-system of Drosophila melanogaster: coming of age. Bioessays 2004; 26:1088–1096.

73. Turk B, and Stoka V. Protease signaling in cell death: caspases versus cysteine cathepsins. FEBS Lett 2007; 581(15):2761–2767.

74. Reid MB. Response of the ubiquitin-proteasome pathway to changes in muscle activity. Am J Physiol Regul Integr Comp Physiol 2005; 288:R1423–1431.

75. Asher G, Reuven N, Shaul Y. 20S proteasomes and protein degradation "by default." Bioessays 2006; 28:844–849.

76. Sun Y. E3 ubiquitin ligases as cancer targets and biomarkers. Neoplasia 2006; 8:645–654.

77. Hurley JH, Lee S, Prag G. Ubiquitin-binding domains. Biochem J 2006; 399:361–372.

78. Kim JH, Park KC, Chung SS, Bang O and Chung CH. Deubiquitinating Enzymes as Cellular Regulators. J Biochem 2003; 134(1):9–18.

79. Murata S. Multiple chaperone-assisted formation of mammalian 20S proteasomes. IUBMB Life 2006; 58:344–348.

80. Hartmann-Petersen R, Gordon C. Proteins interacting with the 26S proteasome. Cell Mol Life Sci 2004; 61:1589–1595.

81. Yano M, Kanesaki Y, Koumoto Y, et al. Chaperone activities of the 26S and 20S proteasome. Curr Protein Pept Sci 2005; 6:197–203.

82. Bennett RG, Hamel FG, Duckworth WC. Insulin inhibits the ubiquitin-dependent degrading activity of the 26S proteasome. Endocrinology 2000; 141:2508–2517.

83. Adegoke OA, McBurney MI, Samuels SE, Baracos VE. Modulation of intestinal protein synthesis and protease mRNA by luminal and systemic nutrients. Am J Physiol Gastrointest Liver Physiol 2003; 284:G1017–1026.

84. Molinari M, Sitia R. The secretory capacity of a cell depends on the efficiency of endoplasmic reticulum-associated degradation. Curr Top Microbiol Immunol 2005; 300:1–15.

85. Meusser B, Hirsch C, Jarosch E, Sommer T. ERAD: the long road to destruction. Nat Cell Biol 2005; 7:766–772.

86. McCracken AA, Brodsky JL. Recognition and delivery of ERAD substrates to the proteasome and alternative paths for cell survival. Curr Top Microbiol Immunol 2005; 300:17–40.

87. Kruse KB, Brodsky JL, McCracken AA. Autophagy: an ER protein quality control process. Autophagy 2006; 2:135–137.

88. Mortimore GE, Poso AR. Intracellular protein catabolism and its control during nutrient deprivation and supply. Annu Rev Nutr 1987; 7:539–564.

89. Godlewski MM, Slupecka M, Wolinski J, et al. Into the unknown – the death pathways in the neonatal gut epithelium. J Physiol Pharmacol 2005; 56(Suppl 3):7–24.

90. Mortimore G, Poso A. Amino acid control of intracellular protein degradation. Methods Enzymol 1998; 166:461–476.

91. Kuma A, Hatano M, Matsui M, et al. The role of autophagy during the early neonatal starvation period. Nature 2004 Dec 23; 432:1032–1036.

92. Kadowaki M, Kanazawa T. Amino acids as regulators of proteolysis. J Nutr 2003; 133:2052S–2056S.

93. Kanazawa T, Taneike I, Akaishi R, et al. Amino acids and insulin control autophagic proteolysis through different signaling pathways in relation to mTOR in isolated rat hepatocytes. J Biol Chem 2004; 279:8452–8459.

94. Miotto G, Venerando R, Marin O, et al. Inhibition of macroautophagy and proteolysis in the isolated rat hepatocyte by a nontransportable derivative of the multiple antigen peptide Leu8-Lys4-Lys2-Lys-beta Ala. J Biol Chem 1994; 269:25348–25353.

95. Goll DE, Thompson VF, Li H, et al. The calpain system. Physiol Rev 2003; 83:731–801.

96. Carragher NO. Calpain inhibition: a therapeutic strategy targeting multiple disease states. Curr Pharm Des 2006; 12:615–638.

97. Lu X, Rong Y, Baudry M. Calpain-mediated degradation of PSD-95 in developing and adult rat brain. Neurosci Lett 2000; 286:149–153.

98. Wendt A, Thompson VF, Goll DE. Interaction of calpastatin with calpain: a review. Biol Chem 2004; 385:465–472.

99. Ou BR, Forsberg NE. Determination of skeletal muscle calpain and calpastatin activities during maturation. Am J Physiol 1991; 261:E677–683.

100. Tanaka K, Harioka T, Murachi T. Changes in contents of calpain and calpastatin in rat liver during growth. Physiol Chem Phys Med NMR 1985; 17:357–363.

101. Raju TN. Epidemiology of late preterm (near-term) births. Clin Perinatol 2006; 33:751–763.

102. American Academy of Pediatrics Committee on Nutrition. Nutritional needs of preterm infants. In: Kleinman R, ed. Pediatric nutrition handbook. Elk Grove: American Academy of Pediatrics; 1998: 55–79.

103. Catzeflis C, Schutz Y, Micheli J. Whole-body protein-synthesis and energy-expenditure in very low birth weight infants. Pediatr Res 1985; 19:679–687.

104. Snyderman S, Boyer A, Kogut M, Holt L. The protein requirement of the preterm infants. The effect of protein intake on the retention of nitrogen. J Pediatr 1969; 74:872–880.

105. Duffy B, Gunn T, Collinge J, Pencharz P. The effect of varying protein quality and energy intake on the nitrogen metabolism of parenterally fed very low birthweight (less than 1600 g) infants. Pediatr Res 1981; 15:1040–1044.

106. Zlotkin SH, Bryan MH, Anderson GH. Intravenous nitrogen and energy intakes required to duplicate in utero nitrogen accretion in prematurely born human infants. J Pediatr 1981; 99:115–120.

107. van den Akker CH, te Braake FW, Wattimena DJ, et al. Effects of early amino acid administration on leucine and glucose kinetics in premature infants. Pediatr Res 2006; 59:732–735.

108. Thureen PJ, Melara D, Fennessey PV, Hay WW Jr. Effect of low versus high intravenous amino acid intake on very low birth weight infants in the early neonatal period. Pediatr Res 2003; 53:24–32.

109. Kadrofske MM, Parimi PS, Gruca LL, Kalhan SC. Effect of intravenous amino acids on glutamine and protein kinetics in low-birth-weight preterm infants during the immediate neonatal period. Am J Physiol Endocrinol Metab 2006; 290:E622–630.

110. Agus MS, Javid PJ, Piper HG, et al. The effect of insulin infusion upon protein metabolism in neonates on extracorporeal life support. Ann Surg 2006; 244:536–544.

111. Pierro A, Carnielli V, Filler R, et al. Characteristics of protein sparing effect of total parenteral nutrition in the surgical infant. J Pediatr Surg 1988; 23:538–542.

112. Jones M, Pierro A, Garlick P. Protein metabolism kinetics in neonates: effect of intravenous carbohydrate and fat. J Pediatr Surg 1995; 30:458–462.

113. Pierro A, Jones M, Garlick P. Nonprotein energy-intake during total parenteral-nutrition – effect on protein-turnover and energy-metabolism. Clin Nutr 1995; 14:47–49.

114. Rubecz I, Mestyan J, Varga P, Klujber L. Energy meabolism, substrate utilization, and nitrogen balance in parenterally fed postoperative neonates and infants. The effect of glucose, glucose + amino acids, lipid + amino acids inflused in isocaloric amounts. J Pediatr 1981; 98:42–46.

115. Kashyap S, Towers HM, Sahni R, et al. Effects of quality of energy on substrate oxidation in enterally fed, low-birth-weight infants. Am J Clin Nutr 2001; 74:374–380.

116. Kashyap S, Ohira-Kist K, Abildskov K, et al. Effects of quality of energy intake on growth and metabolic response of enterally fed low-birth-weight infants. Pediatr Res 2001; 50:390–397.

117. Regan FM, Cutfield WS, Jefferies C, et al. The impact of early nutrition in premature infants on later childhood insulin sensitivity and growth. Pediatrics 2006; 118:1943–1949.

118. Hofman PL, Regan F, Cutfield WS. Prematurity – another example of perinatal metabolic programming?. Horm Res 2006; 66:33–39.

119. Cooke R, Ford A, Werkman S, et al. Postnatal growth in infants born between 700 and 1,500 g. J Pediatr Gastroenterol Nutr 1993; 16:130–135.

120. Carlson S, Ziegler E. Nutrient intakes and growth of very low birth weight infants. J Perinatol 1998; 18:252–258.

121. Schulze K, Kashyap S, Ramakrishnan R. Cardiorespiratory costs of growth in low birth weight infants. J Dev Physiol 1993; 19:85–90.

122. Embleton N, Pang N, Cooke R. Postnatal malnutrition and growth retardation: an inevitable consequence of current recommendations in preterm infants? Pediatr 2001; 107:270–273.

123. Heird W, Dell R, Driscoll J, et al. Metabolic acidosis resulting from intravenous alimentation mixtures containing synthetic amino acids. N Engl J Med 1972; 287:943–948.

124. Johnson J, Albritton W, Sunshine P. Hyperammonemia accompanying parenteral nutrition in newborn infants. J Pediatr 1972; 81:154–161.

125. Denne S, Karn C, Wang J, Liechty E. Effect of intravenous glucose and lipid on proteolysis and glucose production in normal newborns. Am J Physiol 1995; 269:E361–E367.

126. Anderson T, Muttart C, Bieber M, et al. A controlled trial of glucose vs glucose amino acids in premature infants. J Pediatr 1979; 94:947–951.

127. Braake F, van den Akker C, Wattimena D, et al. Amino acid administration to premature infants directly after birth. J Pediatr 2005; 147:457–461.

128. Ridout E, Melara D, Rottinghaus S, Thureen PJ. Blood urea nitrogen concentration as a marker of amino-acid intolerance in neonates with birthweight less than 1250 g. J Perinatol 2005; 25:130–133.

129. Rivera A Jr, Bell EF, Bier DM. Effect of intravenous amino acids on protein metabolism of preterm infants during the first three days of life. Pediatr Res 1993; 33:106–111.

130. Saini J, MacMahon P, Morgan J, Kovar I. Early parenteral feeding of amino acids. Arch Dis Child 1989; 64:1362–1366.

131. van Goudoever J, Colen T, Wattimena J, et al. Immediate commencement of amino acid supplementation in preterm infants: effect on serum amino acid concentrations and protein kinetics on the first day of life. J Pediatr 1995; 127:458–465.

132. van Lingen R, van Goudoever J, Luijendijk I, et al. Effects of early amino acid administration during total parenteral nutrition on protein metabolism in pre-term infants. Clin Sci 1992; 82:199–203.

133. Saenz de Pipaon M, VanBeek RH, Quero J, et al. Effect of minimal enteral feeding on splanchnic uptake of leucine in the postabsorptive state in preterm infants. Pediatr Res 2003; 53:281–287.

134. Torrallardona D, Harris CI, Fuller MF. Lysine synthesized by the gastrointestinal microflora of pigs is absorbed, mostly in the small intestine. Am J Physiol Endocrinol Metab 2003; 284:E1177–1180.

135. Saenz de Pipaon M, Quero J, Wattimena DJ, Sauer PJ. Effect of two amino acid solutions on leucine turnover in preterm infants. Biol Neonate 2005; 87:236–241.

136. des Robert C, Le Bacquer O, Piloquet H, et al. Acute effects of intravenous glutamine supplementation on protein metabolism in very low birth weight infants: a stable isotope study. Pediatr Res 2002; 51:87–93.

137. Kalhan SC, Parimi PS, Gruca LL, Hanson RW. Glutamine supplement with parenteral nutrition decreases whole body proteolysis in low birth weight infants. J Pediatr 2005; 146:642–647.

138. Dallas MJ, Bowling D, Roig JC, et al. Enteral glutamine supplementation for very-low-birth-weight infants decreases hospital costs. J Parenter Enteral Nutr 1998; 22:352–356.

139. Lacey JM, Crouch JB, Benfell K, et al. The effects of glutamine-supplemented parenteral nutrition in premature infants. J Parenter Enteral Nutr 1996; 20:74–80.

140. Neu J, Li N. Pathophysiology of glutamine and glutamate metabolism in premature infants. Curr Opin Clin Nutr Metab Care 2007; 10(Jan):75–79.

141. Parimi PS, Kalhan SC. Glutamine supplementation in the newborn infant. Semin Fetal Neonatal Med 2007; 12(Feb):19–25.

142. Bertolo RF, Brunton JA, Pencharz PB, Ball RO. Arginine, ornithine, and proline interconversion is dependent on small intestinal metabolism in neonatal pigs. Am J Physiol Endocrinol Metab 2003; 284:E915–922.

143. Brunton JA, Bertolo RF, Pencharz PB, Ball RO. Proline ameliorates arginine deficiency during enteral but not parenteral feeding in neonatal piglets. Am J Physiol 1999; 277:E223–231.

144. Amin H, Zamora S, McMillan D, et al. Arginine supplementation prevents necrotizing enterocolitis in the premature infant. J Pediatr 2002; 140:425–431.

145. Zamora SA, Amin HJ, McMillan DD, et al. Plasma L-arginine concentrations in premature infants with necrotizing enterocolitis. J Pediatr 1997; 131:226–232.

146. Chesney R, Helms R, Christensen M, et al. The role of taurine in infant nutrition. Adv Exp Med Biol 1998; 442:463–476.

147. Wharton BA, Morley R, Isaacs EB, et al. Low plasma taurine and later neurodevelopment. Arch Dis Child Fetal Neonatal Ed 2004; 89:F497–498.

148. Lourenco R, Camilo M. Taurine: a conditionally essential amino acids in humans? An overview in health and disease. Nutr Hosp 2002; 17:262–270.

149. Heird WC. Taurine in neonatal nutrition–revisited. Arch Dis Child Fetal Neonatal Ed 2004; 89:F473–F474.

150. Ehrenkranz R, Younces N, Lemons J, et al. Longitudinal growth of hospitalized very low birth-weight infants. Pediatr 1999; 104:280–289.

151. Lucas A. Nutrition, growth, and development of postdischarge, preterm infants. In: Hay W, Lucas A, eds. Posthospital nutrition in the preterm infant. Columbus: Ross Laboratories; 1995: 81–89.

152. Ziegler EE, Thureen PJ, Carlson SJ. Aggressive nutrition of the very low birthweight infant. Clin Perinatol 2002; 29:225–244.

153. Kashyap S, Heird W. Protein requirements of low birthweight, very low birthweight, and small for gestational age infants. In: Raiha N, ed. Nestle nutrition workshop series: Protein metabolism during infancy. New York: Vevey/Raven Press; 1994: 133–151.

154. AAP. Pediatric nutrition handbook, 5th edn. 2004.

155. Chandra R. Immunoglobulin and protein levels in breast milk produced by mothers of preterm infants. Nutr Res 1982; 2:27–30.

156. Faerk J, Skafte L, Petersen S, et al. Macronutrients in milk from mothers delivering preterm. Adv Exp Med Biol 2001; 501:409–413.

157. Lucas A. Enteral nutriton. In: Tsang R, Lucas A, Uauy R, Zlotkin S, eds. Nutritional needs of the preterm infants: scientific basis and practical guidelines. Baltimore: Williams & Wilkins; 1993: 209–223.

158. Schanler R, Hurst N, Lau C. The use of human milk and breastfeeding in premature infants. Clin Perinatol 1999; 26:379–398.

159. Atkinson S. Effects of gestational age at delivery on human milk components. In: Jensen R, ed. Handbook of milk composition. San Diego: Academic Press; 1995: 222–237.

160. Lucas A, Hudson G. Preterm milk as a source of protein for low birth weight infants. Arch Dis Child 1984; 59:831–836.

161. Engelke S, Shah B, Vasan U, Raye J. Sodium balance in very low-birth-weight infants. J Pediatr 1978; 93:837–841.

162. Ronnholm K, Sipila I, Siimes M. Human milk protein supplementation for the prevention of hypoproteinemia without metabolic imbalacne in breast milk-fed, very low-birth-weight infants. J Pediatr 1982; 101:243–247.

163. Greer F, Steichen J, Tsang R. Calcium and phosphate supplements in breast milk-related rickets: results in a very-low-birth-weight infant. Am J Dis Child 1982; 136:581–583.

164. Kuschel C, Harding J. Mulicomponent fortified human milk for promoting growth in preterm infants. Cochrane Review Library 2003.

165. Ehrenkranz R, Gettner P, Nelli C. Nutrient balance studies in premature infants fed premature formula or fortified preterm human milk. J Pediatr Gastroenterol Nutr 1989; 8:58–67.

166. Greer F, McCormick A. Improved bone mineralization and growth in premature infants fed fortified own mother's milk. J Pediatr 1988; 112:961–969.

167. Berseth C, Van Aerde J, Gross S, et al. Growth, efficacy, and safety of feeding an iron-fortified human milk fortifier. Pediatr 2004; 114:e699–e706.

168. Arslanogul A, Moro G, Ziegler E. Adjustable fortification of human milk fed to preterm infants: does it make a difference? J Perinatol 2006:1–8.

169. Morley R, Lucas A. Influence of early diet on outcome in preterm infants. Acta Paediatr Suppl 1994; 405:123–126.

170. Cooke RJ. Adjustable fortification of human milk fed to preterm infants. J Perinatol 2006; 26:591–592.

171. de Boo HA, Cranendonk A, Kulik W, et al. Whole body protein turnover and urea production of preterm small for gestational age infants fed fortified human milk or preterm formula. J Pediatr Gastroenterol Nutr 2005; 41:81–87.

172. Reichman B, Chessez P, Putet G. Diet, fat accretion, and growth in premature infants. N Engl J Med 1981; 305:1495–1500.

173. Heird WC. Determination of nutritional requirements in preterm infants, with special reference to 'catch-up' growth. Semin Neonatol 2001; 6:365–375.

174. Lemons J, Bauer C, Oh W. Very low birth weight outcomes of the National Institute of Child Health and Human Development Neonatal Research Network, January 1995 through December 1996. Pediatrics 2001; 107:1e.

175. Friel J, Andrews W, Matthew J, et al. Improved growth of very low birth weight infants. Nutr Res 1993; 13:611–620.

176. Lucas A, Bishop N, Cole T. Randomized trial of nutrition for preterm infants after discharge. Arch Dis Child 1992; 67:342.

177. Clandinin M, Van Aerde J, Merkel K, et al. Growth and development of preterm infants fed infant formulas containing docosahexaenoic acid and arachidonic acid. J Pediatr 2005; 146:461–468.

178. Thureen PJ. Measuring energy expenditure in preterm and unstable infants. J Pediatr 2003; 142:366–367.

179. Callaghan WM, MacDorman MF, Rasmussen SA, et al. The contribution of preterm birth to infant mortality rates in the United States. Pediatrics 2006; 118:1566–1573.

Chapter 11

Noninvasive Techniques to Monitor Nutrition in Neonates

Dominique Darmaun, MD, PhD • Jean-Christophe Rozé, MD

Use of Indirect Calorimetry to Assess Rates of Energy Expenditure and Substrate Oxidation
Use of Doppler to Determine Organ Blood Flows in Specific Tissues in Neonates
Methods for Measuring Body Composition in Infants
Principles of Isotope Dilution to Assess Nutrient Metabolism in vivo
Use of Stable Isotope Methods to Assess Dietary Intake and Rates of Energy Expenditure
Use of Stable Isotope Methods to Investigate Carbohydrate and Lipid Metabolism
Noninvasive Methods to investigate Whole-Body Protein Turnover in Neonates
Use of Stable Isotope Methods to Assess the Kinetics of Specific Proteins, Amino Acids, or Regional Protein Kinetics

The first month of life is a unique period characterized by a tremendous growth rate (≈25 g/day, i.e., 1 g/h), and a highly dynamic state of protein accretion, substrate turnover, and energy expenditure. Yet the conventional methods used to assess nutrition rely almost exclusively on the determination of substrate concentrations, which only provide static information. For instance, a rise in the concentration of a substrate can be the consequence of either (a) a rise in the production rate (Ra) of that substrate, (b) a decrease in its rate of disappearance (Rd), or (c) a combination of both mechanisms. Improving our understanding of substrate fluxes may help design better strategies to improve nutrient retention and growth in neonates: this has been the main incentive for the development of ethically acceptable, noninvasive techniques to investigate nutrition and metabolism in vivo in infants over the last two decades.

Far from being a comprehensive review, this chapter will briefly review the principles of selected current methods suitable for the assessment of energy and substrate metabolism in vivo in infants, with an emphasis on energy and protein metabolism, as delineated in the chapter outline above.

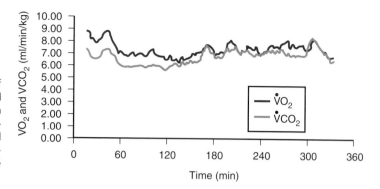

Figure 11-1 Typical time course of oxygen consumption ($\dot{V}O_2$) and carbon dioxide production ($\dot{V}CO_2$) in a 900-g infant, with an average respiratory quotient of 0.93, and $FIO_2-FEO_2 = 0.0148$, with a ventilator flow rate at 5530 mL/min (Rozé et al., personal data).

USE OF INDIRECT CALORIMETRY TO ASSESS RATES OF ENERGY EXPENDITURE AND SUBSTRATE OXIDATION

When performed with appropriate skill, indirect calorimetry (IC) appears to be one way of determining rates of energy expenditure (EE) with acceptable precision in neonates. Indirect calorimetry is based on the determination of respiratory exchange, i.e., of the composition of inspired and expired gases, and flow through the open circuit through a hood (canopy) or the ventilator (Fig. 11-1). Oxygen consumption ($\dot{V}O_2$) and carbon dioxide production ($\dot{V}CO_2$) are calculated using the following equations (1):

$$\dot{V}O_2 = \dot{V}E(FIO_2 - FECO_2 + FICO_2FEO_2 - FIO_2FECO_2)/(1 - FIO_2 - FICO_2)$$

$$\dot{V}CO_2 = \dot{V}E(FECO_2 - FICO_2 + FICO_2FEO_2 - FIO_2FECO_2)/(1 - FIO_2 - FICO_2)$$

where FIO_2 and $FICO_2$ are the O_2 and CO_2 concentrations measured in inspired gas, and FEO_2 and $FECO_2$ are the corresponding concentrations in expired air. $\dot{V}E$ is the flow measured on the expiratory circuit.

Energy metabolism involves the oxidation of substrates and the release of energy, heat, and carbon dioxide. The ratio of the volume of carbon dioxide released ($\dot{V}CO_2$) to the volume of oxygen used ($\dot{V}O_2$) depends on the quality of the "fuel mix" being metabolized, and is described by the respiratory quotient (RQ) calculated as $RQ = \dot{V}CO_2/\dot{V}CO_2$. Energy expenditure is calculated after correction for protein oxidation (usually by nitrogen measurement in collected urine). Energy expenditure (EE, kcal/min) can also be deducted from $\dot{V}CO_2$ and $\dot{V}O_2$ measurements (L/min), without taking into account nitrogen excretion, using the Weir's equation (2):

$$EE = (3.9 \times \dot{V}O_2) + (1.1 \times \dot{V}CO_2)$$

As the oxidation of pure carbohydrate yields an RQ of 1.0, and pure fat oxidation an RQ of 0.7, the relative contribution of fat and carbohydrate to overall energy expenditure can be deduced from the determination of RQ. Thus, under most circumstances, an RQ close to 0.7 is interpreted as indicating undernutrition, whereas an RQ approaching or exceeding 1.0 is considered to be indicative of overfeeding (3). Nevertheless, this interpretation was never intended when the technique was first introduced, and the underlying assumptions lack any scientific proof.

Several studies suggest that 24 h and 48 h EE can be extrapolated from measurements performed over a 6 h period: a 30 min equilibration coupled with variable EE collection periods may facilitate data collection in the clinical care setting. Most studies have used "home made" devices. Yet a calorimeter designed for infants has become commercially available: its design includes a constant internal gas flow, which obviates the need to measure flow rates, and uses the gas dilutional model described by Takala et al. (4). This instrument has been validated for use in preterm infants (5).

The accuracy of IC in measuring $\dot{V}O_2$ has nevertheless been questioned (6). Some limitations indeed exist. First, for mathematical reasons inherent to the Haldane transform algorithm, FiO_2 must be less than 0.50 to avoid the excessive error associated with higher inspiratory oxygen fractions. Secondly, oxygen concentration difference between inspiratory and expiratory circuit can be less than 0.0010 when measurement is performed in very low birth weight infants: as $\dot{V}O_2$ can be less than 6 mL/min in extremely low birth weight neonates, if the flow is >4000 mL/min the oxygen concentration difference between inspiratory and expiratory circuit indeed is less than 0.0010. So, to limit errors, an oxygen analyzer with an accuracy of better than 0.0001 must be used, and every attempt should be made to reduce flow and oxygen fluctuations. Oxygen fluctuations can be reduced by using gas from a gas tank instead of the wall source or by sampling gas samples through a mixing chamber placed in the expired-air inspired-air circuits, instead of directly sampling inspiratory and expiratory gas. Flows lower than 3000 mL/min are exposed to the risk of gas contamination from room air during $\dot{V}O_2$ measurement using a canopy, and this represents a limitation of the method as well. Thirdly, in ventilated babies, the presence of leaks secondary to using an uncuffed tracheal tube leads to underestimation of both $\dot{V}O_2$ and $\dot{V}CO_2$.

During ventilation support (ventilator, CPAP, or oxygen supplementation), $\dot{V}O_2$ measurement remains a challenge: in infants and children who are treated with supplementary oxygen, indirect calorimetry measurements may show large errors in respiratory quotient (RQ) (7, 8). Recently, an adaptation of the commercial device taking gas leaks into account has been proposed to perform measurements in patients undergoing ventilation or CPAP (9). To achieve optimal precision, $\dot{V}CO_2$ measurement is performed during a given period, and $\dot{V}O_2$ is then calculated from $\dot{V}CO_2$ measurement by using RQ. RQ is measured during an another period when flow is limited, and oxygen is taken from a gas tank to optimize RQ measurement.

When a canopy is used for measurements, and under conditions of steady state, $\dot{V}O_2$, $\dot{V}CO_2$, and RQ measurements can be performed with sufficient precision. The relative effects of biological variability, age, weight, and weight gain have important implications for the design and interpretation of energy balance studies in preterm infants. During energy balance studies, either a parallel or a cross-over design may be used. Variation due to biological variability can offset or confound the effects of treatment, and limit the ability to detect changes when using the parallel design, while variation due to a "period" effect, i.e., dietary intake, weight, age, weight gain, limits the precision of the cross-over design (6).

When indirect calorimetry is performed with skill and "art," and with meticulous attention to numerous minute details to limit errors, its use to assess energy expenditure in neonates is legitimate. Indirect calorimetry has been performed in a variety of physiological conditions: enteral or parenteral nutrition, weaning from ventilation (oxygen cost of breathing) (10), or weaning from incubator (11). The most relevant data obtained in infants regard nutrient oxidation during enteral nutrition. For instance, oxygen consumption of growing neonates was found to range between 7 and 8 mL/kg/min in six studies, RQ values of 0.85 or above have been observed, and fat oxidation was calculated to be between 2 and 3 g/kg/day (12).

USE OF DOPPLER TO DETERMINE ORGAN BLOOD FLOWS IN SPECIFIC TISSUES IN NEONATES

Abdominal sonograms can be used to visualize abdominal aorta and superior mesenteric artery, and the data used to measure blood flow mean velocity (if the angle between Doppler and the vessel is less than 20 degrees) and resistance index (which is independent of the angle). Thus, the transcutaneous Doppler flow method has been used to evaluate intestinal circulation in infants (13, 14). Blood flow parameters in the superior mesenteric artery change with vasoconstriction or vasodilatation of the intestinal vascular bed. In cases of severe growth retardation as a result of haemodynamic disturbances, the blood flow changes persist into postnatal life (15, 16). Other factors, including postnatal age, gestational age, birth weight, birth asphyxia, patent ductus arteriosus, and the use of various pharmacological agents or phototherapy have been reported to affect splanchnic blood flow patterns in infants.

Prandial state is a major determinant of mesenteric blood flow regulation. In full-term and larger preterm infants, mesenteric blood flow velocity increases after feedings. Several studies carried out in preterm infants reported a positive correlation between feed tolerance and postprandial superior mesenteric artery blood flow velocity, suggesting that higher postprandial blood flow velocity may be associated with a beneficial physiologic response (17). A rise in time-averaged mean velocity by more than 17% at 60 min has a sensitivity of 100% and a specificity of 70% for the prediction of early tolerance to enteral feeds (13).

METHODS FOR MEASURING BODY COMPOSITION IN INFANTS

Oral or nasogastric administration of ^2H_2O, a stable isotope, followed by urine or saliva sampling, allows for the determination of total body water (TBW) by isotope dilution principles (cf. infra). As labeled water distributes in fat-free mass, TBW, in turn, is used to determine lean body mass, assuming a constant water content in lean body mass (18, 19). Dual X-ray absorptiometry (DXA) has become the method of reference to determine body composition in most populations, and the method has been validated in small animals and human neonates (20–22). It delivers minimal radiation, as the dose of one infant whole-body scan is estimated at 3 μSv (0.3 mrem), and has the capability of measuring bone mineral content as well as body fat mass and lean body mass (22). Because fat-free mass contains virtually all the water and conducting electrolytes in the body, fat-free mass has a much higher electrical conductivity than fat mass: this principle is used to determine fat-free mass by bioelectrical impedance analysis (18). More recently, air-displacement plethysmography (ADP) has been proposed: body density is assessed from the ratio of body mass to body volume (23). Body mass is measured on an electronic scale, and body volume is measured in an enclosed chamber by applying gas laws that relate pressure changes to volumes of air in the enclosed chamber. These air volumes are used to calculate body volume. The percent of fat mass is then calculated from body density using published equations (24). Despite the potential usefulness of body-composition assessment in infants, these methods have not yet gained wide popularity because of their perceived complexity, and, in some cases, the lack of sufficient data regarding validity.

PRINCIPLES OF ISOTOPE DILUTION TO ASSESS NUTRIENT METABOLISM IN VIVO

Isotope dilution methods rely on a simple, robust principle. The analogy can be drawn with the way the unknown volume (V, expressed in L) of a bathtub is measured by diluting a known mass (m, g) of a dye in the tub, and measuring its concentration (c, g/L) after thorough mixing. As $c = m/V$, V can easily be deducted as: $V = m/c$ (Fig. 11-2). Similarly, when the concentration of a substrate S in a sampled pool ([S]) is constant (Fig. 11-2), this implies that the appearance

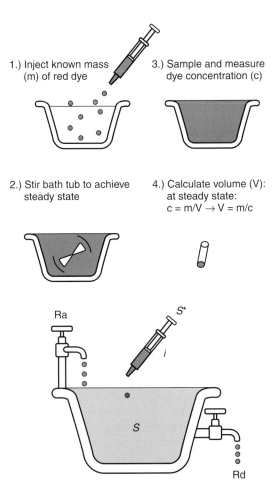

1.) Inject known mass (m) of red dye

2.) Stir bath tub to achieve steady state

3.) Sample and measure dye concentration (c)

4.) Calculate volume (V): at steady state: $c = m/V \rightarrow V = m/c$

Figure 11-2 Top panel: determination of the unknown volume of a bathtub using dye dilution (top), and of a substrate turnover rate (bottom) using isotope dilution principles. Bottom panel: use of a continuous infusion of labeled substrate S* to determine the fluxes of appearance (Ra) and disappearance (Rd) of substrate S into/from a pool. At steady state, and isotopic equilibrium: [S] is constant, so Ra = Rd, and $i/Ra \approx [S^*]/[S]$.

rate (Ra) of S into the pool is exactly matched by the amount of substrate leaving the pool in the same unit of time (rate of disappearance, Rd). If a known, minute amount of labeled substrate S* is infused at a constant rate (i, μmol/kg/min) into the pool, the few molecules of labeled S* entering the pool are continuously diluted by a larger number of molecules of unlabeled S arising from Ra. Once isotopic equilibrium is achieved, [S*]/[S] becomes equal to the ratio of labeled substrate infusion rate (i) to Ra: $[S^*]/[S] \approx i/Ra$.

The only tracers usable in neonates are labeled with stable isotopes, which are "heavier" forms of elements due to the presence of one or several additional neutrons in the nucleus, and are not radioactive. As they are already present at low but significant natural abundance in all tissues and foodstuffs, e.g. $\approx 1.1\%$ for ^{13}C (vs. $\approx 98.9\%$ for "natural" ^{12}C), and are devoid of any known side-effects when in small amounts, stable isotopes can be safely used for metabolic studies in infants, and pregnant women (Table 11-1).

USE OF STABLE ISOTOPE METHODS TO ASSESS DIETARY INTAKE AND RATES OF ENERGY EXPENDITURE

Use of ^2H_2O in Breast-Fed Infants

Conventional determination of milk intake in breast-fed babies is difficult, as it relies on pre- and post-feeding weighing, and can be inaccurate. Over a quarter of a century ago, Coward et al. validated the use of a single dose of ^2H_2O given to a

Table 11-1   Selected Stable Isotopes used in Tracer Studies in Neonates in vivo

Element	Isotope	Natural abundance (%)	Isotope	Natural abundance (%)
Hydrogen	^1H	99.9	^2H	0.01
Carbon	^{12}C	98.9	^{13}C	1.1
Nitrogen	^{14}N	99.6	^{15}N	0.4
Oxygen	^{16}O	99.8	^{18}O	0.2

nursing mother, along with the determination of ^2H-enrichment on two subsequent saliva samples in her infant, as a way to assess daily milk intake in breastfed infants (25, 26).

Intravenous Infusion of Labeled Bicarbonate to Measure Energy Expenditure

As outlined above, the determination of gas exchanges by indirect calorimetry can be laborious and inaccurate in very low birth weight infants. During the routine care of the mechanically ventilated neonate, the clinical practice has been to utilize uncuffed endotracheal tubes because of reduced laryngeal damage, which results in significant air leaks around the tube. Therefore, capture of all expired CO_2 is difficult. The isotopic dilution of CO_2 during the intravenous infusion of $H^{13}CO_3Na$ can be used to determine rates of CO_2 production without the need for the determination of total expired CO_2. In this technique, a 2 h, primed, continuous infusion of $H^{13}CO_3Na$ is administered, with intermittent sampling of breath aliquots from the expiratory circuit of the ventilator or from a ventilated hood. The method was validated against indirect calorimetry in healthy adults (27). As the labeled bicarbonate infusion is short (2 h), it can be immediately followed by a 3 h tracer infusion designed to assess, for instance, the oxidation rate of a substrate, e.g., $[^{13}C]$leucine, since assessment of CO_2 is mandatory to calculate rates of leucine oxidation (cf. infra): such an approach has been applied to investigate very low birth weight preterm infants (28–31).

Use of Doubly Labeled Water to Assess Total Energy Expenditure (TEE)

Upon administration of $^2H_2{}^{18}O$, the deuterium is excreted by the body as water, whereas the oxygen is eliminated faster, since it leaves the body as both CO_2 and water. Assuming body water represents a single compartment, the decline in $^2H_2$-enrichment in body water reflects water output, whereas the decline in ^{18}O-enrichment is faster, as it represents the sum of water output and CO_2 output. The rate of CO_2 production therefore can be calculated by the difference between the two elimination rates (32). Standard equations for indirect calorimetry are then applied. When reviewing measurements of TEE performed using doubly labeled water in >300 healthy infants in the first year of life, Davies et al. showed that estimates of energy intake derived from the measurements of TEE are considerably below the current international recommendations (33). The same technique applied in babies born small for gestational age (SGA) suggests that SGA infants have an ≈20% higher TEE and hence requirement, compared with infants born with a weight appropriate for their gestational age, even when energy expenditure is expressed per unit of fat free mass (34).

USE OF STABLE ISOTOPE METHODS TO INVESTIGATE CARBOHYDRATE AND LIPID METABOLISM

Glucose Metabolism

Three decades ago, Bier et al. were first to determine hepatic glucose production using an infusion of D-[6,6-^{2}H$_2$]glucose in human infants, and showed a nearly linear relationship between estimated brain weight and glucose production from the 1-kg premature infant to the 80-kg adult, suggesting that brain size may be a principal determinant of those factors that regulate hepatic glucose output throughout life (35). Isotope dilution has since been used extensively, for instance, to assess the response of hepatic glucose production to insulin: Farrag et al. found that elevation of plasma insulin (while maintaining plasma glucose at basal level through exogenous glucose – an approach classically termed "euglycemic clamp") was unable to fully suppress endogenous glucose production in neonates, contrary to what happens in adults and older children (36). Glycogenolysis and gluconeogenesis are the two sources that contribute to overall glucose production. Gluconeogenesis can be quantitated using isotope dilution methods: when exogenous glucose was reduced to half normal in very low birth weight (VLBW) infants receiving total parenteral nutrition, the infusion of [2-^{13}C]glycerol showed glycerol to be the main gluconeogenic precursor, as it accounted for 64% of the endogenous glucose production rate; the remaining fraction of gluconeogenesis – originating from precursors other than glycerol, presumably amino acids such as alanine and glutamine – was quantitated from the incorporation of ^{2}H into glucose during the infusion of ^{2}H$_2$O. Taken together, these studies demonstrate that, when receiving insufficient amounts of glucose but ample lipid and amino acid supply, VLBW infants are able to maintain blood glucose concentration through gluconeogenesis, mainly from glycerol (37).

Lactose Synthesis

Lactose – a disaccharide composed of 1 glucose and 1 galactose moiety – is the main carbohydrate in milk. Until recently, its origin had not been delineated in human milk. By combining [U-^{13}C$_6$]glucose and [2-^{13}C]glycerol infusion in lactating mothers, and monitoring the ^{13}C-enrichment in breast milk lactose, Sunehag et al. determined that, in the fed state, virtually all the glucose in milk lactose arises from plasma glucose, whereas only 68% of the galactose arises from glucose, and glycerol contributes to the de novo synthesis of galactose in human breast (38).

Lipid Fuel Kinetics

Over two decades ago, the first infusions of [1-^{13}C]palmitate or [2-^{13}C]glycerol (39) and [^{2}H$_3$] β-hydroxybutyrate (40) demonstrated that in human neonates glycerol, fatty acid and ketone body fluxes measured after 4 h or fasting are in the range observed after >16–24 h of fasting in adults; 75% of transported glycerol was found to be converted to glucose, and represented 5% of hepatic glucose production. More recently, the appearance of ^{2}H in arachidonic acid (20:4 n–6) and docosahexaenoic acid (22:6 n–3) after administration of ^{2}H-labeled linoleic acid (18:2 n–6) and linolenic acid (18:3 n–3), respectively, demonstrated that human infants have the capacity to convert dietary essential fatty acids to their longer-chain polyunsaturated fatty acid derivatives (41), even though this synthesis rate may not be sufficient to cover the infants' requirements. In enterally fed preterm infants, the administration of medium-chain triglycerides was found to decrease the oxidation of ^{13}C-labeled linoleic acid and of long-chain polyunsaturated fatty acids, without compromising endogenous n–6 long-chain polyunsaturated fatty acid synthesis (42).

Lipid Synthesis

Recent studies using a 12 h [^{13}C]acetate infusion showed that the rate of endogenous cholesterol synthesis was approximately three times higher in premature infants than that found in adult subjects, indicating that the cholesterol-synthesizing machinery is well developed in premature infants (43).

Determining the isotope enrichment in the "true" precursor is required to calculate the synthetic rates of complex molecules, and is intrinsically difficult as the precursor pool may be "hidden" or located in poorly accessible tissues, such as liver. The long-chain fatty acid molecules can be viewed as the product of the polymerization of numerous 2-carbon units (acetyl-CoA) precursor molecules (e.g, 8-acetyl-CoA in palmitic acid). Mass isotopomer distribution analysis (MIDA) (44) is an innovative approach in which the pattern of distribution of singly vs. multiply labeled product molecules is first measured using mass spectrometry in the large "polymer" molecule, and used to "back calculate" isotope enrichment in the small precursor subunit molecule, using statistical modeling. Rates of lipoprotein-palmitate lipogenesis measured using MIDA in neonates were found to be similar to those in adult subjects on a normal diet (43).

Over the last decade, the synthesis rate of surfactant phospholipid was measured from the incorporation of ^{13}C into serial tracheal aspirates after a 24 h tracer infusion of either [^{13}C]acetate, [^{13}C]glucose, or [^{13}C$_4$]palmitate (45), or [^{2}H]palmitate (46), whereas the synthetic rate of Surfactant-associated protein B can be assessed by an infusion of [^{13}C]valine (46).

NONINVASIVE METHODS TO INVESTIGATE WHOLE-BODY PROTEIN TURNOVER IN NEONATES

Nitrogen Balance to Investigate Whole-Body Protein Homeostasis

Nitrogen balance has long been the "gold standard" for assessing rates of protein accretion in infants. It relies on the assumption that when body protein mass is in steady state, as it is in a healthy, stable-weight adult, nitrogen (N) losses match nitrogen intake, so that (N intake − N excretion) = 0. As protein gain is a prerequisite for growth, the balance must be positive in a growing infant: (N intake − N excretion) > 0. Net protein gain (g/day) is then estimated as N balance × 6.25, as body protein is assumed to contain 1 g N per 6.25 g protein. Even though the methods for the determination of total urinary nitrogen (usually, chemiluminescence) are robust, and although very valuable data have been acquired with N balance (47), the approach has numerous limitations: (i) N intake is difficult to assess in many instances, for instance in breast-fed infants; (ii) determination of urinary N loss requires urine collection, which is prone to measurement error; (iii) N losses through skin desquamation, feces, or sweat, although significant, are not measurable, and urinary urea N excretion (or even solely urinary urea N) is taken as an estimate of overall N loss; (iv) somewhat disturbingly, N balance often turns out to be positive in healthy, stable-weight adults; and (v) finally, a negative N balance does not provide any insight into the mechanism involved, as it can reflect increased protein breakdown, decreased protein synthesis, or a combination of both mechanisms. Tracers are ideally suited to that task.

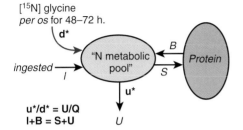

[^{15}N] glycine
per os for 48–72 h.

d*

ingested → I

"N metabolic pool"

B
S

Protein

u*

u*/d* = U/Q
I+B = S+U

U

Figure 11-3 Use of [^{15}N]glycine to assess whole body protein metabolism.

The "End Product" Method

[^{15}N]Glycine was the first stable isotope used for the assessment of protein turnover in vivo (48). Briefly, when [^{15}N]glycine is administered at a constant rate (d^*), the ^{15}N-enrichment in urinary urea reaches steady state after 48–72 h (Fig. 11-3). It is assumed that glycine's N is evenly distributed in the body "nitrogen metabolic pool" and that the fraction of the ^{15}N dose administered that is eventually excreted (u^*) equals the fraction of the "nitrogen pool turnover" excreted as urea (U): $u^*/d^* = U/Q$ (Fig. 11-2). Whole-body N turnover (Q) therefore is quantitated by measuring steady-state ^{15}N-enrichment in urinary urea as follows: $Q = U/(u^*/d^*)$.

Assuming the body N pool is at steady state, the amount of N entering the pool, i.e. the sum of dietary N intake (I) and N released from protein breakdown (B) equals the amount leaving the pool, and directed either toward protein synthesis (S) or oxidation to urea (U). Therefore, $B = Q - I$, and $S = Q - U$ (48).

Even though the determination for ^{15}N by isotope ratio mass spectrometry (IRMS) is accurate and sensitive, the method shares some of the difficulties associated with N balance, and relies on a host of unproven assumptions. For instance, there is no unique "nitrogen metabolic pool" since both anatomical and biochemical compartmentation have been documented for glycine N: (i) as glycine crosses cell membranes poorly, it does not equilibrate between plasma and tissues (e.g., red blood cells) (49); and (ii) glycine's amino-N does not end up evenly distributed among the 20 free amino acids (50). To overcome this obstacle, some authors have used a mixture of several ^{15}N-labeled amino acids (51). In addition, as measurements require a 48 h collection, attempts have been made at using ^{15}N-enrichment in urinary ammonium, another end-product of protein metabolism. Yet the use of either precursor results in different estimates for Q (52)

The "Precursor Amino Acid" Method

Short, 4–6 h intravenous infusion of highly enriched L-[1-^{13}C]leucine (>95% ^{13}C) has become the method of choice to assess whole-body protein kinetics in humans (Fig. 11-4). As leucine is an essential amino acid, the unlabeled free leucine present in plasma can only arise from exogenous leucine supplied by dietary (or intravenous) intake (I), or from the release of free leucine by the breakdown of body protein. Therefore $Ra = I + B$. On the other hand, leucine can only undergo oxidation (to CO_2 and urea), or incorporated into protein synthesis (S, or non-oxidative leucine disposal, NOLD). Upon infusion of [^{13}C]leucine, the labeled leucine molecules entering the free leucine pool follow the same fate as unlabeled leucine molecules, and $^{13}CO_2$ appears in breath, due to [^{13}C]leucine oxidation, and in body proteins, due to protein synthesis. The dilution of [^{13}C]leucine in the natural leucine pool is termed [^{13}C]leucine *enrichment*, since [^{13}C]leucine already exists in small amounts at baseline, and tracer infusion merely results in enriching the leucine pool above natural abundance. At steady state, ^{13}C-enrichment in the free leucine pool reflects the ratio of [^{13}C]leucine infusion rate (i), to leucine Ra.

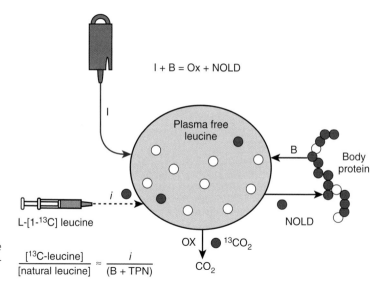

$$I + B = Ox + NOLD$$

Figure 11-4 Use of $[^{13}C]$leucine infusion to assess whole body protein metabolism.

$$\frac{[^{13}C\text{-leucine}]}{[\text{natural leucine}]} \approx \frac{i}{(B + TPN)}$$

Ra (μmol/kg per min) can thus be calculated from the dilution of $[^{13}C]$leucine. Ra = $i[(Ei/Ep)-1]$, where Ei and Ep (mole% excess) are ^{13}C-enrichments in the infused solution and plasma at steady state, respectively, and i is the tracer infusion rate (μmol/kg per min). Since Ra = $I + B$, B can easily calculated as $B = Ra - I$. Assuming leucine concentration is constant over the time course of the experiment (a few hours), Ra = Rd. By collecting expired air, leucine oxidation (Ox) can be determined, and NOLD, an estimate of leucine utilization for protein synthesis, calculated as NOLD = Ra − Ox (53). Absolute rates of whole-body protein synthesis, oxidation, and breakdown (g protein/kg per day) can then be extrapolated, as body protein contains $\approx$610 μmol leucine per g protein. The set up for a $[^{13}C]$leucine infusion involves the placement of two I.V. lines: one short catheter usually placed in an antecubital vein for the infusion of tracer, and a second catheter inserted into a contralateral, superficial vein for blood sampling. During the course of the isotope infusion, the hand is placed in heating pads to produce "arterialized-venous" blood, which more accurately reflects mixed arterial blood (54).

The leucine model relies on several assumptions (Table 11-2), most of which have survived two decades of intense scrutiny, and are considered valid. For instance, protein synthesis obviously does not occur in plasma, but in intracellular space. The true precursor pool used for protein synthesis is t-RNA-bound leucine, and assessing the isotope enrichment in that intracellular pool would pose tremendous ethical and technical difficulties, as it would involve the sampling of tissue biopsy samples, and the labor-intensive extraction of intact t-RNA-bound leucine. Isotope enrichments are instead measured in the plasma α-keto-isocaproate (KIC) pool, the keto acid of leucine, as a surrogate pool for t-RNA-bound leucine. Upon infusion of $[^{13}C]$leucine, labeled leucine is instantaneously transaminated to its

Table 11-2	Some of the Assumptions in the $[^{13}C]$Leucine Model

Absence of isotopic effect
Absence of any metabolic effect of infused tracer
The fraction of $^{13}CO_2$ produced that is recovered in breath is known
Absence of tracer "recycling"
The fate of the tracer (even though labeled on a single carbon) reflects that of the entire molecule
Plasma "pool" reflects intracellular leucine pool

keto-acid (^{13}C-KIC) upon entrance into intracellular space, and KIC is known to freely equilibrate with plasma KIC. As KIC only arises from leucine, and can only be produced inside cells, ^{13}C-KIC should be a suitable surrogate pool for intracellular leucine, and is easy to sample and measure. Plasma ^{13}C-KIC enrichment has been found to have an enrichment slightly ($\approx$10–20%) lower than plasma leucine, and human studies using multiple KIC and leucine tracers (55) and animal studies with tissue biopsies proved KIC to be a reliable reflection of the precursor leucine pool use for protein synthesis. Isotope enrichments are measured using mass spectrometry techniques. Isotope ratio mass spectrometry (IRMS) is used to determine very low enrichments (<0.01 mole% excess) in relatively pure gases (e.g. ^{13}C-enrichment in expired CO_2), whereas gas chromatography–mass spectrometry (GCMS) is used to determine higher enrichments (>0.1 mole% excess) in organic molecules in a complex matrix (e.g., plasma leucine or KIC) (19). Finally, gas chromatography–combustion–isotope ratio mass spectrometry (GC-C-IRMS) combines the capability of GC to resolve multiple "peaks" in plasma with the ability of IRMS to determine very low enrichments: in that approach, GC is used to separate organic molecules in a complex matrix (e.g., plasma leucine), the molecule of interest is converted online to pure gas (e.g., CO_2, through an online 800°C combustion oven), and finally analyzed as a gas by IRMS (56).

Assessment of leucine oxidation requires indirect calorimetry to measure overall CO_2 production (CO_2), and the collection of breath aliquots either from a ventilated hood, or from the expiratory circuit of the ventilator in patients receiving assisted ventilation, to determine $^{13}CO_2$ enrichment. As the recovery of metabolically produced $^{13}CO_2$ is not quantitative over the short time frame of isotope infusion, a correction factor is used to correct for this incomplete recovery (57). Even though recovery is often estimated from literature values at $\approx$80% (53), it should ideally be determined for each specific clinic and the population studied, as it can vary from one patient to the next. One way to measure it is to perform a short, 2 h infusion of labeled bicarbonate immediately before the infusion of labeled leucine (27, 28): an additional advantage of this approach is that it provides an assessment of CO_2, without the need for indirect calorimetry, as described above.

As the collection of breath is still a significant constraint, alternate approaches have been designed. For instance, as leucine oxidation ultimately represents irreversible amino acid wasting, several authors have estimated [^{13}C]leucine oxidation from the determination of urinary N excretion during [^{13}C]leucine infusion without any breath sampling (58).

Alternatively, labeled phenylalanine can be infused instead of labeled leucine (59). As phenylalanine is an essential amino acid, its metabolism is similar to that of leucine, with one exception: upon L-[ring-^{2}H$_4$]phenylalanine infusion, the immediate product of its oxidation is L-[ring-^{2}H$_4$]tyrosine, which can be measured in plasma samples (59). The ratio of [^{2}H$_4$]tyrosine/[^{2}H$_5$]phenylalanine reflects the fraction of tyrosine production arising from phenylalanine oxidation. The main limitation of the latter approach is that it should be combined with an infusion of a separate (e.g. [^{13}C]tyrosine) tracer to trace overall tyrosine Ra.

Finally, even though current GCMS instruments allow for the determination of isotope enrichments in as little as 100 μL of plasma, blood sampling may be hindered by ethical considerations, if a catheter is required for the sole purpose of blood sampling during an isotope infusion, rather than for clinical monitoring. This warrants the search for alternate sampling sites. Similar values for the enrichment of plasma and urinary leucine were observed upon infusion of [^{13}C]leucine (60). More recently, Darling et al. demonstrated the enrichments to differ slightly between plasma and urine for several amino acids, due to the significant presence of D-[^{13}C]amino acids that originate as contaminants from commercially manufactured tracers, as a result of the preferential excretion of D-amino acids in renal tubule. The 100% optical purity of the labeled amino acid should therefore be verified before implementing urine collection (61).

Leucine kinetics have been measured in a variety of conditions to investigate the regulation of protein kinetics in neonates. For instance, insulin was found to suppress proteolysis, and decrease protein synthesis, in VLBW infants (62), as it does in adults. Compared with the conventional "glucose only" infusion, immediate commencement of intravenous amino acid supply on the first day of life was shown to result in improved protein balance through a stimulation of protein synthesis in preterm infants with respiratory distress (63, 64). The response to a graded infusion of intravenous amino acids was measured in clinically stable premature infants in the first week of life: in contrast to the dose-dependent suppression of proteolysis seen in healthy full-term neonates, the endogenous rate of appearance of leucine was unchanged in response to amino acids (65). As glutamine is relatively unstable in solution, conventional amino acid mixtures for parenteral nutrition (PN) are devoid of glutamine. Yet glutamine may be "conditionally essential" in situations associated with major stress, e.g., in VLBW receiving PN: infusion of glutamine-enriched PN was found to decrease leucine oxidation and protein breakdown in PN-fed premature infants (31, 58).

USE OF STABLE ISOTOPE METHODS TO ASSESS THE KINETICS OF SPECIFIC PROTEINS, AMINO ACIDS, OR REGIONAL PROTEIN KINETICS

The methods described so far only provide insight into whole-body protein metabolism. This is obviously a simplistic view, since protein metabolism occurs in various tissues, at widely different rates. For instance, some proteins (such as liver enzymes) only have half-lives of a few minutes, whereas muscle protein turns over at a mere $\approx$1–2% per day. This consideration has led to the pursuit of newer approaches to assess the rates of protein turnover in different tissues or individual proteins.

Upon infusion of any labeled amino acid, the tracer equilibrates in the free amino acid pool in most tissues, and a fraction of the tracer participates in protein synthesis and is incorporated in every protein in the body. The ability to measure relatively low isotopic enrichments in specific proteins by GC-C-IRMS (56) has allowed the determination of the synthetic rates of specific proteins. For instance, serum albumin can be isolated from plasma samples obtained at set times over the course of a 72 h infusion of [^{15}N]glycine. The isolated protein is then hydrolyzed in vitro, and the rise in ^{15}N-enrichment in the albumin-bound glycine residues can be measured. The fraction of albumin synthesized per unit time is termed fractional synthesis rate (FSR), expressed as % per day, and simply calculated by dividing the rise in albumin-bound [^{15}N]glycine enrichment by the time lapsed, and by the enrichment in the precursor free glycine pool. The precursor used for the calculation is either plasma free glycine, or hippurate, another product of glycine metabolism presumably derived from the same intracellular hepatic pool, which can be isolated from urine (66).

The kinetics of non-essential amino acids can be quantified as well through a combined infusion of [^{13}C]leucine, and of a tracer of the non-essential amino acid of interest, e.g., [^{15}N]glutamine. As glutamine is non-essential, two sources contribute to its overall appearance rate (RaGln) in the fasting state: glutamine release from protein breakdown, and glutamine de novo synthesis. Assuming protein breakdown releases free amino acids in proportion to their relative abundance as bound residues in body protein, glutamine release from proteolysis is estimated as

0.421×RaLeu, where RaLeu is postabsorptive leucine appearance rate, and 0.421 is the ratio of glutamine to leucine abundance as bound residues in body protein (both expressed in μmol amino acid/g protein). The fraction of the RaGln that cannot be accounted for by release of glutamine from protein breakdown is attributed to the de novo synthesis of glutamine (67). This approach was used to demonstrate that VLBW infants are able to synthesize glutamine de novo as soon as the 10th day of life (68). Yet another approach was used to determine whether some amino acids classified as non-essential in adults may become essential in infants: Miller et al. monitored the appearance of ^{13}C in non-essential amino acids after administration of [U-^{13}C]glucose, and observed very little ^{13}C-enrichment in plasma cysteine, suggesting cysteine may be a conditionally essential amino acid in neonates (69). Dual isotope techniques have been used to assess regional amino acid kinetics as well. By combining the intravenous infusion of L-[$^{13}C_5$]glutamine, with orogastric infusion of L-[1-^{13}C]glutamine, 46–53% of the glutamine delivered through the enteral route was found to be extracted in the splanchnic tissues (gut plus liver), based on the appearance of the enterally infused tracer into plasma (68). These data suggest glutamine may be used intensively as an energy fuel in neonatal gut.

In summary, over the last two decades, the changes experienced in the noninvasive techniques for investigation of neonatal nutrition and metabolism have been dramatic, and the analogy can be drawn with the advent of cinema after a long era of static, motionless photography. Dynamic fluxes of energy substrates, proteins, and specific nutrients have become accessible to the investigator with ethically acceptable methods. These techniques have produced a tremendous wealth of information on nutrient fluxes in the human neonate. Although most of these techniques are and will remain restricted to research protocols, the physiological information accumulated with these techniques has already impacted significantly on the nutritional strategies for the management of newborn infants, and will continue to do so.

REFERENCES

1. Forsyth JS, Crighton A. An indirect calorimetry system for ventilator dependent very low birthweight infants. Arch Dis Child 1992; 67:315–319.
2. Weir V. New methods for calculating metabolic rate with special reference to protein metabolism. J Physiol 1949; 109:1–9.
3. Lafeber HN. The art of using indirect calorimetry for nutritional assessment of sick infants and children. Nutrition 2005; 21:192–198.
4. Takala J, Keinänen O, Väisänen P, Kari A. Measurement of gas exchange in intensive care: laboratory and cinical validation of a new device. Crit Care Med 1989; 17:1041–1047.
5. Shortland GJ, Fleming PJ, Walter JH. Validation of a portable indirect calorimetry system for measurement of energy expenditure in sick preterm infants. Arch Dis Child 1992; 67:1207–1211.
6. Perring J, Henderson M, Cooke RJ. Factors affecting the measurement of energy expenditure during energy balance studies in preterm infants. Pediatr Res 2000; 48:518–523.
7. Kalhan SC, Denne SC. Energy consumption in infants with broncho-pulmonary dysplasia. J Pediatr 1990; 116:662–664.
8. Thureen PJ, Phillips RE, DeMarie MP, et al. Technical and methodologic considerations for performance of indirect calorimetry in ventilated and nonventilated preterm infants. Crit Care Med 1997; 25:171–179.
9. Bauer K, Ketteler J, Laurenz M, et al. In vitro validation and clinical testing of an indirect calorimetry system for ventilated preterm infants that is unaffected by endotracheal tube leaks and can be used durng nasal continuous positive airway pressure. Pediatr Res 2001; 49:394–401.
10. Rozé JC, Chambille B, Fleury MA, et al. Oxygen cost of breathing in newborn infants with long-term ventilatory support. J Pediatr 1995; 127:984–987.
11. Dollberg S, Mimouni FB, Weintraub V. Energy expenditure in infants weaned from a convective incubator. Am J Perinatol 2004; 21:253–256.
12. Putet G. Lipids as an energy source for the premature and full term neonate. In: Polin AR, Fox WW, Abman SH, eds. Fetal and neonatal physiology, third edn. Saunder; 2004: 415–417.
13. Robel-Tillig E, Knupfer M, Pulzer F, et al. Blood flow parameters of the superior mesenteric artery as an early predictor of intestinal dysmotility in preterm infants. Pediatr Radiol. 2004; 34:958–962.

14. Pezzati M, Dani C, Tronchin M, et al. Prediction of early tolerance to enteral feeding by measurement of superior mesenteric artery blood flow velocity: appropriate- versus small-for-gestational-age preterm infants. Acta Paediatr 2004; 93:797–802.

15. Van Bel F, Van Zwieten PH, Guit GL, Schipper J. Superior mesenteric artery blood flow velocity and estimated volume flow: duplex Doppler US study of preterm and term neonates. Radiology 1990; 174:165–169.

16. Martinussen M, Brubakk AM, Vik T, et al. Relationship between intrauterine growth retardation and early postnatal superior mesenteric artery blood flow velocity. Biol Neonate 1997; 71:22–30.

17. Fang S, Kempley ST, Gamsu HR. Predition of early tolerance to enteral feeding in preterm infants by measurement of superior mesenteric artery blood flow velocity. Arch Dis Child Fetal Neonatal Ed 2001; 85:F42–F45.

18. Raghavan CV, Super DM, Chatburn RL, et al. Estimation of total body water in very-low-birth-weight infants by using anthropometry with and without bioelectrical impedance and H218O. Am J Clin Nutr 1998; 68:668–674.

19. Wolfe RR. Tracers in biomedicine. Wiley; 1992..

20. Picaud JC, Rigo J, Nyamugabo K, et al. Evaluation of dual-energy X-ray absorptiometry for body-composition assessment in piglets and term human neonates. Am J Clin Nutr 1996; 63:157–163.

21. Picaud JC, Nyamugabo K, Braillon P, et al. Dual-energy X-ray absorptiometry in small subjects: influence of dual-energy X-ray equipment on assessment of mineralization and body composition in newborn piglets. Pediatr Res 1999; 46:772–777.

22. Schmelzle HR, Fusch C. Body fat in neonates and young infants: validation of skinfold thickness versus dual-energy X-ray absorptiometry. Am J Clin Nutr 2002; 76:1096–1100.

23. Ma G, Yao M, Liu Y, Lin A, et al. Validation of a new pediatric air-displacement plethysmograph for assessing body composition in infants. Am J Clin Nutr 2004; 79:653–660.

24. Siri WE. The gross composition of the body. Adv Biol Med Phys 1956; 4:239–280.

25. Coward WA, Sawyer MB, Whitehead RG, et al. New method for measuring milk intakes in breast-fed babies. Lancet 1979; 2(8132):13–14.

26. Coward WA, Cole TJ, Sawyer MB, et al. Breast-milk intake measurement in mixed-fed infants by administration of deuterium oxide to their mothers. Hum Nutr Clin Nutr 1982; 36:141–148.

27. Spear ML, Darmaun D, Sager BK, et al. Use of [^{13}C]bicarbonate infusion for measurement of CO_2 production. Am J Physiol 1995; 268:E1123–E1127.

28. Bresson JL, Mariotti A, Narcy P, et al. Recovery of [^{13}C]-bicarbonate as respiratory $^{13}CO_2$ in parenterally fed infants. Eur J Clin Nutr 1990; 44:3–9.

29. Van Goudoever JB, Sulkers EJ, Chapman TE, et al. Glucose kinetics and glucoregulatory hormone levels in ventilated preterm infants on the first day of life. Pediatr Res 1993; 33:583–589.

30. Liet JM, Piloquet H, Marchini JS, et al. Leucine metabolism in preterm infants receiving parenteral nutrition with medium chain- vs. long chain-triacylglycerol emulsions. Am J Clin Nutr 1999; 69:539–543.

31. Des Robert C, Le Bacquer O, Piloquet H, et al. Acute effects of intravenous glutamine supplementation on protein metabolism in very low birth weight infants: a stable isotope study. Pediatr Res 2002; 51:87–93.

32. Schoeller DA. Recent advances from application of doubly labeled water to measurement of human energy expenditure. J Nutr 1999; 129:1765–1768.

33. Davies PSW. Energy requirements for growth and development in infancy. Am J Clin Nutr 1998; 68:939S–943S.

34. Davies PS, Clough H, Bishop NJ, et al. Total energy expenditure in small for gestational age infants. Arch Dis Child Fetal Neonatal Ed 1996; 74:F20.

35. Bier DM, Leake RD, Haymond MW, et al. Measurement of "true" glucose production rates in infancy and childhood with 6,6-dideuteroglucose. Diabetes 1977; 26:1016–1023.

36. Farrag HM, Nawrath LM, Healey JE, et al. Persistent glucose production and greater peripheral sensitivity to insulin in the neonate vs. the adult. Am J Physiol 1997; 272:E86–E93.

37. Sunehag AL, Haymond MW, Schanler RJ, et al. Gluconeogenesis in very low birthweight infants receiving total parenteral nutrition. Diabetes 1999; 48:791–800.

38. Sunehag AL, Louie K, Bier JL, et al. Hexoneogenesis in the human breast during lactation. J Clin Endocrinol Metab 2002; 87:297–301.

39. Bougnères PF, Karl IE, Hillman LS, et al. Lipid transport in the human newborn: palmitate and glycerol turnover and the contribution of glycerol to neonatal hepatic glucose output. J Clin Invest 1982; 70:262–270.

40. Bougnères PF, Lemmel C, Ferre P, et al. Ketone body transport in the human neonate and infant. J Clin Invest 1986; 77:42–48.

41. Salem N Jr, Wegher B, Mena P. Arachidonic and docosahexaenoic acids are biosynthesized from their 18-carbon precursors in human infants. Proc Natl Acad Sci USA 1996; 93:49–54.

42. Rodriguez M, Funke S, Fink M, et al. Plasma fatty acids and [^{13}C]linoleic acid metabolism in preterm infants fed a formula with medium-chain triglycerides. J Lipid Res 2003; 44:41–48.

43. Renfurm LN, Bandsma RH, Verkade HJ, et al. Cholesterol synthesis and de novo lipogenesis in premature infants determined by mass isotopomer distribution analysis. Pediatr Res 2004; 56:602–607.

44. Hellerstein MK, Neese RA. Mass isotopomer distribution analysis: a technique for measuring biosynthesis and turnover of polymers. Am J Physiol 1992; 263:E988–E1001.

45. Bohlin K, Patterson BW, Spence KL, et al. Metabolic kinetics of pulmonary surfactant in newborn infants using endogenous stable isotope techniques. J Lipid Res 2005; 46:1257–1265.

46. Cogo P, Baritussio A, Rosso F, et al. Surfactant-associated protein B kinetics in vivo in newborn infants by stable isotopes. Pediatr Res 2005; 57:519–522.

47. Picaud JC, Putet G, Rigo J, et al. Metabolic and energy balance in small- and appropriate-for-gestational-age, very low-birth-weight infants. Acta Paediatr Suppl 1994; 405:54–59.

48. Picou D, Taylor-Roberts T. The measurement of total protein synthesis and catabolism and nitrogen turnover in infants in different nutritional states and receiving different amounts of dietary protein. Clin Sci 1969; 36:283–296.

49. Darmaun D, Froguel P, Rongier M, et al. Amino acid exchange between plasma and erythrocytes in vivo in humans. J Appl Physiol 1989; 67:2383–2388.

50. Fern EB, Garlick PJ, Waterlow JC. Apparent compartmentation of body nitrogen in one human subject: its consequences in measuring the rate of whole-body protein synthesis with ^{15}N. Clin Sci (Lond) 1985; 68:271–282.

51. Plath C, Heine W, Wutzke KD, et al. ^{15}N Tracer kinetic studies on the validity of various ^{15}N tracer substances for determining whole-body protein parameters in very small preterm infants. J Pediatr Gastroenterol Nutr 1987; 6:400–408.

52. Pencharz P, Beesley J, Sauer P, et al. A comparison of the estimates of whole-body protein turnover in parenterally fed neonates obtained using three different end products. Can J Physiol Pharmacol 1989; 67:624–628.

53. Matthews DE, Motil KJ, Rohrbaugh DK, et al. Measurement of leucine metabolism in man from a primed, continuous infusion of L-[1–^{13}C]leucine. Am J Physiol 1980; 238:E473–E479.

54. Abumrad NN, Rabin D, Diamond MP, et al. Use of a heated superficial hand vein as an alternative site for the measurement of amino acid concentrations and for the study of glucose and alanine kinetics in man. Metabolism 1981; 30:936–940.

55. Horber FF, Horber-Feyder CM, Krayer S, et al. Plasma reciprocal pool specific activity predicts that of intracellular free leucine for protein synthesis. Am J Physiol 1989; 257:E385–E399.

56. Yarasheski KE, Smith K, Rennie MJ, et al. Measurement of muscle protein fractional synthetic rate by capillary gas chromatography/combustion isotope ratio mass spectrometry. Biol Mass Spectrom 1992; 21:486–490.

57. Hoerr RA, Yu YM, Wagner DA, et al. Recovery of ^{13}C in breath from NaH^{13}CO$_3$ infused by gut and vein: effect of feeding. Am J Physiol 1989; 257:E426–E438.

58. Kalhan SC, Parimi PS, Gruca LL, et al. Glutamine supplement with parenteral nutrition decreases whole body proteolysis in low birth weight infants. J Pediatr 2005; 146:642–647.

59. Thompson GN, Pacy PJ, Merritt H, et al. Rapid measurement of whole body and forearm protein turnover using a [^{2}H$_5$]phenylalanine model. Am J Physiol 1989; 256:E631–E639.

60. De Benoist B, Abdulrazzak Y, Brooke OG, et al. The measurement of whole body protein turnover in the preterm infant with intragastric infusion of L-[1–^{13}C]leucine and sampling of the urinary leucine pool. Clin Sci (Lond) 1984; 66:155–164.

61. Darling PB, Bross R, Wykes LJ, et al. Isotopic enrichment of amino acids in urine following oral infusions of L-[1–^{13}C]phenylalanine and L-[1–^{13}C]lysine in humans: confounding effect of D-[^{13}C]amino acids. Metabolism 1999; 48:732–737.

62. Poindexter BB, Karn CA, Denne SC. Exogenous insulin reduces proteolysis and protein synthesis in extremely low birth weight infants. J Pediatr 1998; 132:948–953.

63. Rivera A Jr, Bell EF, Bier DM. Effect of intravenous amino acids on protein metabolism of preterm infants during the first three days of life. Pediatr Res 1993; 33:106–111.

64. Van Goudoever JB, Colen T, Wattimena JL, et al. Immediate commencement of amino acid supplementation in preterm infants: effect on serum amino acid concentrations and protein kinetics on the first day of life. J Pediatr 1995; 127:458–465.

65. Poindexter BB, Karn CA, Leitch CA, et al. Amino acids do not suppress proteolysis in premature neonates. Am J Physiol 2001; 28:E472–E478.

66. Yudkoff M, Nissim I, McNellis W, et al. Albumin synthesis in premature infants: determination of turnover with [^{15}N]glycine. Pediatr Res 1987; 21:49–53.

67. Kuhn KS, Schuhmann K, Stehle P, et al. Determination of glutamine in muscle protein facilitates accurate assessment of proteolysis and de novo synthesis-derived endogenous glutamine production. Am J Clin Nutr 1999; 70:484–489.

68. Darmaun D, Roig JC, Auestad N, et al. Glutamine metabolism in very low birth weight infants. Pediatr Res 1997; 41:391–396.

69. Miller RG, Jahoor F, Jaksic T. Decreased cysteine and proline synthesis in parenterally fed, premature infants. J Pediatr Surg 1995; 30:953–957.

Chapter 12

Nutritional Requirements of the Very Low Birth Weight Infant

Patti J. Thureen, MD • William W. Hay, Jr., MD

Differences between Fetal and Neonatal Nutrition
Current Understanding of Specific Nutrient Requirements of the Very Preterm Infant
Scientifically Based Approaches for Providing Parenteral and Enteral Nutrition to Low Birth Weight Infants

---

Due to advances in perinatal care, very preterm infants between 23 and 26 weeks of gestation and 500 and 1000 g birth weight are surviving at increased rates. Most of their body growth and the associated development of functional capacity, therefore, take place outside of the uterus. Nutrition to support this growth and development must be provided by intravenous and enteral routes rather than by the placenta. Many advances in intravenous and enteral nutrition of preterm infants have been developed over the past several years, but the increasing survival at lower birth weights, the degree of immaturity of the surviving infants, and the increasing dependence on extrauterine nutrition of these vulnerable infants are providing renewed interest in the absolute importance of postnatal nutrition. Extremely low birth weight infants (ELBW) (defined as <1000 g in weight) have unique nutritional metabolic substrate requirements for energy balance and growth, predicted by a high protein turnover rate, high metabolic rate, and high glucose utilization rate. The ELBW infant has endogenous energy reserves of only about 200 kcal, enough to maintain energy balance for only 3–4 days without an exogenous energy supply. Thus the ELBW infant is extremely vulnerable to inadequate nutritional intake. Growth and development of sensitive organs, particularly the brain, clearly are dependent on unique, though variable, mixes of specific nutrients, provided at optimal rates and by safe and efficacious routes. There also is abundant evidence from animal experiments and human observational studies that prolonged undernutrition during critical periods of development (between 22 and 40 weeks post-conceptional age for humans) adversely affects long-term growth and neuro-developmental and cognitive outcomes. Nationally, nutritional strategies for very preterm infants are resulting in postnatal growth failure from which the neonate does not recover by hospital discharge (1–3). Nutritional practices in preterm infants vary considerably and there are no definitive regimens that have been shown to safely provide nutrition, growth, and development of these infants. Despite the advances in nutrition of these infants, therefore, we now are at a new threshold of determining what nutrients we should provide to these infants, at what

DIFFERENCES BETWEEN FETAL AND NEONATAL NUTRITION

The currently recommended standard for providing comprehensive postnatal nutrition to very preterm infants is one that meets the unique nutritional requirements of the growing human fetus and duplicates normal in utero human fetal growth and development (5). This long-standing recommendation by the American Academy of Pediatrics has not included guidelines about how this should be achieved, however, and there are no data in the literature to support or refute this recommendation. Therefore, appreciating the differences between normal fetal nutrition and commonly used postnatal nutritional practices in very preterm neonates may be a useful first step to developing nutritional strategies to meet this standard for postnatal growth in very preterm neonates.

Protein

Amino acid uptake by the fetus is far in excess of that needed to meet accretion requirements; the excess amino acids are oxidized, contributing significantly to fetal energy production (6, 7). In contrast, amino acids usually are infused into the preterm neonate in the first several weeks of life at low rates that are significantly less than required to provide for normal rates of fetal protein accretion.

Carbohydrate

Glucose delivery to the fetus is determined by the maternal glucose concentration and occurs at rates that reflect fetal glucose utilization for energy production (8). Fetal glucose utilization also occurs at relatively low plasma insulin concentrations that only reach neonatal levels towards the end of the third trimester of gestation (9). In contrast, glucose usually is infused into the preterm newborn at higher rates than the fetus receives in utero, frequently producing hyperglycemia and plasma insulin concentrations that are significantly higher than those seen in the fetus (10).

Fat

At 50–60% of gestation there is little fetal lipid uptake (11), indicating that energy metabolism is not dependent on fat early in the third trimester. Instead, fetal fat accumulation only gradually increases towards term (12). At this early stage of development fetal lipid uptake involves primarily the essential fatty acids which are necessary for membrane development, particularly in cells of the central nervous system and in red blood cells. During the later part of the third trimester fetal lipid uptake and deposition in adipose tissue increase markedly, producing a term fetus with 12–18% body weight as fat (12). In contrast, in the very preterm newborn infant lipid is commonly provided as an energy source in amounts that exceed in utero delivery rates, contributing to adipose tissue production much earlier in development and in excess of rates that occur gradually over the third trimester of fetal development (13). Clearly, current nutritional practices in preterm infants (high energy intakes of lipid and glucose accompanied by low protein intakes) contrast with the nutrient supplies that the normally growing fetus receives (high amino acid uptake with just sufficient uptakes of glucose and lipid) (Table 12-1). The risks and benefits of these different nutritional patterns for the very preterm infant are not known. Improved understanding of specific nutrient requirements at

Table 12-1	Fetal vs. Preterm Neonatal Nutrition

Normal fetal nutrition
1. Amino acids are actively transported by the placenta into the fetus at rates greater than the fetus uses for net protein accretion
2. The excess amino acid supply is oxidized for energy
3. Glucose and lipids are taken up and used by the fetus at rates that meet energy needs

Contrasting "customary" ELBW/VLBW nutrition
1. Glucose is infused intravenously into the infant at rates higher than the infant uses for oxidative metabolism
2. The excess glucose infusion produces hyperglycemia
3. Amino acids are infused at rates less than needed for normal rates of protein accretion and growth

early gestational ages is required, therefore, to develop optimal parenteral and enteral nutritional strategies for extremely preterm neonates.

CURRENT UNDERSTANDING OF SPECIFIC NUTRIENT REQUIREMENTS OF THE VERY PRETERM INFANT

Current knowledge of the nutritional requirements of preterm infants has been extrapolated from both animal and human fetal research as well as the growing body of literature from neonatal studies (Table 12-2).

Glucose

The very preterm infant has high energy requirements produced by the relatively large body proportions of very metabolically active organs (heart, liver, kidney, and brain) at this early stage of development (14, 15). Thus the very preterm infant requires a large and continuous supply of glucose for energy metabolism.

Table 12-2	General Principles of Early Postnatal Nutrient Requirements of the Very Preterm Infant

1. Metabolic and nutritional requirements do not stop with birth, and in the preterm newborn are equal to or greater than those of the fetus
2. Intravenous feeding is always indicated when normal metabolic and nutritional needs are not met by normal enteral feeding, within hours, not days, of birth
3. **Glucose:** 5–7 mg/min/kg beginning at birth, increasing to 10–11 mg/min/kg (38–42 kcal/kg/day) for full intravenous nutrition; adjust frequently to keep plasma glucose concentration > 60 and < 120 mg/dL
4. **Lipid:** to meet additional energy (and EFA) needs; 2–3 g/kg/day = 18–27 kcal/kg/day
5. **Amino acids:** infuse at rates just higher than the infant can use, but at rates appropriate for the developmental stage of protein turnover and growth: 3–4 g/kg/day at 23–30 weeks gestational age, 2.5–3 g/kg/day at 30–36 weeks gestational age, 2–3 g/kg/day at 36–40 weeks gestational age
6. **Oxygen:** Remember that blood oxygen content (percent saturation times hemoglobin concentration) directly affects growth, regardless of the PaO_2
7. **Minimal enteral feeding (MEF)**, also called "priming", "trophic", or "non-nutritive" feedings: generally breast milk and/or formula at intakes of 5 to 25 mL/kg/day are safe to start on postnatal day 1 in stable preterm infants, even as early as 24 weeks gestation, do not increase the risk of NEC, and do promote gut growth and development in contrast to intravenous nutrition

Because glycogen content is relatively limited in the very preterm infant, unless glucose is supplied directly, glucose deficiency and hypoglycemia commonly develop in these infants.

The minimal fetal glucose requirement has been measured directly in fetal sheep and is approximately 9 mg/min/kg between mid-gestation and the start of the third trimester (16). However, at term the fetal glucose requirement falls to about half this rate. Similar rates of glucose utilization have been estimated from endogenous glucose production rates in both the stable very preterm infant with sufficient glycogen stores and in the term infant (17–20). Teleologically, this could be interpreted as the minimum glucose supply rate necessary to maintain adequate energy supply to the brain, because glucose is the principal energy substrate of the fetal brain. Glucose intake needed to support the energy costs of protein synthesis and deposition probably adds an additional glucose requirement of approximately 2–3 mg/min/kg. Thus, very preterm neonates usually require 9–10 mg/min/kg of glucose to meet all of their glucose utilization needs (21). This total supply is variably provided by endogenous glucose production and intravenous infusion. A common and usually successful starting rate for intravenous glucose infusion in the very preterm infant is ~5–7 mg/kg/min, which allows for the variable rate of endogenous glucose production to provide for additional glucose needs. Total glucose requirements and starting intravenous infusion rates usually decrease to 5–6 mg/min/kg and 3–4 mg/kg/min, respectively, by term gestation.

From a clinical standpoint, the minimal glucose intake is that which maintains an "acceptable" glucose concentration, a value that varies among clinicians and their institutions. If it is assumed that the fetal glucose concentration is the appropriate reference for preterm infants of the same gestational age, then a reasonable normoglycemic range for the preterm infant can be obtained by measuring the plasma glucose concentration in the fetus at similar gestational ages. Several studies have reported normal fetal glucose concentrations in umbilical venous blood obtained at the time of cordocentesis (22, 23). From these data it can be extrapolated that the lower limit of normal glucose concentration over the gestational age range 24–32 weeks is >3 mM (~ 54 mg/dL), which is considerably higher than current definitions of neonatal hypoglycemia. Whether or not this lower limit of glucose concentration should be maintained in preterm infants has not been tested, but needs to be, as a recent retrospective study indicated that neurodevelopment was progressively impaired in preterm infants with an increasing number of days in which they had recurrent low glucose concentrations (<2.6 mmol/L [47 mg/dL]) (24).

The upper limit of the normal glucose concentration has not been defined in preterm infants, although many references use the value of 120 mg/dL (6.7 mmol/L) (25). Common clinical practice is to tolerate glucose concentrations of up to 150–200 mg/dL, but the safety and consequences of this practice are unknown. In the first few days of life in extremely preterm neonates, hyperglycemia probably results from endogenous glucose production in response to stress-reactive hormones, especially the catecholamines epinephrine and norepinephrine, as well as glucagon (26). Catecholamines inhibit insulin secretion and diminish insulin's action to promote glucose utilization in peripheral tissues. Along with glucagon and cortisol, they also increase rates of glycogen breakdown and the release of amino acids into the circulation that then are available for increased rates of gluconeogenesis. Beyond the first week of life and with improvement in physiological condition, hyperglycemia in preterm infants more likely is due primarily to excessive glucose infusions rates. Less commonly, it also could be a harbinger of infection or other disease processes associated with a systemic inflammatory response (10).

The upper limit for the rate of intravenous glucose administration is that above which glucose exceeds the energy needs of the body and the metabolic capacity for glucose oxidation. Under these conditions the excess glucose infused and taken up by cells is converted to fat. Glucose conversion to fat is an energy-inefficient process that results in increased energy expenditure, increased oxygen consumption, and increased carbon dioxide production. The latter has the potential to produce CO_2 retention that may exacerbate existing lung disease, particularly in infants with chronic lung disease of prematurity or bronchopulmonary dysplasia (27). The rate of glucose administration that exceeds the maximal glucose oxidative capacity is not completely known in neonates, but probably is above 11–13 mg/kg/min ($\sim$18 g/kg/day). This value may be lower if lipid also is given (19, 28).

Fat

The most remarkable aspect of lipid development during late fetal life in humans is the deposition of large amounts of body fat, up to12–18% of body weight (12). The biological value of this adiposity is not clear, nor are the mechanisms that produce it. Whether this developmental growth pattern of high fat deposition over the last third of pregnancy should be recapitulated in preterm infants of the same gestational age is not known. Because such infants are currently fed diets high in carbohydrate and lipids, they usually meet or exceed normal rates of intrauterine fat deposition in adipose tissue.

Although fatty acids are not readily oxidized in the fetus, fat oxidation does develop after birth, even in very preterm infants (29). Failure to provide sufficient non-protein energy will lead to increased rates of lipolysis and oxidation of endogenously released fatty acids. This problem applies particularly to potentially excessive oxidation of essential fatty acids, as these very preterm infants have very little adipose tissue and thus a ready supply of non-essential fatty acids. This could lead to deleterious alterations in the amount and structure of critical membranes of cells of the developing central nervous system and potentially to abnormal neurological outcome. The roles of, requirements for, and appropriate balance of the $\omega-3$ and the $\omega-6$ essential polyunsaturated fatty acids series remain to be determined, although there is increasing evidence that increased supply of $\omega-3$ end products, particular docosahexaenoic acid, has beneficial effects on selected aspects of development (30, 31).

In terms of minimal lipid intake in the ELBW infant in the early neonatal period, intravenous lipid is primarily administered to prevent essential fatty acid (EFA) deficiency and, if tolerated, to serve as an energy substrate. Unfortunately, metabolism of lipids infused intravenously may be impeded in this population by both an immaturity of mechanisms of triglyceride and fatty acid metabolism and by clinical conditions, such as infection, surgical stress, and malnutrition, that, via excessive catecholamine secretion and reduced insulin secretion and concentration, inhibit lipid clearance from the circulation (32). Thus, despite recognized needs for lipids for both membrane structural development and energy expenditure, hyperlipemia is a common complication of lipid emulsion infusions as part of intravenous nutrition in the more stressed and unstable of these infants, much as hyperglycemia is a common complication of dextrose infusion for intravenous nutrition despite high glucose needs. Excessive fatty acid supply also contributes to hyperglycemia, by at least two major metabolic processes. Fatty acids act competitively with glucose by providing carbon that substitutes for glucose carbon oxidation (29), and the oxidation of fatty acids in the liver produces co-factors that promote gluconeogenesis. Fatty acids also inhibit insulin action in the liver, thereby releasing the normal suppression of hepatic glucose production provided by insulin (33).

In terms of the upper limit of fat intake early in the neonatal course, clinical practices vary widely because of unresolved controversies surrounding adverse effects of intravenous lipid administration, for example the possible contributions to pulmonary disease and impaired bilirubin metabolism that have been noted in various studies using a large variety of intravenous lipid infusion rates (34, 35). Later in the neonatal course, fat is the primary energy source of the neonate, and current enteral and parental recommendations are that it should account for 40–50% of total energy intake.

Amino Acids and Protein

Maximal weight-specific protein gain throughout life occurs prior to 32 weeks gestation. Thus, amino acid requirements are high in the fetus and very preterm infant in order to provide for the exceptionally high fractional protein synthetic and growth rates at this early developmental age (36). Infants who receive only supplemental glucose lose 1% of protein stores each day, and this may be even greater in very preterm newborns (37, 38). If the target nutritional intake in the very preterm newborn is to achieve fetal protein accretion rates, then early amino acid administration is critical to avoiding protein malnutrition. The quantity of postnatal amino acid administration that is required to produce fetal rates of protein accretion has not been determined, but appears to be at least 3 g/kg/day.

Protein accretion also is affected by energy intake. Energy is required for both protein metabolism and deposition. Not only are relative protein accretion rates higher in the ELBW infant, but so also are relative protein synthetic and breakdown rates, both of which are energy-dependent processes. Synthesis-to-gain ratios in ELBW infants may be as high as 5:1. It has clearly been shown in preterm infants that at the same protein intake, increasing energy intake increases protein accretion rate up to a maximal energy intake of 100–120 kcal/kg/day. This relationship, however, is curvilinear, with most of the effect of energy on protein gain taking place at less than 50–60 kcal/kg/day (39). Such observations support the need for much higher protein intakes than these infants normally receive and indicate that protein gain will be greatest with protein, not energy, intake. In the first days of life in the ELBW infant when energy intolerance may be an issue, the minimum energy required to metabolize protein is not known.

Many unique amino acid entry rates and plasma concentrations are present in the normal fetus and probably contribute to important aspects of fetal metabolic development (7). As with the essential fatty acids, while many of the individual amino acids have been shown to have specific roles in various aspects of fetal metabolism and growth, there has been insufficient study of which of these are truly essential for normal development and which are of primary importance for stimulation of protein accretion and growth of lean body mass. Furthermore, to date, no amino acid mix or dietary protein source has been studied specifically to determine whether or not such unique plasma amino acid concentrations should be mimicked in the preterm infant.

Energy

In order to prevent breakdown of endogenous energy stores, enough energy must be given to at least provide for energy expenditure. From data collected in ventilated ELBW infants in the first days of life, resting metabolic rate is approximately 40 kcal/kg/day (40). Approximately 20% of basal metabolic rate is accounted for by protein metabolism, or about 4–5 kcal per g protein. The energy cost of protein accretion is the sum of the energy stored (4 kcal/g) plus the metabolic cost of protein gain, which is estimated to be approximately 10 kcal/g protein. Therefore, energy intake to meet energy requirements for protein accretion should be at least 10 kcal/g protein gained. Studies indicate that protein growth in most ELBW infants probably occurs when amino acid intake rates are at or above 1.0–1.5 g/kg/day (41–43). Therefore, minimal total energy intake should equal resting metabolic rate plus 10 kcal/kg of infant weight for each g/kg of protein intake above 1 g/kg. For a relatively stable, ventilated ELBW infant in the first days of life, this would give a minimal energy requirement of approximately 50 kcal/kg/day of energy intake at an amino acid intake of 2 g/kg/day, and 60 kcal/kg/day at an amino acid intake of 3 g/kg/day. This theoretical calculation supports the clinical observation that most infants will be in a positive protein balance at 2 g/kg/day of protein intake when given at least 50–60 kcal/kg/day of energy. These estimates are at or above the usual protein intake and less than the usual energy intake that these infants receive, perhaps thereby contributing to their slower rates of growth of lean body mass while they deposit fat in adipose tissue at normal to increased rates.

In the absence of protein intake, glucose is probably a more effective energy substrate in preventing protein breakdown than is fat (28). When amino acids are given, both glucose and lipid are known to be protein-sparing, but the optimal glucose/lipid intake ratio in the ELBW infant is still unclear. Studies in older children and adults have shown the positive effect of both glucose and lipid on nitrogen retention. Though it has been known for over 15 years that the amount and type of energy can affect protein balance in the parenterally fed neonate, based on the few studies done in the neonate receiving exclusive intravenous nutrition, the impact of the composition and amount of the energy source on protein metabolism remains controversial. Optimal glucose/lipid intake ratios that maximize protein accretion have not been determined in the neonatal population. However, it is worth considering that the fetus at comparable gestational age to the ELBW infant uses primarily glucose and not lipid as a non-protein energy source. Furthermore, as discussed above, the fetus also takes up at least twice the amino acid load that it requires for net protein accretion. The balance is oxidized, providing energy. The optimal energy intake, therefore, is most likely one consisting primarily of glucose and amino acids. Such a regimen also would spare essential fatty acids from oxidation, allowing their incorporation into essential developing membranes, especially those in the central nervous system.

Oxygen

Although oxygen usually is not thought of as a nutrient, insufficient oxygen does lead to growth failure by decreasing protein synthesis more than breakdown, producing a deficit in net protein balance and growth. Preterm infants recovering from bronchopulmonary dysplasia also do not grow well when chronically deficient in oxygen (44). Many other studies in both fetuses and neonates define reduced growth rate at low blood oxygen contents from either reduced oxygen supply or anemia (45). The latter point is important, because several recent studies suggest that various forms of oxygen toxicity in preterm infants might be prevented by reducing blood oxygen partial pressure and saturation values to lower ranges than are customarily used, e.g., SaO_2 to 80–90% and PaO_2 to 45–65 torr (46). There is no current consensus about whether such lower oxygen levels, or even normal fluctuations in oxygen levels in the conventional SaO_2 range of 90–99%, will affect metabolism sufficiently to also regulate the synthesis of amino acids into protein and thus the rate of growth.

SCIENTIFICALLY BASED APPROACHES FOR PROVIDING PARENTERAL AND ENTERAL NOURISHMENT TO LOW BIRTH WEIGHT INFANTS

Optimizing nutritional support is critical to avoiding adverse growth and neurological outcomes. Unfortunately, well-controlled prospective studies that validate nutritional regimens for very preterm neonates are rare. It has become clear that the postnatal growth failure seen in very preterm infants must be countered with a combination of early parenteral and enteral nutrition in higher amounts than have been previously used (Table 12-2). This has been called "early aggressive nutrition." Using this approach, intravenous nutrition is initiated in the first hours after birth and then is given in conjunction with initially small, slowly advancing, enteral feedings beginning on the first day of life. The role of intravenous nutrition is to achieve rapid, maximal nutrition and that of early enteral feedings to prime the gut and stimulate normal hormonal homeostasis.

Over the past several years there has been a growing national and international trend towards more aggressive nutritional management of preterm infants that is designed, presumptively, to achieve in utero growth rates, either primarily or by catch up. The principal current controversy in neonatal nutrition is the lack of definable and accurately measurable "ideal" outcomes of controlled variations in nutrition intervention. Research is essential to determine accurate measures of efficacy and safety in response to more aggressive supply of nutrients administered to very preterm infants starting at birth. As a first hypothesis, replicating body composition of the fetus of the same gestational age as the preterm infant could be considered a more desirable nutritional goal than simply achieving the fetal rate of weight gain. Based on the significant variation in clinical practice, attaining a targeted rate of weight gain in very preterm infants is likely to be accomplished by very different nutritional strategies and without consideration of "quality" of weight gain. Both human and animal investigations indicate that under-nutrition, particularly insufficient protein intake, during critical development periods may adversely affect long-term linear growth (contributing to a shorter final height), neurodevelopmental outcomes, and general health (47–49). In contrast, over-feeding and/or positive crossing of growth percentiles may be associated with adverse later life health outcomes such as obesity and type 2 diabetes. These contrasting responses to the amount (over- versus under-nutrition) and the timing of specific approaches to neonatal nutrition raise a number of as yet unanswered questions regarding postnatal nutrition of the very preterm infant.

Parenteral Nutrition

A number of studies in preterm infants have demonstrated that infusion of amino acids with glucose as early as the first day of life decreases protein catabolism. In general, 1.5–2.0 g/kg/day of protein intake is sufficient to avoid catabolism in neonates (41, 42). In terms of the upper limits of protein intake, if the goal is to achieve intrauterine rates of protein deposition, then requirements of 3.8–4.0 g/kg/day of protein intake just to provide sufficient amino acids for protein accretion have been estimated for ELBW. In the first randomized trial of early "low" versus "high" parenteral amino acid intake, it was demonstrated that increased parenteral amino acid intakes for approximately 24 h produced short-term increases in protein growth in preterm infants (43). This prospective, randomized study included 28 infants (mean weight 946 ± 40 g) who received either 1 g/kg/day (low amino acid intake) or 3 g/kg/day (high amino acid intake) in the first days of life. Efficacy was determined by protein balance, and was significantly lower in the 1 g/kg/day group compared to the 3 g/kg/day amino acid intake group by both nitrogen balance and leucine stable isotope methods. In terms of potential toxicity with the higher amino acid intake, there were no significant differences between groups in the amount of sodium bicarbonate administered, the degree of metabolic acidosis, or the blood urea nitrogen (BUN) concentration. When compared with plasma amino acid concentrations of normally growing second- and third-trimester human fetuses who were sampled by cordocentesis the normal fetal amino acid concentrations for both essential and non-essential amino acids were equal to those in the 3 g/kg/day group (except for threonine and lysine, which were significantly lower than seen in the fetus), but were at least twice the concentrations in the 1 g/kg/day group.

Since the publication of the results from this study, initiation of 3 g/kg/day of parenteral amino acid intake in the first 1–2 days of life has become routine in many neonatal intensive care units. Nevertheless, a number of clinicians are hesitant to prescribe this rate of amino acid infusion because of concerns about potential amino acid toxicity. Currently there are no definitive clinical markers of toxicity from protein intake. In general, many clinicians follow BUN levels. However, a recent study in preterm infants showed no correlation between amino acid intake and BUN concentration (50). Although gradually increasing amino acid intake over the first several days of parenteral nutrition is often advocated, there is no evidence that this specifically promotes tolerance of amino acids. Clearly, further studies are needed to determine whether even higher amino acid intakes are safe and efficacious when administered to very preterm neonates.

There has been no study to determine whether or not the unique plasma amino acid concentrations of the fetus should be mimicked in the preterm infant. Currently used intravenous amino acid mixtures designed for normal infants have been shown to promote nitrogen and protein balance more favorably than mixtures more commonly used in adults (51), but they still do not provide normal fetal concentrations of all of the essential amino acids, particularly for threonine and lysine, both essential amino acids and thus perhaps limiting in their control over protein synthesis, unless the entire mixture is infused at rates sufficient to provide these two amino acids at rates necessary to control growth (43). Further, both cysteine and tyrosine are considered indispensable amino acids for the infant and are not part of usual intravenous amino acid mixtures (52), as both tyrosine and cysteine are insoluble and cysteine is unstable in aqueous solution. Consequently, plasma cysteine and tyrosine concentrations of infants receiving cysteine- and tyrosine-free amino acid mixtures are quite low. Greater intakes of the precursors of these two amino acids, methionine and phenylalanine, do not result in greater plasma concentrations of cysteine and tyrosine although they do result in higher plasma concentrations of the precursors (53). Cysteine hydrochloride is soluble and is reasonably stable in aqueous solution for up to 48 h; thus, it is possible to supplement parenteral nutrition infusates with cysteine hydrochloride. However, trials of cysteine supplementation have not shown a clinically significant beneficial effect of parenteral cysteine intake on nitrogen retention (54). Some of the newer parenteral amino acid mixtures contain soluble N-acetyl-L-tyrosine, but its contribution to producing plasma tyrosine in sufficient concentrations for enhancing tyrosine metabolism is questionable as it is rapidly excreted into the urine. Thus there is considerable need to define the requirements and route of delivery for both tyrosine and cysteine in infants requiring parenteral nutrition. Glutamine is considered by many to be a conditionally essential amino acid in the preterm infant (55). It is the most abundant amino acid in plasma and human milk. It is an effective energy source for cells with rapid turnover such as enterocytes and is an important precursor of nucleic acids, nucleotides, and protein. However, like cysteine, it is unstable in aqueous solution and, therefore, is not a component of any parenteral amino acid mixture. Several animal and adult human studies have demonstrated benefits to providing glutamine in parenteral amino acid feeding regimens, including attenuation of gut atrophy associated with fasting, prevention of infection, and possibly decreased mortality. As a result, several parenteral and enteral studies regarding glutamine safety and efficacy have been conducted in preterm infants. A recent review of such studies in very low birth weight infants concluded that glutamine supplementation had no significant effect on decreasing the incidence of sepsis or necrotizing enterocolitis (NEC), risk of death, or long-term development (56). These examples demonstrate that there is considerable room for development of more optimal formulations specifically designed for the unique needs of the very preterm infant.

Glucose administration is often limited in the first days of life by the development of hyperglycemia, with a reported incidence of 20–85% of ELBW infants (10). This hyperglycemia is often attributed to both peripheral and hepatic insulin resistance, the former resulting in decreased peripheral glucose utilization and the latter in ineffective insulin inhibition of hepatic glucose production. In addition to limiting glucose delivery, hyperglycemia may induce an osmotic diuresis, putting the infant at risk of dehydration. The ideal strategy to deal with this early hyperglycemia in very ELBW infants has not been defined, but includes practices such as (i) lowering glucose intake until hyperglycemia resolves or until fluid requirements would result in hypotonic fluid administration, (ii) accepting at least a modest degree of hyperglycemia (<150–200 mg/dL, for example), and (iii) initiating exogenous insulin therapy at rates either to control hyperglycemia alone or to both control hyperglycemia and allow for increased substrate delivery and utilization. The first two strategies prevent adequate early nutrition, and the latter utilizes a therapy whose safety has been questioned because of the development of lactic acidosis in very preterm infants receiving glucose plus insulin (57). Insulin used in the neonate as a nutritional adjuvant has been shown to successfully lower glucose levels and to increase weight gain without undue risk of hypoglycemia (58). However, little is known about the effects of intravenous insulin infusions and relative hyperinsulinemia on the quality of weight gain and increased counter-regulatory hormone concentrations.

Administration of intravenous amino acids has been shown to decrease glucose concentrations in ELBW infants, presumably by enhancing endogenous insulin secretion. In the above study by Thureen et al. (43), an approximate doubling of insulin concentration occurred in the high versus low amino acid intake study group. The lower incidence of neonatal hyperglycemia following the earlier postnatal introduction of parenteral amino acids may be due to increased insulin secretion (39). It is possible, therefore, that a more aggressive approach to early and relatively higher intravenous infusions of amino acids to very preterm ELBW infants might promote endogenous pancreatic insulin secretion that would minimize the incidence and severity of hyperglycemia and reduce or even prevent the need for intravenous insulin infusion.

Minimal intravenous lipid intakes should be targeted to prevent essential fatty acid deficiency (EFA, i.e. deficiency of linoleic and linolenic acids and their end products), particularly in view of its critical role in postnatal brain development (30, 31). EFA deficiency develops by 4–5 days after birth if exogenous fat is not given and can be prevented with as little as 0.5 g/kg/day lipid (estimates range from 0.25 to 1.0 g/kg/day). Because most intravenous lipid emulsions are richer in ω−6 rather than ω−3 essential fatty acids, there is the potential for higher rates of intravenous lipid infusion to lead to greater amounts of vasoactive, prostaglandin-derived products and lesser amounts of critical central nervous system membrane producing products (59) This issue clearly needs further study.

Other benefits of intravenous lipid include its role as a high-density energy source (which can be provided by the peripheral venous route due to its isotonicity with plasma) and as a vehicle for facilitating delivery of fat-soluble vitamins. Intravenous lipids also contribute to early development of gluconeogenesis by promoting the development of enzymes and co-factors in the liver from fatty acid oxidation that increase gluconeogensis (60). Optimal intravenous lipid intake above that which prevents EFA is controversial and has resulted in different lipid administration strategies among neonatal intensive care centers. Early use and/or rapid advancement of lipid emulsions in the preterm infant has been cautious, however, because of concern for potential development of several possible complications, including lipid intolerance, hyperglycemia, potential interference with immune function, impaired bilirubin metabolism, and adverse effects on pulmonary function. There has been no recent evidence, though, that these concerns have been seen with the modest infusion rates of 0.5–1.0 g/kg/day that are commonly used today. A recent review comparing "early" (<5 days of age) versus "late" (>5 day of age) initiation of parenterally administered lipids included five studies in 397 neonates and demonstrated no significant statistical differences between groups in the primary outcomes of growth rates, death, and chronic lung disease or the secondary outcomes, which included several pulmonary disorders (61). The authors concluded that early parenteral lipid administration could not be recommended for benefits of short-term growth or prevention of morbidity and mortality. However, there appears to be no clear contraindication to starting intravenous lipid infusions within the first day of life in most preterm infants, and there is a benefit in terms of ameliorating or preventing EFA deficiency. Clearly there is a critical need for more definitive information regarding the conditions under which intravenous fat administration should be limited.

There also has been recent interest in use of medium-chain triacylglycerides (MCT) instead of, or in combination with, currently used long-chain triacylglyceides (LCT) in preterm neonates. The theoretical advantages of MCT compared to LCT intravenous lipid preparation include: (i) possible enhanced clearance from plasma, (ii) ability to enter hepatic mitochondria without the requirement for carnitine-mediated transport, and (iii) improved immune function. Despite such theoretical advantages, recent studies indicate that LCTs actually are more effective in promoting protein accretion in preterm newborns (62). Thus, there is little reason to use MCT emulsions other than, perhaps, as a supplement to usual intravenous lipid preparations.

Enteral Nutrition

An "early aggressive" approach to nutrition requires early introduction of enteral nutrition in order to (i) provide trophic benefits of nutrient stimulation to the gut, (ii) provide a more comprehensive package of nutrient administration, and (iii) avoid prolonged parenteral nutrition. The most common reason for delayed initiation and limited advancement of enteral feedings in preterm infants is the concern for increasing the risk of necrotizing enterocolitis (NEC). Clearly, there often is reason to cautiously initiate enteral feeding in very preterm infants soon after birth, because of the known immaturity of a number of physiological and hormonal systems at early gestational ages. Early enteral feeding, however, prevents gut atrophy, stimulates maturation of the gastrointestinal (GI) system, may actually enhance eventual feeding tolerance, and may reduce the incidence of NEC, especially when colostrum and human milk are used.

Despite such concerns that early enteral feeding increases the risk of NEC in the preterm infant, there is a paucity of definitive studies to guide early enteral feeding in very preterm neonates. Several small physiological studies give clues to best feeding practices, but don't provide comprehensive strategies for enteral feedings. Meta analyses of enteral feeding practices are often not conclusive because there are an enormous number of variables in existing studies that make comparisons among studies difficult, and generalizations about safety and efficacy problematic. There are a number of enteral feeding trials with a decreased incidence of NEC as the primary outcome, but most of these are underpowered and not definitive.

By 24 weeks of gestation the GI tract is anatomically well developed and most digestive enzymes are present. Sufficient gastric acid secretion is available for intragastric digestion and, although lactase activity is relatively low, it is present in sufficient amounts and activity for moderate lactose digestion except in the most premature infants. The most significant deterrent to successful enteral feeding in the very preterm infant, however, is their limited GI motility (63). Both gastric emptying and intestinal transit times are significantly delayed compared to the term infant and organized gut motility does not begin until 32–34 weeks gestation.

Minimal Enteral Feeding (MEF)

There is no uniform definition for MEF, but it generally refers to small amounts of enteral feedings of breast milk and/or formula at intakes of 5–25 mL/kg/day. Such minimal enteral feedings are also referred to as "priming" feedings because of their role in stimulating many aspects of gut function, "trophic" feedings for their positive impact on gut growth, and "non-nutritive" feedings to indicate that they are not intended to be a primary source of nutrition. Studies in newborn animals indicate that even brief periods of early enteral feeding can significantly increase intestinal mucosal mass compared to animals that are not fed (64). Direct contact of the gut tissue with breast milk has been shown to increase intestinal mass and enhance DNA synthetic rates (65). A series of studies in term and preterm neonates demonstrated that, in response to enteral feeding, there was a significant postnatal increase in secretion and plasma and gut intraluminal concentrations of several gastrointestinal hormones that have various roles in stimulating gut mucosal growth, development, and motility, and influence pancreatic and hepatic metabolism. Even minimal enteral feeding has produced a surge of these enteric hormones that mimics the response seen in healthy term nursing infants, and as little as 12 ml/kg over 6 days significantly increases their concentrations (66).

MEF was first initiated to avoid the deleterious effects induced by absence of enteral nutrient stimulation on gut structure and function without stressing the immature gut. Though not all studies have evaluated the same outcomes, beneficial effects have included shorter time to full enteral feeds, faster weight gain, less feeding intolerance, less need for phototherapy, enhanced serum gastrin concentrations, enhanced maturation of the small intestine function, and shorter hospitalization.

Compared to formula, breast milk appears to confer significant advantage for protection against infection, the development of allergies, and the incidence of NEC in preterm infants. In most centers it is the preferred first feeding for preterm infants. Unfortified breast milk and dilute formula, however, do not provide sufficient protein to sustain in utero rates of growth when they are the sole sources of nutrition and they do not induce normal motor activity as well as more concentrated products. No definite conclusions can be drawn about the relative tolerance of fortified versus regular-strength formula or breast milk, although fortification of breast milk does not appear to delay gastric emptying.

In a series of systematic reviews in the Cochrane Database (18, 67–69) it was concluded that (i) MEF decreased days to full enteral feeding and length of hospitalization, (ii) there is too little information to recommend early versus delayed MEF, and (iii) rapid versus slow rate of feeding advancement results in more rapid weight gain, but there are insufficient data to determine the effect of rate of advancement on the incidence of NEC. Even more recently, a review of trophic feedings concluded the following: (i) for high-risk infants, those receiving trophic feedings had an overall decrease in the number of days to full feeding, total number of days feedings were held, and total length of hospital stay compared to those with no enteral intake; (ii) based on a single trial, when compared to advancing enteral feedings, trophic feedings required more days to reach full enteral feeding and longer hospital stay, but a marginally significant reduction in NEC; and (iii) whether no feedings, trophic feedings, or advancing feedings should be used initially cannot be determined due to limitations of the studies involved.

There have been few studies to define specific clinical situations that contraindicate MEF, other than the general concern for the risk of necrotizing enterocolitis with any enteral feeding. However, understanding normal transitional physiology and clinical conditions associated with gut development indicate several situations in which MEF might be withheld, or at least not advanced. Any condition that is known to decrease gut blood flow may be a contraindication to enteral feeding. Neonatal animal studies suggest that hypotension and asphyxia may predispose to gut injury when enteral feedings are given (70, 71). Physiological studies of enteral nutrition have not been conducted in human preterm neonates in these circumstances, but it is reasonable to assume that in some infants these conditions have compromised GI tract function and integrity. Because there often is no diagnostic means by which to identify these infants, feedings frequently are withheld for several to many days in sick or very preterm neonates.

Summary and Future Challenges

Current nutritional regimens in the vulnerable population of very preterm ELBW neonates produce postnatal growth failure. In order to develop data-based feeding strategies to achieve normal in utero growth rates postnatally, much more information needs to be obtained. Important areas for research include, but are not limited to, safe upper limits of amino acid intake, improved markers for protein toxicity, side-effects and mechanisms of action of insulin when used as a nutritional adjuvant, characterization of the neonatal stress response and its effect on nutritional metabolism, effects of commonly used neonatal medications on specific nutrient metabolism, and incidence of NEC in various enteral feeding strategies. Once these issues have been addressed, then nutritionally related long-term growth and developmental outcomes can be prospectively studied.

Acknowledgements

Supported by: Grant MO1 RR00069 from the General Clinical Research Centers Program, NCRR, NIH (WWH Associate Director); NIH Grants K24 RR018358 (PJT, PI), R01 HD046752 (PJT, PI); and NIH Grants HD42815 (WWH, PI), DK52138 (WWH, PI), HD28794 (WWH, PI), HD07186 (WWH, PI).

REFERENCES

1. Carlson SJ, Ziegler EE. Nutrient intakes and growth of very low-birth weight infants. J Perinatol 1998; 18:252–258.
2. Cooke RJ, Ainsworth SB, Fenton AC. Postnatal growth retardation: a universal problem in preterm infants. Arch Dis Child Fetal Neonatal Ed. 2004; 89:F428–F430.
3. Ehrenkranz R, Younes N, Lemons J, et al. Longitudinal growth of hospitalized very low birthweight infants. Pediatrics 1999; 104:280–289.
4. Embleton NE, Pang N, Cooke PJ. Postnatal malnutrition and growth retardation: an inevitable consequence of current recommendations in preterm infants? Pediatrics 2001; 107:270–27.

5. American Academy of Pediatrics Committee on Nutrition. Nutritional needs of low-birth-weight infants. Pediatrics 1985; 76:976–986.

6. Lemons JA, Adcock EW 3rd, Jones MD Jr, et al. Umbilical uptake of amino acids in the unstressed fetal lamb. J Clin Invest 1976; 58:1428–34.

7. Regnault TRH, Brown LD, Hay WW Jr. Fetal requirements and placental transfer of nitrogenous compounds. In: Polin RA, Fox WW, Abman SH, eds. Fetal and neonatal physiology, 4th edn. Philadelphia: Elsevier (WB Saunders Co); 2007: in press.

8. Hay WW Jr, Meznarich HK. Effect of maternal glucose concentration on uteroplacental glucose consumption and transfer in pregnant sheep. Proc Soc Exp Biol Med 1988; 190:63–69.

9. Aldoretta PW, Gresores A, Carver TD, Hay WW Jr. Maturation of glucose-stimulated insulin secretion. Biol Neonate 1998; 73:375–386.

10. Cowett RM, Farrag HM. Selected principles of perinatal-neonatal glucose metabolism. Semin Neonatol 2004; 9:37–47.

11. Hay WW Jr. Metabolic interrelationships of placenta and fetus. Placenta 1995; 16:19–30.

12. Sparks JW, Girard JR, Battaglia FC. An estimate of the caloric requirements of the human fetus. Biol Neonate 1980; 38:113–119.

13. Sabita U, Thomas EL, Hamilton G, et al. Altered adiposity after extremely preterm birth. Pediatr Res 2005; 57:211–215.

14. Battaglia FC, Meschia G. An Introduction to fetal physiology. Orlando: Academic Press; 1986: 100–135.

15. Battaglia FC, Meschia G. Fetal nutrition. Annu Rev Nutr 1988; 8:43–61.

16. Molina RD, Meschia G, Battaglia FC, Hay WW Jr. Gestational maturation of placental glucose transfer capacity in sheep. Am J Physiol 1991; 261:R697–R704.

17. Kalhan SC, Oliven A, King KC, Lucero C. Role of glucose in the regulation of endogenous glucose production in the human newborn. Pediatr Res 1986; 20:49–52.

18. Kennedy KA, Tyson JE, Chamnanvanikij S. Early versus delayed initiation of progressive enteral feedings for parenterally fed low birth weight or preterm infants. Cochrane Database Syst Rev 2000; (2):CD001970.

19. Denne SC, Karn CA, Wang J, Liechty EA. Effect of intravenous glucose and lipid on proteolysis and glucose production in normal newborns. Am J Physiol. 1995; 269:E361–E367.

20. Sunehag AL, Haymond MW, Schanler RJ, et al. Gluconeogenesis in very low birth weight infants receiving total parenteral nutrition. Diabetes 1999; 48:791–800.

21. Hay WW Jr. Nutrition and development of the fetus: carbohydrate and lipid metabolism. In: Walker WA, Watkins JB, Duggan CP, eds. Nutrition in pediatrics (basic science and clinical applications), 4th edn. Hamilton, Ontario, Canada: BC Decker; 2007: in press.

22. Bozzetti P, Ferrari MM, Marconi AM, et al. The relationship of maternal and fetal glucose concentrations in the human from midgestation until term. Metabolism 1988; 37:358–363.

23. Marconi AM, Paolini C, Mauro B, et al. The impact of gestational age and fetal growth on the maternal-fetal glucose concentration difference. Obstet Gynecol 1996; 87:937–942.

24. Lucas A, Morley R, Cole TJ. Adverse neurodevelopmental outcome of moderate neonatal hypoglycemia. BMJ 1988; 297:1304–1308.

25. Dweck JS, Cassady G. Glucose intolerance in infants of very low birth weight. I. Incidence of hyperglycemia in infants of birth weight 1,100 grams or less. Pediatrics 1974; 53:189–195.

26. Louik C, Mitchell AA, Epstein MF, et al. Risk factors for neonatal hyperglycemia associated with 10% dextrose infusion. Am J Dis Child 1985; 139:783–786.

27. Forsyth JS, Murdock N, Crighton A. Low birthweight infants and total parenteral nutrition immediately after birth. III. Randomised study of energy substrate utilisation, nitrogen balance, and carbon dioxide production. Arch Dis Child 1995; 73:F13–F16.

28. Bresson JL, Narcy P, Putet G, et al. Energy substrate utilization in infants receiving total parenteral nutrition with different glucose to fat ratios. Pediatr Res 1989; 25:645–648.

29. Chessex P, Gagne G, Pineault M, et al. Metabolic and clinical consequences of changing from high-glucose to high-fat regimens in parenterally fed newborn infants. J Pediatr 1989; 115:992–997.

30. Carlson SE. Docosahexaenoic acid and arachidonic acid in infant development. Semin Neonatol 2001; 6:437–444.

31. Carlson SE, Werkman SH, Rhodes PG, Tolley EA. Visual acuity development in healthy preterm infants: effect of marine oil supplementation. Am J Clin Nutr 1993; 58:35–42.

32. Pierro A, Carnielli V, Filler RM, et al. Metabolism of intravenous fat emulsion in the surgical newborn. J Pediatr Surg 1989; 24:95–102.

33. Gilbert M, Pere MC, Baudelin A, Battaglia FC. Role of free fatty acids in hepatic insulin resistance during late pregnancy in conscious rabbits. Am J Physiol 1991; 260:E938–E945.

34. Sosenko IR, Rodriguez-Pierce M, Bancalari E. Effect of early initiation of intravenous lipid administration on the incidence and severity of chronic lung disease in premature infants. J Pediatr 1993; 123:975–982.

35. Prasertsom W, Phillipos EZ, Van Aerde JE, et al. Pulmonary vascular resistance during lipid infusion in neonates. Arch Dis Child 1996; 74:F95–F98.

36. Meier PR, Peterson RG, Bonds DR, et al. Rates of protein synthesis and turnover in fetal life. Am J Physiol 1981; 240:E320–E324.

37. Denne SC. Regulation of proteolysis and optimal protein accretion in extremely premature newborns. Am J Clin Nutr 2007; 85:621S–62.

38. Rigo J, Senterre J. Nutritional needs of premature infants: current issues. J Pediatr 2006; 149:S80–S88.

39. Micheli JL, Schutz Y. Protein. In: Tsang RC, Lucas A, Uauy R, Zlotkin S, eds. Nutritional needs of the preterm infant, scientific basis and practical guidelines. Pawling: Caduceus Medical 1993; 29–46.

40. Thureen PJ, Phillips RE, DeMarie MP, et al. Technical and methodological considerations for performance of indirect calorimetry in sick and recovering preterm infants. Crit Care Med 1997; 25(1):171–179.

41. Rivera A Jr, Bell EF, Bier DM. Effect of intravenous amino acids on protein metabolism of preterm infants during the first three days of life. Pediatr Res 1993; 33:106–111.

42. Thureen PJ, Anderson AH, Baron KA, et al. Protein balance in the first week of life in ventilated neonates receiving parenteral nutrition. Am J Clin Nutr 1998; 68:1136–1228.

43. Thureen PJ, Melara D, Fennessey PV, Hay WW Jr. Effect of low versus high intravenous amino acid intake on very low birth weight infants in the early neonatal period. Pediatr Res 2003; 53:24–32.

44. Groothuis JR, Rosenberg AA. Home oxygen promotes weight gain in infants with bronchopulmonary dysplasia. Am J Dis Child 1987; 141:992–995.

45. Stockman JA II, Clark DA. Weight gain: a response to transfusion in the premature infant. AJDC 1984; 138:831–833.

46. Tin W. Oxygen therapy: 50 years of uncertainty. Pediatrics 2002; 110:615–616.

47. Hack M, Schlechter M, Cartar L, et al. Growth of very low birth weight infants to age 20 years. Pediatrics 2003; 112:e30–38.

48. Lucas A, Morley R, Cole TJ. Randomised trial of early diet in preterm babies and later intelligence quotient. BMJ 1998; 317:1481–1487.

49. Singhal A, Fewtrell M, Cole TJ, Lucas A. Low nutrient intake and early growth for later insulin resistance in adolescents born preterm. Lancet 2003; 361(9363):1089–1097.

50. Ridout E, Diane Melara D, Rottinghaus S, Thureen PJ. Blood urea nitrogen concentration as a marker of amino acid intolerance in neonates with birthweight less than 1250 grams. J Perinat 2005; 25:130–133.

51. Heird WC, Hay WW Jr, Helms RA, et al. Pediatric parenteral amino acid mixture in low birth weight infants. Pediatrics 1988; 81:41–50.

52. Roberts SA, Ball RO, Filler RM, Moore AM, Pencharz PB. Phenylalanine and tyrosine metabolism in neonates receiving parenteral nutrition differing in pattern of amino acids. Pediatr Res 1998; 44:907–914.

53. Wykes LJ, House JD, Ball RO, Pencharz PB. Aromatic amino acid metabolism of neonatal piglets receiving TPN: effect of tyrosine precursors. Am J Physiol 1994; 267:E672–E679.

54. Zlotkin SH, Bryan MH, Anderson GH. Cysteine supplementation to cysteine-free intravenous feeding regimens in newborn infants. Am J Clin Nutr 1981; 34:914–923.

55. Parimi PS, Kalhan SC. Glutamine supplementation in the newborn infant. Semin Fetal Neonatal Med 2007; 12:19–25.

56. Tubman TRJ, Thompson SW, McGuire W. Glutamine supplementation to prevent morbidity and mortality in preterm infants. Cochrane Database Syst Rev 2005; (1):CD001457..

57. Poindexter BB, Karn CA, Denne SC. Exogenous insulin reduces proteolysis and protein synthesis in extremely low birth weight infants. J Pediatr 1998; 132:948–953.

58. Binder ND, Raschko PK, Benda GI, et al. Insulin infusion with parenteral nutrition in extremely low birth weight infants with hyperglycemia. J Pediatr 1989; 114:273–280.

59. Sellmayer A, Koletzko B. Long-chain polyunsaturated fatty acids and eicosanoids in infants-Physiological and pathophysiological aspects and open questions. Lipids 1999; 34:199–205.

60. Sunehag A. The role of parenteral lipids in supporting gluconeogenesis in very premature infants. Pediatr Res 2003; 54:480–486.

61. Simmer K, Rao SC. Early introduction of lipids to parenterally-fed preterm infants. Cochrane Database Syst Rev 2005; (2):CD005256.

62. Liet JM, Piloquet H, Marchini JS, et al. Leucine metabolism in preterm infants receiving parenteral nutrition with medium-chain compared with long-chain triacyglycerol emulsions. Am J Clin Nutr 1999; 69:539–543.

63. Newell SJ. Gastrointestinal function and its ontogeny: how should we feed the preterm infants? Semin Neonatol 1996; 1:59–66.

64. Widdowson E, Colombo V, Artavanis C. Changes in the organs of pigs in response to feeding for the first 24 hours after birth. II. The digestive Tract. Biol Neonate 1976; 28:272–281.

65. Heird WC, Schwarz SM, Hansen TH. Colostrum-induced enteric mucosal growth in beagle puppies. Pediatr Res 1984; 18(6):512–515.

66. Lucas A, Bloom S, Aynsley-Green A. Gut hormones and "minimal enteral feeding". Acta Paediatr Scand 1986; 75:719–723.

67. Kennedy KA, Tyson JE, Chamnanvanikij S. Rapid versus slow rate of advancement of feedings for promoting growth and preventing necrotizing enterocolitis in parenterally fed low-birth-weight infants. Cochrane Database Syst Rev 2000; (2):CD001241.

68. Tyson JE, Kennedy KA. Minimal enteral nutrition for promoting feeding tolerance and preventing morbidity in parenterally fed infants. Cochrane Database Syst Rev 2000; (2):CD000504.

69. Tyson JE, Kennedy KA. Trophic feedings for parenterally fed infants. Cochrane Database Syst Rev 2005; (3):CD000504.pub2.

70. Szabo JS, Mayfield SR, Oh W, Stonestreet BS. Postprandial gastrointestinal blood flow and oxygen consumption: effects of hypoxia in neonatal piglets. Pediatr Res 1987; 21(1):93–98.

71. Crissinger KD, Granger DN. Mucosal injury induced by ischemia and reperfusion in the piglet intestine: influences of age and feeding. Gastroenterology 1989; 97(4):920–926.

Chapter 13

Macro and Micronutrients

Frank R. Greer, MD

Calcium and Vitamin D
Calcium/Vitamin D Deficiency
Vitamin A
Vitamin E
Vitamin K
Iron

Determining the requirements for macro and micronutrients in the neonate has been the subject of many publications, government reports and conferences, indicative of the many controversies and even lack of information for many of these nutrients. The adequate intake (AI) of any given nutrient for the preterm or term newborn infant is the daily intake that meets the nutritional requirement of "medically stable" infants at the specified gestational age or birth weight. For the term infant, the gold standard for determining adequate intake is derived from the mean values of nutrients found in human milk. For the preterm infant, no such gold standard is available, and the adequate intake of a nutrient depends typically on a "factorial approach" using the accumulation of a specific nutrient that occurs in the fetus of the same weight and gestational age. Compared to term infants, nutrient stores are limited in preterm infants, even though the needs (e.g. energy) are very high during the period of transition from fetal to neonatal life, as well as during periods of "medical instability" and subsequent recovery. The nutrient needs are most difficult to achieve during periods of "medical instability." During these periods when there is essentially no growth followed by periods of more rapid growth, the "adequate intake" is a moving target. Thus, for the smaller preterm infants in the NICU, the "adequate intake" may vary considerably over time. In these clinical situations, the range of average intakes is derived from observational, as well as randomized, controlled trials. These average intakes should sustain adequate nutrition and growth over time without abnormal clinical findings, symptoms, or biochemical/functional abnormalities, and are used to define a "reasonable range of intakes." This is often the best that can be done for a given nutrient for any individual neonate. When the exact "adequate intake" for any nutrient is not known, it is very important that a reasonable range of intakes is established and/or re-established as soon as possible in small infants. Given the interaction between genes and early diet and the possible effects on long-term fetal and newborn programming, this may be very important (see Chapter 10).

Historically speaking, though we have done well in meeting the nutritional needs of term infants who are not breast-fed, we have done very poorly with infants whose birth weights are less than 1500 g, as indicated by the growth outcomes from 1993–1994 and 2000–2001, published by the Neonatal Network (Fig. 13-1) (1, 2).

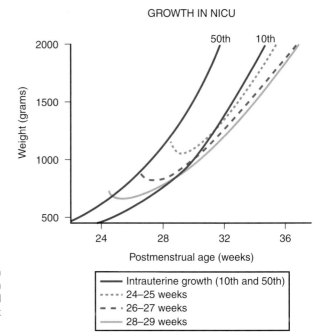

GROWTH IN NICU

Figure 13-1 Growth of pretmature infants in the NICU setting with a birth weight less than 1500 g. From RA Ehrenkranz et al. Longitudinal growth of hospitalized very low birth weight infants. Pediatrics 1999; 104(2 Pt 1):280–289.

These results indicate that the goal of supporting nutrition and growth in the VLBW infant, such that a postnatal growth rate approximating that of a normal fetus at the same gestational age is achieved, remains elusive.

In the following pages, important selected nutrients (both vitamins and minerals) will be reviewed. Controversial issues regarding these nutrients will be highlighted.

CALCIUM AND VITAMIN D

The physiology and requirements of calcium and vitamin D are so closely intertwined that one cannot be discussed without the other. These two nutrients are important in understanding the etiology of the early hypocalcemia of prematurity, osteopenia of prematurity and vitamin D deficiency rickets in older infants.

Though calcium is important for many bodily processes, including muscle contraction, neurotransmission, and enzyme function, its most important function is skeletal support: 99% of the total body calcium is in bone, where it combines with phosphorus to form crystalline hydroxyapatite. Less than 1% exists in the serum, of which 50% is bound to serum albumin, 5% is bound to other anions (HCO_3, citrate, PO_4), and 45% is in the metabolically active form as ionized calcium. Ionized calcium not only plays a role as an intracellular "second" messenger but, equally important, it serves as an extracellular "first" messenger. The discovery of G-protein-coupled extacellular Ca-sensing receptors on the chief cells of the parathyroid gland, renal tubular cells, bone and cartilage cells, placental cytotrophoblasts, as well as intestinal villi, has gone a long way towards revealing the interaction of these tissues in systemic calcium homeostasis, as depicted in Figure 13-2. The Ca-sensing receptor-induced signals specifically modulate cellular functions such as parathyroid hormone secretion from the parathyroid gland and calcium reabsorption in the kidney (3). Thus, it is not surprising that serum Ca is under very tight control, with an elaborate homeostatic mechanism that involves both circulating calciotropic hormones and the extracellular calcium-sensing receptors (Fig. 13-2). A calcium-regulating gene has been described on chromosome 3 in humans, which determines the set point for serum calcium.

Ca^{2+} HOMEOSTATIC SYSTEM

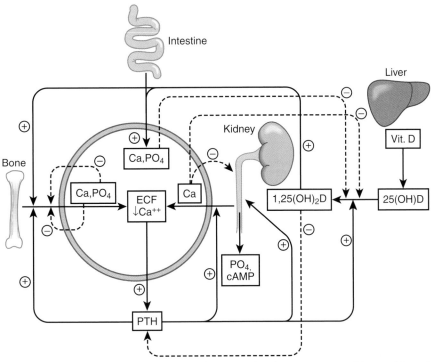

Figure 13-2 Calcium homeostasis showing the intereations between serum calcium, calciotropic hormones, and organ systems.

Mutations of this gene have been described that alter the "calciostat" setting. These include familial hypercalcemia with hypercalciuria and severe neonatal primary hyperparathyroidism (4).

The calciotropic hormones include 1,25-(OH)$_2$-vitamin D, parathyroid hormone (PTH), calcitonin, parathyroid hormone related peptide (PTH-rp), growth hormone and miscellaneous insulin-like growth factors. 1,25-(OH)$_2$-Vitamin D, really a hormone and not a true vitamin, is the physiologically active form of vitamin D. Vitamin D$_3$ (cholecalciferol, the parent compound) can be synthesized in the skin from cholesterol on exposure to UV-B light (Fig. 13-2). It is contained naturally in relatively few foods (e.g. fish oils) but is often a dietary supplement. Once cholecalciferol is released into the circulation, it is converted to 25-OH-vitamin D in the liver, the main circulatory form of the vitamin, whose measurement determines sufficiency of vitamin D. The renal tubular cells subsequently convert 25-OH-vitamin D into 1,25-(OH)$_2$-vitamin D. The mechanism of action of 1,25-(OH)$_2$-vitamin D is similar to that of all steroid hormones. It is transported in the blood bound to vitamin D-binding protein. On entering the cell cytoplasm, it disassociates itself from the vitamin D binding protein and binds to a nuclear vitamin D nuclear receptor (VDR) (Fig. 13-2) All vitamin D target tissues (intestine, kidney, bone, etc.) contain a cytoplasmic VDR for 1,25-(OH)$_2$-vitamin D, which then binds to the DNA in the nucleus to effect gene transcription and the synthesis of a variety of vitamin D-dependent proteins, including Ca-binding proteins (5, 6).

Parathyroid hormone, an 84-amino-acid peptide secreted by the parathyroid gland chief cells, is primarily responsible for maintaining serum calcium. Actions of this hormone include (6):

- renal: inhibition of proximal tubular PO$_4$ reabsorption, increased distal tubular reabsorption of filtered Ca via cyclic AMP;

- renal: stimulates 1-8-hydroxlyation of 25-OH vitamin D to the physiologically active $1,25(OH)_2$-vitamin D;
- bone: stimulates bone resorption of Ca.

Calcitonin is a 32-amino-acid peptide produced by the C cells of the thyroid gland. Its actions are to lower serum Ca by decreasing resorption of Ca from bone as well as decreasing renal Ca resorption resulting in calciuria (6). It is less important than PTH, as its congenital absence does not result in serious disorders of calcium metabolism.

Calcium Requirements

Estimates of the calcium requirements of the preterm infant are based on our knowledge of the exponential accumulation of calcium with increasing gestation in the fetus. A term infant accumulates between 25 and 30 g of calcium, or approximately 1% of body weight. Two-thirds of this calcium is accumulated in the last trimester of pregnancy, a calcium accretion rate of 90–150 mg/kg/day with a peak of 150 mg/kg/day at 36–38 weeks of gestation (7). After the birth of the preterm infant, it is difficult to meet this calcium accretion rate by either parenteral or enteral supplementation. With the present limitations on the amount of Ca that can be added to TPN solutions, retention rates of Ca generally do not exceed 60 mg/kg/day, which impacts on bone mineral content of growing preterm infants (8). With the onset of enteral feedings, intestinal absorption of Ca in the preterm infant becomes a significant consideration. Though there are relatively few good balance studies in this population, it is known that calcium absorption increases with both postconceptional and chronologic (postnatal) age. In growing preterm infants the percent absorption of Ca is between 50% and 80% of intake (8–10). Thus the intake of calcium to meet the intrauterine requirements of calcium accretion of 90–150 mg/kg day would be somewhere between 120 and 200 mg/kg/day (8).

For the term infant, skeletal accretion is somewhere between 60 and 140 mg/day during the first year of life. Based on the average breast milk concentration of Ca (26.4 mg/dL), a retention rate of 61% for Ca and an average intake of 780 mL of human milk, the current recommended adequate intake would be 128 mg/day, an amount easily achieved in breast-fed infants and exceeded by most formula-fed infants (11).

Vitamin D Requirements

In the immediate neonatal period, the major source of vitamin D is of maternal origin until external supplements (parenteral or enteral) are begun, as human milk contains no significant amount. For preterm and full-term infants in the USA, recommended intakes for vitamin D are between 200 and 400 IU day when fed orally, and between 40 and 200 IU when supplied parenterally (8, 11, 12).

CALCIUM/VITAMIN D DEFICIENCY

Early Hypocalcemia of Prematurity (EHP)

EHP, defined as a total serum Ca of less than 7.0 mg% (1.75 mmol/L) or an ionized Ca of < 3.5 mg% (0.9 mmol/L), affects 30–57% of all preterm infants (13, 14). Suggested etiologies of this disorder have included decreased Ca intake (15), vitamin D deficiency and abnormalities of vitamin D metabolism (16–19).

The degree and prevalence of EHP increase with decreasing gestational age, which is more important than the actual birth weight. Most of the decrease in serum Ca occurs during the first 72 h of life, with slow recovery by 7–10 days of age if not treated (20). Typically the hypocalcemia is asymptomatic. Though no adverse effects have been clearly documented, it is difficult to determine the morbidity or mortality from EHP because of other complicating variables that typically occur in the infants with the lowest serum calcium.

There are relatively few studies of the treatment of early hypocalcemia in premature infants, given the frequency of the diagnosis. It has been common practice to maintain serum calcium with either oral supplements or parenteral infusions of calcium, and this can be done with an oral dose of 75–150 mg/kg/day of elemental Ca, or 24–35 mg/kg/day of Ca added to i.v. fluids (15, 20–24). However, the efficacy of this "traditional" therapy has not been demonstrated and it is controversial. One group of investigators has shown that an infusion of a single calcium bolus (18 mg/kg) improves cardiovascular function (increased heart rate, increased blood pressure, improved left ventricular function) in infants with EHP (25, 26), but a subsequent study did not confirm these results (27). Similarly, adverse effects of EHP have been infrequently reported. A single study described heart failure in six newborn infants with hypocalcemia, although only one of these infants was premature (28). A report has also associated hypocalcemia with patent ductus arteriosus (29).

Others have attempted to treat EHP with various vitamin D metabolites, assuming that it would be vitamin D-responsive. It is known that $1,25-OH_2$-vitamin D increases within 24 h of birth in both term and preterm infants, in response to the decline in serum calcium and rising PTH. Thus, renal 1-alpha-hydroxlyation of 25-OH-vitamin D begins at the time of birth, if not before. Nevertheless, numerous investigators have attempted to treat or prevent EHP with supplements of vitamin D or its metabolites, with mixed results. In three studies of small numbers of premature infants ($n = 8$–14), all on oral feedings of formula with birth weights greater than 1000 g, 2 μg/kg/day of oral 25-OH-vitamin D (19) or 0.1 to 1.0 μg/day of $1,25-OH_2$-vitamin D significantly raised serum calcium (18, 30). In one uncontrolled study in infants fed human milk with birth weight >1500 g, oral supplements of 1200 IU vitamin D, 10 μg of 25-OH-vitamin D, or 0.5 μg of $1,25-OH_2$-vitamin D failed to increase serum Ca (31). In a second study using pharmacologic doses of intramuscular $1,25-OH_2$-vitamin D (0.05–3 μg) no changes in serum Ca were noted (32). From these studies, one is unable to conclude that the hypocalcemia of prematurity can be treated or prevented by vitamin D and its metabolites. These infants typically have inappropriately low PTH and elevated calcitonin levels, and it could be hypothesized that calcium is not absorbed from bone secondary to this hypercalcitonemia. Absence of functional PTH receptors in bone as well as the intestine in preterm infants may also confound EHP. Certainly, in the case of VLBW infants who are not on oral feedings of milk, there would be little expected response to $1,25-OH_2$-vitamin D, given its known mechanism of action (Fig. 13-2).

Osteopenia/Rickets of Prematurity

This disease has been associated with deficiencies of both Ca (as well as phosphorus) and vitamin D in the preterm infant. Osteopenia of prematurity is a metabolic bone disease associated with under-mineralization of the skeleton of the premature infant. There may also be an accumulation of under-mineralized osteoid which interrupts the mineralization of the growth plate of bone. Hence, the terms osteopenia and rickets of prematurity are used interchangeably in the literature. In these infants, the extrauterine rate of skeletal mineralization is delayed compared with that of the corresponding in utero fetal skeleton, similar to the delay in the extrauterine growth rate. The most severe complication is bone

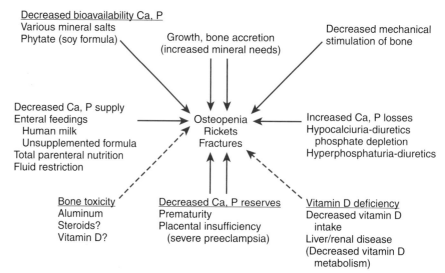

Figure 13-3 Proposed schema for the multiple etiologies of osteopenia of prematurity.

fractures, frequently involving the rib bones, but fractures are not uncommon in long bones as well.

This disorder occurs in virtually every premature infant with a birth weight of less than 1500 g. The more critically ill premature infants have the most significant degree of osteopenia, and the frequency of rickets/fractures is in general inversely correlated with birth weight. When looked for systematically with radiographs, the incidence of fractures in these preterm infants ranges from 20 to 32% (33–35) and increases to 50–60% in infants with a birth weight of <1000 g (36–38).

Details on the histopathology of this disorder are limited (39, 40) and the etiology is multifactorial, as shown in Figure 13-3. As discussed above, a major factor is the limited bone stores of calcium (and phosphorus) at birth and the failure to achieve the intrauterine accretion rate of minerals as noted. Osteopenia occurs even with the use of high-mineral-containing formulas and breast-milk fortifiers specifically designed for VLBW infants.

Recent literature has found evidence that a decrease in "bone loading" plays a very significant role in the development of osteopenia of prematurity (41–45). Bone loading in these infants is limited, largely accomplished by passive or active muscle activity. Increased bone loading (i.e. passive exercise program with range of motion to joints) promotes bone formation, whereas decreased bone loading (decreased physical activity) results in bone resorption. Two lines of evidence support the importance of "bone loading" in preterm infants. First, increased biochemical markers of bone resorption in preterm infants (hydroxyproline, type 1 collagen telopeptide, alkaline phosphatase) have been observed (44–46). Second, studies have demonstrated that organized programs of passive physical activity in premature infants improve measurements of bone mineralization (47–50). Surprisingly, these passive exercise programs may be effective with as little as 5–10 min of movement a day (48).

Vitamin D deficiency, on the other hand, is an unusual cause of bone disease in the preterm infant in a population that is vitamin D "replete." Premature infants with osteopenia generally have normal levels of 25-OHD and increased levels of 1,25-$(OH)_2$D. Daily oral supplements of 2000 IU/day of vitamin D for 6 weeks do not affect the incidence of osteopenia in premature infants (34) and 200–400 IU/day appears to be adequate (51).

Other aspects of clinical care that may affect osteopenia of prematurity are shown in Figure 13-3.

The diagnosis of osteopenia is based on radiologic and laboratory findings. A physical examination is not very helpful unless the disease has progressed to an advanced state and there is tenderness and swelling at fracture sites in the long bones. In older patients, the rachitic rosary of the constochondral junction and craniotabes of the skull may be present. Because the legs of these infants are non-weight-bearing, the more obvious clinical signs of rickets in the lower extremities in older children are not evident.

In most cases, the diagnosis is made from routine X-rays, usually of the chest, where healing rib fractures or severe hypomineralization may be observed. In the more advanced form of the disease, standard radiographs of the wrists and knees may show the classic signs of rickets, but usually not before 2 months of age. However, conventional radiologic measures cannot detect decreases in bone mineral content until a 30–40% loss of bone mineral has occurred (52, 53). Special techniques such as single photon absorptiometry (SPA), dual energy X-ray absorptiometry (DXA) and quantitative computed tomography (QCT) and transmission ultrasound, though they are more sensitive, are in general only used for research purposes in preterm infants (54, 55).

A number of serum biochemical markers have been used to screen for osteopenia of prematurity. These include calcium, phosphorus, alkaline phosphatase, parathyroid hormone, 25-OH-vitamin D, $1,25(OH)_2$-vitamin D and osteocalcin. Urinary values that have been used include fractional excretion of calcium and tubular reabsorption of phosphate as well as calcium/creatinine ratio. A low serum phosphorus (generally < 4.5 mg%) is the single best indicator of mineral deficiency in these infants.

For infants in the USA and Canada, VLBW infants with osteopenia clearly do not need more than 200–400 IU of vitamin D a day, as recommended by the American Academy of Pediatrics Committee on Nutrition and others (11, 12). The high $1,25(OH)_2D$ concentrations and adequate levels of 25-OHD in almost all infants diagnosed with this disorder support this recommendation, which assumes VLBW infants will not be maintained on diets with grossly inadequate concentrations of Ca and P such as unfortified human milk. Increasing vitamin D intakes to 960 IU/day or higher has not proven beneficial (34, 51). Parenteral requirements for vitamin D are less clear, though with the present multivitamin preparations available for infants it is difficult to exceed 400 IU/days without concerns for increased amounts of some of the accompanying vitamins. Nevertheless, preterm infants on long-term TPN have exhibited adequate vitamin D status on solutions supplying as little as 30–35 IU/kg/day (56).

Though there are some indications that a routine passive "exercise" program may be beneficial (47–49), the most important component of prevention and treatment is the supply of adequate amounts of calcium and phosphorus, without which any bone-loading exercises would be ineffective. The logical goal of such therapy would be to attain the intrauterine rate of bone mineralization. To do so would require enteral intakes of ~ 200 mg/kg/day of calcium and 90 mg/kg/day of phosphorus, assuming a 65% absorption of calcium (at best) and an 80% absorption of phosphorus. The special formulas available for VLBW infants will supply these amounts of minerals. Commercial fortifiers for human milk are also available, containing the appropriate amounts of calcium and phosphorus. As noted above, the achievement of the intrauterine accretion of bone mineral in VLBW infants during the first 8 weeks of life is problematic, even with adequate mineral intake. Prevention of severe osteopenia with fractures and rickets is possible with these intakes, however. Catch-up bone mineralization eventually occurs in these infants many months after discharge (57–60).

The prevention and/or treatment of osteopenia in VLBW infants on TPN is subject to the limitations of TPN solutions as discussed above. The concentration of calcium and phosphorus obtainable in these solutions is not likely to achieve the in utero rate of accretion of bone mineral. However, enough can be infused with TPN solutions to prevent overt fractures and rickets in these patients. Solutions containing 60 mg/dL (15 mmol) of calcium and 46 mg/dL (15 mmol) of phosphorus will maintain the desired biochemical and calciotropic hormone indices of mineral homeostasis (56).

Vitamin D Deficiency Rickets in Infants

Cases of rickets in infants secondary to inadequate vitamin D intake and decreased exposure to sunlight continue to be reported in the USA (61–65). This represents an extreme degree of deficiency of the vitamin. The majority of these cases have been reported in infants who are exclusively breast-fed without supplemental vitamin D, as the vitamin D content of human milk is minimal (66). Often infants with rickets have increased skin pigmentation and a history of decreased sunshine exposure, but in many areas of the USA sunshine exposure during the winter months is not effective for the cutaneous synthesis of vitamin D (67). It has been recommended that vitamin D deficiency be prevented in all breast-feeding infants with a vitamin D supplement of 200–400 IU/day until they are receiving adequate amounts of vitamin D from vitamin D-fortified formula or dairy products (11, 12).

VITAMIN A

Physiology/Biologic Mechanisms of Action

The term vitamin A refers to a number of compounds that include both the naturally occurring and synthetically derived retinoids. The biologic activity of vitamin A is diverse. It is essential for vision, growth, healing, reproduction, cell differentiation, and immunocompetency. This multiplicity of effects is due to its mechanism of action through gene regulation. The action is similar to that of steroid hormones, in that a specific retinoic-acid-receptor protein complex becomes bound to nuclear DNA, resulting in regulation of specific genes.

Retinol is the naturally occurring alcohol of the vitamin, formed in vivo from its precursor β-carotene, found in plants and thus plentiful in most diets. Vitamin A is transported in plasma as retinol, bound to retinol-binding protein (RBP), a specific carrier protein synthesized in the liver. For β-carotene there is little specific information on its uptake or its metabolism during the perinatal period. However, β-carotene can meet the fetal and newborn growth requirements for vitamin A.

Ingested carotene and dietary retinyl esters are converted to free retinol in the proximal small intestine after the action of hydrolases from the pancreas and intestinal brush border. These enzymes may have low activity in the premature infant in the early days of life. After solubilization with bile salts into mixed micelles, retinol is absorbed into the intestinal cells, reesterified, and incorporated into chylomicrons that are transported via lymph (thoracic duct) into the circulation, as with all fat-soluble vitamins. Intraluminal bile acids, important for this process, are decreased in premature infants and may lead to inadequate micelle formation and affect retinol absorption (68).

After absorption, chylomicrons, containing lipoprotein-bound retinyl esters, are taken up by the liver, the main storage organ for retinol (90% of body stores) (69). Premature infants are potentially born with low or marginal liver vitamin A stores (70, 71). In one study of 25 preterm infants who died within the first 24 h of life, 37% had liver concentrations less than 20 μg/g (70), compared to the normal adult concentration of 100–300 μg/g (72). The ability of preterm infants to offset an inadequate intake of vitamin A from liver stores is limited.

Following retinol hydrolysis in the liver, the subsequent transport of retinol to other tissues for metabolism is dependent on liver RBP synthesis and secretion (73). After secretion of the RBP-retinol complex, RBP binds with plasma transthyretin, reducing the chance for glomerular filtration and renal catabolism of RBP. The circulating retinol-RBP-transthyretin complex is delivered to target tissues. At the time of birth, plasma RBP concentration was lower in a group of 39 preterm infants (gestational age 24–36 weeks) compared to a group of 32 term infants (2.8 ± 1.2 µg/dL vs. 3.6 ± 1.1 µg/dL, mean $\pm$ SD, $P < 0.001$) (74). In this same study, mean plasma vitamin A was also lower in preterm compared to full-term infants (16.0 ± 6.2 µg/dL vs. 23.9 ± 10.2 µg/dL, $P < 0.001$).

Neonatal Requirements

As noted, even term infants are relatively deficient in Vitamin A at the time of birth compared to older children. Based on the vitamin A content of human milk of 180–600 µg/L (75), the recommended intake for term infants is 400–500 µg/day. This intake is easily met by term infant formulas that contain approximately 600 µg/L.

Recommended supplements for the very low birth weight infant are in the 200–450 µg/kg/day range, whether enteral or parenteral, with 450 µg//kg/day preferred. Most infant formulas for the VLBW infant will easily supply this amount as they contain about 3000 µg/L. Even formulas for preterm infants after discharge contain 1020 µg/L of vitamin A. All of the commercially available human milk fortifiers also contain enough vitamin A to meet the requirements.

The vitamin A content of a typical multivitamin oral supplement used for preterm infants is 450 µg/ml. Thus, the recommended intake for the orally fed preterm infant can be met with preterm infant formula, fortified human milk or multivitamin preparations. Supplementation of premature infants with 450 µg/kg/day results in "normalization" of serum retinol and RBP (76, 77).

Using either of two standard multivitamin preparations for TPN solutions provides 690 µg of vitamin A for term infants. However, administration of vitamin A by this method is very inefficient because of loss of vitamin A by photodegradation and binding to intravenous tubing (78, 79). An in vitro study in this system estimated net vitamin A losses of between 62% and 89%. Shielding TPN solutions from photooxidation reactions is difficult (80, 81).

Vitamin A Deficiency/Toxicity

Vitamin A deficiency is not common in term infants in developed countries. However, what constitutes vitamin A deficiency is less clear in the preterm infant. The "adequate" concentration of serum vitamin A in VLBW infants is not known. Serum concentrations below 20.0 µg/dL (0.70 µmol/L) have been considered as deficient in premature infants, and concentrations below 10.0 µg/dL (0.35 µmol/L) as indicating severe deficiency with depleted liver stores. Unfortunately, a single plasma retinol value does not correlate well with liver stores until they become very low (<10.0 µg/dL (<0.35 µmol/L)) (71, 82, 83) or extremely low (<5 µg/dL (<0.17 µmol/L)) (84). Others have looked at plasma RBP. In one study, a high percentage of preterm infants, up to 77%, had plasma RBP below 3.0 µg/dL, which may be indicative of vitamin A deficiency (74). Both the plasma RBP response (77) and the relative rise in serum retinol concentration (40) following intramuscular vitamin A administration have been described as useful tests to assess functional vitamin A status. This is a better method of confirming actual low vitamin A storage than random plasma concentrations (85). Plasma levels only decline after liver reserves have been depleted. Levels less than 20 µg/dL are considered deficient and <10 µg/dL are associated with signs of deficiency.

In a large study, 25% of infants receiving supplemental vitamin A (1500 µg three times per week) and 54% of controls (receiving approximately 300 µg/day) had vitamin A concentrations below 20.0 µg/dL on day 28 (86). Similar percentages, 22% of those receiving supplemental vitamin A and 45% of controls, had a relative dose response of > 10% following an intramuscular dose of 600 µg. From these data it was suggested than an even higher dose of vitamin A may be required to achieve vitamin A sufficiency in very premature infants (birth weights <1000g) (86).

The studies reviewed above with high-dose vitamin A supplements did not report any vitamin A toxicity (76, 78, 86–89). Dosages used in these studies were roughly twice the recommended RDA for premature infants. Another report states that one oral dose of 15 000 µg given to newborns was associated only with an asymptomatic bulging anterior fontanel in 4–5% of the infants (90). However, clinical assessment of toxicity in preterm infants has not been really studied, so guidelines in this area must be made carefully.

It has been known for years that excess maternal vitamin A may cause congenital anomalies in animal fetuses (91, 92), and retinoic acid seems especially teratogenic (74). Women who take more than 3000 µg of vitamin A per day as a supplement have an increased frequency of birth defects. The highest frequency of defects was related to high consumption before the 7th week of gestation (93). The defects (mostly craniofacial, cardiac, and thymic) resulted in a high mortality rate (94–96).

High Dose Vitamin A Supplementation for the Preterm Infant

One of the more controversial issues is whether or not very large doses of supplemental vitamin A (up to 900 µg/kg/day) may ameliorate bronchopulmonary dysplasia (76, 97, 98). Pertinent to the use of Vitamin A for the amelioration of bronchopulmonary dysplasia in addition to its tissue healing effects is that retinol, retinyl palmitate and retinoic acid are all potential antioxidants. It is clear that intramuscular vitamin A is more effective than the enteral route in premature infants for delivering these large doses (99, 100).

Randomized trials using large doses of parenteral vitamin A ($\geq$ 450 µg/kg/day) to prevent chronic lung disease have been reviewed (97). To date, six randomized trials have been published (76, 86–89, 101), though one of these (86) has a sample size 4-times larger than all the others combined and enrolled the smallest and most premature infants (birthweights 401–1000 g). In this study, VLBW preterm infants were supplemented with 15 000 µg intramuscularly three times a week in addition to the vitamin A in parenteral and enteral feeds.

Overall, the results of these studies are mixed. No study has found a significant effect on mortality, differences in days of assisted ventilation, or length of hospital stay (76, 86–89, 101). The pooled data in a meta-analysis for all six studies showed a trend towards reduction in oxygen use at 1 month in survivors that does not reach statistical significance (97) (RR 0.93 [0.86, 1.01]). The study with largest number of infants reported no significant difference in the combined outcomes of death and oxygen use at 36 weeks (RR 0.89 [0.79, 1.0]) (86). However, there was a significant reduction of oxygen use in the vitamin A group at 36 weeks (RR 0.85 [0.73, 0.98]). The need for supplemental oxygen at 36 weeks postmenstrual age declined from 62% in the unsupplemented controls to 55% in the supplemented infants. Using these data, it would require treatment of 14.5 infants with supplemental vitamin A to benefit one patient (86). Concern has also been expressed for the invasiveness of repeated intramuscular injections of vitamin A in return for this very modest benefit, though no side-effects from the high-dose vitamin A supplements were reported from any of these studies. These included clinical monitoring of anterior fontanel pressure and biochemical evidence of vitamin A toxicity.

VITAMIN E

Physiology/Biologic Mechanism of Action

The term vitamin E refers to eight naturally occurring compounds. Though the biological activities of E vitamers vary considerably, they all show antioxidant capability, with the ability to protect cellular and subcellular membranes from oxidative destruction initiated at the molecular level by lipid peroxidation (102). To be effective, tocopherol must be localized in membrane sites exposed to free radicals. The most abundant and active isomer is α-tocopherol. On the basis of in vivo bioassays, the approximate relative potencies of the other vitamin E isomers compared to dl-α-tocopherol are β 40–50%, γ 10–30%, δ about 1%.

A relatively low concentration of vitamin E is found in fetal tissues until body fat increases in late gestation. Total body content of tocopherol in the human fetus increases from about 1 mg at 5 months gestation to approximately 20 mg at term (103). Although pregnancy is associated with a high maternal concentration of circulating vitamin E proportional to rising plasma lipids, transplacental delivery of tocopherols to the fetus is limited. Administering large doses of vitamin E to women in the last weeks of pregnancy has little effect on cord vitamin E levels (104, 105). The ratio of maternal to fetal tocopherol concentration in blood is approximately 4:1 (106). Neonatal tissues also show a relative paucity of vitamin E isomers. In premature neonates the low proportion of adipose tissue further limits the total body vitamin E content.

The absorption of tocopherols is variable, depending on total lipid absorption, as with the other fat-soluble vitamins (107). Bile salts and pancreatic enzymes are essential to the absorption process (108, 109). In general the efficiency of absorption decreases as larger amounts of tocopherol are consumed (110). Decreased absorption of fat, as seen in the premature neonate, results in a parallel loss of tocopherols (107). Factors important in the absorption of vitamin E by the neonate include gestational age, the fat component of the diet, and the preparation of vitamin E given. Little is known about passage of vitamin E through the absorptive cells of the mucosa as no intestinal transfer proteins have been identified for tocopherol. After micelle formation with bile salts, vitamin E is absorbed, incorporated into chylomicrons and transported with fat along with the other fat-soluble vitamins via lymphatic vessels into the venous system. The concentration of tocopherol in plasma varies depending on the amount of associated lipoproteins.

Liver, adipose tissue, and skeletal muscle are the major storage organs for the vitamin. At the cellular level, it must be integrated into lipid droplets, cellular membranes, and organelles to be effective. It is concentrated wherever there is abundant fatty acid, especially in phospholipid membrane-containing structures (e.g., mitochondrial, microsomal, and plasma membranes). Fat accumulates α-tocopherol and can sequester it (111). When the intake of vitamin E is high, the liver is a major repository, but the tocopherol pool in adipose tissue is much larger. Although adipose tissue is sometimes considered a "store" of vitamin E, the tocopherol present in adipocytes is not readily available to other tissues (112).

In the liver, newly absorbed lipids are incorporated into very-low-density lipoproteins (VLDL). VLDL particles subsequently secreted by the liver are preferentially enriched with α-tocopherol. The liver is responsible for the control and release of α-tocopherol into human plasma (113, 114) via the hepatic cytosolic α-tocopherol transfer protein (TTP) (115). The gene for this protein has been localized to the 8q13.1–13.3 region of chromosome 8 (116). Human deficiencies of this protein have now been reported (117–120).

Vitamin E Requirements

The requirement for the term infant are based on the vitamin E content of mature human milk, which is 2–4 mg/L of α-tocopherol (121). The amount of vitamin E ingested daily (approximately 2 mg of α-tocopherol equivalents in 750 mL of mature milk) appears to be adequate to prevent antioxidant deficiency in the term neonate with normal intestinal absorption. This amount is sufficient to raise blood and tissue levels, but is higher per kilogram than the 10–15 mg recommended for older children and adults (122). It is clear that normal blood and tissue concentrations of tocopherol can be achieved promptly in term neonates fed the usual volume of either breast milk or commercial formula. Commercial formulas for term infants contain 1.3–2.5 mg/L.

The situation is different for premature neonates with lower initial stores, decreased blood concentrations and reduced intestinal absorption. Human milk may not provide sufficient vitamin E and early provision of vitamin E is necessary. It is necessary to give larger amounts (i.e., 6–12 mg//kg/day) when vitamin E supplements are provided enterally (123). In studies of enteral nutrition, a daily dose of 10–25 mg of water-miscible α-tocopherol acetate given to 0.6–1.5 kg neonates was required to produce and maintain normal vitamin E status (124–127). Even some premature neonates on this regimen (10–25 mg/day) may not maintain a plasma tocopherol concentration above 0.5 mg/dL, especially if they receive iron-fortified formula. Special formulas for preterm infants for use in the hospital contain 32–51 mg/L. Those for use after hospital discharge contain 27–30 mg/L. The commercially available human milk fortifiers all contain vitamin E.

In intravenously nourished neonates, 1 mg/kg/d eventually corrects the vitamin E deficiency state, but up to 7–10 days may be required (128–130). Parenteral α-tocopherol acetate at 3 mg/kg/day rapidly corrects low vitamin E levels and abnormal peroxide hemolysis tests within 24 h (131, 132). Once a normal blood concentration of vitamin E is achieved, 1–2 mg/kg/day can be given to maintain vitamin E sufficiency, but without continued provision of tocopherol in the parenterally fed infant, insufficiency quickly develops (132). Current multivitamin solutions for pediatric TPN solutions provide 7 mg/day to term infants when used as recommended.

From studies of parenterally and enterally nourished premature neonates, it is reasonable to conclude that the immediate requirement of such neonates for "deliverable or absorbable" vitamin E is 2–3 mg/kg/day and that 1 mg/kg/day suffices once the initial deficiency state is corrected and tissue stores are established. Using multivitamin solutions available for pediatric TPN solutions, 2.8–3.5 mg of vitamin E (α-tocopherol) are provided when used as recommended.

In summary, it is recommended that premature infants receive 2.8–3.5 mg/kg/day vitamin E parenterally and 6–12 mg/kg/day enterally (133). These intakes are approximated with the present formulas and multivitamin preparations. The American Academy of Pediatrics Committee on Nutrition has recommended that formulas provide a minimum of 1 mg of vitamin E per g of linoleic acid and 0.7 mg per 100 kcal, though the special formulas containing iron for premature infants provide 4–6 mg/100 kcal, because of the higher requirement for vitamin E with these formulas (134).

Laboratory Assessment of Vitamin E Sufficiency

As 90% or more of the circulating vitamin E is normally α-tocopherol, serum or plasma samples can be measured. A concentration of at least 0.5 mg/dL indicates adequate nutritional status (135). However, vitamin E concentration in tissue is the most appropriate parameter to measure to assess vitamin E status, though this is not usually available in infants.

Adequate vitamin E concentration is dependent on the concentration of plasma lipids. Tocopherol data have been expressed as a function of lipid concentration in many studies (136–138). These investigations have demonstrated that, although children have significantly lower levels of plasma vitamin E than adults, a tocopherol/total lipid ratio of 0.6–0.8 mg/g indicates adequate nutritional status (136, 137). This ratio would be important to measure in the very premature infant in whom marked changes in lipid levels occur, ranging from very low at birth to high during intravenous feedings of fatty acids. However, this ratio requires measurement of cholesterol, triglycerides, and phospholipids, and requires considerable amounts of blood for a very small premature infant. Part of the explanation for low circulating tocopherol in premature infants relates to decreased plasma lipids compared to the lipid concentration in adults.

To characterize the apparent vitamin E deficiency of premature neonates, the hydrogen peroxide hemolysis test has been recommended (139). However, a study in premature infants (mean 33 weeks gestation) compared plasma and erythrocyte vitamin E levels, vitamin E to lipid ratios, and two variations of the hydrogen peroxide hemolysis test. The investigators concluded that there was no satisfactory method for the clinical assessment of vitamin E deficiency in the premature infant (140). It is important to differentiate between tocopherol-sufficient and tocopherol-deficient premature neonates, however, as parenteral vitamin E is being advocated in high doses for prophylaxis against neonatal disorders associated with oxygen toxicity (see below).

Vitamin E Deficiency in the Neonate

Several adverse consequences potentially attributable to vitamin E deficiency have been described in the medical literature in infants and children (141–153). Though controversy has surrounded the conditions attributed to human vitamin E deficiency, the deficiency state described in premature infants is the most convincing (123, 124, 131, 139, 140). Some of these investigations have defined methods of correcting or preventing vitamin E deficiency in the critically ill, low birth weight neonate (125–127, 132, 154–156) but, unfortunately, they have also identified toxicity associated with excess doses of tocopherol preparations (157).

The absorption of vitamin E in premature neonates has been studied primarily by the technique of administering large single dosages and measuring the blood concentration sequentially. From these results, it appears that neonates less than 32 weeks gestation have significant malabsorption of tocopherol compared to term neonates and older children (158). Prematurely delivered neonates may show evidence of vitamin E deficiency owing to several factors, including limited tissue storage at birth, intestinal malabsorption, and rapid growth rates that increase nutritional requirements in general. Many premature neonates may not be given enteral or even parenteral vitamin E for several days because of severe respiratory disorders requiring ventilatory assistance. Even when they are given tocopherol supplements, premature neonates with respiratory distress syndrome may have a low blood tocopherol concentration (123, 131, 139, 158, 159).

Oski and Barness have implicated tocopherol deficiency as a responsible factor in hemolytic anemia of prematurity (141). As described in detail elsewhere, the conclusions from hematological studies of vitamin E supplementation in premature neonates differ depending on other variables that influence vitamin E status and requirements (135). Nevertheless, the careful investigations by Gross and Melhorn indicated the following in the preterm infant: (1) an abnormal degree of hemolysis occurs in association with vitamin E deficiency; (2) supplementation of premature neonates with 25 mg of α-tocopherol acetate per day decreases the hemolysis and leads to a modest but significant increase in blood hemoglobin content; and (3) the hemolytic anemia associated with vitamin E deficiency is aggravated by ingestion of iron in iron-fortified formulas (160). It has been established that vitamin E deficiency under certain nutritional dietary conditions contributes to accelerated hemolysis and leads to anemia in premature neonates.

High-Dose Vitamin E Therapy in Preterm Infants/Toxicity

A potential role of vitamin E supplementation in preventing or ameliorating retinopathy of prematurity was proposed in 1949 by Owens and Owens and has remained controversial (161). Tocopherols are concentrated in the retinal tissue, where lipid concentrations are high and clearly can interrupt oxidation reactions that conceivably initiate the injury process. A recent meta-analysis (162) of six randomized controlled trials with a total sample of 704 VLBW infants treated with vitamin E and 714 VLBW controls (144, 145, 163–165) found no difference in the overall incidence of ROP between the two groups. However, there was a significant difference in the incidence of Grade III ROP between the two groups, 2.4% in the vitamin E versus 5.5% in the controls (pooled odds ratio 0.44, 95% CI 0.21–0.81, $P < 0.02$). However, the total number of infants with severe ROP was very small and the authors recommended that further studies be done on the smallest infants (birth weight below 1000 g). It is concluded that at present there is no clear benefit of giving large doses of vitamin E for the intended purpose of preventing severe retinal disease.

Bronchopulmonary dysplasia is another condition of premature neonates that was reported to be preventable by vitamin E therapy (143). Further investigation of the role of vitamin E in bronchopulmonary dysplasia did not lead to confirmation of the original data, by either the same investigators (151) or others (166, 167). The rationale for this proposed effect is again logical, as tocopherols prevent oxidation-related injury of pulmonary membrane systems. However, it cannot be claimed that vitamin E in large doses prevents bronchopulmonary dysplasia in preterm infants.

There are also data supporting the suggestion that vitamin E supplementation, if given in the first 12 h of life, can reduce the incidence of intraventricular hemorrhage (149, 150, 168, 169). The hypothesis is that the effect is related to the vitamin's ability to scavenge free radicals, which then protects brain matrix capillary endothelial cells from hypoxic-ischemic injury. However, vitamin E in large doses cannot be recommended to prevent intraventricular hemorrhage at this time. Further study is required (128).

Serious toxicity has been associated with megavitamin E supplements in premature neonates (157). As reviewed elsewhere (170), the adverse effects may have been attributable to the vehicle used for megavitamin E supplementation rather than the tocopherol preparation per se. Doses of vitamin E exceeding 3.5 mg/kg/day by the parenteral route or 25 mg/kg/day by the enteral route should be regarded as experimental and having potentially more risk than benefit for premature neonates. It must be emphasized there is no compelling evidence to treat the premature infant with pharmacologic doses of vitamin E to prevent any condition.

VITAMIN K

Physiology/Biologic Mechanism of Action

Vitamin K is routinely administered in large quantities at the time of birth to all infants in the USA and Canada. It exists in two forms: (1) vitamin K_1 or phylloquinone, which is the plant form of the vitamin, and (2) vitamin K_2, a series of compounds with unsaturated side-chains of varying length, synthesized by bacteria and collectively referred to as menaquinones. The vitamin functions post-ribosomally as a cofactor in the metabolic conversion of intracellular precursors of vitamin K-dependent proteins to active forms. The coagulation factors II (prothrombin), VII, IX, and X were the first of these proteins to be described. Other vitamin K-dependent proteins in plasma include proteins C, S, and Z. Vitamin K-dependent proteins have been identified in nearly all tissues of the body. These include osteocalcin (bone gla protein), matrix gla protein of the skeleton, and kidney gla protein (171).

All of the known vitamin K-dependent proteins have in common γ-carboxyglutamic acid (Gla), the unique amino acid formed by the post-ribosomal action of vitamin K-dependent carboxylase. These Gla residues are located in the homologous amino-terminal domain with a high degree of amino acid sequence identity present in all vitamin K-dependent proteins (172). They are required for the calcium-mediated action of these proteins and are the location of specific calcium-binding sites. An overview of the current knowledge of vitamin K metabolism can be found in more detail elsewhere (171–174).

There is very little information on menaquinones in the perinatal period. Most of the bacteria comprising the normal intestinal flora of human milk-fed infants do not produce menaquinones, including *Bifidobacterium*, *Lactobacillus* and *Clostridium* species. Bacteria that produce menaquinones include *Bacteroides fragilis* and *Escherichia coli*, which are more common in formula-fed infants. Both phylloquinone and menaquinone are actually more prevalent in the stools of formula-fed infants (all formulas in the USA are fortified with phylloquinone) compared to breast-fed infants (175, 176). In the newborn liver, unlike adults, phylloquinone predominates over menaquinones (81 ± 73 vs. 9 ± 2 pmol/g/liver) (177). Menaquinones are not readily available from the hepatic pool (178), compared to phylloquinone. Little is known about their absorption from the intestinal tract, plasma transport, or clearance from circulation. Most of the gut bacterial pool of menaquinones, located within bacterial membranes, is probably not available for absorption. Thus, at first glance, menaquinones may not appear to be important in human nutrition. However, this view is complicated by the fact that there may be conversion of phylloquinone to menaquinone-4 in humans (174, 179, 180). Menaquinone-4 is utilized in infants, as supplementation with this form of vitamin K has eliminated hemorrhagic disease of the newborn in Japan (181).

Vitamin K_1 has been reported to be present in low (<2 µg/ml) to undetectable concentrations in cord blood (176, 182–184). One study demonstrated that of 156 cord bloods in term infants, none had measurable vitamin K (185). Thus, there is no correlation between maternal and cord blood levels. From all of the available evidence it appears that very small quantities of vitamin K cross the placenta from mother to fetus. Indeed, even maternal pharmacological doses of vitamin K have unpredictable effects on cord blood concentration (176, 182–184).

Vitamin K is absorbed from the intestine into the lymphatic system, requiring the presence of both bile salts and pancreatic secretions (186). The lymphatic system is the major route of intestinal transport of absorbed phylloquinone in association with chylomicrons. Little is known of the existence of carrier proteins. In the neonate, 29% of an oral dose of vitamin K_1 is reportedly absorbed from the intestine (187). The importance of the enterohepatic circulation of vitamin K in the human is unknown. Compared to other fat-soluble vitamins, relatively small amounts of vitamin K have been reported in the liver of the neonate. However, vitamin K is found in relatively high concentrations in liver, heart, and bone compared to other tissues (188, 189). In adult humans it has been demonstrated with labeled vitamin K_1 that the total body pool of vitamin K is replaced approximately every 2.5 h (190). This information is not available for infants.

Neonatal Requirements

Compared to the other fat-soluble vitamins, there is little specific information regarding the infant requirements for vitamin K. Vitamin K is found in the milk fat globules. Human milk generally contains less than 10 μg/L. The concentration is affected by maternal supplements One study found a concentration 3.0 ± 2.3 μg/L (SD) in six mothers delivering between 26 and 30 weeks gestation (191). By supplementing these mothers with 2.5 mg phylloquinone a day orally for 2 weeks the vitamin K concentration of the milk was increased to 64.2 ± 31.4 μg/L (SD) (191). In term infants, supplements of vitamin K to mothers will increase vitamin K in both breast milk and infant serum (192).

Though the official DRI for infants is 2–2.5 μg/d, it seems prudent to continue 1 mg of phylloquinone intramuscularly at birth to infants, given the low vitamin K content of human milk and the limited stores at birth. For preterm infants with birth weights <1000 g, 0.3 mg/kg intramuscularly would be sufficient (193). This amount of vitamin K should sustain the infant at least through the first 2 weeks of life.

As all infant formulas for low birth weight infants contain large amounts of vitamin K (65–100 μg/L), 150 ml/kg per day would supply 9.6–15.0 μg/kg/day. For the very low birth weight infant on vitamin K-supplemented formula, no additional vitamin K is needed. The available human milk fortifiers for the very low birth weight infants in the USA all contain vitamin K. Premature infants on formula or fortified human milk by 40 weeks postconceptional age have plasma vitamin K concentrations and intakes comparable to those of term infants on fortified formula (194).

For term infants on TPN solutions, multivitamin preparations will supply 200 μg per day. Intralipid (20%) contains 70 μg/dL of vitamin K. Thus, infants will also receive approximately 10 μg/kg/day with the typical 3 g/kg/day of Intralipid, which would achieve the RDA.

There would appear to be little justification for term infants on TPN to receive the additional large amounts of vitamin K in the multivitamin preparations. Preterm infants receiving 2 mL of M.V.I. Pediatric or Infuvite receive 80–100 μg/day in addition to the 10/μg/kg/day from 3 g/kg/day of Intralipid. A recent report found very high plasma levels (124.4 ± 101.1 ng/ml, adult normal <1 ng/ml) in preterm infants receiving TPN with multivitamins at 2 weeks of age (194). At present, an oral, liquid vitamin preparation for infants containing vitamin K is unavailable.

Laboratory Assessment of Vitamin K Status

In the neonate the concentrations of the vitamin K-dependent clotting factors (factors II, VII, IX, and X) are generally 25–70% of normal adult concentrations, and there is little difference at the time of birth between 30 and 40 weeks gestational age infants (195, 196). Normal adult concentrations of these factors are not achieved until 6 months of age. Premature infants may show an accelerated postnatal maturation towards adult levels compared to term infants. The prothrombin time has a wider range and variablity in the newborn at birth (11–16 s) compared to the adult (11–14 s), and this persists through the first 6 months of life. In contrast, the activated partial thromboplastin time shows a similar pattern compared to adults through the first 6 months of life (195, 196). Oddly enough, in the neonate, the prophylactic injection of vitamin K_1 does not significantly alter these tests or the measurements of the individual clotting factors (184, 197). Thus, the differences in coagulation between adults and newborns cannot totally be ascribed to vitamin K "deficiency." The coagulation differences may be limited by the availability of precursor proteins for the synthesis of vitamin K-dependent carboxylase enzymes of the vitamin K cycle, rather than the availability of vitamin K_1 itself.

Human vitamin K deficiency results in the secretion of partially carboxylated prothrombin into the plasma, referred to as abnormal prothrombin, or PIVKA-II (protein induced by vitamin K absence or antagonism) (198). PIVKA-II is a heterogeneous molecule. It consists of a mixed pool of partially and completely carboxylated prothrombin (199). Detection rates of PIVKA-II in cord blood have ranged from 10% to 30% (200–203). PIVKA-II values in a large series of full-term newborn infants in the USA at the time of birth have been reported. Of 148 cord bloods, 49/148 (33%) were positive for PIVKA-II (= 0.2 AU/ml) (185). A second study of 13 premature infants (27–36 weeks gestation) and 46 term infants (37–41 weeks) found no correlation between gestation age and PIVKA-II values in cord blood (204). Thirty-one infants (52%) had elevated PIVKA-II in cord blood. Finally, in another report in premature infants (24–36 weeks gestation), PIVKA-II levels were elevated in cord blood in 19/69 samples (27.5%) (194).

The usefulness of this measurement for showing a subclinical vitamin K deficiency is a point of controversy. A number of studies have shown that the initial prophylactic vitamin K administered to the newborn results in near elimination of the measurable PIVKA-II values that were present in cord blood at the time of birth (205–208). Similarly, in preterm infants PIVK-II is not detected at 2 and 6 weeks after birth with high intakes of vitamin K (194). In a study of exclusively breast-feeding infants who received vitamin K prophylaxis at birth (either orally or intramuscularly), there was no significant correlation between measurable PIVKA-II levels and low plasma vitamin K levels during the first 3 months of life (185). In general, normal values and standards of PIVKA-II measurements have not been established. In the newborn infant its usefulness as a predictor of subclinical vitamin K deficiency remains to be demonstrated.

Vitamin K Deficiency

As the vitamin K content of human milk is low and the newborn infant's stores of vitamin K are small, vitamin K deficiency with hemorrhage in the newborn is a worldwide problem. In the USA and Canada it is not a major concern as nearly all infants receive prophylactic vitamin K at the time of birth.

Though human milk does not supply the DRI for vitamin K of 2–2.5 µg/day for exclusively breast-fed infants, these infants generally do not show any signs of deficiency during the first 3 months of life if they received prophylactic vitamin K at birth (185). Formulas for term infants, with added vitamin K, supply 7–9 µg/kg/day, exceeding the RDA.

In the USA, the most common scenario for hemorrhagic disease of the newborn is in an exclusively breast-fed infant who does not receive vitamin K prophylaxis at birth, and may or may not have another disease that compromises vitamin K absorption, such as biliary atresia or α-1-antitrypsin deficiency. In the classic form of the disease, hemorrhage occurs between days 2 and 10 of life, and intracranial hemorrhage is uncommon. It is hallmarked by generalized ecchymoses and gastrointestinal bleeding. Bleeding from a circumcision site or umbilical cord stump is also common. A second form of the disease, late hemorrhagic disease, is less benign. Again, this form occurs mostly in breast-feeding infants between 6 weeks and 6 months of life and the associated intracranial hemorrhage results in devastating neurologic sequelae (209).

High-Dose Vitamin K for Infants/Toxicity

Pharmacologic doses of the vitamin are used in the newborn period for prevention of hemorrhagic disease. Historically, hyperbilirubinemia and kernicterus were reported in premature infants in the 1960s prophylactically treated with large quantities of a highly protein-bound form of the vitamin (menadione), no longer in clinical use (219). In term infants given 1 mg intramuscularly for newborn prophylaxis, there was an association reported with subsequent onset of childhood leukemia, but this initial report has not been confirmed (220).

A number of studies have tried to associate periventricular-intraventricular hemorrhage (PIVH) in the very low birth weight infant with vitamin K deficiency (210–215). Maternal supplements of vitamin K have been given as a result (216–218). However, given the very low transfer rate of vitamin K across the placenta and the mixed outcomes of these studies, one cannot conclude that PIVH in the premature infant is secondary to vitamin K deficiency at birth. In fact, it is clear that many cases of PIVH occur in infants 3 or more days after receiving the customary prophylactic dose of phylloquinone at birth, implying that vitamin K does not prevent PIVH. To date, toxicity from vitamin K has not been reported in the premature infant with the currently available formulations.

IRON

Physiology and Mechanisms of Action

One of the most controversial micronutrients for the newborn infant is iron, whether or not one is addressing the term or preterm infant. This is largely because of the worldwide distribution of iron deficiency, and because iron deficiency has long-term effects on neurodevelopment and behavior that may not be reversible. At the same time, too much iron is toxic, so that the therapeutic:toxic ratio is narrower than for most other nutrients. Controversies in the newborn include: appropriate laboratory measurements to define the deficiency state; the timing of onset of supplementation versus the potential for adverse effects of too much iron for preterm infants; the amount of iron in infant formula; and the timing of onset of supplementation for exclusively human-milk-fed infants.

Iron is a critical nutrient for many biological processes, including DNA replication and gene expression, cell respiration, including ATP formation, as well as transport and delivery of oxygen. It is required for erythropoiesis (hemoglobin formation), is an integral component of many enzymes essential for brain development, and critical for cardiac and skeletal muscle function (myoglobin).

As with calcium and many other minerals, 80% of the iron in the term infant is accumulated by the fetus between 24 and 40 weeks gestation at a rate of 1.6 to 2.0 mg/kg/day. Total body iron at the time of birth is roughly 75 mg/kg of body weight regardless of size of the infant; 75% of the iron is in the red blood cells and 15% in the liver at the time of birth (221–226).

Iron can be absorbed in both the organic and inorganic forms. The organic form, existing as ferritin or as hemoproteins, is highly bioavailable and contained in the liver and muscle of red meat. For newborn infants, not typically fed meat, this is not usually a source of dietary iron. The inorganic or ferrous form of iron, frequently used as a dietary supplement, can be chelated and precipitated by a number of dietary factors, making it much less bioavailable. These dietary factors include phytates, phosphates, tannates, oxalates, and carbonates. Studies with stable isotopes of Fe have measured the amount of inorganic iron absorption in preterm infants to be 34–42% of intake. This is more than the 7–12% of iron intake observed in term infants (227–229). Factors that enhance absorption in preterm infants include postnatal age, iron deficiency, dosing of iron between meals to include formula feeding, and normal vitamin C status (227–233). Factors that suppress Fe absorption include formula feeding (compared to human milk) and red-cell transfusions (234). Gestational age, postconceptional age, and rh-Epo therapy have minimal effect on Fe absorption (229, 230).

The absorption of Fe in adults occurs in the apical surfaces of the enterocytes of the duodenum. Organic or heme iron is transported into the enterocyte via the recently described heme carrier protein 1 (HCP1) (235). The exact pathway after entry into the enterocyte is unknown, though the heme oxygenase enzyme that frees iron from the protoprophyrin ring is known to be present in the microsomal fraction of the enterocyte (236). More is known about the absorption of non-heme iron. One pathway involves the reduction of ferric iron to the ferrous state, at the enterocyte brush border via the enzyme duodenal ferric reductase. Subsequently, divalent metal transporter 1 (DMT1) shuttles the reduced iron across the apical membrane (237).

Once the iron enters the enterocyte, it can be stored as ferritin for later use or sloughed off with the senescent enterocyte. Alternatively, the intracellular non-heme iron can be transported across the basolateral membrane via the non-heme iron transporter, ferroportin, into the circulation. It is an important exporter of intracellular Fe and is present on the basolateral surface of the enterocyte as well as on hepatocytes and macrophages.

Once in the circulation, iron binds to transferrin and is transported to the site of use or storage. Erythrocyte precursors express high levels of transferrin receptor 1 (TfR1) and thus have preferred access to circulating Fe. As red cells become senescent they are taken up by macrophages. Macrophages export the recovered Fe via ferroportin, the same transporter found on duodenal enterocytes. Iron is stored in the liver, which takes up the absorbed Fe from the portal system via TfR1 (238).

The human body is able to prioritize available iron both between and within organs. When iron is deficient, hepatic stores are depleted first, followed by lower-priority tissues such as skeletal muscle and the intestine. With a greater degree of iron deficiency, cardiac iron is compromised, followed by brain iron and finally red-cell iron. Thus, iron deficiency anemia represents a severe form of iron deficiency, and the prioritization of iron for red cells even over the brain accounts for the adverse neurodevelopmental effects of iron deficiency in the infant. Iron is essential for neuronal proliferation, myelination, energy metabolism, neurotransmission and various enzyme systems in the central nervous system (239). Intra-organ prioritization also occurs and this has been demonstrated in the developing rat brain. Within the neonatal rat brain, there is selective hippocampal and cortical vulnerability to perinatal iron deficiency (239).

As iron is prioritized to red cells, clearly its role in the transport of oxygen is its most critical function. Oxygen is reversibly bound to hemoglobin in the high pO_2 environment of the lungs and is released in the relatively low pO_2 environment of the tissues (238). The oxygen affinity is influenced by a number of factors, including the concentration of 2,3-diphosphoglycerate and pH. For the reversible oxygen binding to occur, the iron in the heme moiety must be maintained in the ferrous state. The red cells possess mechanisms to ensure that iron remains in the reduced ferrous state; however, in the face of oxidant drugs or toxins, genetic abnormalities in the red cells or abnormalities in hemoglobin itself, these protective mechanisms fail, resulting in nonfunctional hemoglobin. Muscle oxygen delivery is dependent in part on the tissue concentration of myoglobin. As with hemoglobin, myoglobin synthesis is impaired by iron deficiency. Low muscle myoglobin impairs oxygen delivery just as low hemoglobin concentrations in blood (238).

Neonatal Iron Requirements

From the large volume of available literature, the iron requirement for stable, growing preterm infants, whether feeding human milk or formula, is 2–4 mg/kg/day (240). This recommendation will be tempered by the amount of iron removed by phlebotomy, the number of transfusions of packed red blood cells (delivers 1 mg of elemental Fe per ml), and erythropoietin therapy (increases iron requirements). It seems unlikely that iron supplements are needed in the first 2 weeks of life in preterm infants, as erythropoietin levels are very low during this time. Once full enteral feedings are established, iron supplements may be started. In general this will be after 2 weeks but before 8 weeks of age. Though there are concerns about the oxidant effects of iron on diseases such as BPD and ROP, no study to date has demonstrated a cause-and-effect relationship between enteral iron intake and these oxidant-stress-related diseases. This may be secondary to the premature infant's ability to put iron into ferritin more effectively, or the overall slower delivery and incorporation of enteral iron supplements. Enteral iron supplementation is important, as iron deficiency may also play a role in the anemia of prematurity. Supplementation with 2–3 mg/kg/day of Fe started before hospital discharge in premature infants, even in the pre-erythropoietin era, has been shown to decrease the prevalence and degree of anemia in preterm infants (241–243). There is also good evidence to support iron supplementation after hospital discharge as well (241–243).

For infants maintained exclusively on TPN, iron supplementation is more problematic given the unknown risks of toxicity of intravenous iron in preterm infants. In the infant who is not growing or is receiving frequent transfusions while on TPN therapy, additional iron supplementation is not an issue.

Laboratory Assessment of Iron Deficiency

This has remained one of the most controversial issues in any pediatric age group, even though Fe-deficiency anemia is one of the most serious pediatric nutrient deficiencies on a worldwide basis. Perhaps the simplest measure of Fe deficiency is an increase in the hemoglobin of 1.0 g/dL after a month of appropriate iron intake. A recent WHO report recommended that populations be screened with hemoglobin, ferritin and CRP and/or serum transferrin receptor (244).

Serum ferritin is a sensitive measure of iron stores in healthy subjects (245). A concentration of 1 μg/L of serum ferritin corresponds to 8–10 mg of storage iron. Serum ferritin levels below 12 μg/L are specific for Fe deficiency and denote exhaustion of iron stores (245). However, a low serum ferritin does not indicate the severity of iron deficiency. Even more significantly, ferritin is an acute-phase reactant and its serum levels may be elevated in the presence of chronic inflammation, infection, malignancy, and liver disease (244–246). Hence the WHO's recommendation to always measure a CRP along with the serum ferritin (244). Serum ferritin measurements are readily available from most clinical laboratories. In children, a cut-off value of 10 μg/L has been suggested as opposed to 12 μg/L (247). In premature infants, plasma levels are elevated at birth and generally fall with increasing postnatal age. Thus, the cut-off values for ferritin in these infants may be up to 60 μg/L near the time of birth (246).

Serum transferrin receptor 1 (TfR1) is also a measure of iron status, detecting iron deficiency at the cellular level (248). TfR1 is found on cell membranes and allows iron-binding transferrin to enter the cell. When the iron supply is inadequate, there is an up-regulation of TfR1 to increase the cell's ability to compete for available iron. As the number of membrane receptors is proportional to the receptors found in plasma, an increase in circulating TfR1 is seen with iron-deficiency erythropoiesis or iron-deficiency anemia. When serum ferritin falls below 12 μg/L, the TfR1 beings to rise and is proportional to the deficit in functional iron (248, 249). It is not affected by inflammation like ferritin (249). It is a particularly useful measure of Fe deficiency in pregnancy as it declines rapidly with the mobilization of stores for the fetus and expansion of the mother's red cell mass. Unfortunately, for TfR1 there is no international standard and its measurement is not widely available. Normal values for infants and young children are unknown at this time (244).

Other investigators have advocated measuring the zinc protoporphyrin to hemoglobin ratio. This test effectively measures the Fe incorporation into protoporhyrin IX in red blood cells. When Fe is deficient, Zn is substituted for Fe in the protoporphyrin, and it is a functional measurement of Fe deficiency reflecting the balance between Fe stores and erythropoiesis (250, 251). Though this method shows promise and is relatively easy to measure, there are few data on its use as a diagnostic tool in infants (252, 253).

Thus, in balance, a reliable, sensitive, and specific method of determining Fe status in infants is not yet available.

Iron Deficiency and Toxicity

Though iron-deficiency anemia (IDA) is often equated with iron deficiency, IDA represents a severe form of the deficiency given the prioritization of iron for red blood cells, as discussed above. In other words, in a clinical situation of negative iron balance, iron deficiency occurs long before IDA. A major concern is the relationship of iron deficiency in infancy and early childhood, and later neurobehavioral development (253–260). Many studies have demonstrated an association between early iron deficiency and later cognitive deficits. Lozoff et al. have reported detecting cognitive deficits 10 years after the iron-deficient insult (261). However, in most of these studies there are many confounding variables, though Lozoff et al.'s work would indicate that iron supplementation (both low and high) is associated with improved neuro-development. A recent Cochrane review on this subject, looking at whether treatment of iron-deficiency anemia improved psychomotor development, concluded that there was unclear but plausible evidence (two randomized controlled trials) demonstrating improvement if the treatment extended more than 30 days in very young children (262). Another major concern in young children is that iron deficiency enhances lead absorption and the association between blood lead levels and iron deficiency (263). As childhood lead poisoning causes neurological and developmental deficits, iron deficiency may exacerbate this problem by enhancing lead absorption.

Much attention has been paid to potential iron deficiency in growing premature infants as well as exclusively breast-fed term infants beyond 4 months of life. Infants with intrauterine growth retardation and born to mothers with diabetes may also be at risk for iron deficiency (264, 265). Again, given the confounding variables in studies of these populations of infants, a direct causal relationship between iron deficiency and neurobehavorial deficits has not been made in developed countries.

Iron toxicity has been a major concern of medical care providers for infants. The premature infant has been thought to be at a higher risk for iron-induced oxidant injury, which may play a role in BPD, ROP, PIVH and NEC through tissue damage from iron-induced oxidant injury (266–271). Though some studies made the association of the total number of red blood cell transfusions (with their high Fe loads) and the prevalence of these disease states (266–271), the obvious confounding variable is that the smaller, sicker infants who get these diseases also receive the most transfusions. Interestingly enough, the more conservative transfusion practices of recent years in preterm infants have not impacted on the incidence of BPD,

PIVH, ROP,and NEC. A direct cause and effect of iron intake on these disorders has not been made in preterm infants to date.

REFERENCES

1. Lemons JA, Bauer CR, Oh W, et al. Very low birth weight outcomes of the National Institute of Child Health and Human Development Neonatal Research Network. January 1995 through December 1996. NICH Neonatal Research Network. NICH Neonatal Research Network. Pediatrics 2001; 107:E1.
2. Dusick AM, Poindexter BB, Ehrenkranz RA, et al. Growth failure in the preterm infant: can we catch up? Semin Perinatol 2003; 27:302.
3. Tfelt-Hansen J, Brown EM. The calcium-sensing receptor in normal physiology and pathophysiology: a review. Crit Rev Clin Lab Sci 2005; 42:35.
4. Riccardi D, Gamba G. The many roles of the calcium-sensing receptor in health and disease. Arch Med Res 1999; 30:436.
5. Dusso AS, Thadhani R, Slatopolsky E. Vitamin D receptor and analogs. Semin Nephrol 2004; 24:10.
6. Brown AJ, Dusso A, Slatopolsky EL. Vitamin D. Am J Physiol 1999; 277:F157.
7. Shaw JCL. Evidence of defective skeletal mineralization in low birthweight infants: the absorption of calcium and fat. Pediatrics 1976; 57:16.
8. Atkinson S, Tsang RC. Calcium, magnesium, phosphorus and vitamin D. In: Tsang RC, Uauy R, Kolezko B, Zlotkin SH, eds., Nutrition of the preterm infant: scientific basis and practical guidelines, 2nd edn. Cincinnati, OH, Digital Educational Publishing 2005; 245–276.
9. Hillman LS, Tack E, Covell DG, et al. Measurement of true calcium absorption in premature infants using intravenous ^{44}Ca and oral ^{45}Ca. Pediatr Res 1988; 23:589.
10. Barltrop D, Mole RH, Sutton A. Absorption and endogenous faecal excretion of calcium by low birth-weight infants on feeds with varying contents of calcium and phosphate. Arch Dis Child 1977; 52:41.
11. Standing Committee on the Scientific Evaluation of Dietary Reference Intakes, Food and Nutrition Board, Institute of Medicine: Dietary Reference Intakes. 1997; for calcium, pp. 71–149; vitamin D pp. 250–287.
12. Gartner LM, Greer FR. Section on Breastfeeding and Committee on Nutrition, American Academy of Pediatrics. Prevention of rickets and vitamin D deficiency: new guidelines for vitamin D intake. Pediatrics 2003; 111:908.
13. Rosli A, Fanconi A. Neonatal hypocalcemia. "Early type" in low birth weight newborn. Helv Paediatr 1973; 28:443.
14. Tsang RC, Light IJ, Sutherland JM, et al. Possible pathogenetic factors in neonatal hypocalcemia of prematurity. The role of gestation, hyperphosphatemia, hypomagnesemia, urinary calcium losses, and parathormone responsiveness. J Pediatr 1973; 82:423.
15. Brown DR, Tsang RC, Chen IW. Oral calcium supplementation in premature and asphyxiated neonates. J Pediatr 1976; 89:973.
16. Rosen JF, Roginsky M, Nathenson G, et al. 25-hydroxyvitamin D. Plasma levels in mothers and their premature infants with neonatal hypocalcemia. Am J Dis Child 1974; 127:220.
17. Hillman LS, Haddad GJ. Perinatal vitamin D metabolism III. Factors influencing late gestational human serum 25-hydroxyvitamin D. Am J Obset Gynecol 1976; 125:196.
18. Chan GM, Tsang RC, Chen IW, et al. The effects of 1,25(OH)$_2$ vitamin D supplementation in premature infants. J Pediatr 1978; 93:91.
19. Fleischman AR, Rosen JF, Nathenson G. 25-hydroxycholecalciferol for early neonatal hypocalcemia: Occurrence in premature newborns. Am J Dis Child 1978; 132:973.
20. Brown DR, Steranka BH, Taylor FH. Treatment of early onset neonatal hypocalcemia. Am J Dis Child 1981; 135:24.
21. David L, Salle B, Chopard P, et al. Studies on circulating immunoreactive calcitonin in low birth weight infants during the first 48 hours of life. Helv Paediatr Acta 1977; 32:39.
22. Moya M, Domenech E. Calcium intake in the first five days of life in the low birthweight infant. Effect of calcium supplements. Arch Dis Child 1978; 52:784.
23. Nelson N, Finnstrom O. Blood exchange transfusions in newborns, the effect on serum ionized calcium. Early Hum Dev 1988; 18:157.
24. Salle BL, David L, Chopard JP, et al. Prevention of early neonatal hypocalcemia in low birthweight infants with continuous calcium infusion: Effect on serum calcium, phosphorus, magnesium, and circulating immunoreactive parathyroid hormone and calcitonin. Pediatr Res 1977; 11:1180.
25. Mirror R, Brown DR. Parenteral calcium treatment shortened the left ventricular systolic time intervals of hyocalcemic neonates. Pediatr Res 1984; 18:71.
26. Salsburey DJ, Brown DR. Effect of parenteral calcium treatment on blood pressure and heart rate in neonatal hyocalcemia. Pediatrics 1982; 69:605.
27. Venkataraman PS, Wilson DA, Sheldon RE, et al. Effect of hypocalcemia on cardiac function in very-low-birth-weight preterm neonates. Studies of blood ionized calcium, echocardiography, and cardiac effect of intravenous calcium therapy. Pediatrics 1985; 76:543.
28. Troughton O, Singh SP. Heart failure and neonatal hypocalcemia. BMJ 4: 1972; 76.
29. Hammerman C, Eidelman AI, Gartner LM. Hypocalcemia and the patent ductus arteriosus. J Pediatr 1979; 94:961.

30. Lin CY, Ishida M. Calcium homeostasis in premature infants and treatment of early hypocalcaemia by 1,25-dihydroxycholecalciferol. Eur J Pediatr 1987; 146:383.
31. Salle BL, David L, Glorieux FH, et al. Early oral administration of vitamin D and its metabolites in premature neonates. Effect on mineral homeostasis. Pediatr Res 1982; 16:75.
32. Venkataraman PS, Tsang RC, Steichen JJ, et al. Early neonatal hypocalcemia in extremely premature infants. High incidence, early onset, and refractoriness to supraphysiologic doses of calcitriol. Am J Dis Child 1986; 140:1004.
33. Callenbach JC, Sheehan MB, Abramson SJ, et al. Etiologic factors of rickets in very low-birth-weight infants. J Pediatr 1981; 98:800.
34. Evans JR, Allen AC, Stinson DA, et al. Effect of high-dose vitamin D supplementation on radiographically detectable bone disease of very low birth weight infants. J Pediatr 1989; 115:779.
35. Koo WWK, Sherman R, Succop P, et al. Sequential bone mineral content in small preterm infants with and without fractures and rickets. J Bone Miner Res 1988; 3:193.
36. Lindroth M, Westgren U, Laurin S. Rickets in very-low-birth-weight infants. Acta Paediatr Scand 1986; 75:927.
37. Lyon AJ, McIntosh N, Wheeler K, et al. Radiological rickets in extremely low birthweight infants. Pediatr Radiol 1987; 17:56.
38. Masel JP, Tudehope D, Cartwright D, et al. Osteopenia and rickets in the extremely low birth-weight infants. Australia Radiol 1982; 1:83.
39. Griscom NT, Craig MN, Newhauser EBF. Systemic bone disease developing in small premature infants. Pediatrics 1971; 48:883.
40. Opperheimer SJ, Snodgrass GJAI. Neonatal rickets. Arch Dis Child 1980; 55:945.
41. Frost HM. Perspectives: A proposed general model of the "mechanostat" (suggestions from a new paradigm). Anat Rec 1996; 244:139.
42. Miller ME. The bone disease of preterm birth; a biomechanical perspective. Pediatr Res 2003; 53:10.
43. Rauch F, Schoenau E. Skeletal development in premature infants; a review of bone physiology beyond nutritional aspects. Arch Dis Child Fetal Neonatal Ed 2002; 86:F82.
44. Beyers N, Alhert B, Taijaard JF, et al. High turnover osteopenia in preterm infants. Bone 1994; 15:5.
45. Greer FR, Chen X, McCormick A. Urinary hydroxyproline: Relationships to growth, bone mineral content, and serum alkaline phosphatase in premature infants. J Pediatr Gastroenterol Nutr 1991; 13:176.
46. Mora S, Weber G, Bellini A, et al. Bone modeling alteration in preterm infants. Arch Pediatr Adolesc Med 1994; 148:1215.
47. Moyer-Mileur L, Luetkemeier M, Boomer L, et al. Effect of physical activity on bone mineralization in premature infants. J Pediatr 1995; 127:620.
48. Moyer-Mileur LJ, Brunstetter V, McNaught TP, et al. Daily physical activity program increases bone mineralization and growth in preterm very low birth weight infants. Pediatrics 2000; 106:1088.
49. Nemet D, Dolfin T, Litmanowitz I, et al. Evidence for exercise-induced bone formation in premature infants. Int J Sports Med 2002; 23:82.
50. Aly H, Moustafa MF, Hassanein SM, et al. Physical activity combined with massage improves bone mineralization in premature infants: a randomized trial. J Perinatol 2004; 24:305.
51. Backstrom MC, Maki R, Kuusela A-L, et al. Randomized controlled trial of vitamin D supplementation on bone density and biochemical indices in preterm infants. Arch Dis Child Fetal Neonatal Ed 1999; 80:F161.
52. Greer FR. Determination of radial bone mineral content in low birth weight infants by photon absorptiometry. J Pediatr 1988; 113:213.
53. Mazess RB, Peppler WW, Chesney RW, et al. Does bone measurement of the radius indicate skeletal status? J Nucl Med 1984; 25:281.
54. Chesney RW. The assessment of bone mineral status and mineral dietary adequacy. In: Tsang RC, Mimouni F, eds., Calcium nutriture for mothers and children. Carnation nutrition educational series, vol 3. New York, Glendale/Raven 1992 101–128.
55. Nemet D, Dolfin T, Wolach B, et al. Quantitative ultrasound measurements of bone speed of sound in premature infants. Eur J Pediatr 2001; 160:736.
56. Koo WWK, Tsang RC, Succop P, et al. Minimal vitamin D and high calcium and phosphorus needs of preterm infants receiving parenteral nutrition. J Pediatr Gastroenterol Nutr 1989; 8:225.
57. Schanler RJ, Burns PA, Abrams SA, et al. Bone mineralization outcomes in human milk-fed preterm infants. Pediatr Res 1992; 31:583.
58. Horseman A, Ryan SW, Congdon PJ, et al. Bone mineral content and body size 65 to 100 weeks postconception in preterm and full term infants. Arch Dis Child 1989; 64:1579.
59. Chan GM, Mileur LJ. Posthospitalization growth and bone mineral status of normal preterm infants. Feeding with mother's milk or standard formula. Am J Dis Child 1985; 139:896.
60. Abrams SA, Schanler R, Garza C. Bone mineralization in former very low birth weight infants fed either human milk or commercial formula. J Pediatr 1988; 112:956.
61. Kreiter SR, Schwartz RP, Kirkman HN Jr, et al. Nutritional rickets in African American breast-fed infants. J Pediatr 2000; 137:153.
62. Pugliese MF, Blumberg DL, Hludzinski J, et al. Nutritional rickets in suburbia. J Am Coll Nutr 1998; 17:637.
63. Sills IN, Skuza KA, Horlick MN, et al. Vitamin D deficiency rickets. Reports of its demise are exaggerated. Clin Pediatr (Phila) 1994; 33:491.
64. Ward LM. Vitamin D deficiency in the 21st century: a persistent problem among Canadian infants and mothers. CMAJ 2005; 172:769.

65. Weisberg P, Scanlon KS, Li R, et al. Nutritional rickets among children in the United States: review of cases reported between 1986–2003. Am J Clin Nutr 2004; 80:1697S.

66. Lamin-Keefe CJ. Vitamin D and E in human milk. In: Jensen RD, ed., Handbook of milk composition. San Diego, CA, Academic Press 1995 706–717.

67. Webb AR, Kline L, Hollick MF. Influence of season and latitude on the cutaneous synthesis of vitamin D$_3$: exposure to winter sunlight in Boston and Edmonton will not promote vitamin D$_3$ synthesis in human skin. J Clin Endocrinol Metab 1988; 67:373.

68. Ong DE. Absorption of vitamin A. In: Blomhoff R, ed., Vitamin A in health and disease. New York, Marcel Dekker 1994 37–72.

69. Blomhoff R. Transport and metabolism of vitamin A. Nutr Rev 1994; 52:513.

70. Shenai JP, Chytil F, Stahlman MT. Liver vitamin A reserves of very low birth weight neonates. Pediatr Res 1985; 19:892.

71. Olson JA, Gunning DB, Tilton RA. Liver concentrations of vitamin A and carotenoids, as a function of age and other parameters of American children who died of various causes. Am J Clin Nutr 1984; 39:903.

72. Hugue T. A survey of human liver reserves of retinol in London. Br J Nutr 1982; 47:165.

73. Soprano DR, Blaner WS. Plasma retinol-binding proteins. In: Sporn MB, Roberts AB, Goodman DS, eds., The retinoids, 2nd edn. Orlando, Academic Press 1994 257–282.

74. Shenai JP, Chytil F, Jhaveri A, et al. Plasma vitamin A and retinol binding protein in premature and term neonates. J Pediatr 1981; 99:302.

75. Canfield LM, Giuliano AR, Graver EJ. Carotenoids, retinoids, and vitamin K in human milk. In: Jensen RD, ed., Handbook of milk composition. San Diego, CA, Academic Press 1995 693–705.

76. Shenai JP, Kennedy KA, Chytil F, et al. Clinical trial of vitamin A supplementation in infants susceptible to bronchopulmonary dysplasia. J Pediatr 1987; 111:269.

77. Shenai JP, Rush MG, Stahlman MT, et al. Plasma retinol binding protein response to vitamin A administration in infants susceptible to bronchopulmonary dysplasia. J Pediatr 1990; 116:607.

78. Howard L, Chu R, Feman S, et al. Vitamin A deficiency from long-term parenteral nutrition. Ann Intern Med 1980; 93:576.

79. Silvers KM, Sluis KB, Darlow BA, et al. Limiting light-induced lipid peroxidation and vitamin loss in infant parenteral nutrition by adding multivitamin preparations to intralipid. Acta Paediatr 2001; 90:242.

80. Laborie S, Lavoi JC, Pineault M, et al. Contribution of multivitamins, air, and light in the generation of peroxides in adult and neonatal parenteral nutrition solutions. Ann Pharmacother 2000; 34:440.

81. Chessex P, Laborie S, Lavoie JC, et al. Photoprotection of solutions of parenteral nutrition decreases the infused load as well as the urinary excretion of peroxidies in premature infants. Semin Perinatol 2001; 25:55.

82. Olson JA. Serum levels of vitamin A and carotenoids as reflectors of nutritional status. J Natl Cancer Inst 1984; 73:1439.

83. Meyer KA, Popper H, Steigmann F, et al. Comparison of vitamin A of liver biopsy specimens with plasma vitamin A in man. Proc Soc Exp Biol Med 1942; 49:589.

84. Montreewasuwat N, Olson JA. Serum and liver concentrations of vitamin A in Thai fetuses as a function of gestational age. Am J Clin Nutr 1979; 32:601.

85. Zachman RD, Samuels DP, Brand JM, et al. Use of the intramuscular relative dose response test to predict bronchopulmonary dysplasia in premature infants. Am J Clin Nutr 1996; 63:123.

86. Tyson JE, Wright LL, Oh W, et al. Vitamin A supplementation for extremely-low-birth-weight infants. N Engl J Med 1999; 340:1962.

87. Bental RY, Cooper PA, Cummins RR, et al. Vitamin A therapy-effects on the incidence of bronchopulmonary dysplasia. S Afr J Food Sci Nutr 1994; 6:141.

88. Paragaroufalis C, Cairis M, Pantazatou E, et al. A trial of vitamin A supplementation in infants susceptible to bronchopulmonary dysplasia (abstract). Pediatr Res 1988; 23:518A.

89. Wardle SP, Hughes A, Chen S, et al. Randomized controlled trial of oral vitamin A supplementation in preterm infants to prevent chronic lung disease. Arch Dis Child Fetal Neonatal Ed 2001; 84:F9.

90. Agaoestina T, Humphrey JH, Taylor GA, et al. Safety of one 52-μmol (50,000 IU) oral dose of vitamin A administered to neonates. Bull World Health Org 1994; 72:859.

91. Robens JR. Teratogenic effects of hypervitaminosis A in the hamster and guinea pig. Toxicol Appl Pharmacol 1970; 16:88.

92. Geelan JCA. Hypervitaminosis A-induced teratogensis. CRC Crit Rev Toxicol 1979; 6:351.

93. Rothman KJ, Moore LL, Singer MR, et al. Teratogenicity of high vitamin A intake. N Engl J Med 1995; 333:1369.

94. Lammer EJ, Chen DT, Hoar RM, et al. Retinoic acid embryopathy. N Engl J Med 1985; 313:837.

95. Benke PJ. The isotretinoin teratogen syndrome. JAMA 1984; 251:3267.

96. Lott IT, Bocian M, Pribram HW, et al. Fetal hydrocephalus and ear anomalies associated with maternal use of isotretinoin. J Pediatr 1984; 105:597.

97. Darlow BA, Graham PJ. Vitamin A supplementation for preventing morbidity and mortality in very low birthweight infants (Cochrane Review). The Cochrane Library, Issue 2. Oxford, Update Software 2001.

98. Robbins ST, Fletcher AB. Early vs. delayed vitamin A supplementation in very-low-birth-weight infants. J Parenter Enteral Nutr 1993; 17:220.

99. Rush MG, Shenai JP, Parker RA, et al. Intramuscular versus enteral vitamin A supplementation in very low birth weight neonates. J Pediatr 1994; 125:458.

100. Schwartz KB, Cox JM, Clement L, et al. Possible antioxidant effect of vitamin A supplementation in premature infants. J Pediatr Gastro Nutr 1997; 25:408.

101. Pearson E, Bose C, Snidow T, et al. Trial of vitamin A supplementation in very low birth weight infants at risk for bronchopulmonary dysplasia. J Pediatr 1992; 121:420.

102. Burton GW, Traber GW. Vitamin E. antioxidant activity, biokinetics and bioavailability. Annu Rev Nutr 1990; 10:357.

103. Dju MY, Mason KI, Filer LI. Vitamin E (tocopherol) in human fetuses and placentae. Etudes Neonatales 1952; 1:46.

104. Cruz CS, Wimberley PD, Johansen K, et al. The effect of vitamin E on erythrocyte hemolysis and lipid peroxidation in newborn premature infants. Acta Paediatr Scand 1983; 72:823.

105. Mino M, Nishimo H. Fetal and maternal relationship in serum vitamin E level. J Nutr Sci Vitaminol 1973; 19:475.

106. Farrell PM. Vitamin E. In: Shils M, Young V, eds., Modern nutrition in health and disease. Philadelphia, Lea & Febeger 1988 340.

107. Farrell PM, Zachman RD, Gutcher GR. Fat soluble vitamins A, E, and K in the premature infant. In: Tsang RC, ed., Vitamin and mineral requirements in preterm infants. New York, Marcel Dekker 1985 63–98.

108. Bieri JG, Farrell PM. Vitamin E. Vitam Horm 1976; 34:31.

109. Farrell PM, Bieri JG, Fratantoni JF, et al. The occurrence and effects of human vitamin E deficiency: A study in patients with cystic fibrosis. J Clin Invest 1977; 60:233.

110. Losowky MS, Kelleher J, Walker BE. Intake and absorption of tocopherol. Ann NY Acad Sci 1972; 203:212.

111. Bieri JG, Evarts RP. Effect of plasma lipid levels and obesity on tissue stores of α-tocopherol. Proc Soc Exp Biol Med 1975; 149:500.

112. Bieri JG. Kinetics of tissue α-tocopherol depletion and repletion. Ann NY Acad Sci 1972; 203:181.

113. Traber MG, Burton GW, Hughes L, et al. Discrimination between forms of vitamin E by humans with and without genetic abnormalities of lipoprotein metabolism. J Lipid Res 1992; 33:1171.

114. Traber MG, Sokol RJ, Kohlschutter A, et al. Impaired discrimination between stereoisomers of α-tocopherol in patients with familial isolated vitamin E deficiency. J Lipid Res 1993; 34:201.

115. Traber MG. Determinants of plasma vitamin E concentrations. Free Rad Biol Med 1994; 16:229.

116. Doerfllinger N, Linder C, Puahchi K, et al. Ataxia with vitamin E deficiency: refinement of genetic localization and analysis of linkage disequilibrium by using new markers in 14 families. Am J Hum Genet 1995; 56:1116.

117. Sokol RJ, Kayden HJ, Bettis DB, et al. Isolated vitamin E deficiency in the absence of fat malabsorption – familial and sporadic cases: characterization and investigation of causes. J Lab Clin Med 1988; 111:548.

118. Ben Hamida C, Doerflilnger N, Belal S, et al. Localization of Friedreich ataxia phenotype with selective vitamin E deficiency to chromosome 8q by homozygosity mapping. Nature Genet 1993; 5:195.

119. Ben Hamida M, Belal S, Sirugo G, et al. Friedreich's ataxia phenotype not linked to chromosome 9 and associated with selective autosomal recessive vitamin E deficiency in two inbred Tunisian families. Neurology 1993; 43:2179.

120. Ouahchi K, Arita M, Kayden H, et al. Ataxia with isolated vitamin E deficiency is caused by mutations in the α-tocopherol transfer protein. Nature Genet 1995; 9:141.

121. Lammi-Keefe CJ. Vitamin D and E in human milk. In: Jensen RD, ed., Handbook of milk composition. San Diego, CA: Academic Press 1995 706–717.

122. Food and Nutrition Board, Institute of Medicine, Dietary Reference Intakes for Vitamin C, Vitamin E, Selenium, and Carotinoids. Washington DC, National Academy Press 2000 186–283.

123. Huijbers WAR, Schrijver J, Speek AJ, et al. Persistent low plasma vitamin E levels in premature infants surviving respiratory distress syndrome. Eur J Pediatr 1986; 145:170.

124. Gross SJ, Gabriel E. Vitamin E status in preterm infants fed human milk or infant formula. J Pediatr 1985; 106:634.

125. Hittner HM, Speer ME, Rudolph AJ, et al. Retrolental fibroplasia and vitamin E in the preterm infant – comparison of oral versus intramuscular administration. Pediatrics 1984; 73:238.

126. Ronnholm KAR, Dostalova L, Simes MA. Vitamin E supplementation in very-low-birth-weight infants: Long-term follow-up at two different levels of vitamin E supplementation. Am J Clin Nutr 1989; 49:121.

127. Friedman CA, Wender DF, Temple DM, et al. Serum alpha-tocopherol concentrations in preterm infants receiving less than 25 mg/kg/day alpha-tocopherol acetate supplements. Dev Pharmacol Ther 1988; 11:273.

128. Laro MR, Wojewardine K, Wald NJ. Is routine vitamin E administration justified in very low-birthweight infants? Dev Med Child Neurol 1990; 32:442.

129. Farrell PM. Vitamin E deficiency in premature infants. J Pediatr 1979; 95:869.

130. Banagale RC, Bray JJ, Erenberg AP. Serum free tocopherol levels in premature infants (PI) receiving total parenteral nutrition (TPN). Pediatr Res 1981; 15:492A.

131. Phillips B, Franck LS, Greene HL. Vitamin E levels in premature infants during and after intravenous multivitamin supplementation. Pediatrics 1987; 80:680.

132. Gutcher GR, Farrell PJM. Early intravenous correction of vitamin E deficiency in premature infants. J Pediatr Gastroenterol Nutr 1985; 4:604.

133. Greene HL, Hambridge KM, Schanler R, et al. Guidelines for the use of vitamins, trace elements, calcium, magnesium, and phosphorus in infants and children receiving total parenteral nutrition:

report of the Subcommittee on Pediatric Parenteral Nutrient Requirements from the Committee on Clinical Practice Issues of The American Society for Clinical Nutrition. Am J Clin Nutr 1988; 48:1324.

134. American Academy of Pediatrics, Committee on Nutrition. Nutritional Needs of Preterm Infant, Pediatric Nutrition Handbook, 5th edn. American Academy of Pediatrics 2003 23–46.

135. Farrell PM. Vitamin E. A comprehensive treatise. In: Machlin LJ, ed., Human health and disease. New York, Marcel Dekker 1980 519–620.

136. Farrell PM, Levine SL, Murphy MD, et al. Plasma tocopherol levels and tocopherol-lipid relationships in a normal population of children as compared to health adults. Am J Clin Nutr 1978; 31:1720.

137. Horwitt MK, Harvey CC, Dahm CH Jr, et al. Relationship between tocopherol and serum lipid levels for determination of nutritional adequacy. Ann NY Acad Sci 1972; 203:223.

138. Sokol RJ, Heubi JE, Iannacone ST, et al. Vitamin E deficiency with normal serum vitamin E concentrations in children with chronic cholestasis. N Engl J Med 1984; 310:1209.

139. Gutcher GR, Raynor WJ, Farrell PM. An evaluation of vitamin E status in premature infants. Am J Clin Nutr 1984; 40:1078.

140. Van Zoeren-Grobben D, Jacobs NJM, Houdkamp E, et al. Vitamin E status in preterm infants: Assessment by plasma and erythrocyte vitamin E-lipid ratios and hemolysis tests. J Pediatr Gastro Nutr 1998; 26:73.

141. Oski FA, Barness LA. Vitamin E deficiency: A previously unrecognized cause of hemolytic anemia in the premature infant. J Pediatr 1967; 70:211.

142. Horwitt MK, Bailey P. Cerebellar pathology in an infant resembling chick nutritional encephalomalacia. Arch Neural Psychiatr 1959; 95:869.

143. Ehrenkranz RA, Bonta BW, Ablow RC, et al. Amelioration of bronchopulmonary dysplasia after vitamin E administration: A preliminary report. N Engl J Med 1979; 229:564.

144. Johnson L, Schaffer D, Quinn G, et al. Vitamin E supplementation and the retinopathy of prematurity. Ann NY Acad Sci 1982; 393:473.

145. Hittner HM, Godio LB, Rudolph AJ, et al. Retrolental fibroplasia: Efficacy of vitamin E in a double-blind clinical study of preterm infants. N Engl J Med 1981; 305:1365.

146. Hittner HM, Godio LB, Speer MI, et al. Retrolental fibroplasia: Further clinical evidence and ultrastructural support for efficacy of vitamin E in the preterm infants. Pediatrics 1983; 71:423.

147. Kretzer FL, Hittner JM, Johnson AT, et al. Vitamin E and retrolental fibroplasia: ultrastructural support of clinical efficacy. Ann NY Acad Sci 1982; 393:145.

148. Sokol RJ. Vitamin E deficiency and neurologic disease. Am Rev Nutr 1988; 8:351.

149. Chiswick ML, Johnson M, Woodhall C, et al. Protective effect of vitamin E (dl-alpha-tocopherol) against intraventricular hemorrhage in premature babies. Br Med J 1983; 287:81.

150. Speer ME, Blifeld C, Rudolph AJ, et al. Intraventricular hemorrhage and vitamin E in the very low-birth-weight infant: Evidence of efficacy of early intramuscular vitamin E administration. Pediatrics 1984; 74:1107.

151. Ehrenkranz RA, Ablow RC, Warshaw JB. Effect of vitamin E on the development of oxygen-induced lung injury in neonates. Ann NY Acad Sci 1982; 393:452.

152. Phelps DL, Rosenbaum AL, Isenberg SJ, et al. Tocopherol efficacy and safety for preventing retinopathy of prematurity: A randomized, controlled, double-masked trial. Pediatrics 1987; 79:489.

153. Bell EF. Prevention of bronchopulmonary dysplasia: Vitamin E and other antioxidants. In: Farrell PM, Tausing LM, eds., Bronchopulmonary dysplasia and related chronic respiratory disorders. Report of the Nineteenth Ross Conference on Pediatric Research. Columbus, OH: Ross Laboratories 1986 77–82.

154. Greene HL, Moore MEC, Phillips B, et al. Evaluation of a pediatric multiple vitamin preparation for total parenteral nutrition. II. Blood levels of vitamins A, D, and E. Pediatrics 1986; 77:539.

155. Bougle D, Boutroy MJ, Heng J, et al. Plasma kinetics of parenteral tocopherol in premature infants. Dev Pharmacol Ther 1986; 9:310.

156. Knight ME, Roberts RJ. Disposition of intravenously administered pharmacologic doses of vitamin E in newborn rabbits. J Pediatr 1986; 108:145.

157. Balistreri WF, Farrell MK, Bove KE. Lessons from the E-ferol tragedy. Pediatrics 1986; 78:503.

158. Melhorn DK, Gross S. Vitamin E-dependent anemia in the premature infant. II. Relationships between gestational age and absorption of vitamin E. Pediatrics 1971; 79:581.

159. Gutcher GR, Lax AM, Farrell PM. Tocopherol isomers in intravenous lipid emulsions and resultant plasma concentrations. J Parent Enteral Nutr 1984; 8:269.

160. Gross S, Melhorn DK. Vitamin E, red cell lipids and red cell stability in prematurity. Ann NY Acad Sci 1972; 203:141.

161. Owens WC, Owens EU. Retrolental fibroplasia in premature infants. Am J Ophthalmol 1949; 32:1631.

162. Taju TNK, Langenberg P, Bhutani V, et al. Vitamin E prophylaxis to reduce retinopathy of prematurity: A reappraisal of published trials. J Pediatr 1997; 131:844.

163. Milner RA, Watts JL, Paes B, et al. RLF in <1500 gram neonates. Part of a randomized clinical trial of the effectiveness of vitamin E, Retinopathy of Prematurity Conference. Columbus, OH: Ross Laboratories 1981 703–716.

164. Finer NN, Schindler RF, Grant G, et al. Effect of intramuscular vitamin E on frequency and severity of retrolental fibroplasia. A controlled trial. Lancet 1982; 1:1087.

165. Puklin JE, Simon RM, Ehrenkranz RA. Influence on retrolental fibroplasia of intramuscular vitamin E administration during respiratory distress syndrome. Ophthalmology 1982; 89:96.

166. Saldanha RL, Cepeda EE, Poland RL. The effect of vitamin E prophylaxis on the incidence and severity of bronchopulmonary dysplasia. J Pediatr 1982; 101:89.

167. Watts JL, Milner R, Zipursky A, et al. Failure of supplementation with vitamin E to prevent bronchopulmonaory dysplasia in infants <1500 g birthweight. Eur Respir J 1991; 4:188.

168. Chiswick M, Gladman G, Sinba S, et al. Vitamin E supplementation and periventricular hemorrhage in the newborn. Am J Clin Nutr 1991; 53:370.

169. Fish WH, Cohen M, Franzek E, et al. Effect of intramuscular vitamin E on mortality and intracranial hemorrhage in neonates of 1,000 grams or less. Pediatrics 1990; 85:578.

170. Slagle TA, Gross SJ. Vitamin E. In: Tsang RC, Nichols BL, eds., Nutrition during infancy. Philadelphia, Hanley & Belfus 1988 277–288.

171. Greer FR, Zachman RD. Neonatal vitamin metabolism. Fat soluble. In: Cowett RM, ed., Principles of perinatal-neonatal metabolism. New York, Springer 1998 943.

172. Suttie JW. Synthesis of vitamin K-dependent proteins. FASEB J 1993; 7:445.

173. Dowd P, Ham SW, Naganathan S, et al. The mechanism of action of vitamin K. Annu Rev Nutr 1995; 15:419.

174. Ferland G. The vitamin K-dependent proteins: An update. Washington: Nutrition Reviews; August 1999:1–9.

175. Fujita K, Kakuya F, Ito S. Vitamin K_1 and K_2 status and fecal flora in breast fed and formula fed 1-month-old infants. Eur J Pediatr 1993; 152:852.

176. Greer FR, Mummah-Schendel LL, Marshall S, et al. Vitamin K_1 (phylloquinone) and vitamin K_2 (menaquinone) status in newborn during the first week of life. Pediatrics 1988; 81:137.

177. Kayata S, Kindberg C, Greer FR, et al. Vitamin K_1 and K_2 in infant human liver. J Pediatr Gastroenterol Nutr 1989; 8:304.

178. Suttie JW. The importance of menaquinones in human nutrition. Annu Rev Nutr 1995; 15:399.

179. Thijssen HHW, Drittij-Reijnders MJ. Vitamin K distribution in rat tissue: dietary phylloquinone is a source of tissue menaquinone-4. Brit J Nutr 1994; 72:415.

180. Thijssen HH, Drittij MJ, Vermeer C, et al. Menaquinone-4 in breast milk is derived from dietary phylloquinone. Brit J Nutr 2002; 87:219.

181. Matsuzaka T, Muneyoshi Y, Tsuji Y. Prophylaxis of intracranial hemorrhage due to vitamin K deficiency in infants. Brain Dev 1987; 9:305.

182. Pietersma-deBruyn ALJM, Van Haard PMM. Vitamin K_1 in the newborn. Clin Chim Acta 1985; 150:95.

183. Shearer MJ, Barkhan P, Rahim S, et al. Plasma vitamin K_1 in mothers and their newborn babies. Lancet 1982; 2:460.

184. Mandelbrot L, Guillaumont M, Leclercq M, et al. Placental transfer of vitamin K_1 and its implication in fetal hemostasis. Thromb Haemost 1988; 60:39.

185. Greer FR, Marshall SP, Severson RR, et al. A new mixed-micellar preparation for oral vitamin K prophylaxis. Comparisons with an intramuscular formulation in breast-fed infants. Arch Dis Child 1998; 79:300.

186. Blomstrand R, Forsgren L. Vitamin K_1 ^3H in man: its intestinal absorption and transport in the thoracic duct lymph. Int Z Vitam Forschung 1968; 38:45.

187. Sann L, Leclercq M, Guillaumont M, et al. Serum vitamin K_1 concentrations after oral administration of vitamin K_1 in low birth weight infants. J Pediatr 1985; 107:608.

188. Thijssen JW, Drittij-Reijnders MJ, Fischer MAJG. Phylloquinoine and menaquinone-4 distribution in rats: Synthesis rather than uptake determines menaquinone-4 organ concentrations. J Nutr 1996; 126:537.

189. Hodges SJ, Bejui J, Leclercq M, et al. Detection and measurement of vitamins K_1 and K2 in human cortical and trabecular bone. J Bone Miner Res 1993; 8:1005.

190. Bjornsson TD, Meffin PG, Swezey SE, et al. Disposition and turnover of vitamin K_1 in man. In: Suttie JW, ed., Vitamin K metabolism and Vitamin K-dependent proteins. Baltimore, University Park Press 1980 328–332.

191. Bolisetty S, Gupta GG, Salonikas C, et al. Vitamin K in preterm breastmilk with maternal supplementation. Acta Paediatr 0998; 87:96.

192. Greer FR, Marshall S, Suttie JW. Improving the vitamin K status of breast-feeding infants with maternal vitamin K supplements. Pediatrics 1997; 99:88.

193. Dietary reference intakes for vitamin A, vitamin K, arsenic, boron, chromium, copper, iodine, manganese, molybdenum, silicon, vanadium and zinc. Food and Nutrition Board, Institute of Medicine. Washington, DC: National Academic Press; 2002.

194. Kumar D, Greer FR, Super DM, et al. Vitamin K status of premature infants. Implications for current recommendations. Pediatrics 2001; 108:1117.

195. Andrew M, Paes B, Milner R, et al. Development of the human coagulation system in the full-term infant. Blood 1987; 70:165.

196. Andrew M, Paes B, Milner R, et al. Development of the human coagulation system in the healthy premature infant. Blood 1988; 72:1651.

197. Göbel U, Sonnenschein-Kosenow S, Petrich C, et al. Vitamin K deficiency in the newborn. Lancet 1977; 2:187.

198. Von Kries R, Greer FP, Suttie JW. Assessment of vitamin K status of the newborn infant. J Pediatric Gastroenterol Nutr 1993; 16:231.

199. Liska DJ, Suttie JW. Location of gamma-carboxyglutamy residues in partially carboxylated prothrombin preparations. Biochemistry 1988; 27:8636.

200. Von Kries R, Shearer MJ, Widdershoven J, et al. Des-gamma-carboxyprothrombin (PIVKA-II) and plasma vitamin K_1 in newborns and their mothers. Thromb Haemost 1992; 68:383.

201. Bovill EG, Soll RF, Lynch M, et al. Vitamin K_1 metabolism and the production of descarboxypro-thrombin and protein C in the term and premature neonate. Blood 1993; 81:77.

202. Motahara K, Endo F, Matsuda I. Effect of vitamin K administration on a carboxyprothrombin (PIVKA-II) levels in newborns. Lancet 1985; 2:242.

203. Motohara K, Takayi S, Endo F, et al. Oral supplementation of vitamin K for pregnant women and effects on levels of plasma vitamin K and PIVKA-II in the neonate. J Pediatr Gastroenterol Nutr 1990; 11:32.

204. Greer FR, Costakos DT, Suttie JW. Determination of des-gamma-carboxy-prothrombin (PIVKA II) in cord blood of various gestational ages with the STAGO antibody – a marker of vitamin K deficiency? Pediatr Res 1999; 45:283.

205. Widdershoven J, Lambert W, Motohara K, et al. Plasma concentrations of vitamin K_1 and PIVKA-II in bottle-fed and breast-fed infants with and without vitamin K prophylaxis at birth. Eur J Pediatr 1988; 148:139.

206. Cornelissen E, Kollée L, DeAbreu R, et al. Effects of oral and intramuscular vitamin K prophylaxis on vitamin K_1, PIVKA-II and clotting factors in breast-fed infants. Arch Dis Child 1992; 67:1250.

207. Cornelissen E, Kollée L, DeAbreu R, et al. Prevention of vitamin K deficiency in infancy by weekly administration of vitamin K. Acta Pediatr 1983; 82:656.

208. Cornelissen E, Kollée L, van Lith T, et al. Evaluation of a daily dose of 25 mg vitamin K_1 to prevent vitamin K deficiency in breast-fed infants. J Pediatr Gastroenterol Nutr 1993; 16:301.

209. Greer FR. Vitamin K deficiency and hemorrhage in infancy. Clin Perinatol 1995; 22:759.

210. Gray OP, Ackerman A, Fraser AJ. Intracranial hemorrhage and clotting defects in low-birth-weight infants. Lancet 1968; 1:545.

211. Cole VA, Durbin M, Olaffson A, et al. Pathogenesis of intraventricular haemorrhage in newborn infants. Arch Dis Child 1974; 49:722.

212. Setzer ES, Webb IB, Wassenaar JW, et al. Platelet dysfunction and coagulopathy in intraventricular hemorrhage in the premature infant. J Pediatr 1982; 100:599.

213. MacDonald MM, Johnson ML, Rumack CM, et al. Role of coagulopathy in newborn intracranial hemorrhage. Pediatrics 1984; 74:26.

214. Beverly DW, Chance GW, Inwood MJ, et al. Intraventricular haemorrhage and haemostasis defects. Arch Dis Child 1984; 59:444.

215. Van de Bor M, Van Bel F, Lineman R, et al. Perinatal factors and periventricular haemorrhage in preterm infants. Am J Dis Child 1986; 140:1125.

216. Pomerance JJ, Teal JG, Gogolok JF, et al. Maternally administered antenatal vitamin K_1: effect on neonatal prothrombin activity, partial thromboplastin time, and intraventricular hemorrhage. Obstet Gynecol 1987; 70:235.

217. Morales WJ, Angel JL, O'Brien WF, et al. The use of antenatal vitamin K in the prevention of early neonatal intraventricular hemorrhage. Am J Obstet Gynecol 1988; 159:774.

218. Kazzi NJ, Ilagan NB, Liang KC, et al. Maternal administration of vitamin K does not improve coagulation profile of preterm infants. Pediatrics 1989; 84:1045.

219. Committee on Nutrition American Academy of Pediatrics. Vitamin K compounds and their water-soluble analogues: Use in therapy and prophylaxis in pediatrics. Pediatrics 1961; 28:501.

220. Klebanoff MA, Read JS, Mills JL, et al. The risk of childhood cancer after neonatal exposure to vitamin K. N Engl J Med 1989; 329:905.

221. Widdowson EM, Spray CM. Chemical development in utero. Arch Dis Child 1951; 26:205.

222. Dallman PR, Siimes MA. Iron deficiency in infancy and childhood: a report for the international nutritional anemia consultative group. Washington, DC, The Nutrition Foundation 1979.

223. Shaw JCL. Parenteral nutrition in the management of sick low birth weight infants. Pediatr Clin N Am 1973; 20:333.

224. Oski FA, Naiman JL. The hematologic aspects of the maternal-fetal relationship. In: Oski FA, Naiman JL, eds., Hematologic problems in the newborn, 3rd edn. Philadelphia, PA, WB Saunders 1982 32–55.

225. Singla PN, Gupta VK, Agarwal KN. Storage iron in human foetal organs. Acta Paediatr Scand 1985; 74:701.

226. Petry C, et al. Placental transferring receptor in diabetic pregnancies with increased iron demand. Am J Physiol 1994; 121:109.

227. Shaw JC. Iron absorption by the premature infant. The effect of transfusion and iron supplements on the serum ferritin levels. Acta Paediatr Scand 1982; 299(suppl):83.

228. Zlotkin SH, Lay DM, Kjarsgaard J, et al. Determination of iron absorption using erythrocyte iron incorporation of two stable isotopes of iron (57Fe and 58 Fe) in VLBW premature infants. J Pediatr Gastronenterol Nutr 1995; 21:190.

229. Widness JA, Lombard KA, Ziegler EE, et al. Erythrocyte incorporation and absorption of 58Fe in premature infants treated with erythropoietin. Pediatr Res 1997; 41:416.

230. Moody GJ, Schanlelr RJ, Abrams SA. Utilization of supplemental iron by premature infants fed fortified human milk. Acta Pediatr 1999; 88:763.

231. McDonald MC, Abrams SA, Schanler RJ. Iron absorption and red blood cell incorporation in premature infants fed an iron-fortified infant formula. Pediatr Res 1998; 44a:508.

232. American Academy of Pediatrics Committee on Nutrition. Nutritional needs of preterm infants. In: Kleinman RE, ed., Pediatric nutrition handbook. Elk Grove Village, IL, American Academy of Pediatrics 1989 55–87.

233. Formon SJ, Nelson SE, Ziegler EE. Retention of iron by infants (In process, citation). Annu Rev Nutr 2000; 20:273.

234. Dauncey MJ, Davies CG, Shaw JC, et al. The effect of iron supplements and blood transfusion on iron absorption by low birth weight infants fed pasteurized human breast milk. Pediatr Res 1978; 12:899.

235. Shaveghi M, Latunde-Dada GO, Oakhill JS, et al. Identification of an intestinal heme transporter. Cell 2005; 122:789.

236. Rouault TA. The intestinal heme transporter revealed. Cell 2005; 122:649.

237. Andrews NC. Understanding heme transport. N Engl J Med 2005; 353:2508.

238. Andrews NC. Iron deficiency and related disorders, Wintrobe's Clinical Hematology, 11th edn. Philadelphia, Lippincott Williams & Wilkins 2004 979–1009.

239. Siddappa A, Rao R, Wobken K, et al. Iron deficiency alters iron regulatory protein and iron transport protein expression in the perinatal rat brain. Peds Res 2003; 53:800.

240. Raghavendra R, Georgieff M. Microminerals. In: Tsang RC, Uauy R, Koletzko B, Zlotkin SH, eds., Nutrition of the preterm infant: scientific basis and practical guidelines. Cincinnati, OH: Digital Educational Publishing 2005 277–310.

241. Doyle JJ, Zypursky A. Neonatal blood disorders. In: Sinclair JC, Bracken MR, eds., Effective care of the newborn infant. Oxford, UK: Oxford University Press 1992 425–451.

242. Friel JK, Andrews WL, Aziz K, et al. A randomized trail of two levels of iron supplementation and developmental outcome in low birth weight infants. J Pediatr 2001; 139:254.

243. Hall RT, Wheller RE, Benson J, et al. Feeding iron-fortified premature formula during initial hospitalization to infants less than 1800 grams birth weight. Pediatrics 1993; 92:409.

244. Report of a Joint World Health Organization/Centers for Disease Control and Prevention Technical Consultation on the Assessment of Iron Status at the Population Level: Assessing the iron status of populations. Geneva, Switzerland, April 2004.

245. Institute of Medicine Food and Nutrition Board, Dietary Relevance Intakes: vitamin A, vitamin K, arsenic, baron, chromium, copper, iodine and iron. Washington DC, National Academy Press 2003 300–306.

246. Kling PJ, Winzerling JJ. Iron status and the treatment of the anemia of prematurity. Clin Perinatol 2002; 29:283.

247. Dallman PR, Siimes MA, Stekel A. Iron deficiency in infancy and childhood. Am J Clin Nutr 1980; 33:86.

248. Beguin Y. Soluble transferring receptor for the evaluation of erythropoiesis and iron status. Clin Chim Acta 2003; 329:9.

249. Skikne BS, Flowers CH, Cook JD. Serum transferring receptor: a quantitative measure of tissue iron deficiency. Blood 1990; 1:870.

250. Juul SE, Zernan JC, Strandjord TP, et al. Zinc protoporhyrin/heme as an indicator of iron status in NICU patients. J Pediatr 2003; 142:273.

251. Winzerling JJ, Kling PJ. Iron-deficient erythropoiesis in premature infants measured by blood zinc protoporhyrin/heme. J Pediatr 1002; 139:134..

252. Miller SM, McPherson RJ, Juul SE. Iron sulfate supplementation decreases zinc protoporphyrin to heme ratio in premature infants. The Journal of Pediatrics 2006; 148:44.

253. Kling PJ. The zinc protoporphyrin/heme ratio in premature infants: Has it found its place? J Pediatr 2006; 148:9.

254. Oski FA, Honig AS. The effect of therapy on the developmental scores of iron-deficient infants. J Pediatr 1978; 92:21.

255. Lozoff B, Brittenham GM, Viteri FE, et al. The effects of short-term oral iron therapy on developmental deficits in iron-deficient anemic infants. J Pediat 1982; 100:351.

256. Aukett MA, Parks YA, Scott PH, et al. Treatment with iron increases weight gain and psychomotor development. Arch Dis Child 1986; 61:849.

257. Lozoff B, Brittenham GM, Wolf AW, et al. Iron deficiency anemia and iron therapy effects on infant developmental tests performance. Pediatrics 1987; 79:981.

258. Walter T, DeAndraca I, Chadud P. Iron deficiency anemia: adverse effects on infant psychomotor development. Pediatrics 1989; 84:7.

259. Idjradinata P, Pollitt E. Reversal of developmental delays in iron-deficient anaemic infants treated with iron. Lancet 1993; 2:1.

260. Armony-Sivan R, Eidelman AI, Lanir A, et al. Iron status and neurobehavioral development of premature infants. J Perinatol 2004; 24:757.

261. Lozoff B, Jimenez E, Hagen J, et al. Poorer behavioral and developmental outcome more than 10 years after treatment for iron deficiency in infancy. Pediatrics 2000; 105:E51.

262. Martins S, Logan S, Gilbert R. Iron therapy for improving psychomotor development and cognitive function in children under the age of three with iron deficiency anaemia (Cochrane Review), The Cochrane Library, Issue 1. Chichester, UK, John Wiley & Sons 2004.

263. Wright RO, Tsaih SW, Schwartz J, et al. Association between iron deficiency and blood lead level in a longitudinal analysis of children following in an urban primary care clinic. J Pediatr 2003; 142:9.

264. Black LS, deRegnier RA, Long J, et al. Electrographic imaging of recognition memory in 34–38 week gestation intrauterine growth restricted newborns. Exp Neurol 2004; 190:S72.

265. Siddappa AM, Georgieff MK, Wewerka SW, et al. Iron deficiency alters auditory recognition memory in newborn infants of diabetic mothers. Pediatr Res 2004; 55:1034.

266. Jansson LT. Iron, oxygen stress, and the preterm infant. In: Lonnerdal B, ed., Iron metabolism in infants. Boca Raton, FL, CRC Press 1990 73–85.

267. Lackmann GM, Hesse L, Tollner U. Reduced iron-associated anti-oxidants in premature newborns suffering intracerebral hemorrhage. Free Radic Biol Med 1996; 20:407.

268. Inder TE, Clemett RS, Austin NC, et al. High iron status in VLBW infants is associated with an increased risk of retinopathy of prematurity. J Pediatr 1997; 131:541.

269. Cooke RW, Drury JA, Yoxall CW, et al. Blood transfusion and chronic lung disease in preterm infants. Eur J Pediatr 1997; 156:47.

270. Hess L, Eberl W, Schlaud M, et al. Blood transfusion: Iron load and retinopathy of prematurity. Eur J Pediatr 1997; 156:4565.

271. Romagnoli C, Zecca E, Gallini F, et al. Do recombinant human erythropoietin and iron supplementation increase the risk of retinopathy of prematurity? Eur J Pediat 2000; 159:627.

Chapter 14

Diverse Roles of Lipids in Neonatal Physiology and Development

Nancy Auestad, PhD

Physiology and Metabolism of Lipids
Lipid Metabolism and Physiology in the Fetus and Newborn
Relevance of Physiologic Differences to Disease Process

Infants born prematurely are faced with physiological and nutritional challenges that for some infants persist long after leaving the neonatal intensive care unit. Achieving a rate of growth and body composition corresponding to that in utero is the gold standard against which the nutritional adequacy of dietary regimens for preterm infants is often evaluated. Lipids play important and very diverse roles in postnatal growth and development. Fat is the major energy component in human milk and infant formula for both full-term and preterm infants, providing 40–55% of the daily energy requirements. As consitutents of cell membranes, phospholipids and other complex lipids have both structural and functional roles. Individual fatty acids have very distinctive roles in fetal and postnatal physiology. This is particularly significant through the most rapid period of perinatal growth, which includes the transition from fetal to postnatal life.

Glucose in the major energy substrate in utero, but after birth a major switch occurs. The fatty acids in human milk and infant formula then become the primary sources of energy for growth and development. Humans cannot synthesize the $n-3$ and $n-6$ polyunsaturated fatty acids and must obtain them from the diet. The fetus acquires these and other fatty acids transplacentally, but after birth, fatty acids from human milk or infant formula are absorbed across the intestinal lumen or provided by parenteral nutrition. The functional maturation of the gastrointestinal system is critical for the digestion of dietary fat and the absorption of fatty acids in infants born prematurely. In utero, adipose tissue stores are laid down largely in the last 10 weeks of gestation. In the first weeks after birth, fatty acids from adipose help support energy requirements and accretion of long-chain $n-6$ and $n-3$ fatty acids in the central nervous system. Infants born prematurely often have limited adipose stores, and, therefore, in the immediate postnatal period rely on dietary fatty acids to a greater extent than term infants. This paper examines these and other aspects of lipids in fetal and postnatal life with an emphasis on infants born prematurely. The impetus is to identify knowledge gaps that with additional research may improve nutrition strategies for these infants.

PHYSIOLOGY AND METABOLISM OF LIPIDS

Lipids by definition are ubiquitous in biological systems and have multiple physiological roles. This section provides an overview of the different types of lipids and their functions, the absorption of dietary fats, lipid transport systems, and a brief synopsis of the diverse functions of fatty acids.

Lipids are a heterogeneous class of compounds that are insoluble in water and soluble in organic solvents. Lipids are typically classified according to their structural features and hydrophobic properties. Neutral lipids, which include triglycerides and sterol esters, are hydrophobic. Complex lipids typically contain three or more distinct components (e.g. glycerol, fatty acids and sugar; glycerol, fatty acids, and/or a phosphate-amine group) and have both hydrophobic and hydrophilic properties. They are often subdivided further as phospholipids (e.g. phosphatidylcholine, phosphatidylethanolamine) and glycerolipids (e.g. sphingolipids, ceremides, and gangliosides). Triglycerides, the most common lipids in the diet of both infants and adults, contain three fatty acyl chains esterified to each of the three hydroxyl groups on a glycerol backbone. Triglycerides are stored in adipose tissue, the major storage fat in the body. Monoglycerides and diglycerides are formed in lipid digestion and as intermediates in lipid metabolism. Phophsolipids contain two fatty acyl chains esterified to two of the three hydroxyl groups of the glycerol backbone. The third hydroxyl group is esterified to phosphate, which in turn is esterified to choline, ethanolamine, serine, or inositol, forming phosphatidylcholine, phosphatidylethanolamine, phosphatidylserine, and phosphatidylinositiol. Phospholipids are the most abundant lipid components in most cell membranes, and adipose tissue is a major storage pool for triglycerides. Sphingolipids resemble the structure of phosphoglycerides except that they contain sphinogsine, an amino alcohol with a long unsaturated hydrocarbon chain, and one other fatty acyl chain instead of the glycerol backbone with two fatty acyl chains. Common sphingolipids include sphingomeylin, cerebrosides, and sulfatides. Another major group of lipid compounds are the sterols, of which cholesterol is the most common. The functional attributes of fatty acids are determined by their carbon chain length, degree of unsaturation, and location of double bonds. Fatty acids are often depicted using a nomenclature that identifies the number of carbon atoms, the number of double bonds, and the number of carbon atoms from the terminal methyl group to the first double bond (Table 14-1). For example, linoleic acid (18:2 n–6) contains 18 carbon atoms and 2 double bonds, with the first double bond starting at the sixth carbon from the terminal methyl group. The most common fatty acids are shown in Table 14-1. The numeric nomenclature (e.g. 18:2 n–6) is used here when referring to fatty acids in tissues and in metabolic pathways, and the common name (e.g. linoleic acid) or abbreviation (e.g. LA) is used when referring to fatty acids in the diet.

Dietary lipids are utilized to support energy requirements, are structurally and biologically significant components of cell membranes, and facilitate the absorption of fat-soluble vitamins (A, D, E, and K). Dietary lipids include triglycerides, phospholipids, sterol esters and sterols as well as other complex lipids. The digestion, absorption, transport, storage and utilization of lipids require special carriers in the body because of their hydrophobic characteristics.

Two fatty acids are classified as essential in the diet, linoleic acid (LA; 18:2 n–6) and α-linolenic acid (ALA, 18:3 n–3). All other fatty acids can be obtained from the diet, formed de novo, or are formed from other fatty acids. For example, DHA (22:6 n–3) can be obtained directly from the diet or formed from 18:3 n–3 by a series of elongation and desaturation steps and β-oxidation (Fig. 14-1). ARA, EPA and DHA, which are among the important structural and physiologically important components of cell membranes, are considered *physiologically* essential. At present,

Table 14-1 Classification of Common Fatty Acids	
Numeric nomenclature (common abbreviation)	Trivial name
Saturated fatty acids	
Medium-chain-length fatty acids	
6:0	Caparoic
8:0	Caprylic
10:0	Capric
12:0	Lauric
14:0	Myristic
Long-chain saturated fatty acids	
16:0	Palmitic
18:0	Stearic
Monounsaturated fatty acids	
16:1 $n-7$	Palmitoleic
18:1 $n-7$	Vaccenic
18:1 $n-9$	Oleic
20:3 $n-9$	Mead acid
22:1 $n-9$	Eurcic
Polyunsaturated fatty acids	
Omega-6 fatty acids	
18:2 $n-6$ (LA)	Linoleic
18:3 $n-6$ (GLA)	γ-Linoleic
Long-chain polyunsaturated fatty acids (LCPUFA)	
20:3 $n-6$ (DGLA)	Dihomo-γ-linoleic
20:4 $n-6$ (ARA)	Arachidonic
22:4 $n-6$	-
22:5 $n-6$	-
Omega-3 fatty acids	
18:3 $n-3$ (ALA)	α-linolenic
Long-chain polyunsaturated fatty acids (LCPUFA)	
20:4 $n-3$	-
20:5 $n-3$ (EPA)	Eicosapentaenoic
22:5 $n-3$ (DPA)	Docosapentaenoic
22:6 $n-3$ (DHA)	Docosahexaenoic

The nomenclature $n-7$, $n-9$, $n-6$, and $n-3$ is interchangeable with $\omega-7$, $\omega-9$, $\omega-6$ and $\omega-3$, respectively.

however, there is not consensus about classifying ARA, EPA or DHA as essential or conditionally essential in the diet. The emphasis of research on the $n-6$ and $n-3$ polyunsaturated fatty acids in recent years highlights their biological importance in many physiological systems, including cardiovascular, immunological and central nervous systems.

Lipid Digestion and Absorption

More than 98% of the fatty acids in human milk and infant formula are present in the form of triglycerides (1). In digestion, the fatty acids from human milk and infant formula are absorbed as 2-monoglycerides and free fatty acids after the milk fat is emulsified and hydrolyzed through digestion. Fat digestion begins with the action of lingual lipase, which is formed by the serous glands of the tongue. Lingual lipase initiates the hydrolysis of triglycerides to fatty acids, primarily those at the $sn-3$ position. In the stomach gastric lipases, which are formed in the gastric mucosa, promote further digestion by preferentially cleaving short- and medium-chain-length fatty acids on triglycerides. Both lingual and gastric lipases appear by 26 weeks of gestation, are active at gastric pH and do not require bile salts. Fat digestion continues in the duodenum with the formation of micelles. Pancreatic

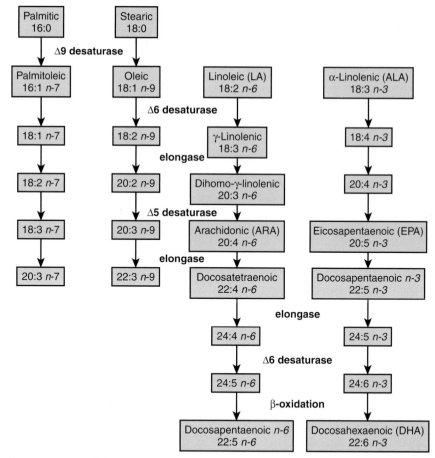

Figure 14-1 Metabolic pathways of fatty acid elongation and desaturation.

lipase hydrolyzes triglycerides in lipid droplets at the $sn-1$ and $sn-3$ positions to free fatty acids and 2-monoglycerides. Bile, which consists of bile salts, phospholipids, and cholesterol, emulsifies fats, a necessary step in the formation of micelles. Colipase, also formed in the pancreas, facilitates the shuttling of the free fatty acids and 2-monoglycerides from the lipid droplet into micelles. In human breast milk, another lipase, bile-salt stimulated lipase, nonselectively converts 2-monoglycerides to glycerol and free fatty acids, a process that increases absorptive efficiency.

Lipid absorption occurs to a large extent by passive diffusion of fatty acids and 2-monoglycerides from micelles across the unstirred water layer and into the intestinal lumen. The peristaltic, churning action of the intestine helps to facilitate this process. Intestinal fatty acid binding proteins assist in shuttling fatty acids and 2-monoglycerides across the intestinal mucosa. In humans, fat absorption is estimated to be about 95% efficient. In infants born prematurely, the efficiency of fat absorption depends on the maturity of the gastrointestinal system and the fat in the diet. For example, fat and calcium absorption is lower in infants fed formula containing palm-olein oil (2), which is present in some infant formulas to match human milk levels of palmitic acid. Absorption efficiencies also are influenced by fatty acid chain length and the degree of fatty acid unsaturation (3). Fatty acids with fewer than 12 carbons are absorbed passively and efficiently by the gastric mucosa and are taken up to a large extent by the portal vein.

Phospholipids are consumed in the diet in much lower amounts than triglycerides by both infants and adults. Phospholipids are also secreted into the intestine in bile. Both dietary and biliary phospholipids are digested after phospholipase A2, a pancreatic enzyme secreted in bile, hydrolyzes fatty acids in the *sn*−2 position. The resulting free fatty acids and lysophosphoglycerides are absorbed through a process similar to that described above for the digestion products of triglycerides.

Cholesterol similarly originates from the diet and from bile. Cholesterol requires bile acids for micellar solubilization and absorption, with a typical absorption efficiency much lower (40–65%) than that for the digestion products of triglycerides and phospholipids. The absorption of dietary cholesterol is facilitated by the intracellular enzyme acyl-coenzyme Acholesterol acyltransferase. Cholesterol is found at low levels in human milk and is not present in infant formulas that use vegetable oils as the exclusive sources of fat.

Transport and Metabolism of Lipids

After absorption into the intestinal epithelium, the free fatty acids and 2-monoglycerides are reassembled into triglycerides and packaged along with phospholipids and cholesterol into chylomicrons. Chylomicrons are transported through the lymphatic system to the superior vena cava by way of the thoracic duct and released into the circulation. The triglycerides in the core of the chyolmicron are hydrolyzed by lipoprotein lipase, releasing the fatty acids at the capillary surface of tissues. This results in the movement of the fatty acids into tissues and the subsequent formation of triglyceride-depleted chylomicron remnants. These remnants then pick up cholesterol esters from HDL, and these particles are rapidly taken up by the liver. This system for transporting fatty acids of dietary origin is called the exogenous transport system.

An endogenous transport system also exists for the interorgan transport of fatty acids that originate internally. Lipids are transported from the liver to peripheral tissues, are moved from the peripheral tissues to the liver, and are moved from adipose stores to different organs. The movement of lipids from the liver to peripheral tissues involves the concerted actions of VLDL, IDL, LDL and HDL. VLDL particles, like chylomicrons, consist of a large hydrophobic core of triglycerides and cholesterol esters and a surface lipid layer consisting of mainly phospholipids and cholesterol. VLDL are assembled in the liver, and deposition of lipids into peripheral tissues is their primary function. After secretion into the circulation, VLDL are acted upon by lipoprotein lipase, which hydrolyzes triglycerides to free fatty acids. The free fatty acids originating from chylomicrons or VLDL can be used as energy substrates, structural components of membrane phospholipids or converted back to triglycerides and stored. Triglycerides from both chylomicrons and VLDL also undergo hydrolysis by hepatic lipase. VLDL particles are converted through hydrolysis of triglycerides to denser, smaller cholesterol- and triglyceride-rich remnants (IDL), which are cleared from plasma through hepatic lipoprotein receptors or may be converted to LDL particles. LDL is the major cholesterol-carrying lipoprotein.

The return of lipids from the peripheral tissues to the liver is often referred to as "reverse cholesterol transport." HDL particles participate in this process by acquiring cholesterol from tissues and other lipoproteins and transporting it to the liver for excretion. The transfer of fatty acids from adipose stores to organs for oxidation is another interorgan transport function. Fatty acids derived largely from adipose tissue triglyceride hydrolysis are secreted into plasma, where they bind to albumin. The albumin-bound fatty acids are removed in a concentration gradient-dependent manner by metabolically active tissues and are used primarily as energy substrates.

Over the past 20 years, few studies have focused on lipid transport over the perinatal period (4–8), and these will not be discussed in subsequent sections. Clearly, more research is needed.

Lipid Utilization

Fatty acids are incorporated into cell membrane lipids (e.g. phospholipids; cardiolipids), used as energy substrates and stored in the form of triglycerides largely in adipose. Some long-chain $n-6$ and $n-3$ fatty acids are precursors of biologically active metabolites that are involved in cell signaling, gene regulation, and other metabolically active systems. The role of the long-chain polyunsaturated fatty acids ARA and DHA in infant growth and development has been a major focus of infant nutrition research over the past two decades.

Lipids are integral components of cell membranes. A considerable amount of research on lipid physiology has focused on two fatty acids, ARA and DHA. ARA is found in cell membranes throughout the body and is a precursor to series-2 eicosanoids, series-3 leukotrienes and other metabolites that are involved in cell signaling pathways and gene regulation (9). DHA is often described by its structural and functional roles in cell membranes (10). It is found in high concentrations in the gray matter in the brain and in the rods and cones of the retina. Depletion studies in animals fed diets lacking total $n-3$ fatty acids consistently have shown that the 22-carbon long-chain $n-6$ fatty acid, 22:5 $n-6$, substitutes structurally, but not functionally, for 22:6 $n-3$ (11–13). When tissue 22:6 $n-3$ levels are inadequate, deficits in visual and learning behaviors are found. Modulating the amount of 22:6 $n-3$ in tissues has been shown to influence neurotransmitter function, ion channel activity, signaling pathways and gene expression (9, 10, 14, 15).

LIPID METABOLISM AND PHYSIOLOGY IN THE FETUS AND NEWBORN

Major shifts in lipid metabolism occur at birth. The route by which fatty acids are acquired, the role of fatty acids as energy substrates, and their significance in adipose tissue stores all change after birth. The fetus acquires fatty acids from the mother by transfer across the placenta, and when infants are born prematurely this supply is cut off. After birth, the capacity for acquiring energy substrates and nutrients then depends on the maturation and functional capacity of the gastrointestinal system. Preterm infants who are able to tolerate enteral feedings absorb fatty acids across the intestinal lumen after the digestion of the fat in human milk or infant formula. Those who are fed parenterally obtain fatty acids in the form of intravenous lipids.

During fetal development, the primary energy substrate is glucose followed by lactate, and surplus amino acids. Fatty acids play only a minor role as energy substrates in the fetus, but after birth fatty acids become major energy substrates. In the fetus, adipose tissue is laid down to a large extent late in the third trimester (Fig. 14–2). Infants born prematurely, thus, have limited adipose reserves at birth. After birth fatty acids in adipose stores are utilized for energy and for accretion into newly formed cell membranes. Preterm infants who are born with inadequate adipose reserves have to rely more on dietary and/or parenteral lipids in the perinatal period to meet fatty acid requirements than do full-term infants. In the perinatal period, large amounts of fatty acids are needed to support the rapid rate of growth, especially that of the brain.

The formation of neural membranes involves the deposition of large amounts of fatty acids for the formation of phospholipids along with sterols and complex lipids (10, 16, 17). The gray matter of brain is enriched in both 22:6 $n-3$ and 20:4 $n-6$, and the rods and cones of the retina are similarly enriched in 22:6 $n-3$. About half of the fatty acids in the the rod outer segment are 22:6 $n-3$. Since mammals cannot form $n-6$ and $n-3$ fatty acids de novo, these must be obtained from the diet either preformed as DHA and ARA or as their parent fatty acids, ALA and

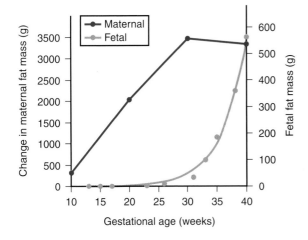

Figure 14-2 Change in maternal (Hytten, 1974) and fetal (Widdowson, 1968) body fat with gestational age during the fetal period 9 (weeks to term) when the fetus is dependent on the placenta for its supply of nutrients. From Haggarty P. European Journal of Clinical Nutrition 55:1563, 2004. © Nature Publishing Group.

LA, respectively. Most infant formulas now contain preformed sources of ARA and DHA. DHA supplements for women who are pregnant or nursing also have become available.

A major focus of research on infant lipid requirements over the past two decades has been the role of the long-chain $n-6$ and $n-3$ fatty acids, specifically 22:6 $n-3$ and 20:4 $n-6$, in visual and cognitive development. These fatty acids are found in human milk, with DHA levels ranging from about 0.1% to more than 1% of total fatty acids (1). ARA levels are less variable, typically ranging from about 0.3 to 0.7% total fatty acids.

Fetal Development

Transplacental Flux of Fatty Acids

The fetus acquires fatty acids from the mother mainly by transplacental flux and to a lesser extent by de novo synthesis (18). Since mammals cannot synthesize the biologically essential $n-6$ and $n-3$ fatty acids de novo, the fetus must obtain these fatty acids from the mother as the 18-carbon parent fatty acids (18:2 $n-6$, 18:3 $n-3$) and/or their long-chain counterparts (20:4 $n-6$, 20:5 $n-3$, 22:6 $n-3$) (Fig. 14-1). The placenta and the fetal liver and brain have the capacity to convert 18:2 $n-6$ to 20:4 $n-6$ and 18:3 $n-3$ to 20:5 $n-3$ and 22:6 $n-3$ (19–21).

A growing body of evidence suggests, however, that the fetus relies largely on transplacental flux of the preformed long-chain $n-6$ and $n-3$ polyunsaturated fatty acids to meet $n-6$ and $n-3$ fatty acid requirements for tissue accretion (20, 22). In the fetus, the circulating levels of the long-chain $n-6$ and $n-3$ fatty acids, primarily 20:4 $n-6$ and 22:6 $n-3$, are *higher* than in the maternal circulation. 18:2 $n-6$ and 18:3 $n-3$ are *lower* in the fetal circulation. Biomagnification is a term that has been used to describe this uphill gradient of 20:4 $n-6$ and 22:6 $n-3$ from the mother to the fetus.

Nutrient transfer is a major function of the human hemochorial placenta, which is unique for mammals in that the fetal chorion is in direct contact with the maternal blood (23). Preferential transfer of $n-6$ and $n-3$ fatty acids involves selective uptake by the syncytiotrophoblast, intracellular metabolic channeling of individual fatty acids, and selective export to the fetal circulation (20, 24). Fatty acids move across the microvillous and basal membranes by simple diffusion or by selective transport facilitated by fatty acid binding proteins. The selective transport of fatty acids and other nutrients from the maternal to fetal plasma involves active transporters that are found on the surface of both maternal and fetal placental membranes (25).

Convincing evidence that a placental plasma membrane fatty acid binding protein (p-FABP$_{pm}$) preferentially binds the n–6 and n–3 fatty acids has been published (24, 26, 27). Studies with human placental membranes have helped identify binding specificity for the n–6 and n–3 fatty acids and interactions among fatty acids for binding (20, 24, 26–28). Insight into the binding kinetics of the placental binding protein, pFABP$_{pm}$, comes from ex vivo studies designed with a fatty acid mixture based on the patterns of maternal plasma fatty acid composition in the third trimester (20). The fatty acid mixture included 16:0, 18:0, 18:1 n–9, 18:3 n–3, 18:2 n–6, 20:4 n–6, and 22:6 n–3. Palmitic acid (16:0) did not bind to the pFABP$_{pm}$, and binding of 18:0 and 18:1 n–9 was low. Among the n–3 fatty acids, 83% of 22:6 n–3 in the mixture bound to the pFABP$_{pm}$, and binding of 18:3 n–3 was not detected. Among the n–6 fatty acids, 98% of the 20:4 n–6 and 23% of 18:2 n–6 bound to the pFABP$_{pm}$. Selectivity of individual fatty acids for transplacental flux to the fetus appears to be influenced by the plasma fatty acid composition of the mother and the abundance of placental FABP binding sites (29, 30).

Maternal fatty acids increase in plasma during the third trimester of pregnancy in response to fetal demands for long-chain n–6 and n–3 fatty acids (22, 31, 32) (Fig. 14-3). Trans fatty acids appear to compete with n–6 and n–3 binding sites in human placental membranes, and high circulating maternal 18:2 n–6 levels may negatively influence both maternal and neonatal n–3 fatty acid status (28, 29, 33). Placental FABP polymorphisms (34) and metabolic conditions, such as insulin-dependent diabetes mellitus (35) and gestational diabetes (36, 37), are associated with low levels of 20:4 n–6 and 22:6 n–3 in cord blood.

Leptin has been detected in the placenta, amniotic fluid and fetal plasma as early as the 18th week of gestation (38–40). Placentally derived leptin appears to play a role in stimulating the mobilization of fatty acids from maternal adipose tissue to the fetus. Placental leptin production increases with increasing fetal to placental weight ratio, and it has been suggested that the placenta may modulate its own substrate supply in response to fetal demands (22). It is estimated that 95% of the leptin formed in the placenta is directed to the maternal plasma, with only 5% directed to the fetus (38). Leptin is also produced by white adipose tissue in the fetus, and this appears to be independent of placental leptin production (38). It has been suggested that umbilical leptin levels are independent of placental leptin production and may be a marker of fat mass in human fetuses (38). Small for gestational newborn infants have lower serum leptin concentrations, and intrauterine growth retardation is associated with decreased circulating leptin concentrations in both newborns and their mothers (41).

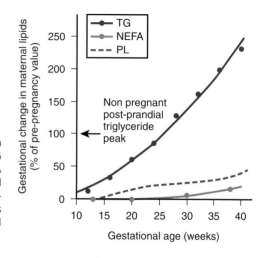

Figure 14-3 Percentage change with state of gestation in the concentration of maternal circulating plasma TG (Darmady and Postle, 1982), PL (Al et al. 1995) and NEFA (McDonald et al. 1975) relative to prepregnancy value: typical maximum value for the increase in plasma triglyceride in a non-pregnant individual following a high fat meal (Frayn, 1996) is indicated. From Haggarty P. European Journal of Clinical Nutrition, 55:1563, 2004. © Nature Publishing Group.

Adipose

More than 90% of adipose deposition in the fetus occurs in the last 10 weeks of gestation (22) (Fig. 14-2). Quantitative estimates of the rate of fetal fat deposition have been made using ultrasound in both healthy pregnancies (42–44) and when gestational diabetes is present (42–44). Although total fat mass represents only 12–14% of the newborn's birth weight, it accounts for about 46% of the variance in neonatal weight (42–44). Ultrasonographic measurement of fetal fat deposition may be a sensitive marker of disproportionate fetal growth and thus may be useful diagnostically. Normative rates of fetal deposition of lean and fat mass have been estimated at 4-week intervals from 19 weeks gestation to term in 36 nonsmoking healthy women with a normal prepregnancy body mass index. Subcutaneous fat mass increased about 10-fold between 19 weeks gestation and term, with the greatest rate of deposition occurring in the last 10 weeks. Lean body mass, which included peripheral muscle, the abdominal area, and head area, increased 5–7-fold between 19 weeks gestation and term. Consistent with other reports, this study found a linear deposition pattern for lean body mass at the whole body level. The growth pattern, however, was distinct for each of the lean body mass compartments. An accelerating rate of growth was found for peripheral muscle, a linear rate was found for the abdominal area, and a slight deceleration was found for the head area.

Fetal fat mass accretion is significantly greater in pregnancies with gestational diabetes than in otherwise healthy pregnancies (44) and has been shown to be influenced by maternal glucose tolerance (43). Increased fat mass in fetuses of mothers with moderately abnormal oral glucose tolerance, but which does not meet the diagnostic criteria for gestational diabetes, has been reported (43). Gestational age, maternal postprandial (1-h) glucose values, and prepregnancy body mass index were associated with the rate of fat deposition. No associations between maternal glucose tolerance and growth of lean body mass in the fetus, on the other hand, were found. There also is a growing body of literature reporting lower circulating levels of both 20:4 *n*–6 and 22:6 *n*–3 in infants born to women with type 1 diabetes, type 2 diabetes or gestational diabetes (37, 45, 46). The implications of these shifts in lipid metabolism need further investigation, particularly in relation to central nervous system development and the potential for early programming and disease risk later in life (47, 48)

Fetal adipose growth also is influenced by both maternal and fetal endocrine status (49, 50). During late gestation, high levels of uncoupling protein 1 (UCP1), which is unique to brown adipose tissue, are formed. In addition to increases in UCP1, IGF-I and IGF-II levels also increase. Restriction of maternal nutrition leads to reduced adipose tissue deposition, but with no effect on UCP1. Increased maternal food intake, on the other hand, leads to increased levels of UCP1 as well as the short form of the prolactin receptor.

The exponential increase in fetal adipose deposition in the third trimester occurs concurrently with the onset of the brain growth spurt (51) and the accretion of the polyunsaturated fatty acids, especially 22:6 *n*–3 and 20:4 *n*–6, in the central nervous system (16). Although the relative percentage of 22:6 *n*–3 and 20:4 *n*–6 in fetal brain and adipose is similar (Table 14-2), the absolute amount of 22:6 *n*–3 and 20:4 *n*–6 deposition in brain is small when compared with that in fetal adipose tissue (22). By term gestation, it has been estimated that approximately 50-fold more 22:6 *n*–3 is stored in the adipose tissue than in the fetal brain.

Central Nervous System

More than 30 years ago, Dobbing and colleagues (1973) showed that the rate of brain growth was fastest from mid-gestation through about the second year after

Table 14-2 Maternal and Fetal 20:4 n−6 and 22:6 n−3 Levels in Diet, Plasma, Adipose and Brain

	MATERNAL (% TOTAL FATTY ACIDS)		FETAL (% TOTAL FATTY ACIDS)	
	ARA (20:4 *n*−6)	DHA (22:6 *n*−3)	ARA (20:4 *n*−6)	DHA (22:6 *n*−3)
Diet	0.5	0.4	–	–
Plasma phospholipid	11.7	1.7	16.6	6.6
Adipose (at birth)	0.1	0.1	9.1	1.6
Brain (at birth)	–	–	8.9	4.1

Adapted from Haggarty P. Effect of placental function on fatty acid requirements during pregnancy. Eur J Clin Nutr 2004; 58:1559.

birth (51, 52). This period, often referred to as the brain growth spurt (51, 52), is when the central nervous system is particularly vulnerable to nutritional insult (53). Neural development, whether described anatomically, biochemically, or physiologically, occurs as a sequential, ordered and integrated process. Key events in neural development include neural induction followed by neurogenesis, migration of neuroblasts, formation of axons and dendrites, dendritic arborization, synaptogenesis, gliogenesis, myelination and programmed cell death. Region-specific growth patterns are coordinated over the entire span of brain development.

The accretion of fatty acids in the formation of membrane-rich neuronal and glial cells during perinatal brain development is particularly high. In the early 1980s, Clandinin and colleagues estimated that the accretion rates for *n*–6 and *n*–3 fatty acids in the third trimester human fetus are 552 mg/day and 67 mg/day, respectively (54). DHA (22:6 *n*–3) accounts for the majority of *n*–3 fatty acids and 20:4 *n*–6, 22:4 *n*–6 and 22:5 *n*–6 account for the majority of *n*–6 fatty acids in brain. Martinez and colleagues later described the patterns of accretion of individual fatty acids, including the *n*–6 and *n*–3 fatty acids, in brain phospholipids through fetal and postnatal development (16).

Maternal DHA (22:6 n–3) Supplementation

The extent to which the maternal dietary intake of the long-chain *n*–6 and *n*–3 fatty acids may affect neurodevelopment is germane to understanding fetal requirements and the requirements of preterm infants for these fatty acids. Associations between maternal plasma and fetal umbilical plasma concentrations of 20:4 *n*–6 and 22:6 *n*–3 were first reported by Al et al. (55). Since then, several studies have examined associations between maternal 22:6 *n*–3 status (56) or the effects of DHA supplementation (57–61) on cord blood and neurodevelopment in infants (Table 14-3). Most (57–61), but not all (61), studies found no measurable effects of maternal DHA supplementation on infant visual or cognitive development. Women were given different DHA supplements (e.g. cod liver oil, algal oil, fish oil), the sample sizes varied, and the usual dietary intake of fish, the main dietary source of DHA, often was not reported. In these supplementation studies, pregnant women were randomized to the DHA supplement or to a placebo around midgestation or later, after the large increase in maternal adipose stores (Fig. 14-2). The large increase in the mobilization of 22:6 *n*–3 from maternal adipose to the fetus in the third trimester may overshadow the contribution from maternal dietary DHA to the circulating plasma pool in the latter half of pregnancy, except perhaps at very high dietary intakes of DHA and EPA (61, 62). Supplementing pregnant women with up to 1300 mg/day of DHA supplementation led to only modest increases in

Table 14-3 Maternal DHA (22:6 n−3) Supplementation

MATERNAL SUPPLEMENTATION

Reference	Total (n)	Period	EPA (mg/day)	DHA (mg/day)	Source of DHA	Maternal DHA (% change)	Infant DHA (% change)	Main developmental results
A. Prenatal supplementation								
Connor et al. 1996 (157)	31	3rd TM	800	1300	Fish oil	–	Cord, 20% ↑	–
Malcolm et al. 2003; Sanjurjo et al. 2004 (58, 60)	20	3rd TM	40	200	Fish oil	–	Cord, 6% ↑	–
Malcolm et al. 2003; Montgomery et al. 2003 (58, 59, 158)	100	2nd and 3rd TM	40	200	Fish oil	Plasma 20% ↑	–	No effect on visual function (ERG; VEP) 2, 6, and 16 weeks PN
Smuts et al. 2003 (57)	350	3rd TM	–	150	High-DHA eggs		Cord, 6% ↑	Length of gestation ↑ by 6 days; No effect on habituation and attention tests at 2, 4, 8, 12 and 18 months PN (subset, n = 70)
B. Postnatal supplementation								
Gibson et al. 1997 (67)	50	B–4 months	–	200 / 400 / 600	Algal oil	HM 200%↑ / – / –	Plasma 30% ↑ / – / –	No effect on visual function (VEP) at 4 weeks PN
Jensen et al. 2005 (64)		B–4 months	–	1000 / 200	Algal oil	HM 500% ↑	Plasma 200% ↑ / Plasma 35% ↑	No effect on visual and cognitive outcomes from 2 weeks to 18 months; Higher scores on psychomotor index at 30 months
Lauritzen et al. 2004 (63)	175	B– 4 months	310	710	Fish oil	300% ↑	–	No effect on visual (VEP) acuity at 2, 4 months
C. Pre- and postnatal supplementation								
Helland et al. 1998, 2001, 2003 (61, 62, 159)	590	2nd TM to 4 months PN	820	1200	Cod liver oil	Plasma 400% ↑ / HM 300% ↑	Cord, 25% ↑ / Infant, 50% ↑	No effect on cognitive function at 2 and 6 weeks and 6 and 9 months; Higher IQ at 4 years

TM, trimester; B, birth; PN, postnatal; HM, human milk.

maternal or cord blood 22:6 n–3 levels (Table 14-3). Maternal DHA supplementation leads to increased human milk and infant plasma levels of DHA, but similarly there is limited evidence for enhanced visual and cognitive development (63–67). Studies in which pregnant women are supplemented with DHA before or early in the first trimester are lacking.

Maternal plasma 22:6 n–3 is lower in multigravid than in primagravid pregnancies (55, 68), suggesting that the 22:6 n–3 that is mobilized from adipose tissue may not be replenished in the short-term. The 22:6 n–3 status of newborn multiplets also is significantly lower than that of singletons (55, 68). Although recommendations for women to consume 300 mg of DHA daily to help ensure adequate availability of this fatty acid to the fetus have been published (http://www.issfal.org.uk/Welcome/AdequateIntakes.asp), more research is needed to understand the significance of maternal 22:6 n–3 status during gestation on perinatal development.

The usual dietary intake of DHA among women from different populations varies widely and is reflected in human milk (1). Fish is the primary dietary source of DHA, and in countries where fish is eaten more frequently, DHA intakes are higher. The average DHA intake in pregnant women in western Canada, for example, is 160 mg/day (29). While there are not similar data from other populations, it is informative to compare dietary intakes of DHA among different regions globally. The *average* DHA intake in Australia is 105 mg/day (69), in the USA 70 mg/day (U.S.; http://www.ahrq.gov/downloads/pub/evidence/pdf/o3cogn/o3cogn.pdf), in France 570 mg/day (70), and in Japan about 600–1160 mg/day (71, 72).

Preterm Infant Development

Nutrient demands of preterm and intrauterine-growth-restricted infants are high and vary depending on the degree of prematurity, immaturity of organs, adequacy of stores, and whether there are concomitant diseases of prematurity. Infants with lower gestational age and birth weight are at greater risk for medical complications. The initiation and advancement of feedings may be delayed to reduce the risk of medical complications related to immaturity of the gastrointestinal system and other vital organs. Consequently, the desired growth rates are not always achieved. Physiological stressors such as bouts of hypotension, hypoxia, infection, surgeries, and hypoglycemia may be transient or may lead to complications requiring medical interventions. The risk of potentially serious complications from necrotizing enterocolitis and other pathologies influences decisions about intake volumes and nutritional goals when feeding preterm infants enterally. Potential adverse effects to the central nervous system and other organs from high plasma levels of certain amino acids, glucose, fatty acids and other metabolic products also are considered when making decisions about the introduction and advancement of enteral feedings. Our understanding of basic physiology in perinatal growth and development continues to evolve, as does the nutritional and medical management of preterm infants.

At birth, adaptation to the extrauterine environment triggers a number of physiologic and metabolic changes. The adaptive changes in lipid physiology and metabolism are particularly remarkable. Before birth, glucose is the major energy substrate, placental flux of fatty acids involves specific fatty acid binding proteins, there is a biomagnification of long-chain n–6 and n–3 fatty acids across the placenta, and fat is deposited in fetal adipose tissues largely in the last 10 weeks of gestation. After birth, fatty acids become the major energy substrates, the gastrointestinal tract becomes critical in the digestion of the fat in milk and the absorption of fatty acids, and infant adipose stores are mobilized to help support the energy demands and requirements for long-chain n–6 and n–3 fatty acids in central nervous development. For infants born prematurely, the immaturity of the gastrointestinal tract and limited adipose stores are important determinants in the adaptation to the extrauterine environment. The thermoregulatory effects and physical cushioning of delicate organs by adipose tissue are also important.

It is well established that preterm infants have greater energy requirements than infants born at term. This comprises energy that is expended, stored and lost. Expended energy is energy that supports basal metabolic rate, energy utilized in activity, energy for new tissue synthesis, thermoregulation or "cold stress," and the thermic effect of food. Stored energy includes energy in both adipose stores and lean body mass. Energy is lost mainly from incomplete digestion and absorption of macronutrients. The estimated average energy cost of growth for preterm infants is 3.0–4.5 kcal/g (73). Average energy intakes of 105–130 kcal/kg/day are typically recommended. About half of the energy is from fat. Infants with bronchopulmonary dysplasia or who are small for gestational age or extremely low birth weight may have even higher energy needs (73).

Fat, the major energy substrate in both human milk and infant formula, comprises 40–55% of the total energy available. For infants born prematurely and for whom sufficient amounts of human milk are not available, preterm infant formulas are the best substitute. Preterm infant formulas, which are more nutrient- and energy-dense than human milk and full-term infant formulas, were designed to achieve growth at rates comparable to those of the reference fetus (74). Most preterm infant formulas provide 24 kcal/fl oz. Human milk fortifiers are also available to enhance the nutritional density of human milk. Preterm infants who are not able to tolerate enteral feedings may be given parenteral lipids as part of their nutritional regimen.

Digestion and Absorption of Dietary Fat

Fat digestion and absorption may be limiting in infants born prematurely because the activity of pancreatic lipase may not be fully developed, bile acid concentrations may be below the critical micellar concentration, the absorptive capacity of enterocytes may be immature, and enterohepatic circulation may be underdeveloped. Human milk lipase, sometimes called bile-salt-dependent lipase, is unique to human milk and has been shown to enhance the digestion of fat in human milk (75, 76). The presence of this lipase in human milk may account for, at least in part, greater fat absorption in preterm infants fed human milk compared with some infant formulas (77).

The maturation of the absorptive capacity for fatty acids and 2-monoglycerides across the intestinal lumen has been proposed as critical for the bioavailability of fatty acids postnatally (78). This is suggested from studies that examined the maturation of fat absorption in preterm infants using ^{13}C tracer methodology. In a study with term and preterm infants, serum concentrations of 1-^{13}C-palmitate were measured after enteral administration of tri-^{13}C-palmitoylglycerol. The authors concluded that maturation of fat digestion and absorption in infants is explained largely by the capacity to absorb fatty acids, which becomes fully mature at around 46 weeks gestation in both term and preterm infants. It is not clear, at present, the extent to which the maturation of lipase activity and bile formation for the solubilization of fatty acids into micelles and intraluminal digestion of fat to fatty acids and 2-monoglycerides may affect intestinal absorption of fatty acids in preterm infants.

Preterm Human Milk

The total fat and the fatty acid composition of human milk from mothers delivering prematurely, like that of women delivering at term, is variable (1). Estimates of total fat content vary from about 45 to 60% of total energy. Many studies report that human milk from women giving birth prematurely has higher levels of medium- and intermediate-chain-length fatty acids (C10:0, C12:0, C14:0) than human milk from women delivering at term (61, 62, 79–84). n–6 and n–3 fatty acid levels in preterm and full-term human milk are highly variable, with *average* DHA levels varying over 10-fold and ARA levels over 3-fold, with even greater variability among individual women.

This variability in the levels of the n–6 and n–3 fatty acids, especially LA and DHA, is highly influenced by the usual fats in the maternal diet. DHA levels in milk are notably higher in countries where fish is a major source of protein in the diet (1) and have been shown to follow dose-response kinetics, with higher maternal dietary DHA associated with higher milk DHA levels (66).

Caloric Density of Human Milk and Infant Formula

Increasing the caloric density of human milk or formulas for preterm infants to meet energy requirements for growth of infants born prematurely is often clinically indicated. Non-protein energy substrates, which include fat, are often used to increase the energy density of human milk or formula. Health care professionals may also add nutrient modules to human milk or infant formula (85). The addition of these modules to enteral feedings, however, can alter the balance of nutrients. It is, therefore, important to assess the nutritional impact of modifying the infant diet and to carefully monitor the infant when providing nutrient modules. Research with preterm infants weighing less than 1500 g at birth has found that, regardless of whether the extra calories were added to standard preterm formula as carbohydrate or as fat, specifically medium chain triglycerides (MCTs), the increased weight gain was due to increased fat deposition, not increased lean body mass (86). Further research is needed to optimize nutritional regimens for preterm infants for optimal deposition of lean body mass and fat mass while supporting adequate growth.

Growth and Energy

MEDIUM-CHAIN TRIGLYCERIDES

Many preterm infant formulas contain MCTs at levels up to about 60% of the total fat. MCTs were initially added to preterm infant formulas to enhance fat and calcium absorption and to provide a readily available source of energy for infants with compromised gastrointestinal function (74). Infants fed preterm infant formulas with up to about 60% of fat as MCTs had better fat absorption than those fed formulas with lower levels of MCTs (74, 87). Subsequent studies, however, have found no differences in fat absorption between infants fed preterm formula with 40–50% of fat as MCT and those fed formula with lower levels (88, 89). Additional research on specific subpopulations of preterm infants may help to clarify the role of dietary MCT on fat absorption. Higher calcium absorption also has been found with increasing levels of MCT in preterm formulas (90).

MCTs in preterm infant formulas help regulate energy balance. Medium-chain-length fatty acids (MCFAs) are released from MCTs by gastric lipases and are absorbed directly through the gastric mucosa (88). It is well established that MCFAs are more readily oxidized for energy than the LCFAs (91). Significantly lower glucose oxidation (92) and increased lipogenesis have been reported in preterm infants fed formula with higher levels of MCT (92, 93). Others report that preterm infant formulas containing 40% MCT spare the oxidation of 18:2 n–6 (94). Increased energy intake and a higher metabolic rate, cheek skin temperature, and total sleep time also have been reported in preterm infants fed formula with up to 63% MCT. (95). It is noteworthy that infants fed formula with MCT have higher urinary dicarboxylic acids, but this is considered clinically insignificant and is a normal response to increased MCT intake (96–100).

A systematic review of preterm infant growth as reported in studies with preterm infants fed formula with high vs. low MCT levels was conducted in 2003 by the Cochrane Database Systematic Review (101). This report concluded that there are no differences in short-term growth, gastrointestinal intolerance, or necrotizing enterocolitis in infants fed formulas containing long-chain triglycerides or MCTs. However, only eight studies, each with small sample sizes, met the criteria for inclusion in this review. Further research with larger sample sizes was suggested.

Although MCFA levels are higher in human milk from mothers delivering prematurely than those delivering at term, many preterm infant formulas contain higher levels than in human milk. An Expert Panel review of the lipid requirements for preterm infants recommended that the amount of MCT in preterm infant formula not exceed 50% of the total fat, but did not recommend a minimum amount (102). There were no concerns about the safety of including MCT in preterm formula and some research suggests specific benefits. Further research on the adaptive changes in the gastrointestinal and metabolic systems of infants born prematurely will help to better understand the role of MCT in the diet of preterm infants.

LONG-CHAIN n–6 AND n–3 FATTY ACIDS

The long-chain n–6 and n–3 fatty acids ARA and DHA were added to preterm formula to help support visual and neural development. Growth, an important determinant of short- and long-term health, has been monitored in the studies of formulas supplemented with DHA or both DHA and ARA. The initial studies with preterm infants fed formulas with added DHA found evidence of slower growth beginning at around 2–4 months gestation-corrected age (103–107). Associations between 20:4 n–6 status and growth were reported (103). Subsequent studies with preterm formulas supplemented with both ARA and DHA or with DHA alone have found no evidence of slower growth (108–111), and one study reported better growth (110). Increased lean body mass and reduced fat mass, without differences in growth, also have been reported in preterm infants fed ARA- and DHA-supplemented formulas (112). More research is needed to better understand the role of ARA and DHA on growth and body composition in preterm infants.

Adipose

After birth, infant adipose tissue is readily mobilized to help support energy needs and requirements for long-chain n–6 and n–3 fatty acids in the immediate postnatal period (50). These changes are nutritionally sensitive, and may be mediated in part by rapid changes in prolactin and leptin secretion after birth. Exposure to the extrauterine environment and activation of UCP 1 results in the mobilization and oxidation of brown fat and increased heat production (50). Within a few hours after birth, adipose tissue stores of the long chain n–6 and n–3 fatty acids, notably 20:4 n–6 and 22:6 n–3, are also liberated (34). It has been estimated that adipose reserves in term infants are depleted in the first 2 months after birth if infant formula does not supply preformed DHA (113). For preterm infants with negligible adipose reserves, hepatic lipid stores may help support requirements for neural tissue accretion, but only for a few days (114). Adipose tissue also provides a cushion that protects internal organs.

Central Nervous System

A major focus of perinatal lipid research over the past two decades has been understanding the dietary requirements for polyunsaturated fatty acids, particularly the long-chain n–6 and n–3 fatty acids ARA and DHA. Interruption of normal gestation by premature birth cuts off the provision of the n–3 and n–6 fatty acids from the mother to the fetus. After birth, infants obtain these fatty acids through human milk or infant formula preformed as ARA and DHA and as their 18-carbon precursors, LA and ALA, respectively. Human milk also contains small amounts of other long-chain polyunsaturated fatty acids, including EPA (20:5 n–3). Infants who are not be able to tolerate enteral feedings and are receiving intravenous lipids as part of a parenteral nutrition regimen obtain the n–6 and n–3 fatty acids primarily as linoleic acid and α-linolenic acid (53).

Neurodevelopmental outcomes related to the addition of ARA and DHA to preterm and full-term infant formulas and in human breast milk have been of particular interest. Human milk and infant formulas contain LA and ALA and comparatively lower levels of ARA and DHA. The central nervous system is enriched in both 20:4 n–6 and 22:6 n–3, and the retina is particularly enriched in 22:6 n–3. Low levels of 18:2 n–6 and negligible amounts of 18:3 n–3 are present. More than a decade of clinical research with infants fed formulas with or without added ARA and/or DHA led to the addition of DHA and ARA to formulas for both preterm and term infants. Many excellent reviews of this and related research have been published (10, 33, 102, 114–122). The reader is directed to these reviews for comprehensive summaries of the studies published to date.

Providing adequate amounts of n–6 and n–3 fatty acids for accretion in brain comparable to that of the fetus without compromising growth is an important goal in the nutritional management of preterm infants. Human milk n–6 and n–3 fatty acid composition has served as a guide from which to design blends of different fats containing n–6 and n–3 fatty acids for infant formula. The DHA levels in formulas studied clinically with preterm infants have varied from about 0.25% to 1.0% of total fatty acids. ARA levels, when included, varied from about 0.40% to 0.72% of total fatty acids. It is well established that increasing the amounts of DHA in human milk or formula leads to higher levels of 22:6 n–3 in plasma and RBC of infants (66). Beneficial effects on the development of the visual system and central nervous system in preterm infants have been generally consistent across studies (110, 123), although some effects were transient (104, 124, 125) and others were found only in subpopulations (111).

It has been suggested that human milk levels of DHA may not be sufficient to meet the requirements for accretion of 22:6 n–3 in the central nervous system of preterm infants (53). A recent study examined DHA intakes at up to 1% total fatty acids in both human milk and formulas for preterm infants (123). Visual function was measured at 2 and 4 months gestation corrected age in preterm infants fed diets with 0.3% or 1.0% fatty acids as DHA. Visual evoked potential latency and acuity were found to be age-dependent. There were only small effects of diet and no further benefits of increasing DHA levels above 0.3% of fatty acids, a level that is similar to that in current preterm infant formulas.

Whether the effects of dietary DHA on visual and neural development persist past the first year has not been studied to date. An epidemiological study of visual function in over five hundred 10–12–year-old children found that those who were born prematurely had near and distance acuities and contrast sensitivity that were lower than in those born at term (126). Multivariate analyses that included infant diet (human milk, preterm formula without DHA and AA, term formula, and unknown diet), birth weight, gestational age, small for gestational age, and several clinical diagnoses (cerebral palsy, strabismus at 6 months, retinopathy of prematurity, cranial ultrasound abnormality) were not able to identify specific factors that predicted long-term visual outcome. Retinopathy of prematurity was surprisingly a poor predictor of outcome. DHA levels in human milk were not reported.

Additional studies are needed to assess the effects of DHA in human milk and preterm infant formula on visual and neural development past the first year. It is possible, also, that other components in human milk may further enhance central nervous system development (53, 127).

Immune

The immune system is immature at birth, and infants, especially those born prematurely, are highly susceptible to infection when exposed to a wide range of pathogens. Cell-mediated immune responses are attenuated during active viral infection, and the formation of virus-specific immunological memory is inefficient in preterm infants. In the fetus, systemic humoral immunity depends on the transplacental transfer of IgG. Both premature birth and intrauterine growth restriction interrupt the normal acquisition of IgG by the fetus. After birth, nutrient-immune interactions can influence the postnatal development of both innate and adaptive immune functions. This includes maturation of specific lymphocyte responses in conjunction with the formation of immunoregulatory and protective proteins following pathogen exposure.

Dietary n–6 and n–3 fatty acids are known to mediate inflammatory and immune responses through multiple mechanisms (128, 129). There exists a large body of research on the role of n–3 fatty acids and inflammatory and immune responses in adults, animal models and cell culture systems. Both 20:4 n–6 and 20:5 n–3 are precursors for prostaglandins and leukotrienes that regulate normal inflammatory processes, and 22:6 n–3 can affect inflammatory responses and T-cell signaling (130, 131).

The n–6 and n–3 fatty acids play a role in the phenotypic maturation of immune cells and the development of functionally competent immunological responses, including the maturation of cytokine markers on T-lymphocytes (130, 132–138). It has been suggested also that neonatal T cell responses to allergens and antigens are distinctively different from those in later life (139). CD4(+) T cell cultures derived from infants showed high levels of apoptosis compared to adult-derived allergen-responsive T-cell cultures. Infant CD4(+) T cells in culture also exhibited an initial burst of short-lived cellular immunity and T-cell memory responsiveness, but with limited intensity and duration (139).

A comparison of the major lymphocyte subpopulations in infants born prematurely (gestational age < 32 weeks; 32–37 weeks), term newborns and adults not surprisingly found that preterm infants born at less than 32 weeks gestation had the most immature lymphocyte phenotypes (136). No differences, however, were found between infants born at 32–37 weeks gestation and those born at term. Infants born prematurely also had a very low percentage of memory helper T lymphocytes (CD45RO(+)CD4(+)) (135). Peripheral blood lymphocyte populations, cytokine production, and antigen maturity were recently studied in a randomized, controlled trial with preterm infants fed a preterm formula, with or without added DHA and ARA from 14 to 42 days after birth (132). The preterm infants fed the ARA and DHA supplemented formula had a higher proportion of antigen mature CD45RO(+)CD4(+) cells, improved IL-10 production, and reduced IL-2 production compared with those fed the unsupplemented formula. In addition, the immune cell responses of the ARA- and DHA-supplemented infants were similar to those of full-term infants fed human milk-fed.

The immune system of the fetus is maintained in a tolerogenic state to prevent adverse immune responses and rejection of the fetus by the mother. Placental IL-10 suppresses the formation of immunologically potent interferon gamma (INF-γ)) by fetal immune cells, and INF-γ down-regulates the formation of proallergic cytokines (e.g. IL-4, IL-13). Although this favors immune tolerance in utero, it can foster an allergic immune response postnatally. Allergic disease and asthma are influenced by both genetic and early environmental exposure related to immune responsiveness (140, 141). Reduced respiratory function in the first months after birth, and prenatal and postnatal factors, such as maternal age and environmental tobacco smoke, are known environmental risk factors for allergic disease. Associations between fetal growth restriction, but not gestational age at birth, and risk for atopic disease and asthma have been reported (142). Intrauterine and early postnatal exposure to allergens has been suggested as primary sensitization events. Lifestyle and diet later in life are thought to be secondary to the effects of the immunological programming during pregnancy and early infancy. Associations between *n*–6 and *n*–3 fatty acid status in the perinatal period and the development of atopic disease have been suggested (140, 141, 143). Observational (144, 145) and fish oil supplementation studies (146–149) suggest that the *n*–3 fatty acids EPA and DHA may help reduce the risk of atopic and allergic disease. More research is clearly needed.

One theory of immune regulation involves homeostasis or skewing between T-helper 1 (Th1) and T-helper 2 (Th2) activity. Th1 cells drive cellular immunity by mounting responses to eliminate viruses and intracellular pathogens and stimulate delayed-type hypersensitivity skin reactions. Th2 cells influence humoral immunity by up-regulating antibody production to fight extracellular organisms. It appears, however, that the cellular mechanisms by which the long-chain *n*–3 fatty acids 20:5 *n*–3 and 22:6 *n*–3 modulate allergic immune responses do not involve skewing of T-cell responses (143, 150). This is in contrast to other nutrients (plant sterols, probiotics, selenium and zinc) and hormones (melatonin, progesterone) that have been shown to influence the Th1/Th2 balance.

Fatty acid effects on the immune system are mediated through membrane fatty acid effects that involve eicosanoid responses (128), endocannabinoid effects (151), cell signaling and gene regulation responses (9, 152), lipid rafts (15, 153), and vascular and intracellular cell adhesion molecules (154, 155). A better understanding of the specific underlying mechanisms that shape the immune response and how polyunsaturated fatty acids may interact to help strengthen the immune system in the perinatal periods is needed.

RELEVANCE OF PHYSIOLOGIC DIFFERENCES TO DISEASE PROCESS

The transition from fetal to postnatal life involves a major shift in metabolism from glucose as the major energy substrate to fat, which makes up about 50% of the daily caloric intake from human milk or infant formula. The fetus acquires lipids and other nutrients transplacentally, while the newborn relies on a functional gastrointestinal system for the digestion and absorption of nutrients in human milk or infant formula. There is also a transition in the pattern of *n*–6 and *n*–3 fatty acid acquisition after birth from that obtained transplacentally. Transplacental flux of 20:4 *n*–6 and 22:6 *n*–3 is greater than that for their 18-carbon precursors, 18:2 *n*–6 and 18:3 *n*–3, respectively. After birth, human milk and infant formula provide greater amounts of the 18-carbon long-chain *n*–6 and *n*–3 fatty acids than ARA and DHA, respectively. Adipose tissue is formed largely in the last 10 weeks of gestation, and after birth, especially in the early postnatal period, helps support energy needs and requirements for the long-chain *n*–3 and *n*–6 fatty acids for the central nervous system. Infants born prematurely have limited adipose stores and organ development may not be fully mature. Adaptation to postnatal life depends to a large extent on the functional maturity of the gastrointestinal tract for the digestion and absorption of lipids.

The intestinal tract is especially vulnerable to damage that may lead to complications such as feeding intolerance and necrotizing enterocolitis. Lower gestational age and birth weight are associated with increased risk for diseases of prematurity. Clinical markers used to assess health (or absence of disease) include markers of nutritional status, such as anthropometric and physiological measures, or functional outcomes associated with physical growth and neurodevelopment. Clinical nutritional assessment includes evaluating the infant's general condition, feeding tolerance, and signs or symptoms of nutrient deficiency or excess. Low adipose and nutrient stores from premature birth or intrauterine growth retardation, the need for parenteral nutrition, periods of energy restriction, and high nutrient requirements may affect overall growth and development.

The method of enteral feeding chosen for each infant is typically based on gestational age, birth weight, and clinical condition. Structural anomalies and patency of the infant's gastrointestinal tract and airways are considered before starting enteral feedings. Specific considerations when feeding preterm infants include at which age to initiate feeding, type of feeding (formula or human milk), method of delivery, feeding frequency, and rate of advancement. Some infants are fed parenterally before starting on enteral feedings. In other words, feeding regimens are determined according to a number of criteria and thus may differ widely among infants born prematurely or with intrauterine growth restriction. A detailed discussion of feeding methods is beyond the scope of this paper, and the reader is referred to an excellent review (156).

Preterm infants who are born with an underdeveloped gastrointestinal system and have limited adipose reserves are at increased risk for poor growth. After enteral feedings are initiated, feeding intolerance may lead to reduced energy intake, nutritional deficits, and fat malabsorption with symptoms of essential fatty acid deficiency. Feeding intolerance may be caused by an immature gastrointestinal tract, immature digestive enzymes, medical complications such as necrotizing enterocolitis or sepsis, hyperosmolar feedings, high feeding volumes or medications. Symptoms of feeding intolerance include increased periods of apnea and bradycardia associated with feedings, large gastric residuals, increased abdominal girth or abdominal distention, vomiting, or stools that are positive for blood or reducing substances. A poor sucking reflex or inability to establish a functional suck and swallow pattern also may limit the infant's capacity to consume adequate amounts of energy and nutrients. Gastrointestinal priming in the first few days (i.e. feeding a low volume of human milk or formula) has been shown to stimulate intestinal function and improve tolerance of enteral feedings. The ability to provide adequate nutrition support, of which dietary lipids are just one component, is essential for optimal growth and development.

Fat malabsorption may lead to essential fatty acid deficiency as well as deficiencies in the fat-soluble vitamins, namely vitamin E, vitamin D, vitamin K and vitamin A. These are among the nutritional deficiencies most commonly reported in infants born prematurely (i.e. calcium, phosphorus, vitamin D, vitamin E, iron, zinc, carnitine, essential fatty acids, and protein). Fat malabsorption may be identified by stools that are large, bulky, oily and unusually foul-smelling. If there is pancreatic insufficiency or bile acids are insufficient, the stools may appear white, gray, or clay-colored. Clinical signs of essential fatty acid deficiency include scaly dermatitis, thrombocytopenia, increased risk of infection, poor growth, and alopecia.

Temperature control may be difficult during the newborn period, especially for infants with intrauterine growth restriction and those born prematurely. Neonates adapt to cold stress by producing heat at the expense of calories needed for growth. During cold stress, the breakdown of brown fat stores provides a metabolic source of nonshivering heat production. Heat may also be generated by crying or moving. The metabolism of brown adipose tissue for the production of heat occurs only in the newborn period. Smaller and less mature infants are born with inadequate adipose stores, a larger body surface area per unit of weight, and a higher body water content. This allows greater water loss and consequently greater heat loss. Dysregulation of temperature control is more common in preterm infants than full-term infants.

Interruption of normal gestation by premature birth cuts off the provision of the n–3 and n–6 fatty acids from the mother to the fetus. After birth, infants obtain these fatty acids through human milk or infant formula preformed as ARA and DHA and as their 18-carbon precursors, LA and ALA, respectively. Accretion of 20:4 n–6 and 22:6 n–3 in the brain and 22:6 n–3 in the retina begins around mid-gestation and continues well after birth. Visual and neurodevelopmental benefits in preterm infants fed preformed sources of ARA and DHA have been demonstrated in the first year after discharge from the hospital. While not clinically significant to the diagnosis or treatment of preterm infants in the neonatal intensive care unit, these fatty acids help support visual and neural development longer-term. Recent reports of lower circulating levels of both 20:4 n–6 and 22:6 n–3 in infants born to women with type 1 diabetes, type 2 diabetes or gestational diabetes (37, 45, 46) are disconcerting, particularly given the numbers of young women at risk for gestational and type 2 diabetes.

Emerging evidence suggests that the long-chain n–6 and n–3 fatty acids may be important in immune system development. The research to date, however, is limited and many questions remain. Among them is identifying the optimum balance between the specific long-chain n–6 and the long-chain n–3 fatty acids (143) that may facilitate maturation of both adaptive and humoral immune function. Infants born prematurely are at increased risk of sepsis, thus enhancing immunological development in the perinatal period has obvious clinical benefits. Allergic disease and asthma are influenced by both genetics and early environmental exposure (140, 141), and immunological programming may occur during pregnancy and early infancy (137).

In summary, there are striking differences in lipid physiology and metabolism between the fetus and infants born prematurely. Dietary fats are important energy substrates postnatally. The long-chain n–6 and n–3 fatty acids, which are acquired postnatally, preformed as ARA and DHA or are formed *in situ* from the dietary essential fatty acids, LA and ALA, are important for central nervous system development and appear to be involved in immune system development. Infants born prematurely rely on a functional gastrointestinal system to support adequate intakes of energy for growth and for n–6 and n–3 fatty acid accretion central nervous system development. Significant advances in our understanding of both fetal and postnatal physiology and in the nutritional and medical management of infants born prematurely have been made in recent years, but knowledge gaps still remain. Further advances will help us to improve the quality of the nutritional regimens for preterm infants.

REFERENCES

1. Jensen RG. Lipids in human milk. Lipids 1999; 34:1243.
2. Koo WW, Hockman EM, Dow M. Palm olein in the fat blend of infant formulas: effect on the intestinal absorption of calcium and fat, and bone mineralization. J Am Coll Nutr 2006; 25:117.
3. Hamosh M, Mehta NR, Fink CS, et al. Fat absorption in premature infants: medium-chain triglycerides and long-chain triglycerides are absorbed from formula at similar rates. J Pediatr Gastroenterol Nutr 1991; 13:143.
4. Diaz M, Leal C, Ramon Y, Cajal J, et al. Cord blood lipoprotein-cholesterol: relationship birth weight and gestational age of newborns. Metabolism 1989; 38:435.
5. Kalra A, Kalra K, Agarwal MC, et al. Serum lipid profile in term and preterm infants in early neonatal period. Indian Pediatr 1988; 25:977.
6. Mortaz M, Fewtrell MS, Cole TJ, et al. Cholesterol metabolism in 8 to 12-year-old children born preterm or at term. Acta Paediatr 2003; 92:525.
7. Pardo IM, Geloneze B, Tambascia MA, et al. Atherogenic lipid profile of Brazilian near-term newborns. Braz J Med Biol Res 2005; 38:755.

8. Singhal A, Cole TJ, Fewtrell M, et al. Breastmilk feeding and lipoprotein profile in adolescents born preterm: follow-up of a prospective randomised study. Lancet 2004; 363:1571.
9. Clarke SD. The multi-dimensional regulation of gene expression by fatty acids: polyunsaturated fats as nutrient sensors. Curr Opin Lipidol 2004; 15:13.
10. Innis SM. Perinatal biochemistry and physiology of long-chain polyunsaturated fatty acids. J Pediatr 2003; 143:S1.
11. Connor WE, Neuringer M. The effects of n–3 fatty acid deficiency and repletion upon the fatty acid composition and function of the brain and retina. Prog Clin Biol Res 1988; 282:275.
12. Jeffrey BG, Mitchell DC, Gibson RA, et al. n–3 fatty acid deficiency alters recovery of the rod photoresponse in rhesus monkeys. Invest Ophthalmol Vis Sci 2002; 43:2806.
13. Lim SY, Hoshiba J, Salem N Jr. An extraordinary degree of structural specificity is required in neural phospholipids for optimal brain function: n–6 docosapentaenoic acid substitution for docosahexaenoic acid leads to a loss in spatial task performance. J Neurochem 2005; 95:848.
14. Uauy R, Mena P, Rojas C. Essential fatty acids in early life: structural and functional role. Proc Nutr Soc 2000; 59:3.
15. Ma DW, Seo J, Switzer KC, et al. n–3 PUFA and membrane microdomains: a new frontier in bioactive lipid research. J Nutr Biochem 2004; 15:700.
16. Martinez M. Tissue levels of polyunsaturated fatty acids during early human development. J Pediatr 1992; 120:S129.
17. Clandinin MT, Chappell JE, Heim T, et al. Fatty acid utilization in perinatal de novo synthesis of tissues. Early Hum Dev 1981; 5:355.
18. Berghaus TM, Demmelmair H, Koletzko B. Fatty acid composition of lipid classes in maternal and cord plasma at birth. Eur J Pediatr 1998; 157:763.
19. Clandinin MT, Wong K, Hacker RR. Synthesis of chain elongation-desaturation products of linoleic acid by liver and brain microsomes during development of the pig. Biochem J 1985; 226:305.
20. Dutta-Roy AK. Transport mechanisms for long-chain polyunsaturated fatty acids in the human placenta. Am J Clin Nutr 2000; 71:315S.
21. Su HM, Huang MC, Saad NM, et al. Fetal baboons convert 18:3 n–3 to 22:6 n–3 in vivo. A stable isotope tracer study. J Lipid Res 2001; 42:581.
22. Haggarty P. Effect of placental function on fatty acid requirements during pregnancy. Eur J Clin Nutr 2004; 58:1559.
23. Fuchs R, Ellinger I. Endocytic and transcytotic processes in villous syncytiotrophoblast: role in nutrient transport to the human fetus. Traffic 2004; 5:725.
24. Dutta-Roy AK. Cellular uptake of long-chain fatty acids: role of membrane-associated fatty-acid-binding/transport proteins. Cell Mol Life Sci 2000; 57:1360.
25. Knipp GT, Audus KL, Soares MJ. Nutrient transport across the placenta. Adv Drug Deliv Rev 1999; 38:41.
26. Campbell FM, Taffesse S, Gordon MJ, et al. Plasma membrane fatty-acid-binding protein in human placenta: identification and characterization. Biochem Biophys Res Commun 1995; 209:1011.
27. Larque E, Demmelmair H, Berger B, et al. In vivo investigation of the placental transfer of (13)C-labeled fatty acids in humans. J Lipid Res 2003; 44:49.
28. Campbell FM, Gordon MJ, Dutta-Roy AK. Preferential uptake of long chain polyunsaturated fatty acids by isolated human placental membranes. Mol Cell Biochem 1996; 155:77.
29. Elias SL, Innis SM. Infant plasma trans, n–6, and n–3 fatty acids and conjugated linoleic acids are related to maternal plasma fatty acids, length of gestation, and birth weight and length. Am J Clin Nutr 2001; 73:807.
30. Haggarty P, Ashton J, Joynson M, et al. Effect of maternal polyunsaturated fatty acid concentration on transport by the human placenta. Biol Neonate 1999; 75:350.
31. Kuhn DC, Crawford M. Placental essential fatty acid transport and prostaglandin synthesis. Prog Lipid Res 1986; 25:345.
32. Innis SM. Essential fatty acids in growth and development. Prog Lipid Res 1991; 30:39.
33. Innis SM. Essential fatty acid transfer and fetal development. Placenta 2005; 26 Suppl A:S70.
34. Haggarty P. Placental regulation of fatty acid delivery and its effect on fetal growth—a review. Placenta 2002; 23(Suppl A):S28.
35. Kuhn DC, Crawford MA, Stuart MJ, et al. Alterations in transfer and lipid distribution of arachidonic acid in placentas of diabetic pregnancies. Diabetes 1990; 39:914.
36. Wijendran V, Bendel RB, Couch SC, et al. Maternal plasma phospholipid polyunsaturated fatty acids in pregnancy with and without gestational diabetes mellitus: relations with maternal factors. Am J Clin Nutr 1999; 70:53.
37. Wijendran V, Bendel RB, Couch SC, et al. Fetal erythrocyte phospholipid polyunsaturated fatty acids are altered in pregnancy complicated with gestational diabetes mellitus. Lipids 2000; 35:927.
38. Lepercq J, Challier JC, Guerre-Millo M, et al. Prenatal leptin production: evidence that fetal adipose tissue produces leptin. J Clin Endocrinol Metab 2001; 86:2409.
39. Hoggard N, Crabtree J, Allstaff S, et al. Leptin secretion to both the maternal and fetal circulation in the ex vivo perfused human term placenta. Placenta 2001; 22:347.
40. Hoggard N, Haggarty P, Thomas L, et al. Leptin expression in placental and fetal tissues: does leptin have a functional role? Biochem Soc Trans 2001; 29:57.
41. Yildiz L, Avci B, Ingec M. Umbilical cord and maternal blood leptin concentrations in intrauterine growth retardation. Clin Chem Lab Med 2002; 40:1114.
42. Bernstein IM, Goran MI, Amini SB, et al. Differential growth of fetal tissues during the second half of pregnancy. Am J Obstet Gynecol 1997; 176:28.

43. Parretti E, Carignani L, Cioni R, et al. Sonographic evaluation of fetal growth and body composition in women with different degrees of normal glucose metabolism. Diabetes Care 2003; 26:2741.

44. Larciprete G, Valensise H, Vasapollo B, et al. Fetal subcutaneous tissue thickness (SCTT) in healthy and gestational diabetic pregnancies. Ultrasound Obstet Gynecol 2003; 22:591.

45. Min Y, Lowy C, Ghebremeskel K, et al. Unfavorable effect of type 1 and type 2 diabetes on maternal and fetal essential fatty acid status: a potential marker of fetal insulin resistance. Am J Clin Nutr 2005; 82:1162.

46. Ghebremeskel K, Thomas B, Lowy C, et al. Type 1 diabetes compromises plasma arachidonic and docosahexaenoic acids in newborn babies. Lipids 2004; 39:335.

47. Plagemann A. Perinatal programming and functional teratogenesis: impact on body weight regulation and obesity. Physiol Behav 2005; 86:661.

48. Garg M, Thamotharan M, Rogers L, et al. Glucose metabolic adaptations in the intrauterine growth-restricted adult female rat offspring. Am J Physiol Endocrinol Metab 2006; 290:E1218.

49. Groh-Wargo S. Recommended enteral nutrient intakes. In: Groh-Wargo S, Thompson M, Cox J, eds., Nutritional care for high-risk neonates, 3rd edn. Los Angeles: Bonus Books; 2000: 231.

50. Symonds ME, Mostyn A, Pearce S, et al. Endocrine and nutritional regulation of fetal adipose tissue development. J Endocrinol 2003; 179:293.

51. Dobbing J, Sands J. Quantitative growth and development of human brain. Arch Dis Child 1973; 48:757.

52. Dobbing J, Sands J. Comparative aspects of the brain growth spurt. Early Hum Dev 1979; 3:79.

53. Georgieff MK, Innis SM. Controversial nutrients that potentially affect preterm neurodevelopment: essential fatty acids and iron. Pediatr Res 2005; 57:99R.

54. Clandinin MT, Chappell JE, Leong S, et al. Intrauterine fatty acid accretion rates in human brain: implications for fatty acid requirements. Early Hum Dev 1980; 4:121.

55. Al MD, van Houwelingen AC, Hornstra G. Long-chain polyunsaturated fatty acids, pregnancy, and pregnancy outcome. Am J Clin Nutr 2000; 71:285S.

56. Colombo J, Kannass KN, Shaddy DJ, et al. Maternal DHA and the development of attention in infancy and toddlerhood. Child Dev 2004; 75:1254.

57. Smuts CM, Huang M, Mundy D, et al. A randomized trial of docosahexaenoic acid supplementation during the third trimester of pregnancy. Obstet Gynecol 2003; 101:469.

58. Malcolm CA, McCulloch DL, Montgomery C, et al. Maternal docosahexaenoic acid supplementation during pregnancy and visual evoked potential development in term infants: a double blind, prospective, randomised trial. Arch Dis Child Fetal Neonatal Ed 2003; 88:F383.

59. Montgomery C, Speake BK, Cameron A, et al. Maternal docosahexaenoic acid supplementation and fetal accretion. Br J Nutr 2003; 90:135.

60. Sanjurjo P, Ruiz-Sanz JI, Jimeno P, et al. Supplementation with docosahexaenoic acid in the last trimester of pregnancy: maternal-fetal biochemical findings. J Perinat Med 2004; 32:132.

61. Helland IB, Smith L, Saarem K, et al. Maternal supplementation with very-long-chain n–3 fatty acids during pregnancy and lactation augments children's IQ at 4 years of age. Pediatrics 2003; 111:e39.

62. Helland IB, Saugstad OD, Smith L, et al. Similar effects on infants of n–3 and n–6 fatty acids supplementation to pregnant and lactating women. Pediatrics 2001; 108:E82.

63. Lauritzen L, Jorgensen MH, Mikkelsen TB, et al. Maternal fish oil supplementation in lactation: effect on visual acuity and n–3 fatty acid content of infant erythrocytes. Lipids 2004; 39:195.

64. Jensen CL, Voigt RG, Prager TC, et al. Effects of maternal docosahexaenoic acid intake on visual function and neurodevelopment in breastfed term infants. Am J Clin Nutr 2005; 82:125.

65. Boris J, Jensen B, Salvig JD, et al. A randomized controlled trial of the effect of fish oil supplementation in late pregnancy and early lactation on the n–3 fatty acid content in human breast milk. Lipids 2004; 39:1191.

66. Makrides M, Neumann MA, Gibson RA. Effect of maternal docosahexaenoic acid (DHA) supplementation on breast milk composition. Eur J Clin Nutr 1996; 50:352.

67. Gibson RA, Neumann MA, Makrides M. Effect of increasing breast milk docosahexaenoic acid on plasma and erythrocyte phospholipid fatty acids and neural indices of exclusively breast fed infants. Eur J Clin Nutr 1997; 51:578.

68. Al MD, van Houwelingen AC, Hornstra G. Relation between birth order and the maternal and neonatal docosahexaenoic acid status. Eur J Clin Nutr 1997; 51:548.

69. Meyer BJ, Mann NJ, Lewis JL, et al. Dietary intakes and food sources of omega-6 and omega-3 polyunsaturated fatty acids. Lipids 2003; 38:391.

70. Astorg P, Arnault N, Czernichow S, et al. Dietary intakes and food sources of n–6 and n–3 PUFA in French adult men and women. Lipids 2004; 39:527.

71. Kuriki K, Nagaya T, Tokudome Y, et al. Plasma concentrations of (n–3) highly unsaturated fatty acids are good biomarkers of relative dietary fatty acid intakes: a cross-sectional study. J Nutr 2003; 133:3643.

72. Yamada T, Strong JP, Ishii T, et al. Atherosclerosis and omega-3 fatty acids in the populations of a fishing village and a farming village in Japan. Atherosclerosis 2000; 153:469.

73. Groh-Wargo S. Recommended enteral nutrient intakes. In: Groh-Wargo S, Thompson M, Cox J, eds., Nutritional care for high-risk neonates, 3rd edn. Los Angeles: Bonus Books; 2000: 231.

74. Roy CC, Ste-Marie M, Chartrand L, et al. Correction of the malabsorption of the preterm infant with a medium-chain triglyceride formula. J Pediatr 1975; 86:446.

75. Hamosh M. Bile-salt-stimulated lipase of human milk and fat digestion in the preterm infant. J Pediatr Gastroenterol Nutr 2 Suppl 1983; 1:S248.

76. Liao TH, Hamosh P, Hamosh M. Fat digestion by lingual lipase: mechanism of lipolysis in the stomach and upper small intestine. Pediatr Res 1984; 18:402.

77. Hamosh M. Digestion in the newborn. Clin Perinatol 1996; 23:191.

78. Rings EH, Minich DM, Vonk RJ, et al. Functional development of fat absorption in term and preterm neonates strongly correlates with ability to absorb long-chain fatty acids from intestinal lumen. Pediatr Res 2002; 51:57.

79. Kovacs A, Funke S, Marosvolgyi T, et al. Fatty acids in early human milk after preterm and full-term delivery. J Pediatr Gastroenterol Nutr 2005; 41:454.

80. Genzel-Boroviczeny O, Wahle J, Koletzko B. Fatty acid composition of human milk during the 1st month after term and preterm delivery. Eur J Pediatr 1997; 156:142.

81. Bitman J, Wood DL, Mehta NR, et al. Comparison of the cholesteryl ester composition of human milk from preterm and term mothers. J Pediatr Gastroenterol Nutr 1986; 5:780.

82. Bitman J, Wood DL, Mehta NR, et al. Comparison of the phospholipid composition of breast milk from mothers of term and preterm infants during lactation. Am J Clin Nutr 1984; 40:1103.

83. Bitman J, Wood L, Hamosh M, et al. Comparison of the lipid composition of breast milk from mothers of term and preterm infants. Am J Clin Nutr 1983; 38:300.

84. Al-Tamer YY, Mahmood AA. Fatty-acid composition of the colostrum and serum of fullterm and preterm delivering Iraqi mothers. Eur J Clin Nutr 2004; 58:1119.

85. Davis A, Baker S. The use of modular nutrients in pediatrics. J Parenter Enteral Nutr 1996; 20:228.

86. Romera G, Figueras J, Rodriguez-Miguelez JM, et al. Energy intake, metabolic balance and growth in preterm infants fed formulas with different nonprotein energy supplements. J Pediatr Gastroenterol Nutr 2004; 38:407.

87. Rey J, Schmitz J, Amedee-Manesme O. Fat absorption in low birthweight infants. Acta Paediatr Scand Suppl 1982; 296:81.

88. Hamosh M, Bitman J, Liao TH, et al. Gastric lipolysis and fat absorption in preterm infants: effect of medium-chain triglyceride or long-chain triglyceride-containing formulas. Pediatrics 1989; 83:86.

89. Sulkers EJ, von Goudoever JB, Leunisse C, et al. Comparison of two preterm formulas with or without addition of medium-chain triglycerides (MCTs). I. Effects on nitrogen and fat balance and body composition changes. J Pediatr Gastroenterol Nutr 1992; 15:34.

90. Sulkers EJ, Lafeber HN, Degenhart HJ, et al. Comparison of two preterm formulas with or without addition of medium-chain triglycerides (MCTs). II. Effects on mineral balance. J Pediatr Gastroenterol Nutr 1992; 15:42.

91. Sulkers EJ, Lafeber HN, Sauer PJ. Quantitation of oxidation of medium-chain triglycerides in preterm infants. Pediatr Res 1989; 26:294.

92. Sulkers EJ, Lafeber HN, van Goudoever JB, et al. Decreased glucose oxidation in preterm infants fed a formula containing medium-chain triglycerides. Pediatr Res 1993; 33:101.

93. Carnielli VP, Rossi K, Badon T, et al. Medium-chain triacylglycerols in formulas for preterm infants: effect on plasma lipids, circulating concentrations of medium-chain fatty acids, and essential fatty acids. Am J Clin Nutr 1996; 64:152.

94. Rodriguez A, Raederstorff D, Sarda P, et al. Preterm infant formula supplementation with alpha linolenic acid and docosahexaenoic acid. Eur J Clin Nutr 2003; 57:727.

95. Telliez F, Bach V, Leke A, et al. Feeding behavior in neonates whose diet contained medium-chain triacylglycerols: short-term effects on thermoregulation and sleep. Am J Clin Nutr 2002; 76:1091.

96. Baumgart S, Pereira GR, Bennett MJ. Excretion of dicarboxylic acids in preterm infants fed medium- or long-chain triglycerides. J Pediatr 1994; 125:509.

97. Henderson MJ, Dear PR. Dicarboxylic aciduria and medium chain triglyceride supplemented milk. Arch Dis Child 1986; 61:610.

98. Whyte RK, Whelan D, Hill R, et al. Excretion of dicarboxylic and omega-1 hydroxy fatty acids by low birth weight infants fed with medium-chain triglycerides. Pediatr Res 1986; 20:122.

99. Wu PY, Edmond J, Auestad N, et al. Medium-chain triglycerides in infant formulas and their relation to plasma ketone body concentrations. Pediatr Res 1986; 20:338.

100. Wu PY, Edmond J, Morrow JW, et al. Gastrointestinal tolerance, fat absorption, plasma ketone and urinary dicarboxylic acid levels in low-birth-weight infants fed different amounts of medium-chain triglycerides in formula. J Pediatr Gastroenterol Nutr 1993; 17:145.

101. Klenoff-Brumberg HL, Genen LH. High versus low medium chain triglyceride content of formula for promoting short term growth of preterm infants. Cochrane Database Syst Rev 2003; CD002777.

102. Klein CJ. Nutrient requirements for preterm infant formulas. J Nutr 2002; 132:1395S.

103. Carlson SE. Arachidonic acid status of human infants: influence of gestational age at birth and diets with very long chain n–3 and n–6 fatty acids. J Nutr 1996; 126:1092S.

104. Carlson SE, Werkman SH, Tolley EA. Effect of long-chain n–3 fatty acid supplementation on visual acuity and growth of preterm infants with and without bronchopulmonary dysplasia. Am J Clin Nutr 1996; 63:687.

105. Carlson SE, Cooke RJ, Werkman SH, et al. First year growth of preterm infants fed standard compared to marine oil n–3 supplemented formula. Lipids 1992; 27:901.

106. Carlson SE, Werkman SH, Peeples JM, et al. Arachidonic acid status correlates with first year growth in preterm infants. Proc Natl Acad Sci USA 1993; 90:1073.

107. Ryan AS, Montalto MB, Groh-Wargo S, et al. Effect of DHA-containing formula on growth of preterm infants to 59 weeks postmenstrual age. Am J Human Biol 1999; 11:457.

108. Vanderhoof J, Gross S, Hegyi T. A multicenter long-term safety and efficacy trial of preterm formula supplemented with long-chain polyunsaturated fatty acids. J Pediatr Gastroenterol Nutr 2000; 31:121.

109. Innis SM, Adamkin DH, Hall RT, et al. Docosahexaenoic acid and arachidonic acid enhance growth with no adverse effects in preterm infants fed formula. J Pediatr 2002; 140:547.

110. Clandinin MT, Van Aerde JE, Merkel KL, et al. Growth and development of preterm infants fed infant formulas containing docosahexaenoic acid and arachidonic acid. J Pediatr 2005; 146:461.

111. O'Connor DL, Hall R, Adamkin D, et al. Growth and development in preterm infants fed long-chain polyunsaturated fatty acids: a prospective, randomized controlled trial. Pediatrics 2001; 108:359.

112. Groh-Wargo S, Jacobs J, Auestad N, et al. Body composition in preterm infants who are fed long-chain polyunsaturated fatty acids: a prospective, randomized, controlled trial. Pediatr Res 2005; 57:712.

113. Farquharson J, Cockburn F, Patrick WA, et al. Effect of diet on infant subcutaneous tissue triglyceride fatty acids. Arch Dis Child 1993; 69:589.

114. Fleith M, Clandinin MT. Dietary PUFA for preterm and term infants: review of clinical studies. Crit Rev Food Sci Nutr 2005; 45:205.

115. Alessandri JM, Guesnet P, Vancassel S, et al. Polyunsaturated fatty acids in the central nervous system: evolution of concepts and nutritional implications throughout life. Reprod Nutr Dev 2004; 44:509.

116. Heird WC. Biochemical homeostasis and body growth are reliable end points in clinical nutrition trials. Proc Nutr Soc 2005; 64:297.

117. Heird WC, Lapillonne A. The role of essential fatty acids in development. Annu Rev Nutr 2005; 25:549.

118. Innis SM. Polyunsaturated fatty acids in human milk: an essential role in infant development. Adv Exp Med Biol 2004; 554:27.

119. Makrides M, Gibson RA, Udell T, et al. Supplementation of infant formula with long-chain polyunsaturated fatty acids does not influence the growth of term infants. Am J Clin Nutr 2005; 81:1094.

120. McCann JC, Ames BN. Is docosahexaenoic acid, an n–3 long-chain polyunsaturated fatty acid, required for development of normal brain function? An overview of evidence from cognitive and behavioral tests in humans and animals. Am J Clin Nutr 2005; 82:281.

121. SanGiovanni JP, Chew EY. The role of omega-3 long-chain polyunsaturated fatty acids in health and disease of the retina. Prog Retin Eye Res 2005; 24:87.

122. Simmer K, Patole S. Longchain polyunsaturated fatty acid supplementation in preterm infants. Cochrane Database Syst Rev 2004;CD000375.

123. Smithers LG, McPhee AJ, Gibson RA, et al. Visual development of preterm infants fed high dose docosahexaenoic acid. Asia Pac J Clin Nutr 2004; 13:S50.

124. Carlson SE, Werkman SH, Peeples JM, et al. Long-chain fatty acids and early visual and cognitive development of preterm infants. Eur J Clin Nutr 1994; 48 Suppl 2:S27.

125. Carlson SE, Werkman SH, Rhodes PG, et al. Visual-acuity development in healthy preterm infants: effect of marine-oil supplementation. Am J Clin Nutr 1993; 58:35.

126. O'Connor AR, Stephenson TJ, Johnson A, et al. Visual function in low birthweight children. Br J Ophthalmol 2004; 88:1149.

127. O'Connor DL, Jacobs J, Hall R, et al. Growth and development of premature infants fed predominantly human milk, predominantly premature infant formula, or a combination of human milk and premature formula. J Pediatr Gastroenterol Nutr 2003; 37:437.

128. Calder PC, Grimble RF. Polyunsaturated fatty acids, inflammation and immunity. Eur J Clin Nutr 2002; 56 Suppl 3:S14.

129. Harbige LS. Fatty acids, the immune response, and autoimmunity: a question of n–6 essentiality and the balance between n–6 and n–3. Lipids 2003; 38:323.

130. Field CJ, Clandinin MT, Van Aerde JE. Polyunsaturated fatty acids and T-cell function: implications for the neonate. Lipids 2001; 36:1025.

131. Jenski LJ, Bowker GM, Johnson MA, et al. Docosahexaenoic acid-induced alteration of Thy-1 and CD8 expression on murine splenocytes. Biochim Biophys Acta 1995; 1236:39.

132. Field CJ, Thomson CA, Van Aerde JE, et al. Lower proportion of CD45R0 + cells and deficient interleukin-10 production by formula-fed infants, compared with human-fed, is corrected with supplementation of long-chain polyunsaturated fatty acids. J Pediatr Gastroenterol Nutr 2000; 31:291.

133. Cerbulo-Vazquez A, Valdes-Ramos R, Santos-Argumedo L. Activated umbilical cord blood cells from pre-term and term neonates express CD69 and synthesize IL-2 but are unable to produce IFN-gamma. Arch Med Res 2003; 34:100.

134. Gasparoni A, Ciardelli L, Avanzini A, et al. Age-related changes in intracellular TH1/TH2 cytokine production, immunoproliferative T lymphocyte response and natural killer cell activity in newborns, children and adults. Biol Neonate 2003; 84:297.

135. Juretic E, Juretic A, Uzarevic B, et al. Alterations in lymphocyte phenotype of infected preterm newborns. Biol Neonate 2001; 80:223.

136. Juretic E, Uzarevic B, Petrovecki M, et al. Two-color flow cytometric analysis of preterm and term newborn lymphocytes. Immunobiology 2000; 202:421.

137. Herz U, Petschow B. Perinatal events affecting the onset of allergic diseases. Curr Drug Targets Inflamm Allergy 2005; 4:523.

138. Satwani P, Morris E, van de Ven C, et al. Dysregulation of expression of immunoregulatory and cytokine genes and its association with the immaturity in neonatal phagocytic and cellular immunity. Biol Neonate 2005; 88:214.

139. Thornton CA, Upham JW, Wikstrom ME, et al. Functional maturation of CD4 + CD25 + CTLA4 + CD45RA + T regulatory cells in human neonatal T cell responses to environmental antigens/allergens. J Immunol 2004; 173:3084.

140. Holt PG. Programming for responsiveness to environmental antigens that trigger allergic respiratory disease in adulthood is initiated during the perinatal period. Environ Health Perspect 1998; 106(Suppl 3):795.

141. Prescott SL, Macaubas C, Holt BJ, et al. Transplacental priming of the human immune system to environmental allergens: universal skewing of initial T cell responses toward the Th2 cytokine profile. J Immunol 1998; 160:4730.

142. Steffensen FH, Sorensen HT, Gillman MW, et al. Low birth weight and preterm delivery as risk factors for asthma and atopic dermatitis in young adult males. Epidemiology 2000; 11:185.

143. Prescott SL, Calder PC. n–3 polyunsaturated fatty acids and allergic disease. Curr Opin Clin Nutr Metab Care 2004; 7:123.

144. Nafstad P, Nystad W, Magnus P, et al. Asthma and allergic rhinitis at 4 years of age in relation to fish consumption in infancy. J Asthma 2003; 40:343.

145. Dunstan JA, Mori TA, Barden A, et al. Fish oil supplementation in pregnancy modifies neonatal allergen-specific immune responses and clinical outcomes in infants at high risk of atopy: a randomized, controlled trial. J Allergy Clin Immunol 2003; 112:1178.

146. Mihrshahi S, Peat JK, Marks GB, et al. Eighteen-month outcomes of house dust mite avoidance and dietary fatty acid modification in the Childhood Asthma Prevention Study (CAPS). J Allergy Clin Immunol 2003; 111:162.

147. Mihrshahi S, Peat JK, Webb K, et al. Effect of omega-3 fatty acid concentrations in plasma on symptoms of asthma at 18 months of age. Pediatr Allergy Immunol 2004; 15:517.

148. Mihrshahi S, Vukasin N, Forbes S, et al. Are you busy for the next 5 years? Recruitment in the Childhood Asthma Prevention Study (CAPS). Respirology 2002; 7:147.

149. Peat JK, Mihrshahi S, Kemp AS, et al. Three-year outcomes of dietary fatty acid modification and house dust mite reduction in the Childhood Asthma Prevention Study. J Allergy Clin Immunol 2004; 114:807.

150. Kidd P. Th1/Th2 balance: the hypothesis, its limitations, and implications for health and disease. Altern Med Rev 2003; 8:223.

151. Klein TW, Newton C, Larsen K, et al. The cannabinoid system and immune modulation. J Leukoc Biol 2003; 74:486.

152. Jump DB, Clarke SD. Regulation of gene expression by dietary fat. Annu Rev Nutr 1999; 19:63.

153. Fan YY, McMurray DN, Ly LH, et al. Dietary (n–3) polyunsaturated fatty acids remodel mouse T-cell lipid rafts. J Nutr 2003; 133:1913.

154. De Caterina R, Massaro M. Omega-3 fatty acids and the regulation of expression of endothelial pro-atherogenic and pro-inflammatory genes. J Membr Biol 2005; 206:103.

155. Eschen O, Christensen JH, De Caterina R, et al. Soluble adhesion molecules in healthy subjects: a dose-response study using n–3 fatty acids. Nutr Metab Cardiovasc Dis 2004; 14:180.

156. Wessel J. Feeding methodologies. In: Groh-Wargo S, Thompson M, Cox J, eds., Nutritional care for high-risk neonates, 3rd edn. Los Angeles: Bonus Books; 2000: 321.

157. Connor WE, Lowensohn R, Hatcher L. Increased docosahexaenoic acid levels in human newborn infants by administration of sardines and fish oil during pregnancy. Lipids 1996; 31(Suppl):S183.

158. Malcolm CA, Hamilton R, McCulloch DL, et al. Scotopic electroretinogram in term infants born of mothers supplemented with docosahexaenoic acid during pregnancy. Invest Ophthalmol Vis Sci 2003; 44:3685.

159. Helland IB, Saarem K, Saugstad OD, et al. Fatty acid composition in maternal milk and plasma during supplementation with cod liver oil. Eur J Clin Nutr 1998; 52:839.

Section III

Select Clinical Entities

Chapter 15

Necrotizing Enterocolitis: Pathogenesis, Clinical Care and Prevention

Josef Neu, MD • Martha Douglas-Escobar, MD

Clinical Presentation
Pathogenesis

Necrotizing enterocolitis (NEC) is the most common severe clinical gastrointestinal emergency that affects primarily newborns. Nevertheless, what is termed "NEC" represents a spectrum of intestinal illnesses that presents in all age groups. One manifestation in adults was first described in the 1940s in Germany in chronically starved persons who had eaten a large meal, possibly including poorly cooked meat (1). The syndrome, called *Darmbrand* (burnt intestine), was associated with *Clostridium perfringens* type C, and cases ceased after standards of living and nutrition improved after the war (1). A similar syndrome in children and young adults called pigbel was also recognized as a common condition in the early 1960s in Papua New Guinea, where it was associated with consumption of poorly cooked pork by protein-deficient persons in ceremonial feasts. Bacteriologic evaluation showed that pigbel was caused by *C. perfringens* type C and its β-toxin (2). β-Toxin is highly sensitive to proteolysis, but prolonged protein deprivation preceding pork feasts, and concurrent consumption of sweet potatoes, which contain trypsin inhibitors, reduced levels of proteolytic enzymes to a degree that allows β-toxin absorption by patients. This disease was the leading cause of childhood mortality in Papua New Guinea until a program of vaccination against *C. perfringens* type C β-toxin dramatically reduced disease incidence (3). More recently similar cases of adult NEC have been recognized in North America, but associated with *C. perfringens* type A (4). Another entity related to NEC, sometimes referred to as typhilits or neutropenic enterocolitis, occasionally manifests after chemotherapy or transplantation in patients with cancer, especially leukemias (5).

In the newborn there exists heterogeneity of what has been termed NEC. Compared to preterms, NEC in term and late preterm infants has a greater association with other predisposing factors such as low Apgar scores, chorioamnionitis, exchange transfusions, prolonged rupture of membranes, congenital heart disease and neural tube defects (6).

Another entity, sometimes confused with NEC, spontaneous intestinal perforations, frequently is not accompanied by significant intestinal necrosis, occurs earlier than NEC and is associated with the use of glucocorticoids and indomethacin, but probably not enteral feeding (7, 8). The more classic form of NEC occurs most commonly in infants less than 32 weeks gestation, presents after the first week after birth, has been associated with aggressive enteral feeding, and does not appear to be

Table 15-1 **NEC in Term and Preterm Infants and Spontaneous Intestinal Perforations**

Entity	NEC in term babies	NEC in premature babies	Spontaneous intestinal perforation
Time of presentation	1st week	> after 1st week	1st week
Localization	Proximal Colon and terminal ileum	Proximal Colon and terminal ileum	Terminal ileum in an antimesenteric position
Histology	Coagulation necrosis	Coagulation necrosis	Minimal necrosis
Associated with feedings	No	Yes	No
Other associations	Congenital Heart disease Prolonged rupture of membranes Chorioamnionitis Low Apgars Neural tube defects Exchange transfusion	PDA Prolonged rupture of membranes Colonization of GI tract	Use of early Dexamethasone and possibly indomethacin Use of Vasopressors PDA Prolonged rupture of membranes

associated with primary hypoxia-ischemia (such as might be seen with low Apgar scores). Table 15-1 distinguishes the features of NEC in term infants from those seen primarily in preterms and from isolated intestinal perforations. In this chapter, the focus will primarily be on a more classic form of NEC seen in premature infants.

The incidence of NEC is inversely proportional to gestational age, with 90% of cases occurring in premature babies. The incidence is clearly related to prematurity, with a sharp decrease in incidence around 35–36 weeks of GA or weight >1500 g. The estimated NEC incidence in the USA is 0.3–2.4 cases/1000 births, but increases to 4–13% in neonates less than 1500 g in weight (9–11). The annual incidence of NEC has not changed in over 30 years, partially due to the increasing survival of very premature infants. From 2500 annual cases reported in the USA, 20–60% require surgery and there is an approximate 20–28% mortality (12). Here we will review selected clinical manifestations of NEC, risk factors predisposing to NEC, pathogenesis, current treatment modalities and prophylactic measures that are currently being evaluated that have potential to prevent this devastating disease.

CLINICAL PRESENTATION

Necrotizing enterocolitis is characterized by the following symptoms and pathology: abdominal distention and tenderness, pneumatosis intestinalis, portal venous gas, occult or frank blood in the stools, intestinal necrosis, bowel perforation, sepsis, and shock. Bell and colleagues (13) originally described three levels of NEC, with Stage 1 being suggestive, Stage 2 being definitive, and Stage 3 being severe. Stage 1 is highly nonspecific and may reflect feeding intolerance, sepsis, or gastrointestinal hemorrhage, or simply manifestations of severe prematurity. Stage 1 should not be considered as definitive NEC and is useful primarily to alert the clinician to early signs that may augur the development of NEC. Stage 2 represents definitive NEC, usually diagnosed radiologically by the presence of pneumatosis intestinalis and/or portal venous gas. Stage 2 can usually be treated with medical management. Stage 3 represents severe disease, usually associated with major systemic signs such as shock, abdominal wall erythema, and bowel perforation. Stage 3 usually requires surgical intervention. However, it should be noted that neonates with non-necrotic spontaneous isolated intestinal perforations also present with Stage 3

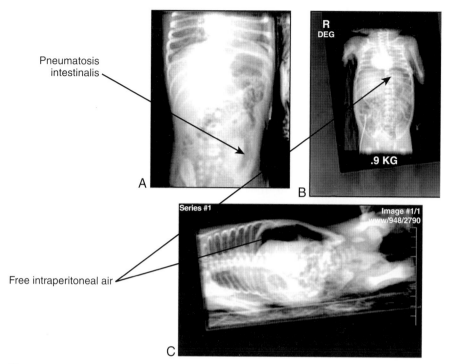

Figure 15-1 Pneumatosis intestinalis (A) and free intraperitoneal air on AP (B) and left lateral decubitus (C) films.

manifestations and can readily be confused with Stage 3 NEC. Thus, even though the Bell's staging system can be useful in terms of management, it is critical to remember that most cases of Stage 1 "NEC" are highly nonspecific and never progress to frank intestinal necrosis. Some cases provide warning signs of increased instability such as mild abdominal distension, increasing apneas and bradycardias, and/or increased feeding intolerance, whereas other cases appear to progress from a perfectly stable-appearing baby to Stage 3 and death within hours. The former frequently permit early intervention that can halt the progression of the disease to a more serious form. The latter occurs so quickly and is so fulminant that it begs for preventative measures that should be provided before the development of symptoms in all at-risk infants.

Radiological Findings

Figure 15-1 shows examples of radiological findings seen with NEC. Left lateral decubitus films usually provide more information than supine films because they can more accurately indicate the existence of pneumoperitoneum. Pneumatosis intestinalis, or gas in the bowel wall, in the appropriate clinical setting is usually diagnostic of NEC. However, it is important to remember that pneumatosis can be associated with other gastrointestinal problems such as Hirschprung's disease, intussusceptions, and atresias. When pneumatosis intestinalis extends into the portal circulation, it is frequently associated with increased severity of disease. Despite this enhanced level of illness, it has recently been suggested that the decision to operate should not be based on portal-venous gas alone (14). Pneumoperitoneum is frequently diagnostic of intestinal perforation with NEC and is considered an indication for immediate surgical intervention, whereas pneumatosis alone, without clinical deterioration of hematological signs or acid-base status, usually is treated medically.

Abdominal ultrasound has also been applied to the diagnosis of NEC (15). Echogenic dots or dense granular echogenicities in the bowel wall can be detected on ultrasonography in patients with early-stage NEC and may be a helpful adjunct in the early diagnosis and monitoring of patients with NEC.

Laboratory Features

We currently do not have a single laboratory feature that provides a definitive diagnosis of NEC. Peripheral hematological studies may reveal abnormally high or low white blood cell counts with a shift toward immature precursors. Progressively decreasing absolute granulocyte counts and thrombocytopenia suggest increasing severity of disease, as do acidosis and severe electrolyte abnormalities. Several inflammatory mediators are found in high concentrations in patients with NEC (16). The use of C-reactive protein (CRP) as an adjunct to abdominal radiographs was evaluated and suggested that CRP becomes abnormal in Stages 2 and 3 NEC (17). In NEC that is only suspected (e.g. Stage 1), normal serial CRPs would indicate that antibiotic therapy should be aborted and there should be an early resumption of feeding. In infants with NEC, persistently elevated CRP after initiation of appropriate risk management suggests associated complications, which might require additional diagnostic and/or surgical procedures.

Pathologic Findings

The pathologic findings of NEC have been described from examinations of bowels from the most severely affected patients who either died or had intestinal perforation requiring bowel resection. The most common involvement is in the terminal ileum and proximal colon. Histologic analysis reveals mucosal edema, hemorrhage, coagulation necrosis, intramural air, and mucosal ulceration

PATHOGENESIS

Much of what we know about the pathogenesis of NEC is derived from epidemiologic studies, individual case evaluations and studies in animals. An ideal animal model that is completely representative of NEC in human premature infants has not yet been developed. The studies thus far suggest a close interplay between genetics, intestinal immaturity (especially the innate immune system), the microbial environment and feeding.

Genetics

The familial and genetic susceptibilities to necrotizing enterocolitis, intraventricular hemorrhage, and bronchopulmonary dysplasia have recently been assessed using logistic-regression techniques. Twin analyses support the theory that intraventricular hemorrhage, necrotizing enterocolitis, and bronchopulmonary dysplasia are familial in origin (18). Given this genetic predisposition, finding a genetic marker that is sensitive, specific and predictive could be a valuable adjunct to prevention. Because of the possibility that inadequate innate immune responses to bacterial antigens in the intestinal flora may play a role in the development of NEC, single nucleotide polymorphisms (SNPs) of CD14, TLR4, and CARD15 (VLBW) were analyzed in very low birthweight infants with and without NEC, but found not to be associated with increased risk (19). Additional evaluation using sophisticated genomic and proteomic array technology may yield important new information about markers of the disease that could identify patients at greatest risk, so that preventive interventions could be instituted in select patients, rather than taking an approach that utilized routine prophylaxis in all patients.

Intestinal Immaturity

As the premature infant matures, several aspects of gastrointestinal development become important in terms of the capability of the GI tract to function as an organ of digestion and absorption. However, the intestine serves not only as a digestive absorptive organ, it is also one of the largest immune organs of the body; it plays a major endocrine and exocrine role and also encompasses neural tissue equivalent to that of the entire spinal cord. As the GI tract develops, tremendous growth occurs, with a doubling of intestinal length in the last trimester of pregnancy; but the surface area increase is even more dramatic, largely because of the villus and microvillus growth during this period of development. Thus the greater the level of prematurity, the greater is the limitation of infants' digestive-absorptive capability and the difficulty in meeting the high nutritional needs, especially during times of stress.

Physicochemical Environment and Barrier Function

The development of the innate and adaptive immune systems of human infants remains largely unexplored. Several aspects of the innate immune system are not only beginning to emerge as critical in short-term diseases during the immediate neonatal period, but also appear to play a role during later life. The innate intestinal barrier is critical in terms of preventing bacterial translocation and initiating the inflammatory response, which might affect not only the well-being of the intestine but distal organs such as the lung and central nervous systems as well (20–22).

One of the first lines of defense against ingested pathogens and toxins is luminal digestion in the stomach and duodenum. Immature physicochemical luminal factors include a lower hydrogen ion output in the stomach (23) and low pancreatic proteolytic enzyme activity (24). A relatively low enterokinase activity and subsequent low tryptic activity are likely to suppress the hydrolysis of toxins that have the ability to damage the intestine. Thus, immature luminal digestion can predispose to entry of pathogens from the environment and allow colonization by pathogens in the distal gastrointestinal tract. In fact, recent studies suggest that further decreasing the already low acid output of the stomach by use of H2 blockers in premature neonates is associated with a higher incidence of necrotizing enterocolitis (25).

Barrier function in the immature intestine is discussed in detail in another chapter in this volume (see Ch. 6). Here we will briefly summarize this important aspect of the developing intestine as it relates to NEC. What we know of the barrier function and the inflammatory potential of the intestine comes primarily from studies in animals and cell cultures, but a few studies in human infants are also beginning to provide some clues. Studies in animals have demonstrated that the intestinal mucin blanket seems to be scant in the newborn and has a different composition from that in adults (26), which appears to make the immature intestine more permeable to high molecular weight molecules. This may also facilitate greater bacterial adherence to the epithelium.

Immature neonates have higher intestinal permeability than older children and adults (27). Preterm infants born at less than 33 weeks of gestation have higher serum concentrations of β-lactoglobulin than term infants given equivalent milk feedings (28). The permeability of the preterm human intestine to intact carbohydrate markers such as lactulose exhibits a developmental pattern of increased permeability with maturation (27). Little is currently known about the maturation of tight junction proteins such as occludin and claudins, which constitute the major paracellular barrier of the epithelium (29). If these junction proteins are more susceptible to toxins or other perturbations in the immature intestine, this could offer a convenient target for preventive or therapeutic interventions that stimulate tight junction protein synthesis.

The motility of the small intestine in premature infants is considerably less organized than that in term infants (30).This is caused by an intrinsic immaturity of the enteric nervous system that delays transit, causing subsequent bacterial overgrowth and distension from gases that are the byproducts of fermentation. It is likely that this immature motility contributes to the milieu in which the interaction of nutrients, immature host defenses and other factors initiate the cascade of events, including transgression of microbes or their toxic products through an immature intestinal mucosal barrier, which eventually culminates in an inflammatory cascade leading to NEC (1, 12, 31).

Inflammatory Mediators

Similar to sepsis and adult respiratory stress syndrome, NEC seems to involve a final common pathway that includes the endogenous production of inflammatory mediators involved in the development of intestinal injury (32). Endotoxin lipopolysaccharide (LPS), platelet-activating factor (PAF), tumor necrosis factor (TNF), and other cytokines, together with prostaglandins and leukotrienes and nitric oxide, are thought to be involved in the final common pathway of NEC pathogenesis (12, 32).

Certain bacteria possess endotoxins that instigate the inflammatory cascade by activating PAF, TNF, and interleukin 1. Interleukin 8 (IL-8), a very potent neutrophil attractant chemokine, also appears to be involved in this process (33, 34). Other cytokines that appear to play a role such as IL-12 and IL-18 have also recently been implicated (35). A better understanding of this cascade is critical because interruption and/or prevention of the cascade by nutritional or pharmacologic means could be the key to prevention of NEC. For example, PAF injected into the aorta of adult rats has been found to cause necrosis of the bowel that can be prevented by pretreatment with PAF-acetylhydrolase and can be exacerbated by a nitric oxide synthase inhibitor (12). Certain nutrients such as omega-3 fatty acids (36), glutamine (37), arginine (38) or probiotic bacteria (39) may also play a role in the prevention of NEC via interruption or prevention of the inflammatory cascade.

Microbial Environment

A review of the microbial environment of the GI tract and its relationship to disease is found in Chapter 5 by Claud and Walker in this volume. Here we offer a brief summary. Humans and other mammals are colonized by a vast array of microorganisms, the so-called microbiota of the gastrointestinal tract. The function of this large quantity of microorganisms, comprising mainly commensals and symbionts, is just beginning to be understood. Some of the currently known functions involve luminal digestion of otherwise non-absorbed carbohydrates (40) and secretion of fatty acids such as butyrate that play a role in the maintenance of intestinal barrier function and proliferation (41, 42). A cross-talk exists between microbes and the intestine whereby stimulation of secretion of peptides by Paneth cells (Fig 15-2) promotes angiogenesis and growth and also promotes an environment that prevents the growth of potentially pathogenic microorganisms (40, 43–46).

Several lines of evidence support the thesis that infection is necessary for the development of NEC (47). Bacteria are often isolated from the blood of infants with NEC. However, it can be debated whether these isolated bacteria play the primary role in the pathogenesis of NEC or whether they are mainly intestinal luminal microbes that have transgressed a damaged mucosal barrier. The large variety of

INTESTINAL CRYPT

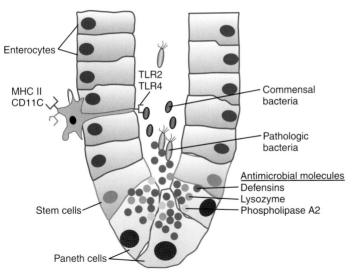

Figure 15-2 Paneth cells are functionally similar to neutrophils: when exposed to bacteria or bacterial products they release antimicrobial molecules into the lumen of the crypt. Stem cells constantly replenish the epithelial cells that migrate and die at the tip of the villi. Paneth cells protect the stem cells and therefore protect the epithelial cell renewal.

bacteria associated with NEC suggests that they are actually bystanders that amplify another process or set of processes. It is also possible that the microorganisms that have been isolated in association with NEC possess a not yet found common pathogenic feature that incites the disease.

The majority of very premature infants in the NICU are started on broad-spectrum antibiotic therapy shortly after birth during a "rule-out-sepsis" workup. This can alter the normal flora with which the neonate would become colonized (48). Rather than becoming colonized with *Lactobacillus, Bifidobacter* or other symbiotic microorganisms, resistant species indigenous to the NICU may colonize the babies' intestines. Whether or how much of a role this has in the pathogenesis of NEC is not known, but certain pathogenic microorganisms have a greater propensity to activate cell surface receptors that transduce signaling molecules such as nuclear factor kappa B (NFκ-B) to the nucleus, which in turn incites a pro-inflammatory response via the synthesis of proinflammatory cyto- and chemokines (44). Furthermore, the provision of antibiotics to rodents has been demonstrated to increase the propensity of the intestine to hemorrhagic colitis (49) and markedly alter the expression of numerous genes associated with intestinal development (50).

The commensal microflora may represent a key regulatory checkpoint for the intestinal inflammatory response. The intestinal epithelium partially relies on Toll-like receptors (TLRs) to act as an interface between the luminal microflora and cellular signal transduction pathways. TLRs are cell surface receptors that recognize specific microbial ligands, from both pathogens and commensals, enabling the innate immune system to recognize non-self, and activating both innate and adaptive immune responses (51). Recent studies suggest that the epithelium and resident immune cells do not simply tolerate commensal microorganisms but are dependent on them (49). This is important not only for disease entities that we see in the NICU such as NEC, which has recently been shown to be decreased with the use of probiotics (52–54), but also for diseases that affect the infant later in life such as allergy and atopy (55). Furthermore, it is possible that TLR agonists such as LPS may actually be useful therapeutic agents in the prevention of NEC and other intestinal pathology.

Table 15-2   Guidelines for Treatment

Bell's Stage (or other signs and symptoms)	Treatment
1. Non-specific signs such as abdominal distension, increased gastric residuals	Consider temporarily withholding enteral feedings, rule-out-sepsis workup, CBC and/or CRP, gastric tube if abdominal distension
2. Pneumatosis intestinalis, portal venous gas, persistence of distended bowel loops with other signs (e.g., grossly bloody stools) and symptoms (decreasing neutrophil and platelet count) of NEC	Withhold feeds, gastric tube to low intermittent suction, 7–10 days of intravenous broad-spectrum antibiotics; close observation with frequent X-rays (esp. left lateral decubitus to rule out perforation)
3. Intraperitoneal free air or other signs of perforation; continued deterioration despite therapy for Stage 2	Surgical intervention

Current Treatment Modalities

Therapy for NEC is highly dependent on its severity. Bell's staging criteria (13) can be highly useful as guidelines. Table 15-2 summarizes one approach. In Stage 1, there is only a suspicion that the disease might be developing. Because of the potentially devastating progression of NEC, extra precautions should be taken. Clinical judgment based on the patient's condition should guide whether and how long the patient should be taken off enteral feedings, whether and how long intravenous antibiotics should be used, and how aggressively the patient is monitored with radiographs and laboratory tests. If a definitive diagnosis is made (Stage 2), the bowel should be decompressed using a large-bore orogastric tube with low intermittent suction. Careful attention needs to be given to fluid and electrolyte status, and systemic antibiotic therapy is started after obtaining blood cultures. When perforation is suspected, or has occurred (Stage 3), intensive support of respiratory and circulatory status is provided, as are frequent monitoring of the abdominal status with left lateral decubitus radiographs and frequent monitoring of acid-base and hematologic status. Clindamycin or metronidazole is used to treat anaerobic infections. If a persistent acidosis with continued deterioration of platelet and white blood cell counts occurs, this may be an indication for surgery even in the absence of overt perforation on radiography.

A review of surgical therapy of NEC is beyond the scope of this chapter. There is considerable controversy whether exploratory laparotomy is preferable to peritoneal drain placement, but current studies do not indicate a clear advantage of one modality over the other, at least in very small prematures (56). Whether there is a difference in long-term neurodevelopmenal outcome of babies treated with one modality versus the other remains controversial and is currently being evaluated.

Of great importance is that NEC is a disease that requires a carefully coordinated approach among neonatologist and pediatric surgeons. Because NEC can be such a rapidly progressive disease, the pediatric surgeons should be notified whenever a definitive or highly suggestive diagnosis of NEC is made, even though most cases of Stage 2 can be managed medically. This will allow for more rapid mobilization for surgery if and when this disease progresses to a surgical emergency.

Prevention

Providing human milk to premature infants has been shown to decrease the incidence of NEC (57, 58). Fresh human milk is composed of numerous immunoprotective factors, such as immunoglobulins, lysozyme, lactoferrin, PAF-acetylhydrolase, macrophages, lymphocytes, and neutrophils. The fatty acid composition and oligosaccharides in human milk may also play an anti-inflammatory and antimicrobial role, respectively. Certain chemokines and cytokines such as IL-10 and TGFβ (59) may play particularly important roles, as may the interactions of human milk components with gut microflora and proteoglycan receptors (60).

Several measures are commonly used to prevent NEC outbreaks. These include careful epidemic precautions when an outbreak of NEC is suspected. Although oral antimicrobial agents have been used for prophylaxis in contacts to interrupt the outbreak (61), the possibility of emergence of resistant organisms limits their routine long-term use.

The aggressive institution of enteral feedings is a risk factor associated with NEC (62, 63). This has, in many cases, caused neonatologists to institute an overly cautious approach to enteral feedings whereby the baby is placed nulla per os (NPO) for several weeks after birth and nourished only by the parenteral route. This approach is known to cause atrophy of the intestinal mucosa and results in overall delayed development of absorptive function, motility, and exocrine hormone secretion, and shifts the intestinal inflammatory response to one that favors the pro-inflammatory cytokines and chemokines over the anti-inflammatory mediators (64). Minimal enteral nutrition is a safe approach that would not be contra-indicated while the infant is on ventilator support, using umbilical catheters, or receiving drugs such as indomethacin or dopamine (65).

Future Directions

As the pathophysiologic cascade for NEC becomes more defined and the tools for investigative science improve our understanding of nutrient-gene interactions and gene polymorphisms, we may begin to develop more targeted therapies for individuals who are most susceptible to NEC.

The potential for prophylaxis of NEC can be found at several levels of the putative pathogenic cascade, but currently it is reasonable to assume that interventions aimed at the more proximal events offer the greatest likelihood of effective prophylaxis when compared to interventions aimed at more distal components of the cascade. For example, nutritional interventions with anti-inflammatory lipids, amino acids such as glutamine and/or arginine, oligosaccharides, or probiotics would offer relatively inexpensive modalities for intervention into the proximal events of the pathophysiologic cascade. Butyrate, a short-chain fatty acid produced by bacterial fermentation, has been found to play a major role in intercellular junction integrity (66). Anti-cytokine therapies aimed at pro-inflammatory mediators are likely to intervene at a point where the process has already begun, and may not be appropriately targeted because several mediators are likely to be involved. Recombinant proteins such as lactoferrin, PAF-acetylhydrolase, epidermal growth factor, erythropoietin, granulocyte colony stimulating factor and other growth factors may also be promising, but are likely to be much more expensive and complicated in terms of potential adverse side-effects. Furthermore, since NEC is multifactorial, a single agent that promotes growth of the intestine or downregulates inflammation will probably not prevent all cases of NEC.

Lastly, we need to underscore the role of human milk in the prevention of NEC (57, 59, 67). Finding ways to obtain and utilize the infant's own mother's milk could have a significant impact in the prevention of NEC, sepsis and feeding intolerance.

Acknowledgement

Supported in part by NIH RO1 HD 38954 to J.N.

REFERENCES

1. Kreft B, Dalhoff K, Sack K. Necrotizing enterocolitis: a historical and current review. Med Klin (Munich) 2000; 95(8):435–441.
2. Murrell TG, Roth L. Necrotizing jejunitis: a newly discovered disease in the highlands of New Guinea. Med J Australia 1963; 50(1):61–69.
3. Lawrence G, Shann F, Freestone DS, Walker PD. Prevention of necrotising enteritis in Papua New Guinea by active immunisation. Lancet 1979; 313(8110):227–230.
4. Sobel J, Mixter CG, Kolhe P, et al. Necrotizing enterocolitis associated with Clostridium perfringens Type A in previously healthy North American adults. J Am Coll Surg 2005; 201(1):48–56.
5. Wagner ML, Rosenberg HS, Fernbach DJ, Singleton EB. Typhlitis: a complication of leukemia in childhood. Am J Roentgenol Radium Ther Nucl Med 1970; 109(2):341–350.
6. Martinez-Tallo E, Claure N, Bancalari E. Necrotizing enterocolitis in full-term or near-term infants: risk factors. Biol Neonate 1997; 71(5):292–298.
7. Stark AR, Carlo WA, Tyson JE, et al. Adverse effects of early dexamethasone treatment in extremely-low-birth-weight infants. N Engl J Med 2001; 344(2):95–101.
8. Attridge JT, Clark R, Walker MW, Gordon PV. New insights into spontaneous intestinal perforation using a national data set: (2) two populations of patients with perforations. J Perinatol 2006; 26(3):185–188.
9. Lemons JA, Bauer CR, Oh W, et al. Very low birth weight outcomes of the national institute of child health and human development neonatal research network, January 1995 through December 1996. Pediatrics 2001; 107(E1).
10. Kliegman RM, Fanaroff AA. Necrotizing enterocolitis. N Engl J Med 1984; 310(17):1093–1103.
11. Neu J. Necrotizing enterocolitis: the search for a unifying pathogenic theory leading to prevention. Pediatr Clin North Am 1996; 43(2):409–432.
12. Hsueh W, Caplan MS, Qu XW, et al. Neonatal necrotizing enterocolitis: clinical considerations and pathogenetic concepts. Pediatr Dev Pathol. 2003; 6(1):6–23.
13. Bell MJ, Ternberg JL, Feigin RD, et al. Neonatal necrotizing enterocolitis: Therapeutic decisions based upon clinical staging. Ann Surg 1978; 187:1–6.
14. Sharma R, Tepas JJ III, Hudak ML, et al. Portal venous gas and surgical outcome of neonatal necrotizing enterocolitis. J Pediatr Surg 2005; 40(2):371–376.
15. Kim W-Y, Kim W, Kim I-O, et al. Sonographic evaluation of neonates with early-stage necrotizing enterocolitis. Pediatr Radiol 2005; 35(11):1056–1061.
16. Markel TA, Crisostomo PR, Wairiuko GM, et al. Cytokines in necrotizing enterocolitis. Shock 2006; 25(4):293–337.
17. Pourcyrous M, Korones SB, Yang W, et al. C-Reactive protein in the diagnosis, management, and prognosis of neonatal necrotizing enterocolitis. Pediatrics 2005; 116(5):1064–1069.
18. Bhandari V, Bizzarro MJ, Shetty A, et al. Familial and genetic susceptibility to major neonatal morbidities in preterm twins. 10.1542/peds.2005–1414. Pediatrics 2006; 117(6):1901–1906.
19. Szebeni B, Szekeres R, Rusai K, et al. Genetic polymorphisms of CD14, toll-like receptor 4, and caspase-recruitment domain 15 are not associated with necrotizing enterocolitis in very low birth weight infants. J Pediatr Gastroenterol Nutr 2006; 42(1):27–31.
20. Speer CP. Inflammatory mechanisms in neonatal chronic lung disease. Eur J Pediatr 1999; 158(Suppl.1):S18–S22.
21. Speer CP. Pre- and postnatal inflammatory mechanisms in chronic lung disease of preterm infants. Paediatr 2004; 5(SupplA):S241–S244.
22. Liu Z, Li N, Neu J. Tight junctions, leaky intestines, and pediatric diseases. Acta Paediatr 2005; 94(4):386–393.
23. Hyman PE, Clarke DD, Everett SL, et al. Gastric acid secretory function in preterm infants. J Pediatr 1985; 106(3):467–471.
24. Antonowicz I, Lebenthal E. Developmental pattern of small intestinal enterokinase and disaccharidase activities in the human fetus. Gastroenterology 1977; 72(6):1299–1303.
25. Guillet R, Stoll BJ, Cotten CM, et al. Association of H2-blocker therapy and higher incidence of necrotizing enterocolitis in very low birth weight infants. Pediatrics 2006; 117(2):e137–e142.
26. Israel EJ. Neonatal necrotizing enterocolitis, a disease of the immature intestinal mucosal barrier. Acta Paediatr Suppl 1994; 396:27–32.
27. Beach RC, Menzies IS, Clayden GS, Scopes JW. Gastrointestinal permeability changes in the preterm neonate. Arch Dis Child 1982; 57(2):141–145.
28. Roberton DM, Paganelli R, Dinwiddie R, Levinsky RJ. Milk antigen absorption in the preterm and term neonate. Arch Dis Child 1082; 57(5):369–372.
29. Nusrat A, Turner JR, Madara JL. Molecular physiology and pathophysiology of tight junctions. IV. Regulation of tight junctions by extracellular stimuli: nutrients, cytokines, and immune cells. Am J Physiol Gastrointest Liver Physiol 2000; 279(5):G85107.
30. Berseth CL. Gastrointestinal motility in the neonate. Clin Perinatol 1996; 23(2):179–190.
31. Martin CR, Walker WA. Intestinal immune defences and the inflammatory response in necrotising enterocolitis. Semin Fetal Neonat Med Inflamm Perinat Dis 2006; 11(5):369–377.
32. Markel TA, Crisostomo PR, Wairiuko GM, et al. Cytokines in necrotizing enterocolitis. Shock 2006; 25(4):329–337.
33. Nanthakumar NN, Fusunyan RD, Sanderson I, Walker WA. Inflammation in the developing human intestine: A possible pathophysiologic contribution to necrotizing enterocolitis. Proc Natl Acad Sci USA 2000; 97(11):6043–6048.

34. Edelson MB, Bagwell CE, Rozycki HJ. Circulating pro- and counterinflammatory cytokine levels and severity in necrotizing enterocolitis. Pediatrics 1999; 103(4Pt.1):766–771.

35. Halpern MD, Holubec H, Dominguez JA, et al. Up-regulation of IL-18 and IL-12 in the ileum of neonatal rats with necrotizing enterocolitis. Pediatr Res 2002; 51(6):733–739.

36. Teitelbaum JE, Walker WA. Review: the role of omega 3 fatty acids in intestinal inflammation. J Nutr Biochem 2001; 12(1):21–32.

37. Dilsiz A, Ciftci I, Aktan TM, et al. Enteral glutamine supplementation and dexamethasone attenuate the local intestinal damage in rats with experimental necrotizing enterocolitis. Pediatr Surg Int 2003; 19(8):578–582.

38. Amin HJ ZS, McMillan DD, Fick GH, et al. Arginine supplementation prevents necrotizing entero-colitis in the premature infant. J Pediatr 2002; 140(4):389–391.

39. Millar M, Wilks M, Costeloe K. Probiotics for preterm infants? Arch Dis Child Fetal Neonatal Ed 2003; 88(5):F354–F358.

40. Hooper LV, Gordon JI. Commensal host-bacterial relationships in the gut. Science 2001; 292:1115–1118.

41. Sanderson IR, Naik S. Dietary regulation of intestinal gene expression. Annu Rev Nutr 2000; 20:311–338.

42. Yoo J, Nichols A, Mammen J, et al. Bryostatin-1 enhances barrier function in T84 epithelia through PKC-dependent regulation of tight junction proteins. Am J Physiol Cell Physiol 2003; 285(2):C300–C309.

43. Haller D, Bode C, Hammes WP, et al. Non-pathogenic bacteria elicit a differential cytokine response by intestinal epithelial cell/leucocyte co-cultures. Gut 2000; 47(1):79–87.

44. Neish AS. The gut microflora and intestinal epithelial cells: a continuing dialogue. Microbes Infect 2002; 4(3):309–317.

45. Stappenbeck TS, Hooper LV, Gordon JI. Developmental regulation of intestinal angiogenesis by indigenous microbes via Paneth cells. Proc Natl Acad Sci USA 2002; 99(24):15451–15455.

46. Porter EM, Bevins CL, Ghosh D, Ganz T. The multifaceted Paneth cell. Cell Mol Life Sci 2002; 59(1):156–170.

47. Bell MJ, Shackelford P, Feigin RD, et al. Epidemiologic and bacteriologic evaluation of neonatal necrotizing enterocolitis. J Pediatr Surg 1979; 14(1):1–4.

48. Kosloske AM. Epidemiology of necrotizing enterocolitis. Acta Paediatr Suppl 1994; 396:2–7.

49. Rakoff-Nahoum S, Paglino J, Eslami-Varzaneh F, et al. Recognition of commensal microflora by toll-like receptors is required for intestinal homeostasis. Cell 2004; 118(2):229–241.

50. Schumann A, Nutten S, Donnicola D, et al. Neonatal antibiotic treatment alters gastrointestinal tract developmental gene expression and intestinal barrier transcriptome. Physiol Genomics 2005; 23(2):235–245.

51. Takeda K, Kaisho T, Akira S. Toll-like receptors. Annu Rev Immunol 2003; 21:335–376.

52. Lin HC, Su BH, Chen AC, et al. Oral probiotics reduce the incidence and severity of necrotizing enterocolitis in very low birth weight infants. Pediatrics 2005; 115(1):1–4.

53. Vinderola G, Matar C, Perdigon G. Role of intestinal epithelial cells in immune effects mediated by gram-positive probiotic bacteria: involvement of toll-like receptors. Clin Diagn Lab Immunol 2005; 12(9):1075–1084.

54. Bin-Nun A, Bromiker R, Wilschanski M, et al. Oral probiotics prevent necrotizing enterocolitis in very low birth weight neonates. J Pediatr 2005; 147(2):192–196.

55. Kalliomaki M, Salminen S, Arvilommi H, et al. Probiotics in primary prevention of atopic disease: a randomised placebo-controlled trial. Lancet 2001; 357(9262):1076–1079.

56. Moss RL, Dimmitt RA, Barnhart DC, et al. Laparotomy versus peritoneal drainage for necrotizing enterocolitis and perforation. N Engl J Med 2006; 354(21):2225–2234.

57. Lucas A, Cole TJ. Breast milk and neonatal necrotising enterocolitis. Lancet 1990; 336(8730):1519–1523.

58. McGuire W, Anthony MY. Donor human milk versus formula for preventing necrotising entero-colitis in preterm infants: systematic review. Arch Dis Child Fetal Neonatal Ed 2003; 88(1):F11–F14.

59. Fituch CC, Palkowetz KH, Goldman AS, Schanler RJ. Concentrations of IL-10 in preterm human milk and in milk from mothers of infants with necrotizing enterocolitis. Acta Paediatr 2004; 93(11):1496–1500.

60. Newburg DS. Innate Immunity and Human Milk. J. Nutr 2005; 135(5):1308–1312.

61. Egan EA, Nelson RM, Mantilla G, Eitzman DV. Additional experience with routine use of oral kanamycin prophylaxis for necrotizing enterocolitis in infants under 1,500 grams. J Pediatr 1977; 90(2):2–331.

62. Anderson DM, Kliegman RM. The relationship of neonatal alimentation practices to the occurrence of endemic necrotizing enterocolitis. Am J Perinatol 1991; 8(1):62–67.

63. Berseth CL, Bisquera JA, Paje VU. Prolonging small feeding volumes early in life decreases the incidence of necrotizing enterocolitis in very low birth weight infants. Pediatrics 2003; 111(3):529–534.

64. Kudsk KA. Current aspects of mucosal immunology and its influence by nutrition. Am J Surg 2002; 183(4):390–398.

65. Neu J, Zhang L. Feeding intolerance in very-low-birthweight infants: what is it and what can we do about it? Acta Paediatr Suppl 2005; 94(449):93–99.

66. Mariadason JM, Kilias D, Catto-Smith A, Gibson PR. Effect of butyrate on paracellular permeability in rat distal colonic mucosa ex vivo. J Gastroenterol Hepatol 1999; 14(9):873–879.

67. Schanler RJ. The use of human milk for premature infants. Pediatr Clin North Am 2001; 48(1):207–219.

Chapter 16

Short Bowel Syndrome

J. Marc Rhoads, MD

Causes and Epidemiology
Pathophysiology and the Adaptive Response
Prevention
Complications
Treatment of SBS
Remaining Questions

CAUSES AND EPIDEMIOLOGY

Short bowel syndrome (SBS) is defined as a condition in which the absorptive capacity of the small intestine is insufficient to maintain hydration and provide sufficient nutrition for growth of the infant. SBS usually results from intestinal resection. All patients with short bowel syndrome require artificial means of nutritional support for a period, either parenteral nutrition (PN) or enteral nutrition provided as specific formulae, often infused enterally. Most children with SBS were born with congenital defects of bowel formation or rotation or were delivered prematurely, subsequently developing necrotizing enterocolitis (NEC). SBS is a relatively common, often lethal, and highly costly medical problem in North America. A recent retrospective cohort study from Toronto estimated the incidence and mortality rates of SBS. They found an incidence of 24.5 per 100 000 live births. The SBS case fatality rate was 37.5% and the cause-specific and proportional mortality rates (for children less than 4 years old) were 2.0 of 100 000 population per year (1). Mortality rates and costs in Europe are comparable to those in North America. In Graz, Austria, the overall related mortality in infants with SBS ranged from 15 to 25%; the annual costs/patient were between $100 000 and $150 000 in US dollars (2).

The leading causes of SBS and relative frequency are listed in Table 16-1 and shown in Figure 16-1. NEC has been reported to cause about 50% of cases, with atresia, volvulus, and gastroschisis combining to account for about 40%.

PATHOPHYSIOLOGY AND THE ADAPTIVE RESPONSE

The most important single factor affecting severity of malabsorption in SBS is the length of bowel resected (3). Under normal conditions, the small intestine receives 185 mL/kg from salivary, gastric, and pancreaticobiliary secretions, in addition to about 100 mL/kg of milk and other fluids. Of this 285 mL/kg, all but about 60 mL/kg are absorbed in the small intestine (based on ileostomy studies) (4). Additionally, about 90% of the total caloric intake is absorbed in the small intestine, the remainder coming from colonic fermentation of malabsorbed carbohydrate to metabolizable short-chain fatty acids in the colon. Thus, the small intestine under

Table 16-1   Causes of Short Bowel Syndrome in Infants

Surgical
Necrotizing enterocolitis
Intestinal atresia: jejunal, ileal, multiple (Christmas tree/apple peel deformity)
Midgut volvulus (secondary to malrotation; secondary to adhesive bands)
Gastroschisis
Omphalocele
Meconium ileus
Thrombotic disorders (inherited or sepsis-related)
Trauma (e.g. swimming pool accidents, nonaccidental trauma)
Hirschsprung's disease (total intestinal aganglionosis, aganglionosis of distal small
   bowel and colon)
Radiation with ischemia
Congenital
Congenital short bowel syndrome

normal conditions has to absorb more than 80% of the salt and water it sees. If the small intestine could not adapt to resection, even the loss of 50% would lead to dehydration and death.

In addition to the length of small intestine, there are other factors of major importance to functional absorptive capacity. These include the preservation of the ileocecal "valve" or sphincter; the functional capacity of the remaining small and large intestine; and the ability of the remaining gut to undergo adaptive changes.

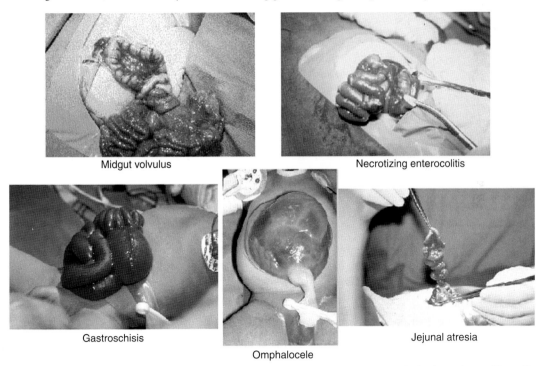

Midgut volvulus   Necrotizing enterocolitis

Gastroschisis   Jejunal atresia

Omphalocele

Figure 16-1 Common causes of short bowel syndrome in infants. Note that in *midgut volvulus* the entire small bowel is at risk from the twist around the base of the mesentery. In this case there is venous congestion of the bowel which is promptly resolved after detorsion.

Necrotizing enterocolitis typically results in focal areas of gangrene (as seen here), but can involve extensive areas resulting in short bowel syndrome. In *gastrochisis* the defect is to the right of the umbilicus and the bowel is not covered. In complicated gastrochisis there may be an atresia and loss of bowel length. *Ompahalocele* is a covered abdominal wall defect with the umbilical cord at the base of the defect.

The *jejeunal atresia* shown is a very proximal jejunal atresia with short bowel syndrome. The proximal small bowel mesentery is absent; the limited amount of distal ileum survived because of collateral vessels from the colonic blood supply.

Photographs of surgical cases were kindly provided by Dr. Vincent Adolph, Ochsner Clinic Foundation, Department of Surgery, Division of Pediatric Surgery.

The ileocecal sphincter provides a mechanical barrier to bacterial migration into the small intestine but also assists in regulating the exit of fluid and nutrients into the colon. Furthermore, loss of this functional barrier predisposes the host to bacterial sepsis, even though it probably does not influence the ultimate goal of achieving full enteral tolerance (5). Loss of the ileocecal sphincter results in many instances in the development of small bowel bacterial overgrowth, a condition which leads to diarrhea, fat and vitamin (B12) malabsorption via bile salt deconjugation (6), fluid loss, abdominal cramps from gas production, liver injury (7), and intestinal inflammation (8). Many children with SBS have nonspecific immune system activation. In one study, there were elevated concentrations of soluble tumor necrosis factor receptor-II and interleukin-6 in 24-h urine and serum in patients with SBS, compared to age-matched controls, indicating that long-term home total PN may be associated with a persistent low-grade inflammatory state (9).

Critical Importance of the Length of Remaining Bowel

Seminal investigations by Wilmore et al. showed that there is a critical length of small intestine (ligament of Treitz to terminal ileum), below which most infants will be dependent for life on PN. In these original studies, the critical length of small bowel was 40 cm (3, 10). As a consequence, surgical strategy evolved toward saving as many segments of bowel as possible, with some surgeons creating a proximal ostomy with multiple end-end anastomoses (11) and others using a temporary "clip and drop back" technique (12).

Given that 40 cm is 1/6 (17%) of the normal bowel length in full-term infants (13), investigators tested experimentally the critical "percentage of remaining small bowel" in experimental rats. In the animal studies, a reproducible finding was that 20% of the total small intestinal length was required for sustaining life on oral feeding (14–18). However, survival rates significantly improved with heightened experience in managing these patients and in administering PN. A large prospective study by Goulet et al. in Paris showed that about 65% of babies who have a bowel >40 cm and <80 cm long will eventually become PN-independent. Even better, over 90% of those with a bowel >80 cm will come off PN (5). However, considerable inter-individual variation has been found, with a number of infants in the UCLA experience surviving off PN with only 20–30 cm of jejunoileum (19). At the University of North Carolina, we had an infant with 26 cm of bowel who became independent of PN at 9 months of age (20). Even more remarkable, two additional infants have been reported who had all but 12 cm of small intestine resected and managed to become PN-independent (19, 21). A recent series published from Saudi Arabia reported astounding result in eight patients with extreme SBS, most of whom had midgut volvulus with intact ileocecal valve. These included four patients with 0–10 cm of small bowel, one with 10–25 cm of small bowel, and the final three with 25–75 cm. Using a protocol of ad lib oral feeding plus PN (i.e., no gastrostomy or nasogastric feeding), all but two patients were weaned from PN. The final two received PN only on alternate months, and they both had <10 cm of small intestine. The radiologically estimated length of jejunoileum increased during the study by approximately 450% over the first 2.5 years after resection (22).

Most often, children who are PN-dependent become PN-independent by 2–3 years of age; however, those children with bowel lengths <40 cm who have come off PN not infrequently regress back to enteral or parenteral nutrition dependency.

Numerical predictors based on bowel length are less reliable in very premature infants, because infants do not acquire the normal 260–275 cm of small bowel until they reach term. Helpful in making predictions are several relatively large studies of bowel length in stillbirths or infants who died prematurely (13, 23, 24). These reports have shown a mean length at 25 weeks of ∼125 cm and at 30 weeks gestation of ~180 cm. If one estimates that >20% of small bowel is required for survival (see below), an infant of 25 weeks gestation could eventually develop full enteral tolerance with only 25 cm of small intestine, barring complications.

Although studies on bowel length have given relatively reliable predictions for PN independence, the length of time required for enteral tolerance has been impossible to predict. Sondhemier et al. showed that during a 12 year interval, all infants who became PN-independent did so by 36 months of age; our experience during 16 years at the University of North Carolina is identical. The most important predictive factor in the Denver study was percentage enteral tolerance at 12 weeks of age. At this apparently critical time point, the calculated percentage of daily energy given enterally was 42% in the group who became PN-independent, in contrast to 10% in the group who never developed PN independence ($P = 0.0008$) (25). However, rare patients are able to come off PN when they are beyond puberty (26).

In adults, it is well-established that full adaptation hinges on the possession of >60 cm small bowel with an intact colon (27).

Mucosal Adaptation

Mechanism

A reproducible finding in experimental SBS is that the functional absorptive capacity per cm of bowel increases after resection. At the microscopic level, the intestine is thicker, with an increase in villus height and crypt depth of ~30% (28). Additionally, at the ultrastructural level there is an increase in microvillus area of about 20% (28). Thus, in SBS there is hyperplasia, with a veritable increase in the number of enterocytes per cm bowel length.

The immediate adaptive response is nutrient-independent. There is an induction of the immediate early genes zif-268, nup-475, and c-myc 1–3 h following resection, but not following transection (placebo treatment) (29). At 3 days post-resection, adaptation in control mice coincides with increased protein expression of p21(waf1/cip1) and decreased p27(kip1) in the proliferative zone (crypt. Adaptation occurs normally in control and p27(kip1)-null mice; however, mice deficient in both p21(waf1/cip1) and p27(kip1) fail to increase baseline rates of enterocyte proliferation and adaptation (30).

In SBS, the increase in absorption of most nutrients per unit gut length or surface area is global, with increased activity of digestive enzymes, including disaccharidases (lactase, sucrase, maltase). However, adaptation is not global with respect to specific transporters localized to particular regions of the bowel. Vitamin B12 absorption and bile salt transport are localized to the ileum but do not arise de novo in the jejunum after bowel resection (Fig. 16-2).

Mucosal hyperplasia and hypertrophy are produced by the interaction of several factors, including the concentration of luminal nutrients (31), pancreatico-biliary secretions (32, 33), hormones such as glucagon-like peptide-2 (34–36), growth hormone, proglucagon, and insulin-like growth factor-1 (37–39), and prostaglandins (14, 40). Luminal factors that are probably very important include trefoil peptides, epidermal growth factor and polyamines. Recent reviews of trophic factors include those by Jeppesen and Mortensen (41) and Wilmore (42).

At the organ level, in many infants there is an increase in bowel diameter, although it is not clear to the author whether dilatation is a mechanism of adaptation or whether dilation represents prior gut ischemia and/or partial obstruction (43).

Functional Assessments

Few tests are available to assess functional bowel mass. The most difficult and important assessment in the patient with SBS is whether or not the child will remain PN-dependent for life. If the patient is developing significant liver

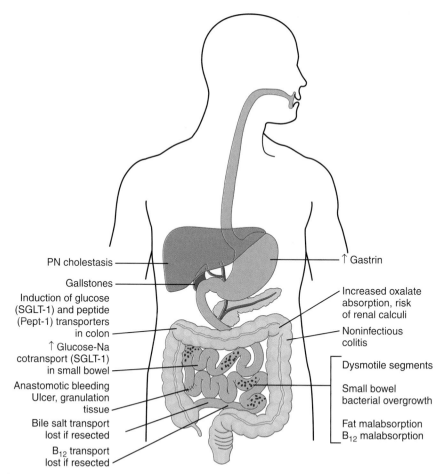

Figure 16-2 Complications of short bowel syndrome. The diagram depicts regional intestinal differences relative to absorption and extraintestinal complications seen in children on chronic parenteral nutrition with short bowel syndrome. Artwork kindly provided by Barbara Siede, Medical Illustrations Dept., Ochsner Clinic Foundation.

impairment because of prolonged PN or losing multiple venous access sites for PN, intestinal transplantation will be considered (44–50).

One useful clinical measurement of adaptation is enteral tolerance (% enteral calories/total calories). This measurement can be made frequently. When full enteral tolerance is reached, there will be little change over time. Thus, a significant (>10%) change in enteral tolerance over time indicates the progression of adaptation.

Two blood tests have been suggested as additional markers for intestinal adaptation. One simple-to-perform assay for intestinal mass reported both in infants (20) and in adults (51, 52) with SBS is serum amino acid level. *Citrulline* (CIT) is an amino acid that is not in the diet or in PN, and is synthesized exclusively in the bowel. Therefore, the CIT level (assuming a steady-state nutritional state) is reflective of enterocyte mass. CIT levels in babies >19 μM are highly predictive of eventual full enteral tolerance (53). In adults, serum CIT correlated not only with small bowel length, but also with protein absorption and with 5-h urinary D-xylose excretion. Additionally, when measured serially in a few subjects, increased absorption was found to parallel an increase in serum CIT level (20, 54).

Another blood test of intestinal adaptation is serum *GLP-2*, which has been shown to be predictive of full enteral tolerance in infants if serum post-prandial levels reach >15 pmol/liter (34). There are few studies of GLP-2 in SBS.

Salt and Water Absorption

In the intestine, water flux follows active salt absorprtion, either nutrient-coupled or linked to anion/cation exchangers. Ninety percent of salt and water absorption takes place in the small intestine under normal conditions (4). There is a gradient of permeability from the proximal to distal intestine, with the "tightest" resistance to passive ion flux in the distal colon and rectum. Therefore, the small intestine is the major absorber, but the colon "has the final say." In patients without a colon, plasma aldosterone levels are exceptionally high; levels return to normal when >50% of the colon is retained in continuity (55). The colon can capture malabsorbed fluid via Na^+/H^+ exchange throughout the colon and aldosterone-activated Na+ channels abundant in the rectum (55, 56). Thus, while the most important variable determining nutrient absorption is the length of small intestine salvaged, the amount of remaining colon is also vitally important to overall Na^+ and fluid and electrolyte balance.

In the jejunum, post-prandial water flux is largely determined by glucose and amino acid-coupled Na^+ absorption. Resection of jejunum in rats results in the appearance in the remaining ileum of a marked increase in glucose-Na^+ cotransport; overall glucose-coupled Na^+ absorption increases 2.5-fold across the remaining small intestine (28). These studies have not been done in humans.

Regional Differences

Of major importance to clinical management are regional differences (Fig. 16-2). The mammalian ileum has greater plasticity than the jejunum, being more capable of villus lengthening and increased transport activity. The stimulatory factor is likely to be the concentration of luminal nutrients rather than how much the bowel has been shortened (33). In health, the *jejunum* has taller villi with greater absorptive surface than the ileum; and mucosal disaccharidases and peptidases are higher in concentration on the jejunal enterocytes than their ileal counterparts. For these reasons, the greatest quantity of salt, nutrient, and water absorption occurs in the jejunum.

As mentioned, the *ileum* is unique to the small intestine in its ability to absorb by active transport vitamin B12 and bile salts. Children with resection of the penultimate ileum (just before the terminal ileum) are at high risk for requiring lifelong B12 shots. When the ileal transporters of taurine or glycine-conjugated bile acids are lost by resection, bile salts trigger cyclic AMP-mediated secretion in the colon (57) and the circulating bile salt pool is depleted, the latter of which impairs fat micellar solubilization and absorption. The hypothesis of an insufficient bile salt pool in SBS has led to recent research looking at whether bile salts, which are cathartics, could be supplemented to enhance fat absorption without triggering diarrhea. One experimental approach has been to administer sarcosine-conjugated bile salts (58, 59). Sarcosine is a dipeptide which is very effectively absorbed in small intestine by a specific transporter in the brush border membrane (60).

Finally, the colon in SBS is capable of increased short-chain fatty acid (SCFA)-driven NaCl absorption (61, 62). This process hinges on the ability of the colon to ferment malabsorbed carbohydrate to butyrate, acetate, and propionate in the colon and is blocked by antibiotic administration (63). Also an essential function of SCFA is to promote small intestinal mucosal hypertrophy (weight, protein and DNA content) by complex mechanisms.

Effect of SBS on Other Gastrointestinal Organs

There is a transient and very significant increase in postprandial but not fasting gastric acid secretion and serum gastrin level after intestinal resection (64). Serum gastrin level, which is usually very high in SBS patients, was not found to correlate with gastric acid output (65). In another study, distal SB resection increased basal and submaximally stimulated gastric acid secretion, but neither proximal nor distal resection altered serum gastrin level (66). Gastric acid and pancreatic enzyme secretions, as well as pancreatic bicarbonate secretion, decreased in one animal study after massive small bowel resection (67).

PREVENTION

Most of the birth defects that produce SBS (e.g. abdominal wall defects, malrotation, and atresias) are not preventable. Much more research is needed in determining environmental toxins and genetic and perhaps even immune factors that contribute to a high rate of birth defects (1 in 28 live births) in our population. On the other hand, it is well-established that the major cause of SBS, NEC, can be prevented by preventing prematurity, slow introduction of enteral feedings, promotion of breast-milk feeding, and strict adherence to hygienic practices in the newborn intensive care unit (68–70). Additionally, NEC is associated with poverty, teenage pregnancy, lack of access to confidential medical care, and socioeconomic factors that need to be addressed by a national public health approach. A consistent observation by the author is that the SBS children living under "disadvantaged" circumstances have a much poorer outcome (for example, more central line infections) than do those in a more socio-economically advantaged environment.

COMPLICATIONS

Medical caretakers experienced in treating infants with SBS will develop an intimate understanding of the medical and *emotional* complications, including suffering, associated with this condition. Recently, a multicenter questionnaire study showed that the quality of life of home PN-dependent children and siblings is not different from that of healthy children, suggesting that these children use effective coping strategies. In contrast, the quality of life of parents (especially mothers) of HPN-dependent children is low (71). *Medical* complications are summarized in Fig. 16-2.

Infection

The most important and frequent complication of SBS is central line-associated septicemia; and the three most important infectious agents (in order of frequency) are Gram-positive cocci, especially coagulase-negative *Staphylococci*; Gram-negative rods; and fungi, especially *C. albicans* (72, 73). The number of infections in these infants gradually declines with increasing postnatal age. Unexpectedly, the number of infections is much lower in infants who are cared for by their biological mothers in their own homes (74).

Thrombosis

The survival of an infant with SBS is predicated on maintaining patency of the central veins into which the cather (Broviac or Hickman) is inserted. However, thrombosis of the veins that are used for catheter sites is almost universal. It is believed that the thrombosis is related to infection, because most lines are removed for this reason. However, some catheters become obstructed with clot spontaneously. Thrombosis may relate to the concentration of dextrose in the PN, and most physicians are careful to provide dextrose concentrations <15% for this reason. Lipid infusion in the catheter may reduce the thrombosis risk (75, 76). After years of PN and central line infection, significant problems with multiple venous obstruction and recanalization are observed (77, 78). Superior vena cava syndrome is often seen, which can lead to macrocephaly and normal pressure hydrocephalus (78). Some have proposed chronic administration of anticoagulants to prevent this complication (79). In a study from Melbourne, investigators treated SBS patients on home PN with oral warfarin. Before commencing anticoagulant therapy, the mean central line "lifespan" was 160 days. Concomitant warfarin therapy was associated with a mean central line patency duration of 352 days. There were no major bleeding events (79).

Cholestasis

Among the earliest findings in infants receiving PN was that the most severe cholestasis occurred in the most premature group, in the infants who were not fed, and in those who developed septicemia (80, 81). Research has identified each macronutrient component of the PN (amino acid, soybean oil, and glucose) as contributing factors. More recently, phytosterols which are present in the soybean emulsion and are present at high levels in human serum of individuals on PN have been found to create a fatty liver in experimental animals (82, 83). Progression of the cholestasis is clearly related to endotoxemia (84, 85). Furthermore, hepatic accumulation of iron admistered in PN may contribute to cause toxicity (86, 87). Copper accumulation in the range of levels seen in Wilson disease is not unusual in PN-dependent patients, but copper overload seems independent of duration of PN and may be a sign rather than a cause of liver disease (88). Removal of copper from the trace elements added to PN is indicated. However, subsequently hypocupremia can result from complete removal of copper, and hypocupremia causes neutropenia (88). Although cholestasis may be initiated by PN in children with SBS, we have found that cholestasis does not always resolve after PN is discontinued. In children who are not fully enterally tolerant in whom PN has been discontinued, the acidosis associated with malabsorption may cause the cholestasis to worsen for weeks after PN has been discontinued. The cholestasis may take several months to resolve after PN is discontinued.

In most patients with SBS, the composition of bile is altered toward a bile salt-depleted, lithogenic bile. Up to 25% of infants with SBS will develop cholelithiasis (89, 90). In relatively large adult series, about 40% develop cholelithiasis (91). One study indicated effective gallbladder emptying with bolus feeding, but not with continuous feeding, the latter of which is used most often in SBS patients (92).

For more than a decade, pediatricians have suspected that the specific amino acid composition used affects liver function in neonates on PN. A preparation designed to normalize serum amino acid levels containing increased cysteine and supplemental taurine (Trophamine, TA) (93) was developed for premature infants, but preliminary comparisons with standard amino acid formulations did not show a difference (94). Recently, a meta-analysis showed that within specific subgroups of neonatal patients, taurine supplementation protected against PN-associated cholestasis (95). A relatively large controlled trial in very low birth weight infants and post-surgical infants supported this conclusion. The use of standard amino acids was associated with a greater than 2-fold increase in the incidence of PN-cholestasis compared to periods of exclusive TA use (90).

One treatment that we have used in infants with SBS is oral ursodeoxycholic acid (UDCA), because of its efficacy in other cholestatic conditions. Recently, a trial investigating very low birth weight infants from Taipei showed that patients who received UDCA therapy with doses of 10–30 mg/kg/day had a shorter duration of cholestasis than the control group (63 vs. 92 days, $P = 0.006$). Furthermore, the peak serum levels of direct bilirubin also were significantly lower in the treatment group.

Attempts to reduce the severity of cholestasis with intravenous cholecystokinin have been largely unsuccessful. In a recent multicenter study in which a total of 243 neonates were enrolled, CCK-octapeptide did not significantly affect conjugated levels, or secondary outcome measures, including incidence of sepsis, time to achieve 50% or 100% of energy intake via the enteral route, number of ICU and hospital days, mortality rate, and incidence of biliary sludge or cholelithiasis (96). What could become the most important recent new advance in parenteral nutrition is the replacement of soybean intralipid with an omega-3 fatty acid preparation that improves cholestasis. A group in Boston initially reported two infants with intestinal failure and chronic cholestasis who had either resolution or improvement of their cholestasis has shortly after commencing the new fish oil preparation (97). These investigators have spearheaded a multicenter trail to confirm efficacy.

D-Lactic Acidosis

D-Lactate is produced by *Lactobacilli* and *Bacteroides* and other Gram-positive bacteria in the intestine. Its serum concentration in normal children is zero, whereas in children with SBS it averages around 500 μM (98) but can exceed a concentration of 141 mM (99)! When infants with SBS develop hyperchloremic metabolic acidosis, enceophalopathy, hypotension, and decompensation, septicemia is the first condition suspected. However, these findings may be caused by D-lactic acidosis. D-Lactic acidosis can be recurrent and it can also be lethal. It is treated by (most importantly) reducing oral intake of calories and particularly of carbohydrates (99, 100) and by administering oral, rather than intravenous, antibiotics such as vancomycin, aimed at lowering the high fecal counts of Gram-positive anaerobic bacteria such as *Lactobacilli* (101). These *Lactobacilli* constitute more than 60% of the fecal organisms in children with SBS (102).

Noninfectious Colitis of SBS

Noninfectious colitis is another common complication in many children with SBS, manifested by diarrhea with blood in the stools (103). This complication appears directly related to "pushing" forward the feedings in the face of diarrhea. When dietary changes are unsuccessful, administering sulfasalazine at 25–50 mg/kg/day or prednisone at 1 mg/kg/day sometimes results in resolution (103). The author has encountered one child who went on to develop ulcerative colitis.

Renal Disease

It is common for infants with SBS to have kidney hypertrophy on ultrasound, and renal calculi occur in ~25% of adult patients with SBS who have a colon. The pathogenesis seems to require a colon in continuity, with hyperoxaluria resulting from calcium soap formation in the colon and hyperabsorption of calcium oxalate from the colon (91, 104). Long-term follow-up of adults on PN has shown a profound 3.5% reduction in creatinine clearance per year, mostly unattributable to infection and aminoglycoside administration (105). In children and rats with SBS, focal renal tubulointerstitial fibrosis has also been reported and appears to result from arginine deficiency (106).

Hypergastrinemia

Gastric acid hypersecretion consequent to extensive small bowel resection is especially important in the first few months post-resection and probably results from excessive gastrin production by stomach antral G-cells, as well as decreased small bowel degradation of the hormone. It may result in maldigestion as well as duodenal ulcers and is managed by pharmacological acid blockade (107).

Mortality

Recent research has identified predictive features for mortality in pediatric SBS. A large cohort of children from Michigan ($n = 80$) was found to have increased mortality if serum conjugated bilirubin was >2.5, with a relative risk of 22.7 ($P < 0.005$), or if the percent of normal small bowel length for post-conceptual age was <10%, with a relative risk of 5.7 ($P < 0.003$). Presence of an ileo-cecalvalve was predictive of weaning, with an odds ratio of 3.9 ($P < 0.0005$) compared with absence of the ileocecal valve (108). Similarly, the previously cited series of Parisian infants found that the duration of PN before enteral sufficiency was correlated with presence of the ileocecal valve and length of bowel (109).

TREATMENT OF SBS

Parenteral nutrition

Parenteral nutrition was the discovery that allowed almost miraculous survival of infants with the intestine resected (110). It is beyond the scope of this review to describe the history and optimal formulation of PN in the treatment of SBS. There are two excellent and recent reviews of this subject (111, 112).

Diet

Careful attention to fluid and electrolyte balance is necessary in all infants with SBS, but particularly in those with ostomies, in whom quantitation of losses of Na, K, Cl, and Zn is very useful in formulating PN. Zinc losses from a jejunostomy may double an infant's normal requirements and a low serum level may impair normal absorption in the remaining bowel (43). It is also generally recommended that children with ileostomy or jejunostomy be re-connected to remaining colon as soon as the infant is deemed healthy enough to tolerate re-anastomosis.

Enteral feedings are administered early after surgery, to exert a trophic effect. Additionally total PN produces an increase in intestinal permeability mostly related to sepsis and liver disease (113). Most pediatric gastroenterologists recommend continuous feeding instead of bolus feedings, because the infants may experience a vicious cycle of large-volume feeding and malabsorptive diarrhea. Furthermore, a study of patients with diarrhea showed that fat, nitrogen, and trace element absorption increased by ~30% with continuous feedings compared with bolus feeding (114). Continuous feeding is controversial, however, because bolus feedings are significantly more likely to produce gallbladder contractions, which may prevent gallstones (92). Furthermore, infants on continuous feeding take longer to develop the oropharyngeal coordination necessary for feeding (115), and speech therapists recommend bolus feedings at least twice daily, even in children on continuous infusion. Our practice is to turn off the continuous infusion for 1 h three times daily, and at these times we give an oral feeding equivalent to 1 h of infused feeding.

The optimal components of the diet have been studied, but an optimal formula has not emerged. One retrospective series from Andorsky *et al.* showed that enteral feeding with *breast milk or an amino acid-based formula* correlated with a shorter duration of PN requirement (116). Some centers advocate amino acid-based formulae to minimize the risk of protein-associated colitis, while others advocate *protein hydrolysates* which have a lower osmolarity. None of these formulae has lactose, which is poorly tolerated. Glucose polymers such as corn syrup solids carry no "osmotic penalty"; otherwise stated, long-chain glucose polymers deliver a quantity of glucose with only one reducing equivalent per chain.

Fat is an important source of calories in SBS, and animal studies have shown that long-chain triglycerides (LCT) have a trophic effect. Specifically, polyunsaturated long-chain fats (such as a fish oil called menhaden oil) are more trophic in rats than diets containing short-chain or saturated fat (117). In patients with a colon present, a high-carbohydrate diet reduced fecal calorie loss and increased energy absorption, compared to a diet high in fat. A recent review summarizes data suggesting that patients with a colon receive different diets than those without a colon (118). Specifically, it is recommended for those *with a colon* that 50–60% of calories be provided as complex carbohydrates, fat given as both MCT and LCT, and oxalates restricted in the diet because of the risk of renal stones (see below). For those *without a colon*, the authors advocate 40–50% of calories from complex carbohydrates, only LCT, and no oxalate restriction. Both groups of patients are recommended to receive oral rehydration and soluble fiber.

Protein is well absorbed, probably because of lower concentrations in formulae and because of a large maximal velocity of peptide (di- and tripeptide) transporters and many different classes of amino acid transporters. There may be disadvantages to feeding formulae containing intact protein to infants with SBS. As mentioned, a high proportion of these infants develop colitis, documented colonoscopically, with cow-milk protein feeding (103). It is unclear whether the colitis results from cow-milk protein sensitization or from malabsorption of bile acids. Animal studies have also suggested that excessive short-chain fatty acids, combined with a low intraluminal pH (<5.0), can produce mucosal damage and inflammation. Both acetate and lactate at p. 4.0 produced significantly greater injury than similarly acidified NaCl (119).

Solid foods are felt to be well-tolerated and we recommend initiation at the normal ages. Meats and complex carbohydrates, e.g. potatoes and cooked vegetables, are well-tolerated. Refined carbohydrates such as candy bars are discouraged.

Pharmacologic treatment

Cholestyramine

The bile salt resin binder cholestyramine (and in older children colestid pills) can produce a dramatic decrease in diarrhea. However, the benefit pertains only to those children who have suboptimal ileal bile salt absorption due to resection. We use 240 mg/kg/day divided into three doses. In cases with extensive resection, there is the potential risk of bile salt binding worsening the malabsorption. Hyperchloremic acidosis has been reported but is rare. Bile salt resins are anion binders which may reduce absorption of anticonvulsants and other drugs.

Antidiarrheal Drugs

Loperamide (0.1 mg/kg/dose TID or QID) can be modestly helpful but does not actually increase salt and water absorption (120). It changes the motor function of the intestine, which results in increased capacitance of the gut and a delay in the passage of fluid through the intestine, but no change in the volume of fluid passed per rectum.

Glutamine + Growth Hormone

Most elemental formulae based on amino acids rather than peptides have been enriched with high concentrations of glutamine (GLN). GLN is the primary metabolic fuel of the gut, a precursor of purines and pyrimidines, and a trophic "signal" to the enterocyte (121). In fact, GLN dosing activates mitogen-activated protein kinases (MAPKs) and enterocyte proliferation much in the same way that growth factors such as epidermal growth factor (EGF) activate MAPKs and proliferation (122). In humans, glutamine reduces the frequency of systemic infections and may also reduce the translocation of intestinal bacteria and toxins, but the latter has not been demonstrated (123), although many rodent studies support this hypothesis (124–126). However, circulating GLN levels are normal and often above normal in patients with SBS, probably because the GLN-metabolizing intestinal cells and lamina propria leukocytes are reduced in number in children with SBS.

Although GLN individually has not been shown to be effective in treating SBS, many trials have been conducted looking at the combination of GLN, growth hormone (GH), and a high-carbohydrate/low-fat (HCLF) diet. The rationale is that GLN + GH more potently stimulates enterocyte mitogenesis and is more trophic (127, 128). A recent meta-analysis of GLN + GH (0.14 mg/kg/day) + HCLF diet which included 13 controlled trials and 258 patients showed that, compared with standard treatment, this combination had a beneficial effect on body weight, stool output, lean body mass, carbohydrate and nitrogen absorption, D-xylose absorption, and the ability to come off PN (129). Only a few pediatric patients have been treated, but growth hormone (0.3 mg/kg per week subcutaneously) plus glutamine (at the homeopathic dose of 30 mg/day) was found to increase height percentile and seemed to facilitate PN independence (130).

The use of fiber and probiotics is controversial. Fiber may promote a deterioration in children missing the colon or with no ileocecal valve. Probiotics may not be beneficial in patients who already have small bowel bacterial overgrowth and, on rare occasions, probiotics have been associated with septicemia in such children (131).

Treatment of infants with SBS with standard pediatric medications, such as antibiotics, is problematic because of erratic absorption in children with SBS. Furthermore, one commonly used parenteral antibiotic is contraindicated, because it can form crystals in the gallbladder. Ceftriaxone treatment has been reported to lead to cholelithiasis and sludge formation resulting from crystallization of the drug itself in the gallbladder (132).

Skin Care

One of the most "irritating" aspects of nursing care is treating the infants' perianal dermatitis and skin excoriation (pun intended). As enteral feedings are advanced and the child is observed to improve, this problem escalates. The author has queried whether the ulcerated groin and buttock are the portal of entry for Gram-negative septicemia. Skin breakdown is probably produced by both bile salt malabsorption (because bile salts are powerful detergents) and excessive SCFA production from malabsorbed carbohydrates. Papulae may also signify high levels of fecal *Candida*. The pH of stools in these infants is often in the 4.0–5.0 range. Perianal dermatitis in SBS may not respond to zinc oxide, antifungals, or to bile salt binders, such as cholestyramine. Combinations of all three can be beneficial. However, the author's experience is that the best therapy is stoma powder as the first application, with overlying application of a combination cream with cholestyramine + zinc oxide + antifungal (clotrimazole or nystatin). This treatment should be applied each time the infant has a stool.

Criteria for discharge from hospital have been established by Sondheimer (43). These include (a) good weight gain on a stable regimen; (b) availability of outpatient pharmacy and nursing services; (c) parental competence, motivation and compliance; (d) ability of the child to tolerate at least 6 h without intravenous nutrition; and (e) adequate financial resources for clinic appointments and long-distance phone calls.

Monitoring

Monitoring children on PN has been reviewed elsewhere (73, 111); occasionally it is also helpful to check serum aldosterone levels to document that sufficient salt and fluid is being administered. We also monitor every 6 months levels of iron (and ferritin) and copper, which are hepatotoxic, as well as the selenium level, an anti-oxidant which can be supplemented if needed (133). For children weaned off PN, the most important clinical variables are body weight and height; serum electrolytes and protein/albumin/prealbumin are also very useful. Many centers also monitor urinary oxalate levels, with renal ultrasounds and a low-oxalate diet administered as needed.

Intermittent bone mineral density testing and vitamin D status are helpful. Recently, children with short bowel syndrome were found to have decreased bone mineral content compared with control subjects; however, it was not significant when adjusted for differences in weight and height (134). Because it is not known whether these children will have normal bone accretion during puberty, some have advocated periodic monitoring and calcium/vitamin D supplementation.

REMAINING QUESTIONS

There are many questions that plague neonatologists and pediatric gastroenterologists who manage infants with SBS. Many of these have been underscored by Goulet et al. (135). Physicians do not know the optimal formula to provide, how to best administer the formula (bolus versus continuously), or how to compose PN in such a manner to avoid hepatic injury. Additionally, we wonder whether enteral antibiotics are beneficial (to prevent bacterial overgrowth, which prolongs adaptation in children (8)) or detrimental (by predisposing to fungemia and *C. difficile* infections). Dietary fiber is said to be helpful in adults with SBS but has been associated with abdominal distension and D-lactic acidosis.

Formulae rich in medium-chain triglycerides (MCTs) are hydrolyzed more rapidly than long-chain triglycerides (LCTs) and are water-soluble, reaching the portal circulation by traversing the enterocytes directly; however, they can produce osmotic diarrhea. MCTs malabsorbed in the human small bowel can traverse the colon, unlike malabsorbed LCTs (62). However, in animal models MCTs are not as trophic as LCTs, the latter of which stimulate pancreatic and biliary secretions (136). Most experts advocate administering both MCTs and LCTs enterally. In fact, recent research suggests that combining them in the parenteral nutrition (using "structured triacylyglycerols" with MCT + LCT) is safe and well tolerated on a long-term basis, and it may be associated with a reduction in liver dysfunction in humans (137, 138). Structural triacylglycerols also provide for better preservation of mucosal mass in animals (139).

Surgically, there is benefit from tapering enteroplasty to improve transit from dilated segments with poor peristalsis; however, there is no proven role for placement of reversed segments or intussuscepted "valves" (reviewed in ref. 135). Bowel lengthening can be beneficial. However, there is controversy about when to perform these technically difficult lengthening procedures and which technique is the most efficacious. The Bianchi procedure consists of dividing the intestine along its longitudinal axis (reviewed in ref. 138), while the serial transverse enteroplasty (STEP) is a newer technique with promising preliminary results (141, 142).

With respect to small intestinal transplantation, research has not yet pinpointed the clinical features that identify when bowel failure becomes irreversible. It is not established whether transplantation is to be recommended universally, given that <50% of survivors will live more than 10 years after transplant (143), according to data up to 2005, although improvements in immunosuppression may improve these numbers. At the current time, the best approach appears to be a multidisciplinary one where enteral feeding is maximized, infection is minimized, home family-administered therapy is promoted, strictures are dilated or resected, dilated segments are subjected to enteroplasty, and (in cases where there has been no progression of absorption) bowel lengthening is performed. When these measures have been taken and the child fails to progress, multidisciplinary evaluation which includes psychologist, social worker, as well as gastroenterologist, dietician, and surgeon should determine whether transplantation is to be undertaken.

Another important question is whether there will be a long-term sequelae of "fully adapted SBS." For example, is there an increased risk of colon cancer, inasmuch as high concentrations of bile salts are mitogens associated with transformation of cultured colonic epithelial cells (144, 145)? Conversely, SBS patients have low serum lipid levels. Are they at lower risk for cardiovascular disease later in life?

REFERENCES

1. Wales PW, de Silva N, Kim J, et al. Neonatal short bowel syndrome: population-based estimates of incidence and mortality rates. J Pediatr Surg 2004; 39(5):690–695.
2. Schalamon J, Mayr JM, Hollwarth ME. Mortality and economics in short bowel syndrome. Best Pract Res Clin Gastroenterol 2003; 17(6):931–942.
3. Wilmore D. Short bowel syndrome. A comprehensive approach to patient management. I. Pathophysiology following massive intestinal resection. J Kans Med Soc 1969; 70(5):233–237.
4. Rhoads JM, Powell DW. Chapter 7: Diarrhea. In: Walker WA, Durie PR, Hamilton JR, et al, eds., Pediatric Gastrointestinal Disease, 1st edn. Toronto, ON: B.C. Decker; 1991: 62–78.
5. Goulet OJ, Revillon Y, Jan D, et al. Neonatal short bowel syndrome. J Pediatr 1991; 119(1 (Pt 1)):18–23.
6. Stewart BA, Karrer FM, Hall RJ, Lilly JR. The blind loop syndrome in children. J Pediatr Surg 1990; 25(8):905–908.
7. Lichtman SN, Sartor RB, Keku J, Schwab JH. Hepatic inflammation in rats with experimental small intestinal bacterial overgrowth. Gastroenterology 1990; 98(2):414–423.
8. Kaufman SS, Loseke CA, Lupo JV, et al. Influence of bacterial overgrowth and intestinal inflammation on duration of parenteral nutrition in children with short bowel syndrome. J Pediatr 1997; 131(3):356–361.
9. Ling PR, Khaodhiar L, Bistrian BR, et al. Inflammatory mediators in patients receiving long-term home parenteral nutrition. Dig Dis Sci 2001; 46(11):2484–2489.
10. Wilmore D. Short bowel syndrome. II. Patient management following massive intestinal resection. J Kans Med Soc 1969; 70(6):280–282.
11. Weber TR, Tracy T Jr, Connors RH. Short-bowel syndrome in children. Quality of life in an era of improved survival. Arch Surg 1991; 126(7):841–846.
12. Vaughan WG, Grosfeld JL, West K, et al. Avoidance of stomas and delayed anastomosis for bowel necrosis: the 'clip and drop-back' technique. J Pediatr Surg 1996; 31(4):542–545.
13. Touloukian RJ, Smith GJ. Normal intestinal length in preterm infants. J Pediatr Surg 1983; 18(6):720–723.
14. Hart MH, Grandjean CJ, Park JH, et al. Essential fatty acid deficiency and postresection mucosal adaptation in the rat. Gastroenterology 1988; 94(3):682–687.
15. de Miguel E, Gomez de Segura IA, Bonet H, et al. Trophic effects of neurotensin in massive bowel resection in the rat. Dig Dis Sci 1994; 39(1):59–64.
16. Taylor RG, Fuller PJ. Humoral regulation of intestinal adaptation. Baillieres Clin Endocrinol Metab 1994; 8(1):165–183.
17. Rokkas T, Vaja S, Murphy GM, Dowling RH. Aminoguanidine blocks intestinal diamine oxidase (DAO) activity and enhances the intestinal adaptive response to resection in the rat. Digestion 1990; 46(Suppl 2):447–457.
18. Vanderhoof JA, Kollman KA. Lack of inhibitory effect of octreotide on intestinal adaptation in short bowel syndrome in the rat. J Pediatr Gastroenterol Nutr 1998; 26(3):241–244.
19. Dorney SF, Ament ME, Berquist WE, et al. Improved survival in very short small bowel of infancy with use of long-term parenteral nutrition. J Pediatr 1985; 107(4):521–525.
20. Rhoads JM, Plunkett E, Galanko J, et al. Serum citrulline levels correlate with enteral tolerance and bowel length in infants with short bowel syndrome. J Pediatr 2005; 146(4):542–547.
21. Holt D, Easa D, Shim W, Suzuki M. Survival after massive small intestinal resection in a neonate. Am J Dis Child 1982; 136(1):79–80.
22. Rossi L, Kadamba P, Hugosson C, et al. Pediatric short bowel syndrome: adaptation after massive small bowel resection. J Pediatr Gastroenterol Nutr 2007; 45:213–221.
23. Weaver LT, Austin S, Cole TJ. Small intestinal length: a factor essential for gut adaptation. Gut 1991; 32(11):1321–1323.
24. FitzSimmons J, Chinn A, Shepard TH. Normal length of the human fetal gastrointestinal tract. Pediatr Pathol 1988; 8(6):633–641.
25. Sondheimer JM, Cadnapaphornchai M, Sontag M, Zerbe GO. Predicting the duration of dependence on parenteral nutrition after neonatal intestinal resection. J Pediatr 1998; 132(1):80–84.

26. Quiros-Tejeira RE, Ament ME, Reyen L, et al. Long-term parenteral nutritional support and intestinal adaptation in children with short bowel syndrome: a 25-year experience. J Pediatr 2004; 145(2):157–163.

27. Messing B, Crenn P, Beau P, et al. Long-term survival and parenteral nutrition dependence in adult patients with the short bowel syndrome. Gastroenterology 1999; 117(5):1043–1050.

28. Schulzke JD, Fromm M, Bentzel CJ, et al. Ion transport in the experimental short bowel syndrome of the rat. Gastroenterology 1992; 102(2):497–504.

29. Sacks AI, Warwick GJ, Barnard JA. Early proliferative events following intestinal resection in the rat. J Pediatr Gastroenterol Nutr 1995; 21(2):158–164.

30. Stehr W, Bernal NP, Erwin CR, et al. Roles for p21waf1/cip1 and p27kip1 during the adaptation response to massive intestinal resection. Am J Physiol Gastrointest Liver Physiol 2005 Dec 8.

31. Weser E. Intestinal adaptation to small bowel resection. Am J Clin Nutr 1971; 24(1):133–135.

32. Ulshen MH, Herbst CA. Effect of removal of pancreaticobiliary secretions on adaptation to short bowel in orally nourished rats. Am J Clin Nutr 1984; 39(5):762–770.

33. Ulshen MH, Herbst CA. Effect of proximal transposition of the ileum on mucosal growth and enzyme activity in orally nourished rats. Am J Clin Nutr 1985; 42(5):805–814.

34. Sigalet DL, Martin G, Meddings J, et al. GLP-2 levels in infants with intestinal dysfunction. Pediatr Res 2004; 56(3):371–376.

35. Scott RB, Kirk D, MacNaughton WK, Meddings JB. GLP-2 augments the adaptive response to massive intestinal resection in rat. Am J Physiol 1998; 275(5 Pt 1):G911–G921.

36. Drucker DJ. Glucagon-like peptide 2. J Clin Endocrinol Metab 2001; 86(4):1759–1764.

37. Lund PK. Molecular basis of intestinal adaptation: the role of the insulin-like growth factor system. Ann N Y Acad Sci 1998; 859:18–36 Nov 17.

38. Vanderhoof JA, McCusker RH, Clark R, et al. Truncated and native insulinlike growth factor I enhance mucosal adaptation after jejunoileal resection. Gastroenterology 1992; 102(6):1949–1956.

39. Lund PK, Ulshen MH, Rountree DB, et al. Molecular biology of gastrointestinal peptides and growth factors: relevance to intestinal adaptation. Digestion 1990; 46(Suppl 2):66–73.

40. Vanderhoof JA, Park JH, Grandjean CJ. Reduced mucosal prostaglandin synthesis after massive small bowel resection. Am J Physiol 1988; 254(3 Pt 1):G373–G377.

41. Jeppesen PB, Mortensen PB. Enhancing bowel adaptation in short bowel syndrome. Curr Gastroenterol Rep 2002; 4(4):338–347.

42. Wilmore DW. Growth factors and nutrients in the short bowel syndrome. JPEN J Parenter Enteral Nutr 1999; 23(5 Suppl):S117–S120.

43. Sondheimer JM. Neonatal Short Bowel Syndrome. In: Thureen PJ, Hay WW, eds., Neonatal Nutrition and Metabolism, 2nd edn. Cambridge, UK: Cambridge University Press; 2006: x–xx.

44. Kocoshis SA. Small bowel transplantation in infants and children. Gastroenterol Clin North Am 1994; 23(4):727–742.

45. Langnas AN, Shaw BW Jr, Antonson DL, et al. Preliminary experience with intestinal transplantation in infants and children. Pediatrics 1996; 97(4):443–448.

46. Atkison P, Williams S, Wall W, Grant D. Results of pediatric small bowel transplantation in Canada. Transplant Proc 1998; 30(6):2521–2522.

47. Sudan DL, Kaufman SS, Shaw BW Jr, et al. Isolated intestinal transplantation for intestinal failure. Am J Gastroenterol 2000; 95(6):1506–1515.

48. Tzakis AG, Todo S, Reyes J, et al. Intestinal transplantation in children under FK 506 immunosuppression. J Pediatr Surg 1993; 28(8):1040–1043.

49. Langnas AN, Dhawan A, Antonson DL, et al. Intestinal transplantation in children. Transplant Proc 1996; 28(5):2752.

50. Kocoshis SA, Beath SV, Booth IW, et al. Intestinal failure and small bowel transplantation, including clinical nutrition: Working Group report of the second World Congress of Pediatric Gastroenterology, Hepatology, and Nutrition. J Pediatr Gastroenterol Nutr 2004; 39(Suppl 2):S655–S661.

51. Crenn P, Coudray-Lucas C, Thuillier F, et al. Postabsorptive plasma citrulline concentration is a marker of absorptive enterocyte mass and intestinal failure in humans. Gastroenterology 2000; 119(6):1496–1505.

52. Crenn P, Vahedi K, Lavergne-Slove A, et al. Plasma citrulline: A marker of enterocyte mass in villous atrophy-associated small bowel disease. Gastroenterology 2003; 124(5):1210–1219.

53. Becker RM, Wu G, Galanko JA, et al. Reduced serum amino acid concentrations in infants with necrotizing enterocolitis. J Pediatr 2000; 137(6):785–793.

54. Jianfeng G, Weiming Z, Ning L, et al. Serum citrulline is a simple quantitative marker for small intestinal enterocytes mass and absorption function in short bowel patients. J Surg Res 2005; 127(2):177–182.

55. Ladefoged K, Olgaard K. Sodium homeostasis after small-bowel resection. Scand J Gastroenterol 1985; 20(3):361–369.

56. Rajendran VM, Kashgarian M, Binder HJ. Aldosterone induction of electrogenic sodium transport in the apical membrane vesicles of rat distal colon. J Biol Chem 1989; 264(31): 18638–18644 Nov 5.

57. Binder HJ, Filburn C, Volpe BT. Bile salt alteration of colonic electrolyte transport: role of cyclic adenosine monophosphate. Gastroenterology 1975; 68(3):503–508.

58. Heydorn S, Jeppesen PB, Mortensen PB. Bile acid replacement therapy with cholylsarcosine for short-bowel syndrome. Scand J Gastroenterol 1999; 34(8):818–823.

59. Gruy-Kapral C, Little KH, Fordtran JS, et al. Conjugated bile acid replacement therapy for short-bowel syndrome. Gastroenterology 1999; 116(1):15–21.

60. Mackenzie B, Loo DD, Fei Y, et al. Mechanisms of the human intestinal H+-coupled oligopeptide transporter hPEPT1. J Biol Chem 1996; 271(10):5430–5437.

61. Nordgaard I, Hansen BS, Mortensen PB. Importance of colonic support for energy absorption as small-bowel failure proceeds. Am J Clin Nutr 1996; 64(2):222–231.

62. Jeppesen PB, Mortensen PB. Colonic digestion and absorption of energy from carbohydrates and medium-chain fat in small bowel failure. J Parenter Enteral Nutr 1999; 23(5 Suppl):S101–S105.

63. Aghdassi E, Plapler H, Kurian R, et al. Colonic fermentation and nutritional recovery in rats with massive small bowel resection. Gastroenterology 1994; 107(3):637–642.

64. Wolf SA, Dozois RR, Telander RL, Go VL. Effect of proximal gastric vagotomy on gastric acid hypersecretion and hypergastrinemia after massive small bowel resection in dogs. Surgery 1977; 81(6):627–632.

65. Rius X, Guix M, Garriga J, et al. Parietal cell volume, hypergastrinemia, and gastric acid hypersecretion after small bowel resection. Experimental study. Am J Surg 1982; 144(2):269–272.

66. Sainz A, Lanas A, Esteva F, et al. Increased gastric acid secretion after massive small bowel resection is related to a decrease in enterogastrones. Eur Surg Res 1995; 27(1):31–38.

67. Seal AM, Debas HT, Reynolds C, et al. Gastric and pancreatic hyposecretion following massive small-bowel resection. Dig Dis Sci 1982; 27(2):117–123.

68. Reber KM, Nankervis CA. Necrotizing enterocolitis: preventative strategies. Clin Perinatol 2004; 31(1):157–167.

69. Neu J, Weiss MD. Necrotizing enterocolitis: pathophysiology and prevention. JPEN J Parenter Enteral Nutr 1999; 23(5 Suppl):S13–S17.

70. Kliegman RM, Walker WA, Yolken RH. Necrotizing enterocolitis: research agenda for a disease of unknown etiology and pathogenesis. Pediatr Res 1993; 34(6):701–708.

71. Gottrand F, Staszewski P, Colomb V, et al. Satisfaction in different life domains in children receiving home parenteral nutrition and their families. J Pediatr 2005; 146(6):793–797.

72. O'Keefe SJ, Burnes JU, Thompson RL. Recurrent sepsis in home parenteral nutrition patients: an analysis of risk factors. J Parenter Enteral Nutr 1994; 18(3):256–263.

73. Moukarzel AA, Haddad I, Ament ME, et al. 230 patient years of experience with home long-term parenteral nutrition in childhood: natural history and life of central venous catheters. J Pediatr Surg 1994; 29(10):1323–1327.

74. Melville CA, Bisset WM, Long S, Milla PJ. Counting the cost: hospital versus home central venous catheter survival. J Hosp Infect 1997; 35(3):197–205.

75. Fujiwara T, Kawarasaki H, Fonkalsrud EW. Reduction of postinfusion venous endothelial injury with intralipid. Surg Gynecol Obstet 1984; 158(1):57–65.

76. Matsusue S, Nishimura S, Koizumi S, et al. Preventive effect of simultaneously infused lipid emulsion against thrombophlebitis during postoperative peripheral parenteral nutrition. Surg Today 1995; 25(8):667–671.

77. Mulvihill SJ, Fonkalsrud EW. Complications of superior versus inferior vena cava occlusion in infants receiving central total parenteral nutrition. J Pediatr Surg 1984; 19(6):752–757.

78. Fonkalsrud EW, Ament ME, Berquist WE, Burke M. Occlusion of the vena cava in infants receiving central venous hyperalimentation. Surg Gynecol Obstet 1982; 154(2):189–192.

79. Newall F, Barnes C, Savoia H, et al. Warfarin therapy in children who require long-term total parenteral nutrition. Pediatrics 2003; 112(5):e386.

80. Pereira GR, Sherman MS, DiGiacomo J, et al. Hyperalimentation-induced cholestasis. Increased incidence and severity in premature infants. Am J Dis Child 1981; 135(9):842–845.

81. Sondheimer JM, Bryan H, Andrews W, Forstner GG. Cholestatic tendencies in premature infants on and off parenteral nutrition. Pediatrics 1978; 62(6):984–989.

82. Ellegard L, Sunesson A, Bosaeus I. High serum phytosterol levels in short bowel patients on parenteral nutrition support. Clin Nutr 2005; 24(3):415–420.

83. Clayton PT, Whitfield P, Iyer K. The role of phytosterols in the pathogenesis of liver complications of pediatric parenteral nutrition. Nutrition 1998; 14(1):158–164.

84. Latham PS, Menkes E, Phillips MJ, Jeejeebhoy KN. Hyperalimentation-associated jaundice: an example of a serum factor inducing cholestasis in rats. Am J Clin Nutr 1985; 41(1):61–65.

85. Trauner M, Fickert P, Stauber RE. Inflammation-induced cholestasis. J Gastroenterol Hepatol 1999; 14(10):946–959.

86. Ben Hariz M, Goulet O, De Potter S, et al. Iron overload in children receiving prolonged parenteral nutrition. J Pediatr 1993; 123(2):238–241.

87. Zambrano E, El-Hennawy M, Ehrenkranz RA, et al. Total parenteral nutrition induced liver pathology: an autopsy series of 24 newborn cases. Pediatr Dev Pathol 2004; 7(5):425–432.

88. Blaszyk H, Wild PJ, Oliveira A, et al. Hepatic copper in patients receiving long-term total parenteral nutrition. J Clin Gastroenterol 2005; 39(4):318–320.

89. Sondheimer JM, Bryan H, Andrews W, Forstner GG. Cholestatic tendencies in premature infants on and off parenteral nutrition. Pediatrics 1978; 62(6):984–989.

90. Wright K, Ernst KD, Gaylord MS, et al. Increased incidence of parenteral nutrition-associated cholestasis with aminosyn PF compared to trophamine. J Perinatol 2003; 23(6):444–450.

91. Nightingale JM, Lennard-Jones JE, Gertner DJ, et al. Colonic preservation reduces need for parenteral therapy, increases incidence of renal stones, but does not change high prevalence of gall stones in patients with a short bowel. Gut 1992; 33(11):1493–1497.

92. Jawaheer G, Shaw NJ, Pierro A. Continuous enteral feeding impairs gallbladder emptying in infants. J Pediatr 2001; 138(6):822–825.

93. Zlotkin SH. TrophAmine. Pediatrics 1988; 82(3):388–390.

94. Forchielli ML, Gura KM, Sandler R, Lo C. Aminosyn PF or trophamine: which provides more protection from cholestasis associated with total parenteral nutrition? J Pediatr Gastroenterol Nutr 1995; 21(4):374–382.

95. Spencer AU, Yu S, Tracy TF, et al. Parenteral nutrition-associated cholestasis in neonates: multivariate analysis of the potential protective effect of taurine. J Parenter Enteral Nutr 2005; 29(5):337–343.

96. Teitelbaum DH, Tracy TF Jr, Aouthmany MM, et al. Use of cholecystokinin-octapeptide for the prevention of parenteral nutrition-associated cholestasis. Pediatrics 2005; 115(5):1332–1340.

97. Gura KM, Duggan CP, Colliner SB, et al. Reversal of parenteral nutrition-associated liver disease in two infants with short bowel syndrome using parenteral fish oil: implications for future management. Pediatrics 2006; 118:e197–e201.

98. Bongaerts G, Tolboom J, Naber T, et al. D-lactic acidemia and aciduria in pediatric and adult patients with short bowel syndrome. Clin Chem 1995; 41(1):107–110.

99. Mayne AJ, Handy DJ, Preece MA, et al. Dietary management of D-lactic acidosis in short bowel syndrome. Arch Dis Child 1990; 65(2):229–231.

100. Karton M, Rettmer RL, Lipkin EW. Effect of parenteral nutrition and enteral feeding on D-lactic acidosis in a patient with short bowel. J Parenter Enteral Nutr 1987; 11(6):586–589.

101. Stolberg L, Rolfe R, Gitlin N, et al. d-Lactic acidosis due to abnormal gut flora: diagnosis and treatment of two cases. N Engl J Med 1982; 306(22):1344–1348 Jun 3.

102. Bongaerts G, Bakkeren J, Severijnen R, et al. Lactobacilli and acidosis in children with short small bowel. J Pediatr Gastroenterol Nutr 2000; 30(3):288–293.

103. Taylor SF, Sondheimer JM, Sokol RJ, et al. Noninfectious colitis associated with short gut syndrome in infants. J Pediatr 1991; 119(1 (Pt 1)):24–28.

104. Nightingale JM. Hepatobiliary, renal and bone complications of intestinal failure. Best Pract Res Clin Gastroenterol 2003; 17(6):907–929.

105. Buchman AL, Moukarzel A, Ament ME, et al. Serious renal impairment is associated with long-term parenteral nutrition. J Parenter Enteral Nutr 1993; 17(5):438–444.

106. Hebiguchi T, Kato T, Yoshino H, et al. Extremely short small bowel induces focal tubulointerstitial fibrosis. J Pediatr Gastroenterol Nutr 2001; 32(5):586–592.

107. Meyers WC, Jones RS. Hyperacidity and hypergastrinemia following extensive intestinal resection. World J Surg 1979; 3(5):539–544.

108. Spencer AU, Neaga A, West B, et al. Pediatric short bowel syndrome: redefining predictors of success. Ann Surg 2005; 242(3):403–409.

109. Goulet O, Baglin-Gobet S, Talbotec C, et al. Outcome and long-term growth after extensive small bowel resection in the neonatal period: a survey of 87 children. Eur J Pediatr Surg 2005; 15(2):95–101.

110. Vargas JH, Ament ME, Berquist WE. Long-term home parenteral nutrition in pediatrics: ten years of experience in 102 patients. J Pediatr Gastroenterol Nutr 1987; 6(1):24–32.

111. Shulman RJ, Phillips S. Parenteral nutrition in infants and children. J Pediatr Gastroenterol Nutr 2003; 36(5):587–607.

112. Goulet O. Parenteral nutrition in pediatrics. Indications and perspectives. Acta Gastroenterol Belg 1999; 62(2):210–215.

113. D'Antiga L, Dhawan A, Davenport M, et al. Intestinal absorption and permeability in paediatric short-bowel syndrome: a pilot study. J Pediatr Gastroenterol Nutr 1999; 29(5):588–593.

114. Parker P, Stroop S, Greene H. A controlled comparison of continuous versus intermittent feeding in the treatment of infants with intestinal disease. J Pediatr 1981; 99(3):360–364.

115. Premji S, Chessell L. Continuous nasogastric milk feeding versus intermittent bolus milk feeding for premature infants less than 1500 grams. Cochrane Database Syst Rev 2001; 1:CD001819.

116. Andorsky DJ, Lund DP, Lillehei CW, et al. Nutritional and other postoperative management of neonates with short bowel syndrome correlates with clinical outcomes. J Pediatr 2001; 139(1):27–33.

117. Vanderhoof JA, Park JH, Herrington MK, Adrian TE. Effects of dietary menhaden oil on mucosal adaptation after small bowel resection in rats. Gastroenterology 1994; 106(1):94–99.

118. DiBaise JK, Young RJ, Vanderhoof JA. Intestinal rehabilitation and the short bowel syndrome: part 2. Am J Gastroenterol 2004; 99(9):1823–1832.

119. Argenzio RA, Meuten DJ. Short-chain fatty acids induce reversible injury of porcine colon. Dig Dis Sci 1991; 36(10):1459–1468.

120. Schiller LR, Santa Ana CA, Morawski SG, Fordtran JS. Mechanism of the antidiarrheal effect of loperamide. Gastroenterology 1984; 86(6):1475–1480.

121. Rhoads M. Glutamine signaling in intestinal cells. J Parenter Enteral Nutr 1999; 23(5 Suppl):S38–S40.

122. Rhoads JM, Argenzio RA, Chen W, et al. Glutamine metabolism stimulates intestinal cell MAPKs by a cAMP-inhibitable, Raf-independent mechanism. Gastroenterology 2000; 118(1):90–100.

123. De-Souza DA, Greene LJ. Intestinal permeability and systemic infections in critically ill patients: effect of glutamine. Crit Care Med 2005; 33(5):1125–1135.

124. Ding LA, Li JS. Effects of glutamine on intestinal permeability and bacterial translocation in TPN-rats with endotoxemia. World J Gastroenterol 2003; 9(6):1327–1332.

125. Margaritis VG, Filos KS, Michalaki MA, et al. Effect of oral glutamine administration on bacterial tanslocation, endotoxemia, liver and ileal morphology, and apoptosis in rats with obstructive jaundice. World J Surg 2005; 29(10):1329–1334.

126. Kim JW, Jeon WK, Kim EJ. Combined effects of bovine colostrum and glutamine in diclofenac-induced bacterial translocation in rat. Clin Nutr 2005; 24(5):785–793.

127. Ziegler TR. Glutamine is essential for epidermal growth factor-stimulated intestinal cell proliferation. J Parenter Enteral Nutr 1994; 18(1):84–86.

128. Rhoads JM, Argenzio RA, Chen W, et al. L-glutamine stimulates intestinal cell proliferation and activates mitogen-activated protein kinases. Am J Physiol 1997; 272(5 Pt 1):G943–G953.

129. Zhou Y, Wu XT, Yang G, et al. Clinical evidence of growth hormone, glutamine and a modified diet for short bowel syndrome: meta-analysis of clinical trials. Asia Pac J Clin Nutr 2005; 14(1):98–102.

130. Ladd AP, Grosfeld JL, Pescovitz OH, Johnson NB. The effect of growth hormone supplementation on late nutritional independence in pediatric patients with short bowel syndrome. J Pediatr Surg 2005; 40(2):442–445.

131. Land MH, Rouster-Stevens K, Woods CR, et al. Lactobacillus sepsis associated with probiotic therapy. 115 ed. 2005; 178–181.

132. Ozturk A, Kaya M, Zeyrek D, et al. Ultrasonographic findings in ceftriaxone: associated biliary sludge and pseudolithiasis in children. Acta Radiol 2005; 46(1):112–116.

133. Litov RE, Combs GF Jr. Selenium in pediatric nutrition. Pediatrics 1991; 87(3):339–351.

134. Dellert SF, Farrell MK, Specker BL, Heubi JE. Bone mineral content in children with short bowel syndrome after discontinuation of parental nutrition. J Pediatr 1998; 132(3 Pt 1):516–519.

135. Goulet O, Ruemmele F, Lacaille F, Colomb V. Irreversible intestinal failure. J Pediatr Gastroenterol Nutr 2004; 38(3):250–269.

136. Vanderhoof JA, Grandjean CJ, Kaufman SS, et al. Effect of high percentage medium-chain triglyceride diet on mucosal adaptation following massive bowel resection in rats. J Parenter Enteral Nutr 1984; 8(6):685–689.

137. Rubin M, Moser A, Vaserberg N, et al. Structured triacylglycerol emulsion, containing both medium- and long-chain fatty acids, in long-term home parenteral nutrition: a double-blind randomized cross-over study. Nutrition 2000; 16(2):95–100.

138. Goulet O, Postaire M, De Potter S, et al. Medium-chain triglycerides and long-term parenteral nutrition in children. Nutrition 1992; 8(5):333–337.

139. Linseisen J, Wolfram G. Efficacy of different triglycerides in total parenteral nutrition for preventing atrophy of the gut in traumatized rats. J Parenter Enteral Nutr 1997; 21(1):21–26.

140. Devine RM, Kelly KA. Surgical therapy of the short bowel syndrome. Gastroenterol Clin North Am 1989; 18(3):603–618.

141. Kim HB, Fauza D, Garza J, et al. Serial transverse enteroplasty (STEP): a novel bowel lengthening procedure. J Pediatr Surg 2003; 38(3):425–429.

142. Tannuri U. Serial transverse enteroplasty (STEP): a novel bowel lengthening procedure, and serial transverse enteroplasty for short bowel syndrome. J Pediatr Surg 2003; 38(12):1845–1846.

143. Middleton SJ, Jamieson NV. The current status of small bowel transplantation in the UK and internationally. Gut 2005; 54(11):1650–1657.

144. Weisburger JH, Reddy BS, Barnes WS, Wynder EL. Bile acids, but not neutral sterols, are tumor promoters in the colon in man and in rodents. Environ Health Perspect 1983; 50:101–107.

145. Nagengast FM, Grubben MJ, van Munster IP. Role of bile acids in colorectal carcinogenesis. Eur J Cancer 1995 Jul;31A(7–8):1067–1070.

Chapter 17

Short Bowel Syndrome and Intestinal Tissue Engineering

Mike K. Chen, MD

Short Bowel Syndrome
Intestinal Tissue Engineering
The Future
Summary

Short bowel syndrome is defined as an inadequate amount of intestine to support normal growth and development. In neonates, this is a particularly devastating problem because of their need for nutrients to support maturation of vital organs and somatic growth. Causes of short bowel syndrome include volvulus, malrotation, gastroschisis, intestinal atresia, cystic fibrosis, and necrotizing enterocolotis. If a portion of the small bowel remains, there are surgical options, including procedures that aim to slow the transit time or lengthen the bowel. The results of these procedures are mixed at best. The only technique currently available for providing additional bowel is intestinal transplantation. This also has had limited success due to a shortage of donors, need for long-term immunosuppression, and potential graft versus host disease.

Intestinal tissue engineering offers an innovative way to replace the intestine without being limited by donor shortage and may obviate the need for immunosuppression if the intestine is regenerated from host tissue. Tissue engineering is a relatively novel investigative discipline that combines engineering principles and biology to produce tissues and organs. Predictably, trying to create new bowel is extremely challenging. The alimentary tract may appear to be a simple tubular structure that comprises the esophagus, stomach, small bowel, colon, and rectum, but it is quite a complex organ. Structural similarities unify this organ, but there are distinct cellular and functional differences that define the various parts of the gut. Functions that need to be duplicated in the engineered bowel include coordinated motility, digestion, and absorption. Additionally, the gut is one of the largest immune organs and an engineered bowel must act as a barrier against unwanted entry and have the capacity to generate an immunologic response if microbial invasions occur.

This review will focus on the current knowledge as well as challenges in intestinal tissue engineering. Focus will be placed on small bowel tissue engineering because it is the most vital aspect of nutrient absorption. Other portions of the gut are replaceable whereas the small bowel is not.

Fortunately, there is a tremendous reserve in gut function so that more than half of the small bowel may be resected without significant metabolic or nutritional sequelae (1). In 1967, Rickham defined short bowel syndrome as having 75 cm or less of small bowel (2). Dorney et al. reported that survival is dependent on an absolute minimum of 15 cm with an ileocecal valve and 25 cm without the valve (3). Nevertheless, most authors feel that the absolute length of small bowel required for survival is difficult to define. It is dependent on the length of small and large bowel present and the presence or absence of the ileocecal valve. In general, the ileum adapts better than the jejunum, and infants can adapt better than older children and adults; and therefore, can survive on a much shorter length.

Surgical options for managing these patients include lengthening the bowel, slowing the transit time, and intestinal transplantation. Bianchi devised a technique to split the dilated bowel and anastomose the segments to increase the length. In an uncontrolled report, he showed that a favorable outcome can be achieved if there is a minimum of 40 cm small bowel intact (4). Jaksic and his colleagues also created an ingenious way to serially staple segments of the dilated bowel that results in lengthening of the bowel (5). It may be advantageous in that it is easier to do. Compared to the Bianchi procedure, the STEP procedure does not disturb the small bowel mesentery and so it may be performed multiple times. Both options have had some success in increasing the volume of feeds that can be tolerated but these procedures require that there is a reasonable amount of bowel present that can be augmented. However, the outcome tends to be poor when there is coexisting hepatic dysfunction (6).

The current best solution for providing more intestine is via intestinal transplantation (7). Inherent problems include need for long-term immunosuppression, recurrent rejections, limited number of donors, and potential graft versus host disease. With the need to wait for a size-matched organ, up to 50% of infants and children die while waiting for intestinal transplantation. Recent increase in the use of combined liver and small bowel transplantation has enhanced the number of donors. Nevertheless, because intestinal transplantation is a limited resource with significant morbidities and a high mortality rate, some infants would not be candidates because of other systemic disorders. Graft survival remains at approximately 50% at 5 years.

INTESTINAL TISSUE ENGINEERING

Tissue engineering is a relatively novel field of study but it offers the hope of providing new tissue that is not limited by donor shortage; that may be free of immunologic issues; and that can be synthesized when needed. Current focus in intestinal tissue engineering is on the small bowel since it is the most critical piece of the alimentary tract.

Conceptually, it is important to note that one does not need to create the entire length of normal small bowel to treat patients with short bowel syndrome. As noted earlier, most people are born with more bowel than needed, and infants with short bowel syndrome generally have some residual functional small bowel. The addition of a small amount of absorptive surface may be sufficient to allow them to thrive and grow without being dependent on parenteral nutrition.

The first experiments designed to create more bowel surface were achieved by patching bowel defects using the serosal surface of another piece of intestine. The researchers noted that neomucosa would grow to cover this bare luminal surface (8, 9). This led others to evaluate the use of prosthetic materials as a patch for repairing a defect created in the small bowel. Because the materials

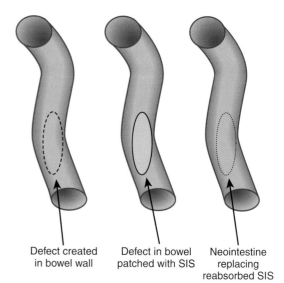

Figure 17-1 Small defects were created on the wall of the bowel and patched with SIS. By 6–8 weeks, the SIS had been resorbed and replaced by neointestine that histologically and functionally resembled native small bowel.

Defect created in bowel wall

Defect in bowel patched with SIS

Neointestine replacing reabsorbed SIS

used were initially nonresorbable, the results were variable. Cogan and his colleagues selected Dacron to patch defects created in the ileum of rabbits (10). The Dacron patch remained intact long enough to allow ingrowth of new intestinal tissue, after which it was extruded. When others tried using a complete tube of polytetrafluoroethylene (PTFE) as an intervening segment in the small bowel, they showed little ingrowth of mucosa (11). The first report on the use of an absorbable patch was by Thompson et al. in 1986 (12). He and his colleagues compared the feasibility of Dacron, PTFE, and polyglycolic acid (PGA) mesh as scaffolds for regenerating neointestine. Neomucosa formation was observed by 2 weeks and by 4 weeks Dacron and PTFE grafts were extruded, whereas PGA meshes were resorbed. The neomucosa was functional as demonstrated by glucose uptake and disaccharidase activity. When a complete Dacron tube was interposed between divided small bowel, no neomucosal growth was observed.

We have also demonstrated that a resorbable biomaterial can be used to patch defects in the small bowel (Fig. 17-1) (13). We used small intestinal submucosa (SIS) because of its demonstrated efficacy in other studies. SIS is an acellular matrix derived from porcine small intestine and it has been used extensively in tissue engineering experiments as well as in clinical care of patients. Matsumoto et al. initially described its utility as a biomaterial in 1966 by inverting the processed small bowel and used it to replace large veins in dogs (14). It has been converted into a commercial product known as Surgisis and is commercially available in variable thickness and sizes.

In our study, the SIS was resorbed and the regenerated neointestine was quite similar to normal small bowel. The SIS lasted long enough for the bowel to grow onto the scaffold. The neointestine was shown to have a mucosa, varying amount of smooth muscle, sheets of collagen, and an outer serosal layer. Placing a tubular configuration of SIS between divided small bowel was unsuccessful. There is no real integrity to the SIS used in our study, and when placed as a tube it either leaked or collapsed on itself and caused obstruction. One of the challenges in fabricating biomaterials for tissue engineering neointestine is to produce a scaffold that can maintain its shape and structure long enough for tissue regeneration to occur prior to breakdown of the material. If the biomaterial is resorbed or degraded prior to completion of the tissue ingrowth, the result is leakage of intraluminal contents, which will lead to sepsis and death. On the other hand, the material cannot be so rigid that it does not allow easy anastomosis and must be malleable so that it can be placed in the peritoneal cavity.

Wang and colleagues fashioned 2-cm-long SIS tubes from Sprague-Dawley rat donors and interposed them in the middle of a 6-cm Thiery-Vella loop in Lewis rats (15). The Thiery-Vella loop is a defunctionalized segment of ileum with both ends brought out to the skin as stomas. This loop took the SIS graft out of continuity with the rest of the intestine to minimize the problems associated with leakage. They placed a silicone stent in the construct to maintain the shape and to keep the SIS from collapsing on itself during the regenerative process. The stent was removed at 3 weeks and the loop was washed with saline. Neomucosa formation was observed at 4 weeks and the SIS graft was completely replaced by regenerated bowel by 12 weeks. Smooth muscle-like cells covered the outer wall and the neo-mucosa morphology appeared similar to native bowel, with the presence of goblet cells, Paneth cells, enterocytes, and enteroendocrine cells. This interesting model protected the SIS graft and allowed the regeneration of a tubular segment of bowel.

Another strategy for producing new tissue is to use donor tissue in combination with a scaffold system as a construct. Vacanti and his colleagues initially reported on the generation of neointestine from minced pieces of fetal intestine in 1988 (16). They modified that initial observation into a model for generating neointestine by using a polymer-organoid construct and implanting this into the omentum of an adult syngeneic rat (17). The small intestine is harvested from neonatal Lewis rats and processed to obtain the intestinal organoids. Tait and his colleagues had observed that these organoids can survive in culture and regenerate (18). The organoids are presumed to contain all the elements present in small bowel, including stem cells, immunocytes, and mesenchyme. The organoids are seeded onto a tubular biomaterial produced from polyglycolic and polylactic acid and the constructs are implanted onto the omentum of an adult Lewis rat. This construct results in the formation of neointestinal cysts attached to a vascular pedicle. The cysts are filled with mucoid material and the histology mirrors that of normal small bowel.

Vacanti and his colleagues have used this model extensively and characterized the cysts to demonstrate their similarity to normal small bowel. They have shown the presence of brush-border enzymes, basement membrane components, electro-physiologic properties, immune ontogeny and lymphangiogenesis (19–21). They also have moved toward therapy with this model by anastomosing the cyst to the native small bowel after massive small bowel resection (22). The rats that were rescued by the neointestinal cysts had increased weight gain and this provides hope that this model may be useful for infants with short bowel syndrome.

In addition to its essential function in food processing and absorption, the small bowel is a vital immune organ. The gastrointestinal (GI) tract contains the largest surface area and is exposed to more than 400 bacterial species and a total of 10^{14} microbial cells (23). The small intestine is exposed to approximately $10^3–10^9$ bacteria per gram of intraluminal content, whereas the colonic mucosa is home to $10^{11}–10^{12}$ bacteria per gram of feces (24). The intestinal surface must provide a barrier against unwanted entry of toxins and organisms. It must efficiently recognize and differentiate between benign commensal bacteria and pathogens. If invasion by pathogens occurs, the gut acts as an immune organ to minimize the incursion and protect the host.

Because the regenerated bowel must be a functional immune organ, Vacanti and colleagues also demonstrated that their model produces neointestinal cysts with an intact mucosal immune system. They showed the presence of an immunocyte population similar to that of native small intestine (20). They anastomosed the neointestinal cyst to the native bowel and revealed that exposure of the mucosa to the luminal content was vital to the regeneration of the immune system. Control neointestinal cysts left unanastomosed had no exposure to luminal contents and only had rudimentary regeneration of the immunocyte population.

Our laboratory has also been successful in producing neointestinal cysts using the intestinal organoid-polymer model. We chose to focus on the practical use of commercially available biomaterials as scaffold for regenerating neointestine. Commercially produced SIS (Surgisis^{R}) and fibrin glue (Tisseel^{R}) were selected because they represent two distinct types of biomaterials and are readily available for clinical use. SIS, as described before, is an extracellular matrix derived from porcine intestine and fibrin glue is most commonly used for controlling hemorrhage. Fibrin glue has been used as a cell delivery vehicle for urothelial and epithelial cells (25). Cartilage structures have been constructed from chondrocytes mixed with fibrin glue (26).

Fibrin glue is composed of natural biological factors including fibrinogen, thrombin, calcium chloride, and fibrinolysis inhibitor (aprotinin). Fibrin glue may represent an ideal biomaterial because it is an easy cell-delivery vehicle; its inherent adhesive property ensures that the seeded cells adhere to the desired surface; the components are easily resorbed and nontoxic; internal matrices formed after the glue sets into an elastic coagulum allow influx of nutrients and also provide scaffolding for the cells to reside upon; the glue and cell construct can be molded to the desired form; undefined inherent growth factors may be present in the fibrin glue mixture; and adding cytokines or growth factors to the construct to enhance tissue regeneration would be easy to accomplish.

Both rats and mice were used in our studies. Small bowel was harvested from neonatal animals and processed to produce intestinal organoids. Approximately 30 000–50 000 organoids were seeded onto each construct. The organoids were placed on SIS, SIS and fibrin glue, or fibrin glue alone. In Vacanti et al.'s studies, they used a tubular construct of polyglycolic acid but our constructs were not shaped into a tube or sphere. Our constructs were left as a folded SIS or a ball of fibrin glue and implanted onto the omentum of an adult syngeneic rat or mouse.

Neointestinal cysts were identified at 6 weeks and the mucosal growth and development were best seen at 10 weeks. Fibrin glue and fibrin glue with SIS produced cysts that had the best histology. Despite not creating a tube or a sphere when forming the constructs, the regenerated cysts had organized architecture similar to normal intestine. Angiogenesis occurred because the cyst was attached to a pedicle that was connected to the omentum (Fig. 17-2). The cysts varied between 2 and 3 cm in diameter and some cysts were as large as 4 cm. The cellular elements within the organoids have the capacity to regulate the regenerative process so that the each layer of the bowel wall is in the proper place. The epithelial cells lined the inner layer forming a mucosa with crypts and villi; mucous was

Figure 17-2 Constructs made by adding intestinal organoids to the biomaterial (SIS or fibrin glue) resulted in pedicled neointestinal cysts measuring up to 3–4 cm.

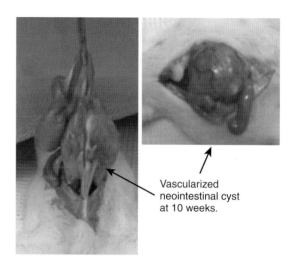

Vascularized neointestinal cyst at 10 weeks.

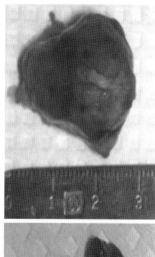

Cyst with serosal covering

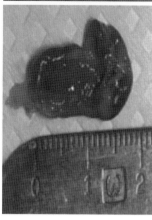

Mucosal lining in the cyst

Figure 17-3 Neointestinal cysts grossly resembled native intestine with a serosal covering and a mucosal lining. Mucoid material was found in the distended cysts. Histologic studies revealed architecture that mirrored normal bowel.

present in the center of the cyst; the submucosa was intact; smooth muscle was present; and there was an appropriate serosal layer (Fig. 17-3).

The ability of these cysts to regenerate from intestinal organoids is a recapitulation of the intestine's ability to repair and regenerate. Numerous enterocyte mitogens have been investigated and they may be used to enhance the growth of new tissue. Indeed, Ramsanahie et al. observed the effects of glucagon-like peptide-2 (GLP-2) on regenerating neointestinal cysts (27). GLP-2 is an endogenous regulatory peptide with a specific potent trophic effect on intestinal mucosal growth and increases the expression of Na^{+}-glucose cotransporter 1 (SGLT1). They found that the administration of GLP-2 enhanced the mucosal growth and increased the expression of SGLT1, suggesting that growth factors may be used to stimulate the regeneration of neointestine. Additionally, the study shows that tissue-engineered tissues are responsive to regulatory factors and can be used as a model to study the effects of exogenously applied components.

THE FUTURE

Although no human studies have been done, one can speculate that current strategies for creating neointestine may be incorporated into the management of patients with short bowel syndrome. One hypothesis would be to harvest small bowel from an infant and process that into intestinal organoids. The organoids can be grown and expanded in culture and then seeded onto a biomaterial such as fibrin glue. The organoid-fibrin glue construct can be implanted back in the child's omentum and allowed to regenerate into a neointestinal cyst. The cyst is then harvested and anastomosed to the native bowel. If the infant has an insufficient amount of bowel, another source may be donor small bowel obtained from a living donor who has a similar genetic makeup. The amount of bowel harvested would be of no consequence to the donor. In this case, immunosuppression may still be required but the therapy would not be limited by donor shortage.

Another potential therapeutic approach would be to anastomose a tubular biomaterial to the native intestine and allow ingrowth to occur. To use the biomaterials currently available, this segment of bowel would have to be taken out of continuity from the native bowel (Thiery-Vella loop). This would allow the neointestine to regenerate on the scaffold without being concerned about the biomaterial breaking down prior to completion of the ingrowth.

Finally, another hypothetical maneuver would be to patch the native bowel with a sheet of biomaterial to expand the luminal surface. After this has occurred, the bowel can be manipulated via a STEP procedure to lengthen the bowel.

SUMMARY

Tissue engineering is a relatively novel field but early investigations are promising. Creating neointestine for infants with short bowel syndrome may be a real therapeutic option in the near future as we continue to enhance our understanding of biomaterials and intestinal growth and renewal.

REFERENCES

1. Jeejeebhoy KN. Therapy of the short-gut syndrome. Lancet 1983; 1:1427.
2. Rickham PP. Massive intestinal resection in newborn infants. Ann R Coll Surg 1967; 41:480.
3. Dorney SA, Ament M, Berquist W, et al. Improved survival in very short small bowel of infancy with use of long term parenteral nutrition. J Pediatr 1985; 107:521.
4. Bianchi A. Experience with longitudinal intestinal lengthening and tailoring. Eur J Pediatr Surg 1999; 9:256.
5. Javid PJ, Kim HB, Duggan CP, et al. Serial transverse enteroplasty is associated with successful short-term outcomes in infants with short bowel syndrome. J Pediatr Surg 2005; 0019:4.
6. Sudan D, Dibaise J, Torres C, et al. A multidisciplinary approach to the treatment of intestinal failure. J Gastrointest Surg 2005; 9:165.
7. Grant D, Abu-Elmagd K, Reyes J, et al. 2003 Report of the Intestine Transplant Registry. Ann Surg 2005; 241:607.
8. Kobold EE, Thal AP. A simple method for management of experimental wounds of the duodenum. Surg Gynecol Obstet 1963; 116:340.
9. Binnington HB, Siegel BA, Kissane JM, et al. A technique to increase jejunal mucosa surface area. J Pediatr Surg 1973; 8:765.
10. Harmon JW, Wright JA, Noel J, et al. Fate of Dacron prostheses in the small bowel of rabbits. Surg Forum 1979; 30:365.
11. Watson LC, Friedman HI, Griffin DG, et al. Small bowel neomucosa. J Pediatr Surg 1980; 28:280.
12. Thompson JS, Kampfe PW, Newland JR, et al. Growth of intestinal neomucosa on prosthetic materials. J Surg Res 1986; 41:484.
13. Chen MK, Badylak SF. Small bowel tissue engineering using small intestinal submucosa as a scaffold. J Surg Res 2001; 99:352.
14. Matsumoto T, Holmes RH, Burdick CO, et al. The fate of inverted segment of small bowel used for the replacement of major veins. Surgery 1966; 60:739.
15. Wang ZQ, Yusuhiro W, Noda T, et al. Morphologic evaluation of regenerated small bowel by small intestinal submucosa. J Pediatr Surg 2005; 40:1898.
16. Vacanti JP, Morse MA, Saltzman WM, et al. Selective cell transplantation using bioabsorbable artificial polymers as matrices. J Pediatr Surg 1988; 23:3.
17. Choi R, Vacanti JP. Preliminary studies of tissue-engineered intestine using isolated epithelial organoid units on tubular synthetic biodegradable scaffolds. Transplant Proc 1997; 29:848.
18. Tait IS, Flint N, Campbell FC, et al. Generation of neomucosa in vivo by transplantation of dissociated postnatal small intestinal epithelium. Differentiation 1994; 56:91.
19. Choi RS, Riegler M, Pothoulakis C, et al. Studies of brush border enzymes, basement membrane components, and electrophysiology of tissue-engineered neointestine. J Pediatr Surg 1998; 33:991.
20. Perez A, Grikscheit TC, Blumberg RS, et al. Tissue-engineered small intestine: ontogeny of the immune system. Transplantation 2002; 74:619.
21. Duxbury MS, Grikscheit TC, Gardner-Thorpe J, et al. Lymphangiogenesis in tissue-engineered small intestine. Transplantation 2004; 77:1162.
22. Grikscheit TC, Siddique A, Ochoa ER, et al. Tissue-engineered small intestine improves recovery after massive small bowel resection. Ann Surg 8200; 240:744.

23. Smith G, Gorbach S. Normal alimentary tract flora. In: Blaser M, Smith J, Ravidin J, eds., Infections of the gastrointestinal tract. New York: Raven; 1995: 53–69.
24. Hao WL, Lee YK. Microflora of the gastrointestinal tract: a review. Methods Mol Biol 2004; 268:491.
25. Bach AD, Bannasch H, Galla TJ, et al. Fibrin glue as matrix for cultured autologous urothelial cells in urethal reconstruction. Tissue Eng 2001; 7:45.
26. Westreich R, Kaufman M, Gannon P, et al. Validating the subcutaneous model of injectable autologous cartilage using a fibrin glue scaffold. Laryngoscope 2004; 114:2154.
27. Ramsanahie A, Duxbury MS, Grikscheit TC, et al. Effect of GLP-2 on mucosal morphology and SGLT1 expression in tissue-engineered neointestine. Am J Physiol Gastrointest Liver Physiol 2003; 235:G1345.

Chapter 18

Adult Consequences of Neonatal and Fetal Nutrition: Mechanisms

Kjersti Aagaard-Tillery, MD, PhD • Nicole Mitchell, MD
• Clotilde desRoberts, MD • Robert H. Lane, MD

EARLY NUTRITION AND ADULT PHENOTYPE

An infant's early nutrition affects the adult phenotype (Table 18-1). As old and intuitive as this concept may be, it has re-entered the consciousness of the research community only in the last 20 years. As a result, the overall interest in the specific experiences and mechanisms through which different perinatal environments lead to adult onset diseases has exploded. This interest is an important research priority because it is an avenue for preventing adult diseases such as diabetes, obesity, and hypertension before they exact a direct toll.

The continuum of early nutrition experienced by humans varies greatly within a single population, let alone between different populations. As a result, the majority of epidemiological studies interested in understanding the adult consequences of fetal and neonatal nutrition have used poor growth, particularly in utero, as a marker of poor nutrition. Therefore, an important assumption of this chapter is that poor nutrition leads to poor growth, in both the fetus and the young child. One of the limits of epidemiological studies on this subject is the focus upon infants who are small for gestational age (SGA), which is typically defined as weight less than the 10th percentile. Infants included in this group may be small for multiple reasons, including normal genetic variation. Furthermore, these studies that focus only upon the SGA infants unavoidably miss infants who are smaller than they should be, but are still above the 10th percentile. Investigations do exist where authors attempt to study intrauterine-growth-retarded infants, and therefore often incorporate measures such as the ponderal index to determine whether an individual's growth is "normal."

Despite these limitations, the epidemiology in this field has been vitally important and often elegant, which is certainly true of the three cohorts (and their respective studies) that have set the standard for understanding the adult consequences of neonatal and fetal nutrition. These cohorts involve the (1) Dutch famine

Table 18-1	Adult Phenotypes Associated with Growth Retardation

Attention deficit disorder
Chronic lung disease
Divorce
Dyslipidemia
Hypertension
Immunodeficiency
Insulin resistance
Neurodevelopmental delay
Neuroendocrine reprogramming
Poor postnatal growth
Renal insufficiency
Schizophrenia

of 1944–1945; (2) the early studies by Barker et al., hence the "Barker Hypothesis"; and (3) the more recent Nurses' Health Study.

The first of these cohorts is the Dutch famine of 1944–1945. This famine occurred as a result of German reprisal for a general railway strike intended to disrupt the transport of German reinforcements toward Allied liberation movements (1, 2). The famine lasted approximately 5 months. Daily rations in Amsterdam dropped from 1800 kcal/day in December of 1943 to 400–800 kcal/day in April of 1945. Although a goal was set for children under the age of 1 and pregnant or lactating women to receive supplemental rations, this was not possible at the height of the famine. After liberation in May of 1945, caloric intake increased to over 2000 kcal/day.

The effects of the famine upon the Dutch population have been examined via multiple sources, including population-based cohorts, military induction records, psychiatric registries, and self reports. One of the more comprehensive studies is the Dutch famine birth cohort study, through which the investigators interviewed 912 individuals who were born at term between November 1st 1943 and February 28th 1947, and assessed socio-economic factors, lifestyle, and medical history (3). Babies exposed to famine conditions early in gestation were not smaller or lighter than non-exposed infants; however, they suffered from an increased incidence of coronary heart disease, hypertension, dyslipidemia, and obesity. Although not quite statistically significant, the adults with coronary heart disease were also more likely to have lower birth weights and smaller head circumferences. Similarly, a cohort born in the Wilhelmina Gasthuis of Amsterdam between November 1943 and February 1947 revealed an association between maternal famine early in pregnancy and an atherogenic lipid profile (higher LDL-HDL cholesterol ratios) (2). Famine early in gestation also altered perceptions of the affected individuals, in that the proportion of people reporting poor self-perceived health was significantly higher in the group of early gestation famine exposure compared to those who had not experienced the in utero famine conditions (4).

Furthermore, babies exposed to the famine in mid-gestation suffered from an increased incidence of obstructive airway disease, as well as an increased incidence of microalbuminuria (5, 6). Interestingly, both of these findings are independent of size at birth. Babies exposed to the famine in late gestation are also more likely to exhibit impaired glucose tolerance, as evidenced by higher 2-h glucose and insulin levels compared to those who had not experienced the in utero famine conditions (7). Furthermore, affective disorders occur more often in those individuals exposed to famine conditions in utero in mid to late gestation (8). Other findings from the Dutch famine cohort that are intriguing, and somewhat frightening, include the associations between experiencing the famine in utero and increased rates of schizophrenia, schizophrenia spectrum disorders, as well as antisocial personality disorder (9).

For all three groups of infants (early, mid, or late gestation exposure) exposed to the Dutch famine, mortality at age 50 was increased. Group-specific mortality for early, mid, or late gestation exposure is 11.5%, 11.2%, and 15.2%, respectively. In contrast, mortality at age 50 for those born after the famine is 7.2%(10).

The second set of studies is the work of Dr. DJ Barker, who, along with his research group, has been a pioneer in the epidemiology of the adult consequences of neonatal and fetal nutrition. As early as 1986, Barker and Osmond noted in the *Lancet* a geographical association between ischemic heart disease in 1968–1978 and infant mortality in 1921–1925 (11). These authors astutely speculated at this time that "poor nutrition in early life increases susceptibility to the affects of an affluent diet."

The observation linking infant mortality and adult disease was continued by the Hertfordshire studies, which for many are still the standard in this area. An initial focus of these studies was a cohort of 5654 men born between 1911 and 1930 in Hertfordshire, England (12). The 1989 manuscript revealed that men with the lowest weights at birth and 1 year of age had the highest death rates from cardiovascular disease. A subset of these men was further used to evaluate the relationship between insulin sensitivity and birth weight. Specifically, 468 men born, raised, and living in east Hertfordshire were studied after ingesting a 75 g glucose drink (13). Men with impaired glucose sensitivity and non-insulin-dependent diabetes were characterized by a lower weight at birth and 1 year of age. Furthermore, the percentage of men with impaired insulin sensitivity decreased as weight increased at 1 year of age; this progression was statistically significant and independent of the adult body mass. This concept, that reduced growth in early life leads to impaired glucose tolerance, has impacted the way multiple clinicians and investigators now approach perinatal metabolism and nutrition.

These investigators and the people of Hertfordshire continue to contribute significantly to our understanding of the relationship between early nutrition and growth and adult diseases. By 2005, the cohort included 37 615 men and women born in Hertfordshire (14). Low birth weight in men from this population increases the risk of cardiovascular disease, whereas low birth weight in women predisposes the affected adults toward cardiovascular and musculoskeletal disease, as well as pneumonia and diabetes. Although there are gender differences, the data suggest that an increase in birth weight by one standard deviation would reduce mortality for both sexes at age 75 by 0.86%.

The third historically significant cohort is the Nurses' Health Study cohort (15, 16). This study was established in 1976 when approximately 122 000 married female registered nurses, ages 30–55, responded to a mailed questionnaire about their life histories. The study has continued through follow-up questionnaires every 2 years eliciting updated histories and medical information. The validity of the self-reported birthweights was assessed via the Nurses' Health Study II, which compared birth certificate weights to the reported weights (17). The Spearman correlation coefficient between the two weights was 0.74. This study added weight to the observations of Barker et al. by noting a significantly increased relative risk for non-insulin-dependent diabetes in women who were low birth weight (< 5.5 lb) when compared to those women of median birth weight (7.1–8.5 lb) (16). The relative risk for women whose weight was <5.5 lb and = 5.5 lb was 1.88 (1.59–2.21) and 1.55 (1.32–1.83) respectively. Adjusting for age, body mass index, and maternal history of diabetes strengthened the association between low birth weight and non-insulin-dependent diabetes. No significant effects on relative risk were noted after adjustment for prematurity, multiple births, maternal age at birth, participant breast-feeding, ethnicity, parental occupation at age 16, paternal diabetes, participant height, parity, cigarette smoking, and physical activity.

The Nurses' Health Study has also been used to investigate the relationship between birth weight and cardiovascular disease in women (18). Non-fatal myocardial infarctions were included as an end point of the study if they met the criteria of the World Health Organization. Non-fatal strokes were included as another end point if they met the criteria of the national survey of stroke. For every 454 g increase in birth weight, a 5% decrease in the risk of non-fatal myocardial infarction was noted, as was an 11% decrease in the risk of non-fatal stroke. As with the above study focusing upon insulin resistance, these findings were largely independent of other key factors such as adult body weight, hypertension, diabetes, lifestyle, and childhood socioeconomic class.

The investigations involving these three cohorts have provided important and seminal insight into the relationship between early growth and nutrition and adult diseases. They have provided an impetus to further studies that identify possible physiological and molecular mechanisms, which may lead to either in utero interventions or postnatal therapies to moderate the impending risks. The following section will focus upon recently identified important biological targets.

DEVELOPMENTAL BIOLOGY OF THE ADULT CONSEQUENCES OF NEONATAL AND FETAL NUTRITION

This section will be divided into two parts. The first part will discuss recent insights into how fetal growth retardation affects phenotype in humans, with animal studies used to focus on possible mechanisms. The discussion is not meant to be all-inclusive, but focuses upon some of the most recent and provocative observations. The second part will discuss recent insights into how growth retardation in the premature infant potentially affects later morbidities, and how dietary interventions may either contribute to or moderate these effects.

Fetus/IUGR

Multiple studies from different regions of the world containing racially distinct cohorts have associated fetal growth retardation with the adult morbidities previously discussed. One of the more recent trends is the realization that the lasting effects of fetal growth retardation are evident in both early life and adulthood. Furthermore, weight gain, and therefore presumably nutrition, modifies the effect of intrauterine growth retardation upon these early results. These findings pertain to issues involving glucose homeostasis, lipid biology, and hypertension; however, an important central theme to this literature, as well as the literature focusing upon adult phenotype, is that cohorts differ, whether it is due to the etiology of fetal growth retardation or the postnatal consequences. As a result, findings between these studies differ slightly, which allows for the wonderful conundrum that multiple mechanisms are likely to be involved.

For example, Mericq et al. followed small for gestational age (SGA) and appropriate for gestational age infants (AGA) through the first 3 years of life (19). Their group measured infants' weights and lengths at 1, 2, and 3 years. At 48 h of life, glucose and insulin levels were measured in these infants, and at 1 and 3 years of life an I.V. glucose tolerance test was assessed after an overnight fast. A calculation of insulin resistance was determined using the homeostasis model. At 48 h of life, SGA infants had decreased insulin levels when compared to AGA infants. At 1 and

3 years of age, SGA infants exhibited increased fasting insulin levels and decreased insulin sensitivity when compared to AGA children.

Similarly, Veening et al. studied 29 SGA and 24 AGA children at approximately 9 years of age with oral glucose tolerance tests (β-cell function) and hyperinsulinemic euglycemic clamp studies (insulin sensitivity) (20). Although in utero growth did not appear to affect glucose tolerance and β-cell function in the two groups, the hyperinsulinemic euglycemic clamp studies revealed decreased insulin sensitivity in the SGA children who experienced catch-up growth and had a body mass index >17 kg/m². The authors concluded that the reduced insulin sensitivity in adulthood may contribute to the enhanced risk of non-insulin-dependent diabetes in adulthood. Arends et al. also found insulin sensitivity to be decreased in short prepubertal SGA children, while, in contrast, the mean acute insulin response was significantly increased in the SGA subjects (21). These findings held true after adjustment for age and body mass index.

Growth retardation also appears to affect cellular energy homeostasis. Chessex et al. compared six SGA infants and thirteen appropriately newborn infants, in terms of energy expenditure (22). Expenditures in the SGA infants increased by 4.8 kcal/kg/day through increased fat oxidation. In contrast, when infant oral glucose disposal was studied in pre-pubertal and early pubertal children (ages 8–14) with a history of IUGR and compared to that of healthy age- and weight-matched control children, lower glucose oxidation characterized the IUGR subjects, though no decrease in overall energy expenditure was noted. Interestingly, lipid oxidation was increased nearly 2-fold, although not significantly based upon variation (23).

The Arends et al. study also noted other differences between SGA and the weight-appropriate counterparts, similar to the large epidemiological studies discussed above. First, systolic blood pressure was significantly increased in the SGA children. Second, although fasting serum free fatty acids, triglycerides, total cholesterol, HDL, and LDL levels were not significantly different between groups, 6 of the 28 children in the SGA group had serum free fatty acids above the normal range. In terms of lipid biology, much of the focus has been on leptin and adiponectin. For example, in a population of 1-year-old SGA infants from Santiago, Chile, SGA infants were characterized by decreased leptin levels (0.29 ± 0.19 nM vs. 0.40 vs. 0.07 nM; $P < 0.05$), as well as a trend towards increased triglycerides ($P = 0.053$) (24).

The next sections will delve into specific mechanisms through which intrauterine growth retardation induces many of these phenotypic changes involving glucose metabolism, lipid homeostasis, and other cardiovascular risk factors. The list is neither exhaustive nor exclusive, and, in fact, evidence continues to accumulate that IUGR adult phenotype is a result of many moderate adjustments that are complementary and probably interdependent (Table 18-2). One theme that becomes evident when looking at the whole body of IUGR physiological studies is that many of the adjustments that are implemented early provide short-term advantages in terms of survival, but also lead to the adult morbidities of diabetes, dyslipidemia, and cardiovascular disease with the passage of time.

Table 18-2   Hormones Linked to the Fetal Origins of Adult Disease

Adiponectin
Androgens
Angiotensin
Leptin
Glucocorticoids
Insulin and its binding proteins

Metabolism

Leptin

Leptin is a 167–amino-acid protein that is produced by adipocytes, which performs multiple functions. Among the most important functions of leptin is the regulation of hypothalamic centers that determine, at least in part, whole-body energy expenditure and fat mass (25). In general, leptin increases energy expenditure and reduces food intake. As a result, humans and rodents lacking either leptin or the leptin receptor develop severe obesity and hyperphagia. In practice, increased serum levels of leptin characterize most obese conditions, and in fact leptin levels typically correlate directly with body fat mass and BMI. The failure of the increased levels of leptin to regulate weight loss suggests a potential state of leptin resistance in many cases of obesity.

In pregnancy, maternal serum leptin levels peak in the second trimester and subsequently plateau (26). At term, maternal leptin levels are approximately 3-times those of a non-pregnant woman. Umbilical cord leptin levels progressively rise starting at 34 weeks gestation and, as expected, umbilical cord leptin levels and ponderal index correlate nicely (27, 28). Placenta does produce leptin, and placental weight also correlates with umbilical cord leptin levels (29, 30). The placental releases 98% of its leptin into the maternal circulation, and 2% in the fetal circulation. Postnatal serum leptin levels in the infant increase after birth. Studies in the rat suggest that this surge moderates the continuing development of hypothalamic regions associated with energy homeostasis (31). The implication of course is that the postnatal surge in leptin functions as an important developmental signal to the hypothalamus and subsequently influences food intake and body weight throughout life.

Within the context of intrauterine growth retardation, maternal serum leptin levels are generally noted to be increased, whereas fetal IUGR serum leptin levels are generally noted to be decreased. For example, Pighetti et al. measured maternal and fetal serum leptin levels in 43 "normal" term pregnancies and 27 pregnancies complicated by asymmetrical IUGR (32). Women from both groups had normal pregravid BMIs (20–27 kg/m^2), and pregnancies complicated by diabetes or hypertension were excluded. In utero, ultrasound identified fetal growth restriction by an abdominal circumference below the tenth percentile, which was confirmed at birth if the birth weight was similarly below the tenth percentile. Finally, a similar proportion of male and female infants appeared in each group. IUGR correlated with increased serum leptin levels in the mothers ($\approx$45 ng/mL vs. 29 ng/mL; $P < 0.01$) and decreased umbilical cord serum levels in the infants ($\approx$8.4 ng/mL vs. 13.1 ng/mL; $P < 0.01$). No significant differences were noted between male and female infants of either group. As expected, umbilical cord serum leptin levels correlated with neonatal birth weight.

Moreover, when Iñiguez et al. measured leptin levels in SGA and appropriately sized infants at 1 and years of age, leptin levels directly correlated with weight and weight gain at both ages and in both genders (33). This correlation is intriguing because of reports associating an increased risk of adult morbidities, such as insulin resistance, in growth-retarded infants who experience the most rapid catch-up growth. Interestingly, leptin levels were also positively associated with fasting insulin levels in both study groups, although the association was stronger in the appropriate-sized controls.

Of course, as with anything in this field, discrepancies exist. Increased umbilical cord serum leptin levels have been noted in at least one study, and another study found no significant differences in leptin levels between the two groups after adjusting for fetal weight (leptin/kg). One cause of the discrepancies may be due to a purported relationship between fetal oxygenation and acid-base status and fetal leptin levels: higher serum leptin levels characterize fetuses suffering from severe distress. Furthermore, a recent study from Mexico noted that, whereas serum leptin levels were decreased in 50 SGA infants relative to 50 appropriately sized infants, logistic regression analysis noted that leptin levels in these infants were not independent of percentage of body fat (34). Gestational age also affects the correlation between fetal growth and umbilical cord serum leptin levels. Before 34 weeks gestation, little relationship exists between umbilical cord serum leptin levels and birth weight.

These discrepancies remind us that leptin is likely to be just one strand of the web, and that the importance of leptin cannot be appreciated without either testing the strength of the strand or identifying other interacting strands. One tool through which to perform these tests is the use of animal models of growth retardation.

A classic and common model of intrauterine growth retardation is undernutrition or malnutrition of the pregnant rat. Multiple variations on the theme exist with this model system, including maternal caloric, caloric-protein, or protein deprivation, respectively. Moreover, moderate controversy exists on whether protein-calorie deprivation is more relevant than protein deprivation with an isocaloric diet, since the latter adds the variable of an increased proportion of either carbohydrate or fat. Considering the wide continuum of human living conditions, all of the variations of this model are relevant and translational, but the differences between the models are important to note when evaluating and applying the data.

In general, maternal under-nutrition or malnutrition results in growth restriction and rapid catch-up growth, such that by early adulthood the body weight of the intrauterine-growth-restricted progeny exceeds that of the control animals. In most studies, these animals develop components of the morbidities afflicting growth-retarded humans, including insulin resistance, dyslipidemia, and hypertension. In a wonderfully methodical study, Fernandez-Twinn et al. reduced maternal protein intake to 50% of controls and measured the circulating levels of several hormones, including leptin, through the pregnancies (35). The low-protein diet significantly reduced both placental and fetal body weights, and at term the low-protein diet also significantly decreased the placental:body weight ratios. In adulthood, the pups that suffer intrauterine low-protein under-nutrition are known to develop diabetes, hyperinsulinemia, and tissue insulin resistance in adulthood. The low-protein diet increased maternal serum leptin levels at day 17 of gestation (term $\approx$21 days) and decreased maternal serum leptin levels at term. No significant differences in perinatal serum leptin levels were noted in the pups suffering the low-protein maternal diet versus the control pups.

To begin the process of defining leptin homeostasis in the postnatal growth-retarded rat, Krechowc et al. used a similar model of maternal food restriction in which dams received 30% of ad libitum food intake versus the controls (36). The growth-retarded pups were cross-fostered, and post-weaning (around 21 days of postnatal life) were fed either ad libitum "normal" rat chow, ad libitum high-fat diet, or 70% of the ad libitum "normal" rat chow diet. The protein/energy ratio, vitamin, and mineral content were identical between the "normal" rat chow and the high-fat chow. At approximately 142 days of age, female rats from each group were injected with either r-rat leptin (2.5 µg/g/day) or saline for 14 days. Leptin sensitivity was measured as the response to body weight and food intake.

As expected, pups in this study from the food-restricted group were significantly growth-restricted. Furthermore, the high-fat diet increased weight gain in both the appropriate-sized rats and the growth-restricted rats, whereas calorie restriction reduced weight gain. Interestingly, although the growth-restricted rats on the high-fat diet caught up in body weight to the appropriately sized rats, they did not catch up in terms of body length. In the growth-restricted progeny fed the "normal" diet, as well as both groups of animal fed the high-fat diet, leptin treatment failed to reduce food intake and only moderately affected weight loss. Furthermore, the leptin resistance in the growth-restricted "normal" diet group occurred in the context of insulin resistance and hypertriglyceridemia.

These findings suggest that prenatal malnutrition may lead to the development of leptin resistance, particularly in adult female rats. Mechanisms responsible for this phenomenon may include cross-talk between the insulin and leptin receptors, as well as hepatic insulin resistance leading to hypertriglyceridemia and subsequent impairment of leptin transport across the blood-brain barrier. Regardless, studies such as these suggest that leptin biology plays a significant role in the effects of early nutrition upon the adult phenotype. Future studies will delve further into "chicken and egg" issues to more clearly differentiate the relative importance of leptin and other molecules produced by adipocytes.

Adiponectin

Adiponectin is also produced by adipocytes, and its receptors adiponectin receptor-1 and adiponectin receptor-2 are found in skeletal muscle and liver, respectively (37). A 244-amino-acid protein is translated from the most abundant mRNA (apM1) found in human adipocytes (38). In mice, administration of adiponectin reduces insulin resistance and serum glucose levels. In humans, serum levels of adiponectin correlate directly with insulin sensitivity, but not with serum lipid profiles or obesity. Furthermore, a diabetes susceptibility locus maps to the adiponectin gene, at human chromosome 3q27 (39).

In the growth-retarded human, the impact of the early malnutrition appears to vary with age. Iñiguez et al. measured leptin levels in 1- and 2-year-old SGA and appropriate-sized infants (33). The SGA infants experienced catch-up growth, such that at 2 years of age only moderate differences existed between the two groups. Although no significant differences existed between SGA infants and the control infants in absolute serum adiponectin levels, differences in adiponectin levels were inversely related to weight gain between 1 and 2 years of age. In contrast to leptin, adiponectin levels were unrelated to insulin levels, and multiple regression analysis found that adiponectin related only to postnatal age. If postnatal age is excluded from the analysis, then determinants of adiponectin levels included lower postnatal body weight ($P < 0.001$) and male gender ($P < 0.03$). Though these findings are not as immediately satisfying as the leptin data from this study, they are thought-provoking based upon many of the gender-specific affects of early growth retardation that have been noted.

In contrast to these findings are those of López-Bermejo et al., who measured adiponectin levels and assessed both insulin resistance and insulin secretion using the homeostasis model of assessment (HOMA) in 32 prepubertal SGA children (mean age 5.4 ± 2.9 years) and appropriately sized children (mean age 5.9 ± 3.0 years) (40). Gestational age adjusted birthweight less than the 10th percentile and greater than the 25th percentile defined the SGA and appropriate sized children, respectively. Exclusion criteria included chromosomal abnormalities, intrauterine infection, gestational diabetes, gestational hypertension, growth hormone deficiency, and abnormal thyroid function.

As expected, SGA infants were lighter and shorter, but had similar BMIs. HOMA analysis of SGA and appropriate-sized children older than 3 years of age demonstrated a tendency towards insulin resistance in the SGA children ($P = 0.046$) after adjustments for sex, age, and BMI standard deviation score. Surprisingly, serum adiponectin levels were significantly higher in the SGA children ($P < 0.0001$), although when the data from the SGA children are broken into BMI quartiles, the findings become more complicated. When compared to the lean SGA children, the higher-quartile SGA children have lower serum adiponectin levels ($P = 0.02$). The higher quartile SGA children were also marked by higher fasting insulin levels ($P = 0.03$), borderline higher HOMA insulin resistance ($P = 0.05$), and higher HOMA β-cell insulin secretion ($P = 0.01$). Finally, in a multiple regression analysis, HOMA insulin resistance explained 35% of the adiponectin variance, and either SGA or birthweight status explained an additional 10 or 15% of adiponectin variance.

These studies differ somewhat from those of Cianfarani et al., who investigated 51 SGA children (mean age 8.6 ± 3.5 years), 17 short appropriate for gestational age children (mean age 10.5 ± 3.6 years), and 24 obese appropriate for gestational age children (10.6 ± 2.6 years) (41). In contrast to the previous study, SGA was defined as birth weight less than the 3rd percentile and appropriate for gestational age was defined as greater than the 10th percentile. The SGA children demonstrated evidence of insulin resistance as measured by HOMA and glucose:insulin ratios ($P < 0.01$ and $= 0.02$, respectively). Furthermore, when compared to both groups of appropriately sized children, SGA children were noted to have lower serum adiponectin levels ($P < 0.0001$). More specifically, in SGA children, adiponectin levels inversely correlated with birth length, age, weight, BMI, and puberty, as well as with fasting insulin and HOMA insulin resistance. Adiponectin levels also differentiated children within the SGA group, in that SGA children who experienced catch-up growth had adiponectin levels that were significantly lower than the SGA children who did not experience catch-up growth. Again, because of the purported predictive value of catch-up growth for adult morbidities, these latter findings suggest that adiponectin may at least be a marker for a higher risk group, if not actually playing a role in the pathophysiology.

The significance of adiponectin levels in the adult pathophysiologies of early malnutrition are further supported by the work of Jaquet et al. (42). This group evaluated 486 SGA young adults (mean age 22.6 ± 4.2 years) and 573 age-matched appropriate for gestational age controls. SGA was defined as less than the 10th percentile, whereas appropriate for gestational age was defined as being between the 25th and 75th percentiles. Mean gestational ages and gender proportions did not significantly differ between the two groups. Although fasting plasma glucose levels did not differ between the SGA and the appropriately sized young adults, higher 2-h glucose levels after a 75 g oral glucose load were seen in the SGA young adults. Furthermore, fasting insulinemia, insulin:glucose ratio, and insulin area under the curve were significantly higher in the SGA group relative to the control group.

As a result, it should not be unexpected that the mean value of serum adiponectin was significantly reduced in the SGA group in comparison to the appropriate for gestational age group. When the levels were adjusted for gender, BMI, waist-to-hip ratio, and oral contraception, the difference was highly significant ($P = 0.008$). Moreover, when insulin resistance markers were taken into account, in addition to the other co-variates, the reduction in adiponectin levels remained significant ($P < 0.01$). Interestingly, in contrast to the control young adults in which the insulin-to-glucose ratio inversely correlated with serum adiponectin levels, the insulin-to-glucose ratio and serum adiponectin levels followed a U-shaped curve across quartiles. In other words, the highest insulin-to-glucose ratio quartile in the SGA group was marked by high serum adiponectin levels. In contrast to the previously discussed study, catch-up BMI was not significantly associated with serum adiponectin concentrations.

In general, early malnutrition and subsequent growth retardation appear to affect serum adiponectin levels. Little has been done at this point using specific rodent models to dissect adiponectin biology within the context of growth retardation. Like leptin, we are still at the point of trying to figure out "chicken and egg" type issues. Whether this is a marker for, or cause of, impending morbidity remains to be seen.

IGF-1

Insulin-like growth factor 1 (IGF-1) is a polypeptide whose homology resembles proinsulin. The bioavailability and subsequent actions of IGF-1 are regulated by binding proteins, which generally moderate the actions of IGF-1 by competing with IGF-1 receptors. Most tissues synthesize IGF-1, and IGF-1 homeostasis appears to have both systemic and paracrine implications, of which the latter are probably unappreciated. In general, IGF-1 levels in human fetuses increase from 18 to 40 weeks of gestation. IGF-1 and IGFBP-3 serum levels slowly increase prior to adolescence, steeply increase during puberty, and decrease thereafter. In contrast, IGFBP-1 serum levels gradually decline prior to adolescence, such that the lowest levels are found in puberty.

IGF-1 and its associated binding proteins are intriguing players in the mechanisms relating early malnutrition to adult disease for several reasons. First, IGF-1 plays a key role in feto-placental growth throughout gestation. Null mutations of IGF-1 in mice reduce fetal size by approximately 40% (43). In humans, IGF-1 gene deletion results in severe prenatal growth failure (44). Second, IGF-1 and IGFBP-3 mediate many of the anabolic and mitogenic actions of growth hormone in postnatal life. Short children have lower IGF-1 and IGFBP-3 levels than tall children. Third, a recent nested case-control study found that low IGF-1 and high IGFBP-3 levels in adulthood predicted increased risk for developing ischemic heart disease (45). Finally, IGF-1 regulates or moderates insulin sensitivity in adulthood. Hepatic IGF-1 is of vital importance for normal carbohydrate metabolism in both mice and humans. In mice, elimination of hepatic IGF-1 production using a Cre/loxP recombination system increases serum levels of insulin without significantly affecting glucose elimination (46). In humans, recombinant IGF-1 is approximately 6% as potent as insulin in the production of hypoglycemia (47). Severe IGF-1 deficiency leads to insulin resistance, which can be reversed with recombinant IGF-1 (48).

Though not as widely recognized, IGF-1 biology also affects glucose homeostasis prior to adulthood. In the following study by Moran et al., the investigators hypothesized that the normal increase in insulin resistance that occurs concomitantly with puberty will be associated with changes in IGF-1, IGFBP-1, and IGFBP-3 levels (49). Euglycemic clamp studies were performed on 357 adolescents (mean age 13.0 ± 1.2 years). IGF-1 levels significantly correlated with insulin sensitivity in both boys ($P = 0.0006$) and girls ($P = 0.02$), although IGF-1 correlated significantly with fasting insulin levels only in girls. IGFBP-1 was negatively associated with insulin resistance in both genders, whereas IGFBP-3 was positively associated with insulin resistance only in boys. The findings of this study are provocative; in that they can be interpreted to suggest that the IGF-1 axis either contributes or responds to the insulin resistance of puberty. Considering the adult data, the latter appears to be more likely.

Multiple investigators find that infants with IUGR or SGA status have lower fetal or cord IGF-1 concentrations when compared to appropriately sized infants. In the fetus, both genetic and environmental factors regulate fetal IGF-1 levels (50). The importance of the latter is supported by the observation that whereas serum IGF-1 levels are similar in discordant monochorionic twins, IGF-1 levels significantly differ in discordant dichorionic twins. This suggests that placental function and subsequent in utero substrate delivery may override genetic determinants of IGF-1 production. Furthermore, placental IGF-1 signaling appears altered in association with poor in utero fetal growth. In a recent study of 14 control and IUGR pregnancies, IUGR reduced both IGF-1 receptor protein levels and IGF-1 signal transduction (51). In contrast, no differences were found in insulin receptor protein levels. The simple conclusion is that IGF-1 homeostasis is certainly altered in both the fetus and the placenta in pregnancies complicated by poor growth. The key question will be which comes first, the poor growth or the altered homeostasis, and the likely answer is that both possibilities occur along the spectrum of the human environmental continuum.

The trend in altered IGF-1 homeostasis continues to be evident in the postnatal period. When comparing IUGR and appropriately sized infants from birth through 6 to 9 months of age, Özkan et al. found that IUGR decreased IGF-1 serum levels and increased serum IGFBP-1, relative to the control infants (52). When the IUGR babies were subdivided into those with and without catch-up growth, the infants without catch-up growth had the lowest IGF-1 values ($P < 0.05$). Finally, birth weight, postnatal weight, and postnatal height correlated directly with IGF-1 and IGFBP-3 levels, but not IGFBP-1 levels. Similarly, when Fattal-Valavski et al. determined IGF-1 levels in pre-adolescent IUGR children (mean age 6.5 ± 2.1 years; $n = 57$) versus control children (7.6 ± 2.8 years; $n = 30$), IGF-1 serum levels were significantly decreased only in the non-catch-up IUGR group (53). Again, significant correlations existed in this study between IGF-1 serum levels and both height and weight percentiles.

Similarly, Barker's group also found that plasma IGF-1 levels correlated positively with height and weight in 200 and 244 preadolescent children from Pune, India, and Salisbury Health District, respectively (54). However, in contrast to the above studies, plasma IGF-1 levels inversely correlated with birth weight (Pune $P = 0.002$; Salisbury $P = 0.003$). Specifically, the highest IGF-1 levels identified children who were below average birth weight and above average weight or height at the time of this study. Furthermore, higher systolic blood pressures were seen in children with the highest IGF-1 levels (Pune $P = 0.01$; Salisbury $P = 0.04$). These findings are particularly intriguing in light of recent observations, which link significant catch-up growth with adult morbidities.

The interaction between birth weight and IGF homeostasis continues into early adolescence. Tenhola et al. investigated the relationship between serum IGF-1 and insulin sensitivity in 55 SGA and AGA age-matched children (55). SGA was defined in this study as birth weight, length, or ponderal index greater than 2 SD below the respective mean for gestational age. Insulin sensitivity was determined by HOMA. After adjusting for BMI, gender, and puberty, SGA increased serum IGF-1 concentrations ($P = 0.006$). In multiple logistic regression analysis, HOMA insulin resistance predicted high serum IGF-1 levels in the SGA children, but not in the appropriately sized control group. Furthermore, the SGA children in the highest IGF-1 quartile had higher BMIs ($P = 0.021$), weight ($P = 0.038$), and weight for height ($P = 0.040$), and well as lower birth weights ($P = 0.077$) versus the SGA children in the lower IGF-1 quartiles.

In adulthood, the relationship becomes even more complicated and, again, genetic and environmental diversity enter the picture, as does the impact of puberty. Verkauskiene et al. investigated a group of young SGA (mean age 22.6 ± 4.3 years) and appropriately sized (mean age 22.6 ± 4.2 years) young adults who were full term (56). Lower birth weight and ponderal index characterized the SGA group. In adulthood, the lower weight and height similarly characterized the SGA group. The SGA adults were also marked by significantly lower mean serum IGF-1 ($P = 0.015$) and IGFBP-3 ($P = 0.04$) levels versus those infants who were appropriately sized at birth. Furthermore, fasting IGF-1 concentrations inversely correlated with age, BMI, smoking, and oral contraceptive use and directly correlated with birthweight and fasting insulin levels.

In contrast to these findings are those of Kajantie et al. and Ben-Shlomo et al. Kajantie et al. investigated 421 subjects who were singleton births between 1924 and 1933 at the Helsinki University Central Hospital (57). Detailed birth records were available for these subjects, including birth weight, length, head circumference, and gestational age, as well as measurements of height and weight between the ages of 7 and 15 years. The average birth weight of these subjects was 3504 ± 422 g (males) and 3342 ± 406 g (females). Fourteen of the subjects were SGA based upon being greater than 2 standard deviations below the norm. When adjusted for sex, current age, and BMI, IGF-1 concentrations did not correlate with any of the measures performed at birth. However, IGFBP-1 did positively correlate with birth weight ($P = 0.03$) and ponderal index at birth ($P = 0.01$). A positive correlation also existed between adult IGFBP-1 concentration and BMI at 7 years of age. Furthermore, serum IGF-1 concentrations were positively associated with adult fasting glucose levels and both systolic and diastolic blood pressures.

Ben-Shlomo et al. investigated 951 individuals from two small towns in South Wales, with birth weights of 3440 ± 490 g (males) and 3300 ± 510 g (females) (58). Anthropometric measures were followed from birth to 5 years of age, as well as to adulthood. Serum IGF-1 and IGFBP-3 levels were measured at approximately 25 years of age. No associations were found between birth weight and either adult IGF-1 or IGFBP-3 levels. Interestingly, the IGF-1:IGFBP-3 ratio showed an inverse relationship with ponderal index at birth, which strengthened with age. Furthermore, the IGF-1:IGFBP-3 ratio also significantly correlated with adult BMI, waist-to-hip ratio, and sagittal abdominal diameter. Poor growth or "downward centile" crossing during childhood was associated with the lower IGF-1 levels, whereas young adults who were tall throughout their life were marked by the highest IGF-I levels. These findings suggest that early adulthood plasma IGF-1 levels associate with patterns of childhood growth.

Childhood malnutrition also probably affects adult IGF-1 biology. Elias et al. utilized a group of 87 post-menopausal women who were exposed to the Dutch famine between the ages of 2 and 20 years (59). These women were divided into moderately exposed and severely exposed based upon weight loss, and 163 unexposed women of similar ages were used as controls. Women who were younger than 2 years at the time of the famine, those who could not be classified to famine exposure, and those who did not reside in occupied Netherlands were excluded. After adjusting for characteristics such as BMI, waist/hip ratio, and cigarette-smoking habits, exposure to famine resulted in a significant increase in IGF-1 ($P = 0.038$) and IGFBP-3 ($P = 0.045$) serum levels.

The relationship between postnatal IUGR and IGF-1 levels is intriguing, although not completely clear, and, if one looks at the trend in the studies by age, IGF-1 appears to gradually increase from the initial low levels in the SGA groups relative to the control groups. This may represent an overcompensation that permits catch-up growth, which is a good thing if you are competing in the world as an adolescent, but the higher IGF-1 levels may have an as yet undefined pathological physiologic effect later in life.

Not all of these effects are necessarily bad, however. Early life events are known to affect hippocampal neurogenesis and increase age-related learning impairments in the rat. Interestingly, IGF-1 regulates the neurotropic response to aging through multiple mechanisms, including increasing mRNA levels of brain-derived neurotropic fats and stimulating hippocampal neurogenesis. Moreover, a recent investigation by Gunnell et al. of 547 white singleton boys and girls found that IGF-1 levels positively correlated with intelligence: for every 100 ng/ml increase in IGF-1, IQ increased by 3.18 points (60).

Furthermore, aging also leads to decreased brain levels of IGF-1. Although the following study uses rats, the findings are worth noting. Darnaudéry et al. exposed pregnant dams from day 14 of pregnancy until term (approximately 21.5 days) to confinement as well as exposure to bright light three times a day (61). After weaning at 21 days, the offspring of stressed and non-stressed dams were housed under identical conditions. At 24 months of age, the progeny of the stressed dams were further divided into two groups: one group received vehicle (NaCl) into the right lateral ventricle for 21 days, the other group received IGF-1 for the same amount of time. Both groups were then exposed to a water maze task. Females whose dams were stressed during pregnancy exhibited learning impairment in the water maze task. IGF-1 infusion restored the performance of spatial learning in the water maze, such that it approximated that of control animals. One of the debates in the field is whether the adult consequences of early life events are a nonspecific response to the early injury, or whether it is in some way teleologically protective, an evolutionary response if you will. Experiments such as these suggest that, at least in some cases, the latter may be true. The possibility exists that we have not appreciated the benefits of the early programming, but have noted the cost, particularly as we have become more sedentary as a species.

To define this toll, initial studies involve the use of IUGR animal models. Investigators have used maternal malnutrition in the rat, as well as another common model of IUGR, bilateral uterine artery ligation of the pregnant rat. This latter model is attractive in that, as in the human, it produces asymmetric IUGR through fetal hypoxia, acidosis, hypoglycemia, and decreased levels of branched-chain amino acids (62, 63), characteristics shared with human infants suffering from uteroplacental insufficiency (64–68). IUGR rat pups in this model are 20–25% lighter than pups from sham-operated controls, and birth weights are normally distributed within and between litters. Furthermore, litter size does not significantly differ between control and IUGR groups. IUGR pups in this model develop early insulin resistance and adult-onset diabetes (69, 70).

A variation in this model is unilateral uterine artery ligation, with pups from the unligated side acting as controls. Vileisis et al. used this model and found that fetal weight correlated with serum glucose ($P < 0.001$), liver IGF-1 protein ($P < 0.001$), and serum IGF-1 protein ($P < 0.001$) levels (71). No correlation was evident for either serum insulin or lung IGF-1 protein. Interestingly, serum fetal glucose concentrations correlated positively with liver ($P < 0.001$) and serum ($P < 0.002$) IGF-1 protein levels, implicating fetal glucose delivery in the regulation of IGF-1 hepatic synthesis.

Using bilateral uterine artery ligation at day 17 of gestation, Houdijk et al. found that neither male nor female animals exhibited catch-up growth in terms of body weight as they reached adulthood, although the female IUGR rats did catch up to controls in terms of nose-anus length (72). As one might expect from the human data in children who do not exhibit significant catch-up growth, no differences were noted between control and IUGR IGF-1 levels at 100 days, regardless of gender. Interestingly, baseline growth hormone levels were significantly decreased ($P < 0.05$), suggesting that IUGR in this model may impact tissue, particularly liver, responsiveness to GH.

When maternal malnutrition is utilized, IGF-1 biology is also affected. In 1991, Bernstein et al. noted that 72 h of maternal fasting decreased serum IGF-1 levels in term rat pups (73). Similarly, Woodall et al. investigated the effects of both protein and caloric malnutrition by restricting pregnant rat intake to 30% of an ad libitum control group. As expected, mean body weights were significantly decreased in the term IUGR fetuses versus controls, and this trend continued through the first 90 days of life. Furthermore, plasma IGF-1 levels were significantly decreased in the IUGR group from the end of gestation ($P < 0.01$) through the first 9 days of life ($P < 0.05$) (74). Woodall et al. also measured mRNA levels of different IGF-1 mRNA transcripts using RNase protection assays (75). IGF-1 mRNA processing involves two different start sites involving exon 1 and exon 2, respectively, as well as different 3′ processing, resulting in Ea and Eb variants. mRNA levels from all start sites were significantly reduced by maternal malnutrition from the end of gestation to day 5 of life and in select start sites up through day of life 15. Expression of Ea IGF-1 mRNA was significantly decreased from the end of gestation to day 5 of life, whereas mRNA levels of Ea were not affected by maternal malnutrition. These investigators also found no difference in growth hormone or growth hormone binding protein mRNA levels, and speculated that their findings suggest a possible post growth hormone receptor defect in IUGR.

These, and other animal studies, have only begun to scratch the surface of the complex relationship between in utero nutrition and IGF-1 biology. The mechanisms regulating IGF-1 gene expression are complex, as suggested by the above studies. A potential mechanism through which IUGR may alter IGF-1 levels is zinc deficiency. Zinc is one of the most abundant divalent ions in living organisms and performs multiple functions secondary to its unique physiochemical properties. Two of zinc's most important properties include (i) the ability to assume multiple coordination numbers and geometries, which make this ion stereochemically adaptable, and (ii) zinc's resistance to oxidation and reduction under physiologic conditions (76, 77).

Zinc deficiency is a world-wide problem, and it is the second most important deficiency in infants (78). In Western societies, zinc deficiency is often associated with a low socioeconomic status (79). The effect of prenatal zinc deficiency is intrauterine growth retardation or IUGR (80–83). The specificity of this effect is suggested by a double-blind study, which found that zinc supplementation significantly reduced the incidence of IUGR and improved most measured indices of fetal health (84). Zinc also plays a significant role in determining postnatal growth. A recent meta-analysis reveals that zinc supplementation improves growth in prepubertal children (85).

Interestingly, dietary intake of zinc significantly contributes to the regulation of IGF-1 levels in both humans and animals, and the liver is considered to be the major source of circulating IGF-1 (86–88). Devine et al. found that zinc was the major determinant of IGF-1 concentrations ($P < 0.033$) in postmenopausal women after 2 years of nutritional supplementation (89). This study controlled for age, weight, and other nutritional intakes, including calcium, iron, protein, and calories. Because of this study's careful design, the authors were able to suggest that zinc intake influences IGF-1 concentrations, even in the face of adequate energy and protein intake. Similarly, although less well controlled because of the ages of the study subjects, several groups have found that zinc supplementation increases serum IGF-1 levels in children (90–93). Unfortunately, in the human literature, studies correlating zinc deprivation to depressed IGF-1 levels are lacking because of the multiple confounding factors that complicate these studies, such as low protein and caloric intake. As a result, the animal literature is necessary to provide further insight.

For example, zinc deprivation of male rats reduces serum IGF-1 levels to 28% of those of control rats which have been fed identical calories and protein through a gastric tube (94). Similarly, Dorup et al. found that zinc deficiency deceased serum IGF-1 levels to 17% of control rat values, while similarly controlling for energy intake (95). Furthermore, when McNall et al. and Ninh et al. compared rats fed a zinc-deficient diet to those fed an appropriate diet, they found that zinc deficiency specifically decreased both serum IGF-1 levels and liver IGF-1 mRNA levels (96, 97).

A controversy exists in the zinc-IGF-1 literature on whether the effect of zinc deficiency upon IGF-1 hepatic expression is due to a dysregulation of the growth hormone (GH) receptor pathway or due to a direct action of zinc upon IGF-1. Two studies respond to this controversy. The first study supplemented *KunMing* mice with zinc and found that, while serum and hepatic IGF-1 mRNA levels increased in these animals, serum and hepatic growth hormone receptor mRNA levels remained unchanged (86). The second study was performed by Ninh et al., who demonstrated that hepatic IGF-1 synthesis requires zinc, and that the lack of a growth-promoting action of growth hormone in zinc-deficient animals resulted from a defect beyond growth hormone binding to its liver receptors (98). In other words, although GH biology certainly plays a role in the regulation of hepatic IGF-1 expression, nutritional zinc also contributes in a fashion independent of the GH pathway. This is particularly true in the developing animal for the following reasons: (i) neither GH receptor mRNA nor specific GH binding is detectable in rat liver until 14–20 days of age (99, 100); (ii) hepatic IGF-1 mRNA levels are not elevated until 3 weeks of age in transgenic mice that are characterized by elevated levels of circulating GH (100); and (iii) liver-specific deletion of IGF-1 in mice reveals that IGF-1 regulates pituitary expression of GH releasing factor, receptor, and secretagogue (101).

Although the above studies demonstrate causal links between zinc nutrition, IGF-1 biology, and growth, conflicting reports exist. Among those is the study by Doherty et al., who performed a double-blind randomized intervention study of 141 children, whose ages fell between 6 months and 3 years, from the Dhaka Shishu Children's hospital in Bangladesh (93). Their weight for age was less than 60% of the National Center for Health Statistics value. Based upon the type of malnutrition (marasmus versus kwashiorkor), the presence of diarrhea, and the numbers of days after recruitment, each child was placed in a standardized feeding regimen, which included vitamin supplementation. Randomization further placed the children into one of three regimens: (i) 1.5 mg/kg elemental Zn for 15 days; (ii) 6 mg/kg elemental zinc for 15 days; and (iii) 6 mg/kg elemental zinc for 30 days.

The diet increased ponderal catch-up growth rapidly, although linear growth was only moderately improved. At baseline, IGF-1 and IGFBP-3 were significantly lower than standard values for healthy, well-nourished European children. During the feeding protocol, IGF-1 and IGFBP-3 increased, reaching a plateau by 15 days. The only difference between the regimens was that IGF-1 was higher in zinc regimen 1 at day 15 ($P = 0.04$). As markers, IGF-1 and IGFBP-3 correlated best with ponderal growth at day 15 and with linear growth at day 90. The authors of this study noted that their lack of differentiation in this particular study may be secondary to either the lower supplementation providing sufficient zinc or the full nutritional supplementation masking the effects of the higher zinc dosing.

The bottom line is that both prenatal and postnatal nutrition affects IGF-1 biology and alters postnatal phenotypic characteristics. On all levels, molecular, endocrinological, and physiological, there is a lot yet to tease out (Table 18-3). One of the more intriguing factors is the relationship between IGF-1 and early growth, particularly in how that relates to adult phenotype. Issues that need to be addressed include the effects of different macro and micro nutrients on both IGF-1 levels and sensitivity.

Cardiovascular

Poor early nutrition and associated decreased growth are strongly associated with cardiovascular disease, with our three historical cohorts providing ample evidence. Multiple mechanisms probably play a role with this grouping of morbidity, so the mechanisms we focus on are neither exclusive nor exhaustive. We focus on two mechanisms, renal morphogenesis and endothelial dysfunction, based upon emerging evidence in both human and animal research (Table 18-4).

RENAL MORPHOGENESIS

Several studies demonstrate that IUGR predisposes the affected neonate towards impaired renal function, as well as an increased risk of adult onset hypertension. Nephrogenesis increases markedly during the third trimester, and is completed by

Table 18-3	Summary – Relationship between Purported Hormones and Nutritional Substrate to Adult Morbidities Discussed in this Chapter
Hormone/nutritional substrate	**Relation to adult morbidities**
Leptin – leptin resistance	Leptin levels correlate with postnatal growth, which may be associated with insulin resistance
Adiponectin	Lower adiponectin levels may be a marker for infants at risk for adult morbidities
IGF-1	Low IGF-1 levels early in life are associated with poor fetal growth; high IGF-1 levels my be associated with the systemic morbidities associated with rapid catch-up growth
Zinc	Prenatal zinc deficiency is associated with poor fetal growth; furthermore, dietary zinc contributes to the regulation of hepatic IGF-1 regulation

34–36 weeks, with 60% of the normal complement of nephrons in the human kidney formed during the third trimester. As a result, the kidney is particularly vulnerable to nutritional insults during this period. Subsequently, human and animal studies have shown that IUGR results in smaller kidneys with decreased nephron numbers. For example, Leroy Hinchliffe et al. have examined post-mortem human kidneys and have remarked upon the decrease in nephron number in IUGR infants (102, 103).

More specifically, Mañalich et al. studied kidneys from SGA and appropriately sized infants who succumbed within 2 weeks of birth secondary to respiratory distress syndrome, infectious complications, cerebral hemorrhage, or perinatal hypoxia-ischemia (104). Gestational ages for these children were 37 ± 1.05 weeks and 38.9 ± 1.29 weeks, respectively. Gender and race were equally distributed between the two groups. A maternal history of essential hypertension and smoking existed in a significantly higher number of the SGA infants than of the appropriately sized infants. Histomorphometric analysis was performed by a renal pathologist who was blinded to the origin of the biopsy. Glomerular number, glomerular volume, and area occupied by glomeruli were measured. A significant positive correlation existed between birth weight and glomeruli number ($r = 0.87$; $P < 0.0001$) and area occupied by glomeruli ($r = 0.935$; $P < 0.0001$), whereas a significant negative correlation existed between birth weight and glomerular volume ($r = 0.84$; $P < 0.001$)

These findings appear relevant when considering the findings of relative hypertension in SGA children early in life. For example, Horta et al. studied a cohort of 749 adolescents from Pelotas, in southern Brazil (105). Approximately 5% of these

Table 18-4	Proposed Factors Involved in the Association between Poor Fetal Growth and Hypertension
Mechanism	**Effect**
Increased renal apoptosis	This may lead to decreased nephron number, which may contribute to the development of hypertension
Vascular endothelial dysfunction (acetylcholine-induced vascular relaxation and/or impaired angiotensin-converting enzyme activity)	This may cause a predisposition toward hypertension

subjects were marked by birth weights of less then 2.5 kg, and SGA was defined as birth weight less than the 10th percentile for gestational age. Investigators gathered anthropometric information on these individuals at birth, 20 months, 42 months, and 15 years. Confounders considered in this study included family income, maternal education, maternal weight and height, maternal age at delivery, maternal smoking, breast-feeding duration, and gender of the child. Once controlling for these and other variables, birth weight was negatively associated with systolic blood pressure. Furthermore, early and late catch-up growth are positively associated with systolic blood pressure in adolescence. On a side note, a separate analysis of this Brazilian cohort noted that catch-up growth in early infancy appeared to provide short-term benefits, in that those SGA children who experienced the greatest catch-up growth experienced fewer hospital admissions and lower mortality between 20 and 42 months. This is consistent with this chapter's theme that much of the SGA or IUGR phenotype is an early adaptation that provides initial benefits, but comes at the cost of later morbidities.

Similarly, Law et al. used the Brompton study cohort to determine the relative effects of SGA and catch-up growth (106). This cohort consisted of 1867 individuals from whom data were collected at birth, 6 months, childhood ($\approx$2–6 years), and young adulthood ($\approx$22 years of life). Of note, only 12 of these individuals weighed less than 2.5 kg at birth. In this cohort, a one kg decrease in birth weight resulted in an increase of 2.7 mmHg (95% CI, 0.4–5.0) and 1.6 mmHg (95% CI, 0.1–3.2) of the young adult systolic and diastolic blood pressures, respectively. Although greater weight gain between 1 and 5 years of life correlated with higher adult systolic blood pressures, weight gain during infancy did not. This latter finding may be due to the association between childhood BMI and adult BMI.

The consequence of the reduced nephron number is more than an amorphous risk factor for hypertension. In Singapore, a nationwide screening program evaluated the effect of low birth weight upon proteinuria and found an 8-fold increased risk of proteinuria in the low birth weight population (107). Furthermore, SGA children with minimal change disease are more likely to relapse, and SGA children afflicted with IGA nephropathy suffer from an increased incidence of arterial hypertension.

The classic rat models of fetal growth retardation, bilateral uterine artery ligation, and maternal malnutrition have been used to assess the renal consequences of growth retardation. Pham et al. used bilateral uterine artery ligation in the Sprague-Dawley rat and found that IUGR decreased glomeruli number by approximately one-third both at term and at 21 days of life ($P < 0.01$ for both) (108). Their data also maintained statistical significance when glomeruli number was standardized with animal weight. Interestingly, these investigators also measured IGF-1 mRNA levels and found them decreased to 38% of control values ($P < 0.01$). Finally, Merlet-Benichou et al. used partial unilateral artery ligation in the rat to induce IUGR, which reduced nephron number by 37% and glomerular filtration rate by 50% (109). Among the groups that used maternal malnutrition, Welham et al. and Vehaskari et al. used low-protein diets to induce IUGR and decrease glomeruli number in IUGR rat kidneys (110, 111).

Using essentially the same model as Pham et al., Schreuder et al. used telemetry to determine whether the uterine artery ligation model induced adult hypertension (112). IUGR and control male rats were studied longitudinally at 6, 9, and 12 months, with the effect of acute stress determined at 6 and 12 months. At all ages, systolic blood pressure was significantly higher in the IUGR group, with a tendency towards a negative correlation ($P = 0.052$). IUGR male rats reacted to stress at 12 months with a significant increase in systolic blood pressure ($P = 0.029$), although a trend also existed at 6 months ($P = 0.072$). Similarly, pulse pressure was not different between the two groups at 6 and 9 months; however, pulse pressure increased in the IUGR animals so that, by 12 months of age, a significant inverse correlation existed between pulse pressure and birth weight. These findings would be consistent with both a decrease in nephron number, as demonstrated by Pham et al., and a change in vascular reactivity.

In summary, both human observations and animal studies demonstrate that the kidney is vulnerable to early nutritional insults. One point of vulnerability may be the dependence of nephrogenesis upon apoptosis. Apoptosis, programmed cell death, is regulated by nutritional and growth factor signals, which are altered in the growth-retarded fetus. Moderation of renal apoptosis is one arena that may be a fruitful intervention in which to minimize the effects of IUGR. On the other hand, apoptosis may also be a "safety valve" through which cells minimize the total amount of necrosis. As with many things in this field, future studies are necessary to determine whether apoptosis is truly undesirable or an immediate adaptation that comes at a later cost.

ENDOTHELIAL DYSFUNCTION

Although reductions in nephron number probably contribute to the hypertensive and cardiovascular complications associated with low birth weight and SGA, other factors are likely to play a role. Biologically and philosophically, this makes sense. Biologically, there is always a reaction or reactions to any particular action. Philosophically, if the adaptations of IUGR are an attempt to increase survival odds, the celestial design committee is unlikely to leave the adaptation to a sole event. In fact, evidence is emerging in both human and animal studies suggesting that endothelial function is altered in the SGA infants.

Vascular endothelial dysfunction has been linked to both hypertension and coronary artery disease. Among the first investigations linking early vascular endothelial dysfunction and low birth weight is a study by Leeson et al., who investigated 333 British children between the ages of 9 and 11 (113). These children resided in four British towns (Bath, Tunbridge, Rochdale, Rhonda). Information available for these children included birth weight, maternal factors, and risk factors such as blood pressure, lipid fractions, preload and postload glucose levels, smoking exposure, and socioeconomic status. To determine endothelial function, a noninvasive ultrasound technique was used to assess the ability of the brachial artery to dilate in response to increased blood flow, which was induced by forearm cuff occlusion and release. The study group consisted of 165 girls and 168 boys. As expected, birth weight showed a graded positive relationship with flow-mediated dilatation (0.027 mm/kg; 95% CI, 0.003–0.051 mm/kg; $P = 0.02$). This relationship was independent of social class, region, ethnic group, and maternal smoking. Furthermore, cardiovascular risk factors such as blood pressure, total and LDL cholesterol, and salivary carnitine levels showed no correlation with flow-mediated dilatation, although HDL cholesterol appeared to be inversely related ($P = 0.05$).

Conceptually, this study was extended by the same group to involve 165 women and 150 men to determine endothelium-dependent and independent vascular responses of the brachial artery (114). The use of a sublingual nitroglycerin spray was used to induce an endothelium-dependent dilatation. These subjects were 20–28 years of age, and mean birth weight was 3.27 kg. Again, a significant positive correlation existed between birth weight and flow-mediated dilatation ($P = 0.04$), but not with nitroglycerin-induced dilatation. Birth length, ponderal index at birth, and placental weight to birth weight ratio were not related to the measures of vascular function, nor did a relationship exist between vascular function and weight at 1 year of age. Because the correlation between birth weight and flow-mediated dilatation was dampened by increasing levels of acquired risk factors, such as smoking, the effect of birth weight appears to be most relevant in those with traditionally lower risk profiles.

One question that typically arises from these types of studies is the extent to which genetics either amplifies or dampens the effects of low birth weight. The best cohort studies deal with this issue statistically, while another option is discordant twin studies. These latter studies have been applied to essentially every aspect of the fetal origins of adult disease paradigm. In the area of vascular endothelial dysfunction, Halvorsen et al. studied 31 twin pairs, of which 21 were monozygotic and 9 were dizygotic (115). Of the monozygotic twins, the gestation of nine pairs was complicated by twin-twin transfusion syndrome. The mean age for the three groups was approximately 8 years. Eight of the 62 twin subjects had a systolic blood pressure above the 90th percentile, and of these eight, seven were from the monozygotic group with a history of poor fetal growth and twin-twin transfusion syndrome. In the monozygotic twin pairs without twin-twin transfusion syndrome, systolic BP was higher and endothelial function more likely to be impaired in the lighter twin.

In terms of the mechanism through which endothelial function is likely to occur, multiple factors are likely to be involved. Two factors for which evidence exist are impaired acetylcholine-induced vascular relaxation and impaired angiotensin-converting enzyme activity. For the former, Martin et al. investigated 40 newborn infants and their mothers 3 days after delivery, as well as 10 healthy age-matched control women (116). The SGA group was made up of 20 infants who were characterized by a birth weight of 2510 ± 270 g and a gestation age of 39 ± 1.3 weeks. The AGA group was made up of 20 infants who were characterized by a birth weight of 3608 ± 460 g and a similar gestation age of 39 ± 1.6 weeks. Gender distribution was similar between the two groups. These investigators induced peripheral vasodilatation through either local application of acetylcholine or local heating, and perfusion differences were assessed by laser Doppler. In response to acetylcholine, SGA infants responded with only a moderate increase in perfusion ($240 \pm 125\%$), whereas the appropriately sized infants responded robustly ($650 \pm 250\%$) ($P < 0.01$). Furthermore, when Martin et al. further divided the SGA group, the lean SGA infants were characterized by lower perfusion increase ($189 \pm 40\%$) versus the symmetrically small SGA infants ($338 \pm 170\%$) ($P < 0.01$). Interestingly, the presence of a family history clouded by cardiovascular disease did not result in changes in perfusion. Furthermore, when comparing either absolute or relative perfusion responses to local heating, no differences were noted between the SGA and the appropriately sized infants. Because acetylcholine vasodilatation is endothelium-dependent, whereas vasodilatation in response to local heat is dependent upon smooth muscle, these findings suggest that acetylcholine endothelial dysfunction is present even at birth.

Another mechanism through which endothelial function dysfunction and cardiovascular morbidity may occur is through the altered function of the angiotensin pathways. Angiotensin-converting enzyme (ACE) plays a key role in the regulation of peripheral blood pressure, and the evidence implicating this pathway derives from both human observation and animal studies. In humans, Forsyth et al. performed a prospective study of full-term infants and measured ACE levels at 1 and 3 months of age (117). Mean birth weight was 3498 ± 506 g. They found a significant negative correlation between ACE activity at both 1 and 3 months and birth weight, $P < 0.001$ and < 0.03, respectively. In rats, Riviere et al. used a 70% caloric-restricted model of maternal nutrition to study the effect upon offspring angiotensin II serum levels, ACE and ACE2 mRNA levels, and ACE activities in multiple tissues (118). ACE2 is a newly described member of the angiotensin pathways that competes with ACE for angiotensin peptide hydrolysis. In their rats, not only was blood pressure moderately increased, but ACE and ACE2 activities were significantly increased in the lung ($P < 0.05$). These authors speculated that increased activity of these enzymes may contribute to the hypertension observed in these animals.

In sheep, several studies emphasize the potential of the angiotensin pathway in mediating cardiovascular disease. Included among these studies is the work of Roghair et al., who used the programming model of antenatal steroid administration in the preterm sheep (119). In this model, a catheterized late-gestation fetus receives betamethasone (10 μg/h) over 48 h, while a control twin receives an identical volume of the 0.9% NaCl vehicle control. Contractile responses of circumflex coronary artery segments were assessed in response to angiotensin, sodium nitroprusside, 8-bromo-cGMP, isoproterenol, and forskolin. The betamethasone-treated twins exhibited a significant increase in angiotensin II coronary artery contractility versus the vehicle-treated controls ($P < 0.05$), but no significant difference to the other vasoactive compounds. Interestingly, mesenteric arteries did not demonstrate the same differential reactivity. Furthermore, increased coronary artery levels of the angiotensin type I receptor differentiated betamethasone-treated and vehicle-treated fetuses ($P < 0.05$).

In contrast to the late-gestation fetus, the early-gestation fetus exposed to glucocorticoids demonstrates aberrant responses to nitric oxide signaling. Segar et al. exposed 27-day-gestation lambs (term = 145 days) to dexamethasone (0.28 mg/kg/day) or vehicle, and subsequently examined the baroreflex function at 10–14 days of postnatal age (120). In these animals, the mean resting blood pressures and hearts were no different between groups; however, though in vivo changes in blood pressure in response to angiotensin II and phenylephrine were similar between the two groups, the dexamethasone-treated lambs displayed a greater increase in blood pressure in response to nitric oxide synthase blockade (23 ± 3 vs. 13 ± 2 mmHg; $P < 0.05$).

These findings are conceptually similar to those of Payne et al., who made rats IUGR by placing a clip upon the abdominal aorta above the iliac bifurcation (121), the latter of which reduces uterine blood flow by approximately 40%. Sham-operated dams were used as control. They subsequently studied nitrite/nitrate production at 4, 8, and 12 weeks of age in aortic endothelium intact vascular strips in the progeny of both groups..

Multiple other mechanisms may be involved in the dysregulation of endothelial function. These studies, along with those involving the kidney, emphasize the complexity of the adaptations that occur in response to early malnutrition. A question that needs to be asked is how vital are these adaptations to fetal survival, and what are the costs of moderating them to minimize the effects upon adult health. The changes in blood pressure regulation may very well ensure survival of the fetus and cost the adult later. As a result, interventions to reverse or change the programming must not be flippantly instituted.

Neuroendocrine Re-Programming

Though these above issues are important, what makes us human is our brain. As a result, the second question parents and physicians ask when looking into a child's future is what the neurological outcome will be. Data existing in humans demonstrate that early malnutrition significantly impacts the brain, and animal models are being used to understand some of the mechanisms that may be involved. This section will discuss the affects upon neuroendocrine re-programming, particularly within the context of the hypothalamic-pituitary adrenal axis (HPA).

Hope exists that changes in HPA may unify many of the phenotypic effects seen in multiple organ systems. Indeed, as with the other systems and organs we have discussed, a significant amount of effort will be necessary to tease apart the effects of the re-programmed HPA axis upon the peripheral tissues versus the effects of the re-programmed peripheral tissues upon the HPA axis. Complicating the issue has been the associations made by multiple groups suggesting that early exposure to high levels of glucocorticoids may trigger many of the events that we see, so again the distinction between cause and effect continues to be blurred.

Of course, the place to start is the Dutch famine studies. Rooij et al. investigated survivors who were born as term singletons at the Wilhelmina Gasthuis in Amsterdam between November 1943 and February 1947 (3). Sixty normoglycemic men and women from this cohort participated in dexamethasone suppression and $ACTH_{1-24}$-stimulation tests, as well as undergoing clinical and anthropometric assessments. Ten men and ten women who were born before the famine, during the famine (defined by any 13 weeks of gestation during which the maternal diet consisted of < 1000 kcal), and after the famine were tested. In general, higher cortisol levels after dexamethasone suppression and a lower cortisol increment after $ACTH_{1-24}$ stimulation characterized men, when compared to the women. As expected, a positive correlation between cortisol levels and waist:hip ratios, 2-h glucose levels, and 2-h insulin concentrations existed.

When comparing cortisol concentration between those who were exposed to famine and those who were not affected, the authors report that no significant differences were found after dexamethasone suppression and $ACTH_{1-24}$ stimulation, including peak cortisol levels, incremental rise, and area under the curve. Adjusting for maternal age, maternal weight gain, birth weight, smoking, and socioeconomic status did not alter the results. In their wisdom, the authors of this study point out that the study sample was small and the variations in cortisol concentration make it difficult to detect differences. Furthermore, these authors note that HPA re-programming may be more evident in those with insulin resistance, as opposed to this normoglycemic population. Finally, the dexamethasone/$ACTH_{1-24}$ stimulation tests assess the adrenal level of the HPA axis, but not the CNS component. As a result, their studies do not exclude the possibility of CNS HPA reprogramming. It is intriguing that, when looking at the data from this study closely, trends exist that suggest an incremental rise in post-dexamethasone cortisol and peak cortisol post $ACTH_{1-24}$ stimulation, as well as an incremental decrease in cortisol increment post $ACTH_{1-24}$ stimulation when comparing exposure to famine in late gestation, mid gestation, and early gestation.

The theme of gender-specific HPA re-programming continues in multiple publications; among the most intriguing is a study by Kajantie et al.. which used a cohort of 7086 singleton individuals who were born between 1924 and 1933 at Helsinski University Hospital to sample for evidence of HPA reprogramming (122). Detailed records of these individuals included birth weight, length, placental weight, head circumference, and gestational age. From the original cohort, 421 individuals underwent measurement of fasting plasma cortisol and corticosteroid binding globulin levels, as well as blood pressure measurement, oral glucose tolerance tests, and body anthropometric assessment.

Similar to the previously discussed study, general gender differences were noted, including higher corticosteroid binding globulin levels in the women ($P < 0.0001$) and higher free cortisol levels in the men ($P < 0.0001$). Furthermore, positive associations between total cortisol and both current BMI ($P = 0.003$) and waist circumference ($P = 0.01$) were also noted, and a positive association between free cortisol index and both diastolic blood pressure ($P = 0.01$) and fasting glucose ($P = 0.02$) were similarly observed. In terms of birth characteristics, a significant positive association between ponderal index in both genders ($P = 0.02$ for men, $P = 0.04$ for women) and free cortisol index occurred. A unique and important finding in this study is that the associations differed based upon gestation age when subgroup analysis was performed.

In infants born before 39 weeks of gestation, both total and free cortisol negatively correlated with birth weight ($P = 0.02$ and 0.09 for birth weight, respectively) and length ($P = 0.001$ and $P = 0.02$). In infants born after 40 weeks of gestation, both total and free cortisol positively correlated with birth weight (($P = 0.06$ and 0.002 for birth weight, respectively) and ponderal index ($P = 0.003$ and 0.003 for birth weight, respectively). Multiple logistic regression analysis was used to test this interaction, which revealed that the interaction between birth weight and gestational age was statistically significant ($P = 0.01$ for total, $P = 0.003$ for free cortisol). In other words, this study suggests that either adult hyper- or hypocortisolism may occur secondary to fetal re-programming, based upon the infant's biological maturity at birth. The meaning of these findings supports the neonatologist's mantra that premature infants are different from full-term infants, and places further legitimacy upon the neonatal community's concern over the re-programming that probably occurs in the NICU.

The animal studies, to date, have focused upon the phenomenon of a fetal overexposure to glucocorticoids, with the general belief that this event programs the newborn to persistent increases in glucocorticoid hormone action. Many of the initial investigations administered dexamethasone to the pregnant animal (rat and sheep), and observed postnatal morbidities in the offspring of these pregnancies. Two of the classic studies came from the Edinburgh laboratories and involve Jonathan Seckl, one of the pioneers in the field. In the first study, pregnant female Wistar rats were given dexamethasone in either week 1, week 2, or week 3 of pregnancy (123). Dexamethasone administration during the third week of pregnancy reduced offspring birth weight ($P = 0.004$) and induced fasting hyperglycemia and hyperinsulinemia ($P = 0.03$). Interestingly, administration of dexamethasone during either the first or second week did not significantly affect either birth weight or postnatal glucose homeostasis.

In a second study, pregnant female Wistar rats were similarly exposed to dexamethasone in the last week of pregnancy and, as previously reported, the offspring of dexamethasone-exposed dams exhibited significant growth retardation (124). Interestingly, gender-specific phenotypes were noted in the adult animals. The male dexamethasone-exposed offspring were characterized by elevated levels of adrenocorticotropic hormone ($P < 0.05$), increased insulin:glucose ratios ($P < 0.05$), and increased levels of corticosterone. In contrast, the female dexamethasone-exposed offspring were characterized by hypertension ($P < 0.05$), elevated levels of plasma angiotensinogen, and increased levels of rennin activity. These results demonstrate once again that many of the phenotypic consequences of early life events are modulated by gender. Obviously, though the fetal effects of the prenatal steroids do not exactly mimic the hypoglycemic and hypoinsulinemic milieu of the IUGR fetus, these studies have been vitally important to our appreciation of the high impact of increased glucocorticoid action upon the fetus.

Two families of molecules play key roles in determining glucocorticoid hormone action. The first family of molecules is the glucocorticoid receptors. Though the product of one gene, multiple receptor subtypes exist based upon multiple promoter and exon variants, and this variation occurs to some extent in human, mice, and rats (125, 126). Though not proven definitively, studies have suggested that the teleological reason for this diversity appears to be allowance for tissue specificity and activity in response to stress. The second family of molecules is the 11β-hydroxysteroid dehydrogenases (11βHSD). 11βHSD1 functions as an 11-oxoreductase, and therefore activates cortisone by converting it to cortisol. 11βHSD2 functions as an 11-dehydrogenase and thereby deactivates cortisol. As a result, 11βHSD2 maintains aldosterone receptor specificity, particularly in the kidney.

Expression of these genes is altered in the two rat models of growth retardation that we have previously discussed. In the model of growth retardation induced by bilateral uterine artery ligation, Baserga et al. have demonstrated that uteroplacental insufficiency and subsequent IUGR increases fetal serum corticosterone levels, as well as gene expression and activation of the hepatic glucocorticoid receptor (127). Conversely, in this model, IUGR significantly decreased hepatic mRNA levels of 11βHSD1 ($P < 0.05$). Similarly, models of maternal malnutrition demonstrate that maternal diet affects the expression of these two gene families. For example, Bertram et al. provided pregnant Wistar dams with either a control diet of 18% casein or a low-protein diet composed of 9% casein throughout the pregnancy (128). As expected, the offspring of the low-protein diet dams were characterized by reduced birth weight and elevated postnatal blood pressure. In terms of the glucocorticoid receptor, mRNA and protein levels of the gene were increased in the kidney at 12 weeks of age ($P < 0.001$ for both mRNA and protein). Furthermore, the offspring of the low-protein diet dams were further characterized by decreased renal mRNA levels of 11βHSD2 at 12 weeks of age ($P < 0.001$).

One of the most interesting findings of the previous study is that the low-protein diet decreased mRNA levels of placental 11βHSD2, without affecting mRNA levels of 11βHSD1. This is consistent with previous reports that 11βHSD2 activity correlates with birth weight, as well as studies that use the 11βHSD inhibitor, carbenoxolone, to decrease birth weight. The importance of placental 11βHSD2 was further supported by a particularly important study by Holmes et al. (129). In this study, 11βHSD2 +/− mice were mated so that each pregnant female would produce +/+, +/− and −/− offspring. These pups were compared to offspring of 11βHSD2 +/+ and −/− matings. The conclusion of this study was that loss of 11βHSD2 activity in the fetoplacental unit early in life results in early life exposure to maternal glucocorticoids and subsequent programming.

What the human and animal studies teach us is that we have a great deal still to learn, but it is reasonable to deduce that glucocorticoid action plays a role in fetal programming, as well as being a target of fetal programming. Glucocorticoid action can be regulated centrally through the HPA axis, peripherally through the degradation of the steroids through aromatases, and locally through the expression of glucocorticoid receptors and the 11βHSD family of genes. This makes sense, because it allows for a great deal of specificity in the action of these powerful hormones, but also adds to the level of difficulty in understanding whether the observed programming is teleologically coordinated.

POSTNATAL NUTRITION – PARTICULARLY WITH THE PRETERM, AND THE POSSIBLE INTERVENTIONS (E.G. DIET)

The studies linking IUGR towards postnatal morbidities and changes in phenotype have increased concern in the neonatal community about the impact of the NICU experience upon the preterm infant, particularly in terms of nutrition. Preterm infants have very limited nutrient reserves at birth, and then they suffer from a variety of stressors such as infection, lung disease, and over-stimulation that increase their metabolic needs. When most preterm infants are discharged home, they are typically growth-restricted. In a large cohort study of preterm infants, Lucas et al. found that three out of four infants at discharge weighed less than the 10th percentile of the population's distributions of birth weights by gestation (130). Similarly, in a multi-center study of more than 24 000 preterm infants from 124 NICUs in North America between 1998 and 2000, the prevalence of extrauterine growth retardation at hospital discharge (<10th percentile) was 28% for weight, 34% for length, and 16% for HC (131)

Following discharge, despite the fact that premature infants consume greater volumes of milk than term infants, and therefore catch up somewhat, poor growth continues to be a significant marker of morbidity (132). For example, poor postnatal growth in preterm humans is associated with an increased risk of neurodevelopmental impairment in later childhood, as well as with less than optimal cognitive and educational outcomes(133).

Prematurity is associated with many of the issues associated with IUGR, including insulin resistance. In a carefully designed study by Hofman et al., insulin sensitivity was measured using glucose-tolerance tests in 72 healthy children, who were 4–10 years of age (134). Fifty of these children were born at less than 32 weeks of age but were appropriately sized; 12 of these children were originally both premature and IUGR. Twenty-two term control and 13 term IUGR infants were also included in the study. The insulin sensitivity for the four groups was as follows (10^{-4} per min per mU per liter): term control, 21.6; term IUGR, 15.1; premature AGA, 14.2 ($P = 0.004$ vs. term controls); and term IUGR, 12.9 ($P = 0.009$). Similarly, Bonamy et al. have observed that prematurity is associated with higher brachial and aortic blood pressures in adolescent girls (135).

Furthermore, how we feed our premature infants when they are in the NICU is a matter of debate at this juncture and, though some studies provide insight, we are still searching for specific answers. For example, O'Connor et al. studied premature infants who were fed (until reaching term) one of the following regimens: predominantly human milk, >50% human milk, <50% human milk, or predominantly formula (136). They found that infants fed predominantly formula weighed 500 g more than infants taking predominantly human milk, a difference that persisted for 6 months. Infants fed the formula were also longer and had larger head circumferences. However, there was a positive association between duration of human milk feeding and the Bayley Mental Index at 12 months chronological age, even after controlling for confounders such as home environment and maternal intelligence. In contrast, Lucas et al., in a large multicenter trial, assigned 502 low birth weight infants to receive either a preterm formula or unfortified donor breast milk as the sole diet (or as a supplement to their mothers' expressed milk) (137). Using Knobloch's developmental screening inventory, this latter study found that the mean developmental quotient was 0.25 standard deviations lower in those infants fed solely unfortified breast milk. This effect was even greater when IUGR infants were fed the unfortified breast milk.

In terms of the impact of postnatal nutrition upon postnatal metabolic phenotype of the NICU graduate, a few studies provide some insight. For example, Singhal et al. determined fasting 32–33 split proinsulin concentrations (a measure of insulin resistance) in 13–16 year olds who were former preterm infants who had been assigned to either a preterm formula (enriched) or banked breast milk/term formula (non-enriched) (138). They found that the teenagers originally fed the non-enriched diets had significantly lower fasting 32–33 split proinsulin levels. Furthermore, the fasting 32–33 proinsulin levels were associated with greater weight gain in the first 2 weeks of life ($P = 0.001$). Similarly, using the same cohort, this Singhal and Lucas research group have observed that feeding with the banked breast milk results in lower blood pressure ($P = 0.001$), a lower LDL:HDL ratio ($P = 0.03$), and a higher leptin to fat mass ratio ($P = 0.007$) (139–141).

The bottom line is that we are slowly becoming aware that our preterm infants are at risk for many of the same issues that the IUGR infants endure. The impact from prematurity has been harder to appreciate because of the confounding factors and the relative youth of neonatology as a field. A pursuit that is going to become of greater import in the next several years is the understanding of how nutrition may modulate the long-term morbidities, and whether we can individualize the nutritional approach based upon the infants' specific risk factors.

MOLECULAR MECHANISMS

Apoptosis

Overview of Apoptosis

Apoptosis and cell cycle arrest in the G1 interval represent two distinct means of cellular growth arrest that result in the inability of a cell to enter S phase. Apoptosis is an evolutionarily conserved mechanism employed by all multicellular organisms in the regulation of growth and differentiation. There are two primary recognized pathways of apoptosis: the intrinsic and extrinsic apoptotic pathways. The intrinsic pathway is signaled by a number of intracellular signals generated in response to hypoxia, DNA damage, *cis* or *trans* activation of oncogenes, or with a limited threshold signal down growth factor cascades. During extrinsic, or activation-induced apoptosis, extracellular agents engage a partially defined cascade of intracellular signal transducers that couple biochemical and gene regulatory signals to induce a series of morphologic changes. Both pathways ultimately result in chromatin condensation and internucleosomal cleavage of DNA (142, 143). In sharp contrast to programmed cell death (apoptosis), cells that become growth-arrested in the G1 phase remain viable, and DNA remains intact. Accumulating evidence suggests that a number of common genes along the p53, calcineurin/calmodulin, and IGF/insulin-inducible pathways are involved in regulating these distinct pathways (144–146). Thus, cellular fate is likely to be determined by a common set of transducing molecules, and subsequent control of cellular proliferation, growth arrest or apoptosis is exerted through the generation or inhibition of additional survival or death signals.

In most cell types, morphologic changes associated with apoptosis ultimately culminate in chromatin condensation, followed by widespread cleavage of nuclear DNA into oligonucleosomal-sized fragments. In addition, early evidence in lymphocytic and transformed cell lines demonstrated that internucleosomal DNA fragmentation is preceded by initial cleavage of chromatin into high-molecular-weight fragments of 200–250 and/or 30–50 kbp (147, 148). This event is subsequently followed by further degradation of the 50-kbp fragments into the characteristic laddering pattern observed following extensive endonucleolytic degradation into oligonucleosomal fragments. Thus the collective data suggest that latent endonucleases capable of internucleosomal cleavage exist in the nuclei of non-apoptotic cells, and that it is probably nuclease derepression which provides cell-specific sensitivity to different apoptotic-inducing agents.

Of interest to our understanding of chromatin remodeling and histone modifications (see below), these processes are further regulated by NADP[H]-dependent histone-modifying enzymes (149). In lymphocytic cells, it has been shown that the exposure of resting lymphocytes to agents capable of either increasing the rate of DNA strand breakage, or inhibiting DNA excision and repair similarly accelerates NAD consumption (150, 151). The formation of intracellular DNA strand breaks activates DNA repair mechanisms that involve the poly(ADP)ribosylation of nuclear proteins via nuclear poly(ADP-ribose) synthetase (147). Nuclear poly(ADP-ribose) synthetase enzyme catalyzes the transfer of the ADP moiety of NAD to existing nuclear proteins, which results in decreased DNA binding affinity and subsequent repression of apoptosis (153).

Signaling for Apoptosis

In response to either intrinsic or extrinsic signals, cells attempt to repair and defend; if unsuccessful they will undergo apoptotic death. Ultimately each of these pathways signal through the tumor suppressor p53, which functions as a key integrator of apoptotic signals. p53 is regarded as the "genome guardianot," and functions to sense and integrate intrinsic cellular damage signals to enable either growth arrest for DNA damage repair, or apoptosis for cell death. Ultimately these signals must collectively converge on the mitochondria to mediate either repair mechanisms or the endonuclease-dependent apoptotic processes as described above.

Prior to convergence proximal to the mitochondria, a critical step in inhibition or induction of apoptosis relies upon the balance of pro- and anti-apoptotic mechanisms. It is now recognized that the BCL2 family of proteins ultimately control the fate of the mitochondria with the differential regulation of their pro-apoptotic arm (pore-forming proteins, e.g., Bax, BAK, BID, PUMA, NOXA, and BIM) and anti-apoptotic arm (e.g., BCL2 and BCL-XL) (154). Coordinate functioning of these proteins is the apoptotic signaling "sensitizer" Myc. Suffice it to say, Myc is capable of sensitizing to apoptosis at any point in the cell cycle in the absence of de novo translation as a result of its ability to function as a transcriptional activator of apoptotic activators or their repressors.

Downstream events enable or repress the relocalization of Bax from its endogenous location in the cytoplasm to the outer mitochondrial membrane. Following relocalization and homo-oligomerization, cytochrome c is released from the mitochondria, which then functions via binding of Apaf-1 and a cascade of cleavage-mediated activation of the caspase family of proteases (155). Ultimately the caspaces converge on critical cellular substrates including poly(ADP-ribose) polymerases (PARP), actin, and pRb.

Apoptosis in Mammalian Development and Nutrition

Apoptosis is important in both placental development and fetal organogenesis. During a normal pregnancy, placental apoptosis typically occurs early (5–7 weeks) as well as in the third trimester. In pregnancies complicated by IUGR, placental apoptosis appears to be increased, which is associated with increased placental levels of p53 and decreased levels of BCL-2 proteins. Because IGF-1 has anti-apoptotic properties, lower levels of IGF-1 or the muted IGF-1 signaling discussed above may be a mechanistic link. Of course, because the placenta secretes placental growth hormone, we are left in the typical conundrum of this field: do lower IGF-1 levels allow increased placental apoptosis, or does increased placental apoptosis lead to decreased IGF-1 levels?

IGF-1 and IGF-2 have been shown to function as survival factors for multiple cell types both in vitro and in vivo, including myoblasts, neurons, cardiac mycotyes, and oligodendrocytes. A number of lines of converging evidence suggest that at the cellular level IGF-1 modulates Myc-sensitization towards apoptosis; this effect is predictable independent of de novo synthesis and cell cycle phase (155). In vivo, IGF-1 and IGF-2 similarly mediate gonadotropin action, including prevention of apoptosis during ovarian folliculogenesis (156).

Recent evidence suggests that there exists a link between nutritional constraints and caloric restriction, epigenetic mechanisms, and mammalian cell survival along the p53 pathway. In the rat, uteroplacental insufficiency resulting in IUGR increases neural and renal apoptosis and alters p53 gene methylation and MDM2 phosphorylation (108, 157, 158). MDM2 both inactivates p53 and is a target of p53's transcriptional factor. As a result, MDM2 serves to provide negative feedback to p53. One of the most important findings in these studies of IUGR and p53 is that the relationship between p53 and MDM2 is disrupted in the fetus, which potentially explains the predisposition of the immature animal to suffer apoptosis versus the postnatal animal.

Furthermore, these changes were further related to alterations in key epigenetic determinants, including DNMT1 (158). Of interest, others have employed an intermittent high-altitude hypoxia model of cardiac ischemia in neonatal rats to examine the influence of neonatal weight on cardiac ischemia (159). In these authors' model, the ability of ischemic preconditioning to induce neonatal cardiac protections under hypoxic conditions was dependent on birth weight: low birth weight animals failed to experience cardiac ischemic protection. Similarly, when in utero stress conditions were induced in pregnant animals with non-conditionable restraints the offspring were marginally growth-restricted (160). However, such a marginal physiologic effect was accompanied by profound alterations along the HPA axis. Furthermore, prenatal stress resulted in a decrease in brain cell proliferation with a concomitant increase in hippocampal caspase activity and BDNF expression (160). Taken together, these studies suggest that in utero insults associated with fetal growth restriction influence p53-dependent and independent apoptotic pathways in an epigenetic-mediated fashion.

Finally, further clues into these processes ex utero have recently emerged. It has long been appreciated that adult caloric restriction delays the onset of numerous age-associated diseases such as cancer, metabolic disorders, and atherosclerotic disease. In lower eukaryotes, restriction manifests as extension of aging, which is thought to result from the cumulative effects of cell loss over time (154). In higher eukaryotes, the cumulative effects of cell loss (apoptosis) have been implicated in degenerative disorders (neural and non-neural), as well as metabolic and atherosclerotic diseases. In their landmark study, Cohen et al. linked these two processes to demonstrate that caloric restriction promotes mammalian cell survival by induction of the SIRT1 Class III histone deacetylase (HDAC), which in turn blocks calorie-restriction-mediated attenuation of apoptosis (154). Of interest to our prior discussion, it has also been well appreciated that mutation in the IGF-1 pathway can extend life-span in a number of organisms in a SIRT1-dependent fashion (161). Similarly, the Sir2 Class III HDAC has now been shown to play an essential role in mediating cardiac myocyte cell survival. Moreover, overexpression of Sir2a protects cardiac myocytes from apoptosis to cause modest hypertrophy (162).

In summary, a number of lines of evidence have converged to bring us to our current understanding that the balance of cellular death and proliferation is under the influence of both the in utero environment, as well as ex utero stress and nutrition conditions. Of interest to the discussion to follow, emerging evidence suggests that the molecular mechanisms regulating these responses are under epigenetic influence. As we will see in our further discussion, the point of convergence between in utero and post-natal nutritional constraints are probably largely influenced by chromatin remodeling and epigenetic influences along the one carbon metabolism pathway, as well as NADPH-, NADP-dependent apoptotic pathways.

Epigenetics

Overview of Epigenetics

While genomic DNA is the template of our heredity, it is the orchestration and regulation of its expression that ultimately results in a complexity and diversity unique among eukaryotic organisms. In recent years, an emerging body of evidence has focused on the role of "epigenetic phenomena" in the modulation of gene expression.

Epigenetic modulation (*epi* meaning *upon*) refers to a heritable change in the pattern of gene expression that is mediated by mechanisms other than alterations in the primary nucleotide sequence, which ultimately produces meaningful patterns of gene expression. Epigenetic phenomena are a fundamental feature of mammalian development that cause heritable and persistent changes in gene expression without altering DNA sequence (163–165). The mechanisms behind these phenomena involve epigenetic determinants of chromatin structure such as DNA methylation and covalent modifications of histones. The methylation of the C-5 position of cytosine occurs in 60–90% of CpG dinucleotides within the vertebrate genome (166). DNA methylation is not random, and stretches of CpG-rich DNA called CpG islands are often unmethylated (166). CpG islands are usually 0.2–1 kb in length and are often found in association with housekeeping and tissue-specific genes (167). DNA methylation of these CpG dinucleotides affects transcription factor binding and results in altered mRNA transcription (168). Paradoxically, CpG methylation in a promoter region generally decreases expression, whereas CpG methylation in a downstream coding region is associated with increased expression (169).

Covalent modifications of histone tails through methylation and acetylation provide a tertiary level of variation through which chromatin structure further regulates transcriptional factor contact points with DNA (170, 171). The effects of methylation of histone H3 and H4 are not straightforward. For example, methylation of histone H3 lysine 9 (K9) generally silences gene expression by contributing to chromatin condensation and gene inactivation; in contrast, methylation of histone H3 lysine 4 (K4) opens chromatin and increases gene expression (170). Similarly, acetylation of histone H3 and H4 generally increases expression by activating chromatin (170, 172). Two mechanisms appear active in this process (171). The first mechanism involves hyperacetylation of histone H3 and H4 over tens of kb and provides an increased potential for transcription. The second mechanism involves "local" acetylation of histone H3 and histone H4 to initiate the transcription of inducible genes. Modification of these epigenetic determinants of chromatin structure is a basic mechanism through which a cell can affect the expression of a gene, or a group of genes, over an extended period.

Epigenetic Modifications, Chromatin Remodeling, and Adult Consequences of in utero Events

Recent animal studies suggest that epigenetic phenomena may be one of the mechanisms that link early life events and latter phenotype. This concept makes sense in the sense that multiple signaling pathways converge upon histones, and that the epigenetic characteristic of persistence allows the link between an early life event and an adult morbidity (173). Both models of IUGR in the rat, maternal malnutrition and uteroplacental insufficiency, have been utilized. Altered epigenetics characteristics have been found in the IUGR kidney, brain, and liver (108, 174).

Because of its ease of use and its relevance within the context of insulin resistance, the majority of work has occurred in the liver. For example, using the model of maternal malnutrition, Lillycrop et al. found that the DNA methylation status and hepatic mRNA levels of the glucocorticoid receptor and peroxisomal proliferator-activated receptor alpha were altered through the first six days of life in the IUGR rat (175).

Using the model of uteroplacental insufficiency, Fu et al. have performed two types of studies. First, this group has focused upon the general characteristics of hepatic chromatin structure and the mechanisms through which these changes occur. In general, IUGR altered hepatocyte levels of methyl-donors (e.g. S-adenosyl methionine), as well as the expression and localization of the chromatin-modifying enzymes, such as Dnmt1 and histone deacetylase I (HDAC1), in a way that was consistent with the decreased DNA methylation and histone hyperacetylation they observed. Second, Fu et al. have demonstrated that IUGR alters the epigenetic characteristics of specific hepatic genes throughout the lifetime of the rat (176). Genes noted to be altered by IUGR in the rat are PPAR gamma co-activator-1, carnitine palmitoyl transferase-1, and dual-specificity phosphatase 5 (DUSP5) (177).

Changes in the latter gene have been noted at up to 120 days of life and, as in the human, are gender-specific.

The latter finding of altered DUSP5 epigenetics and expression was particularly interesting because DUSP5 modulates MAP kinase signaling, an important determinant of both cell survival, which would be important during the initial insult, and hepatic insulin sensitivity, which potentially leads to the morbidity of insulin resistance. For many investigators, the goal has been to identify a specific gene that couples the adaptation to the adult phenotype. As a result, many groups focus upon a specific effector molecule that directly impacts glucose or fat metabolism and subsequently suggest that the affected process is essentially on or off, which directly causes the adult morbidity. The findings of Fu et al. involving DUSP5 suggest a subtle variation in the theme, in that IUGR potentially shifts the sensitivity of Erk signaling by affecting DUSP5 epigenetics and subsequent mRNA expression. This shift in a signaling pathway upstream of several key cellular processes may thereby initiate a relatively coordinated adaptation by the cell.

In summary, data are beginning to emerge that suggest that epigenetic modifications of chromatin structure, such as DNA methylation and histone modifications, may play a role in the postnatal morbidity plaguing the infant with poor growth and nutrition. This is a particularly interesting arena of research because if an intervention affects these epigenetic modifications, a significant change in phenotype is possible. One of the questions that should haunt the field will be whether these changes are good or bad. In other words, if we turn off a "bad" gene by nonspecifically altering chromatin structure through diet, we may be also turning off a "good" gene or turning on a "bad" gene.

REFERENCES

1. Painter RC, Roseboom TJ, Bleker OP. Prenatal exposure to the Dutch famine and disease in later life: an overview. Reprod Toxicol 2005; 20:345–352.
2. Roseboom TJ, van der Meulen JH, Osmond C, et al. Plasma lipid profiles in adults after prenatal exposure to the Dutch famine. Am J Clin Nutr 2000; 72:1101–1106.
3. de Rooij SR, Painter RC, Phillips DI, et al. Hypothalamic-pituitary-adrenal axis activity in adults who were prenatally exposed to the Dutch famine. Eur J Endocrinol 2006; 155:153–160.
4. Roseboom TJ, Van Der Meulen JH, Ravelli AC, et al. Perceived health of adults after prenatal exposure to the Dutch famine. Paediatr Perinat Epidemiol 2003; 17:391–397.
5. Painter RC, Roseboom TJ, van Montfrans GA, et al. Microalbuminuria in adults after prenatal exposure to the Dutch famine. J Am Soc Nephrol 2005; 16:189–194.
6. Lopuhaa CE, Roseboom TJ, Osmond C, et al. Atopy, lung function, and obstructive airways disease after prenatal exposure to famine. Thorax 2000; 55:555–561.
7. Ravelli AC, van der Meulen JH, Michels RP, et al. Glucose tolerance in adults after prenatal exposure to famine. Lancet 1998; 351:173–177.
8. Ravelli GP, Stein ZA, Susser MW. Obesity in young men after famine exposure in utero and early infancy. N Engl J Med 1976; 295:349–353.
9. Susser E, Neugebauer R, Hoek HW, et al. Schizophrenia after prenatal famine. Further evidence. Arch Gen Psychiatry 1996; 53:25–31.
10. Roseboom TJ, van der Meulen JH, Osmond C, et al. Adult survival after prenatal exposure to the Dutch famine 1944–45. Paediatr Perinat Epidemiol 2001; 15:220–225.
11. Barker DJ, Osmond C. Infant mortality, childhood nutrition, and ischaemic heart disease in England and Wales. Lancet 1986; 1:1077–1081.
12. Barker DJ, Winter PD, Osmond C, et al. Weight in infancy and death from ischaemic heart disease. Lancet 1989; 2:577–580.
13. Hales CN, Barker DJ, Clark PM, et al. Fetal and infant growth and impaired glucose tolerance at age 64. BMJ 1991; 303:1019–1022.
14. Syddall HE, Sayer AA, Simmonds SJ, et al. Birth weight, infant weight gain, and cause-specific mortality: the Hertfordshire Cohort Study. Am J Epidemiol 2005; 161:1074–1080.
15. Stampfer MJ, Colditz GA, Willett WC, et al. A prospective study of moderate alcohol drinking and risk of diabetes in women. Am J Epidemiol 1988; 128:549–558.
16. Rich-Edwards JW, Colditz GA, Stampfer MJ, et al. Birthweight and the risk for type 2 diabetes mellitus in adult women. Ann Intern Med 1999; 130:278–284.
17. Troy LM, Michels KB, Hunter DJ, et al. Self-reported birthweight and history of having been breastfed among younger women: an assessment of validity. Int J Epidemiol 1996; 25:122–127.

18. Rich-Edwards JW, Stampfer MJ, Manson JE, et al. Birth weight and risk of cardiovascular disease in a cohort of women followed up since 1976. BMJ 1997; 315:396–400.

19. Mericq V, Ong KK, Bazaes R, et al. Longitudinal changes in insulin sensitivity and secretion from birth to age three years in small- and appropriate-for-gestational-age children. Diabetologia 2005; 48:2609–2614.

20. Veening MA, Van Weissenbruch MM, Delemarre-Van De Waal HA. Glucose tolerance, insulin sensitivity, and insulin secretion in children born small for gestational age. J Clin Endocrinol Metab 2002; 87:4657–4661.

21. Arends NJ, Boonstra VH, Duivenvoorden HJ, et al. Reduced insulin sensitivity and the presence of cardiovascular risk factors in short prepubertal children born small for gestational age (SGA). Clin Endocrinol (Oxf) 2005; 62:44–50.

22. Chessex P, Reichman B, Verellen G, et al. Metabolic consequences of intrauterine growth retardation in very low birthweight infants. Pediatr Res 1984; 18:709–713.

23. Jornayvaz FR, Selz R, Tappy L, Theintz GE. Metabolism of oral glucose in children born small for gestational age: evidence for an impaired whole body glucose oxidation. Metabolism 2004; 53:847–851.

24. Soto N, Bazaes RA, Pena V, et al. Insulin sensitivity and secretion are related to catch-up growth in small-for-gestational-age infants at age 1 year: results from a prospective cohort. J Clin Endocrinol Metab 2003; 88:3645–3650.

25. Zhang Y, Proenca R, Maffei M, et al. Positional cloning of the mouse obese gene and its human homologue. Nature 1994; 372:425–432.

26. Hardie L, Trayhurn P, Abramovich D, Fowler P. Circulating leptin in women: a longitudinal study in the menstrual cycle and during pregnancy. Clin Endocrinol (Oxf) 1997; 47:101–106.

27. Jaquet D, Leger J, Levy-Marchal C, et al. Ontogeny of leptin in human fetuses and newborns: effect of intrauterine growth retardation on serum leptin concentrations. J Clin Endocrinol Metab 1998; 83:1243–1246.

28. Ong KK, Ahmed ML, Sherriff A, et al. Cord blood leptin is associated with size at birth and predicts infancy weight gain in humans. ALSPAC Study Team. Avon Longitudinal Study of Pregnancy and Childhood. J Clin Endocrinol Metab 1999; 84:1145–1148.

29. Masuzaki H, Ogawa Y, Isse N, et al. Human obese gene expression. Adipocyte-specific expression and regional differences in the adipose tissue. Diabetes 1995; 44:855–858.

30. Schubring C, Kiess W, Englaro P, et al. Levels of leptin in maternal serum, amniotic fluid, and arterial and venous cord blood: relation to neonatal and placental weight. J Clin Endocrinol Metab 1997; 82:1480–1483.

31. Bouret SG, Draper SJ, Simerly RB. Trophic action of leptin on hypothalamic neurons that regulate feeding. Science 2004; 304:108–110.

32. Pighetti M, Tommaselli GA, D'Elia A, et al. Maternal serum and umbilical cord blood leptin concentrations with fetal growth restriction. Obstet Gynecol 2003; 102:535–543.

33. Iniguez G, Soto N, Avila A, et al. Adiponectin levels in the first two years of life in a prospective cohort: relations with weight gain, leptin levels and insulin sensitivity. J Clin Endocrinol Metab 2004; 89:5500–5503.

34. Martinez-Cordero C, Amador-Licona N, Guizar-Mendoza JM, et al. Body fat at birth and cord blood levels of insulin, adiponectin, leptin, and insulin-like growth factor-I in small-for-gestational-age infants. Arch Med Res 2006; 37:490–494.

35. Fernandez-Twinn DS, Ozanne SE, Ekizoglou S, et al. The maternal endocrine environment in the low-protein model of intra-uterine growth restriction. Br J Nutr 2003; 90:815–822.

36. Krechowec SO, Vickers M, Gertler A, Breier BH. Prenatal influences on leptin sensitivity and susceptibility to diet-induced obesity. J Endocrinol 2006; 189:355–363.

37. Yamauchi T, Kamon J, Ito Y, et al. Cloning of adiponectin receptors that mediate antidiabetic metabolic effects. Nature 2003; 423:762–769.

38. Maeda K, Okubo K, Shimomura I, et al. cDNA cloning and expression of a novel adipose specific collagen-like factor, apM1 (AdiPose Most abundant Gene transcrip. 1). Biochem Biophys Res Commun 1996; 221:286–289.

39. Saito K, Tobe T, Minoshima S, et al. Organization of the gene for gelatin-binding protein (GBP28). Gene 1999; 229:67–73.

40. Lopez-Bermejo A, Casano-Sancho P, Fernandez-Real JM, et al. Both intrauterine growth restriction and postnatal growth influence childhood serum concentrations of adiponectin. Clin Endocrinol (Oxf) 2004; 61:339–346.

41. Cianfarani S, Martinez C, Maiorana A, et al. Adiponectin levels are reduced in children born small for gestational age and are inversely related to postnatal catch-up growth. J Clin Endocrinol Metab 2004; 89:1346–1351.

42. Jaquet D, Deghmoun S, Chevenne D, et al. Low serum adiponectin levels in subjects born small for gestational age: impact on insulin sensitivity. Int J Obes (Lond) 2006; 30:83–87.

43. Rajkumar K, Barron D, Lewitt MS, Murphy LJ. Growth retardation and hyperglycemia in insulin-like growth factor binding protein-1 transgenic mice. Endocrinology 1995; 136:4029–4034.

44. Woods KA, Camacho-Hubner C, Savage MO, Clark AJ. Intrauterine growth retardation and post-natal growth failure associated with deletion of the insulin-like growth factor I gene. N Engl J Med 1996; 335:1363–1367.

45. Juul A, Scheike T, Davidsen M, et al. Low serum insulin-like growth factor I is associated with increased risk of ischemic heart disease: a population-based case-control study. Circulation 2002; 106:939–944.

46. Isaksson OG, Jansson JO, Sjogren K, Ohlsson C. Metabolic functions of liver-derived (endocrine) insulin-like growth factor I. Horm Res 2001; 55(Suppl 2):18–21.

47. Guler HP, Zapf J, Froesch ER. Short-term metabolic effects of recombinant human insulin-like growth factor I in healthy adults. N Engl J Med 1987; 317:137–140.

48. Woods KA, Camacho-Hubner C, Bergman RN, et al. Effects of insulin-like growth factor I (IGF-I) therapy on body composition and insulin resistance in IGF-I gene deletion. J Clin Endocrinol Metab 2000; 85:1407–1411.

49. Moran A, Jacobs DR Jr, Steinberger J, et al. Association between the insulin resistance of puberty and the insulin-like growth factor-I/growth hormone axis. J Clin Endocrinol Metab 2002; 87:4817–4820.

50. Westwood M, Gibson JM, Sooranna SR, et al. Genes or placenta as modulator of fetal growth: evidence from the insulin-like growth factor axis in twins with discordant growth. Mol Hum Reprod 2001; 7:387–395.

51. Laviola L, Perrini S, Belsanti G, et al. Intrauterine growth restriction in humans is associated with abnormalities in placental insulin-like growth factor signaling. Endocrinology 2005; 146:1498–1505.

52. Ozkan H, Aydin A, Demir N, Erci T, Buyukgebiz A. Associations of IGF-I, IGFBP-1 and IGFBP-3 on intrauterine growth and early catch-up growth. Biol Neonate 1999; 76:274–282.

53. Fattal-Valevski A, Toledano-Alhadef H, Golander A, et al. Endocrine profile of children with intrauterine growth retardation. J Pediatr Endocrinol Metab 2005; 18:671–676.

54. Fall CH, Pandit AN, Law CM, et al. Size at birth and plasma insulin-like growth factor-1 concentrations. Arch Dis Child 1995; 73:287–293.

55. Tenhola S, Halonen P, Jaaskelainen J, Voutilainen R. Serum markers of GH and insulin action in 12-year-old children born small for gestational age. Eur J Endocrinol 2005; 152:335–340.

56. Verkauskiene R, Jaquet D, Deghmoun S, et al. Smallness for gestational age is associated with persistent change in insulin-like growth factor I (IGF-I) and the ratio of IGF-I/IGF-binding protein-3 in adulthood. J Clin Endocrinol Metab 2005; 90:5672–5676.

57. Kajantie E, Fall CH, Seppala M, et al. Serum insulin-like growth factor (IGF)-I and IGF-binding protein-1 in elderly people: relationships with cardiovascular risk factors, body composition, size at birth, and childhood growth. J Clin Endocrinol Metab 2003; 88:1059–1065.

58. Ben-Shlomo Y, Holly J, McCarthy A, et al. An investigation of fetal, postnatal and childhood growth with insulin-like growth factor I and binding protein 3 in adulthood. Clin Endocrinol (Oxf) 2003; 59:366–373.

59. Elias SG, Keinan-Boker L, Peeters PH, et al. Long term consequences of the 1944–1945 Dutch famine on the insulin-like growth factor axis. Int J Cancer 2004; 108:628–630.

60. Gunnell D, Miller LL, Rogers I, Holly JM. Association of insulin-like growth factor I and insulin-like growth factor-binding protein-3 with intelligence quotient among 8- to 9-year-old children in the Avon Longitudinal Study of Parents and Children. Pediatrics 2005; 116:e681–e686.

61. Darnaudery M, Perez-Martin M, Belizaire G, et al. Insulin-like growth factor 1 reduces age-related disorders induced by prenatal stress in female rats. Neurobiol Aging 2006; 27:119–127.

62. Ogata ES, Bussey ME, Finley S. Altered gas exchange, limited glucose and branched chain amino acids, and hypoinsulinism retard fetal growth in the rat. Metabolism 1986; 35:970–977.

63. Ogata ES, Bussey ME, LaBarbera A, Finley S. Altered growth, hypoglycemia, hypoalaninemia, and ketonemia in the young rat: postnatal consequences of intrauterine growth retardation. Pediatr Res 1985; 19:32–37.

64. Economides DL, Nicolaides KH, Campbell S. Metabolic and endocrine findings in appropriate and small for gestational age fetuses. J Perinat Med 1991; 19:97–105.

65. Economides DL, Nicolaides KH, Gahl WA, et al. Plasma amino acids in appropriate- and small-for-gestational-age fetuses. Am J Obstet Gynecol 1989; 161:1219–1227.

66. Nicolaides KH, Economides DL, Soothill PW. Blood gases, pH, and lactate in appropriate- and small-for-gestational- age fetuses. Am J Obstet Gynecol 1989; 161:996–1001.

67. Economides DL, Nicolaides KH, Gahl WA, et al. Cordocentesis in the diagnosis of intrauterine starvation. Am J Obstet Gynecol 1989; 161:1004–1008.

68. Economides DL, Nicolaides KH. Blood glucose and oxygen tension levels in small-for-gestational-age fetuses. Am J Obstet Gynecol 1989; 160:385–389.

69. Simmons RA, Templeton LJ, Gertz SJ. Intrauterine growth retardation leads to the development of type 2 diabetes in the rat. Diabetes 2001; 50:2279–2286.

70. Tsirka AE, Gruetzmacher EM, Kelley DE, et al. Myocardial gene expression of glucose transporter 1 and glucose transporter 4 in response to uteroplacental insufficiency in the rat. J Endocrinol 2001; 169:373–380.

71. Vileisis RA, D'Ercole AJ. Tissue and serum concentrations of somatomedin-C/insulin-like growth factor I in fetal rats made growth retarded by uterine artery ligation. Pediatr Res 1986; 20:126–130.

72. Houdijk EC, Engelbregt MJ, Popp-Snijders C, Delemarre-Vd Waal HA. Endocrine regulation and extended follow up of longitudinal growth in intrauterine growth-retarded rats. J Endocrinol 2000; 166:599–608.

73. Bernstein IM, DeSouza MM, Copeland KC. Insulin-like growth factor I in substrate-deprived, growth-retarded fetal rats. Pediatr Res 1991; 30:154–157.

74. Woodall SM, Breier BH, Johnston BM, Gluckman PD. A model of intrauterine growth retardation caused by chronic maternal undernutrition in the rat: effects on the somatotrophic axis and postnatal growth. J Endocrinol 1996; 150:231–242.

75. Woodall SM, Bassett NS, Gluckman PD, Breier BH. Consequences of maternal undernutrition for fetal and postnatal hepatic insulin-like growth factor-I, growth hormone receptor

and growth hormone binding protein gene regulation in the rat. J Mol Endocrinol 1998; 20:313–326.

76. Dudev T, Lim C. Principles governing Mg, Ca, and Zn binding and selectivity in proteins. Chem Rev 2003; 103:773–788.

77. Vallee BL, Falchuk KH. The biochemical basis of zinc physiology. Physiol Rev 1993; 73:79–118.

78. Loui A, Raab A, Obladen M, Bratter P. Nutritional zinc balance in extremely low-birth-weight infants. J Pediatr Gastroenterol Nutr 2001; 32:438–442.

79. Simmer K, Thompson RP. Zinc in the fetus and newborn. Acta Paediatr Scand Suppl 1985; 319:158–163.

80. Simmer K, Thompson RP. Maternal zinc and intrauterine growth retardation. Clin Sci (Lond) 1985; 68:395–399.

81. Higashi A, Tajiri A, Matsukura M, Matsuda I. A prospective survey of serial maternal serum zinc levels and pregnancy outcome. J Pediatr Gastroenterol Nutr 1988; 7:430–433.

82. Neggers YH, Cutter GR, Acton RT, et al. A positive association between maternal serum zinc concentration and birth weight. Am J Clin Nutr 1990; 51:678–684.

83. Neggers YH, Cutter GR, Alvarez JO, et al. The relationship between maternal serum zinc levels during pregnancy and birthweight. Early Hum Dev 1991; 25:75–85.

84. Simmer K, Lort-Phillips L, James C, Thompson RP. A double-blind trial of zinc supplementation in pregnancy. Eur J Clin Nutr 1991; 45:139–144.

85. Brown KH, Peerson JM, Rivera J, Allen LH. Effect of supplemental zinc on the growth and serum zinc concentrations of prepubertal children: a meta-analysis of randomized controlled trials. Am J Clin Nutr 2002; 75:1062–1071.

86. Yu ZP, Le GW, Shi YH. Effect of zinc sulphate and zinc methionine on growth, plasma growth hormone concentration, growth hormone receptor and insulin-like growth factor-I gene expression in mice. Clin Exp Pharmacol Physiol 2005; 32:273–278.

87. Murphy LJ, Bell GI, Friesen HG. Tissue distribution of insulin-like growth factor I and II messenger ribonucleic acid in the adult rat. Endocrinology 1987; 120:1279–1282.

88. D'Ercole AJ, Stiles AD, Underwood LE. Tissue concentrations of somatomedin C: further evidence for multiple sites of synthesis and paracrine or autocrine mechanisms of action. Proc Natl Acad Sci USA 1984; 81:935–939.

89. Devine A, Rosen C, Mohan S, et al. Effects of zinc and other nutritional factors on insulin-like growth factor I and insulin-like growth factor binding proteins in postmenopausal women. Am J Clin Nutr 1998; 68:200–206.

90. Nakamura T, Nishiyama S, Futagoishi-Suginohara Y, et al. Mild to moderate zinc deficiency in short children: effect of zinc supplementation on linear growth velocity. J Pediatr 1993; 123:65–69.

91. Ninh NX, Thissen JP, Collette L, et al. Zinc supplementation increases growth and circulating insulin-like growth factor I (IGF-I) in growth-retarded Vietnamese children. Am J Clin Nutr 1996; 63:514–519.

92. Hershkovitz E, Printzman L, Segev Y, Levy J, Phillip M. Zinc supplementation increases the level of serum insulin-like growth factor-I but does not promote growth in infants with nonorganic failure to thrive. Horm Res 1999; 52:200–204.

93. Doherty CP, Crofton PM, Sarkar MA, et al. Malnutrition, zinc supplementation and catch-up growth: changes in insulin-like growth factor I, its binding proteins, bone formation and collagen turnover. Clin Endocrinol (Oxf) 2002; 57:391–399.

94. Roth HP, Kirchgessner M. Influence of alimentary zinc deficiency on the concentration of growth hormone (GH), insulin-like growth factor I (IGF-I) and insulin in the serum of force-fed rats. Horm Metab Res 1994; 26:404–408.

95. Dorup I, Flyvbjerg A, Everts ME, Clausen T. Role of insulin-like growth factor-1 and growth hormone in growth inhibition induced by magnesium and zinc deficiencies. Br J Nutr 1991; 66:505–521.

96. Ninh NX, Thissen JP, Maiter D, et al. Reduced liver insulin-like growth factor-I gene expression in young zinc-deprived rats is associated with a decrease in liver growth hormone (GH) receptors and serum GH-binding protein. J Endocrinol 1995; 144:449–456.

97. McNall AD, Etherton TD, Fosmire GJ. The impaired growth induced by zinc deficiency in rats is associated with decreased expression of the hepatic insulin-like growth factor I and growth hormone receptor genes. J Nutr 1995; 125:874–879.

98. Ninh NX, Maiter D, Lause P, et al. Continuous administration of growth hormone does not prevent the decrease of IGF-I gene expression in zinc-deprived rats despite normalization of liver GH binding. Growth Horm IGF Res 1998; 8:465–472.

99. Mathews LS, Enberg B, Norstedt G. Regulation of rat growth hormone receptor gene expression. J Biol Chem 1989; 264:9905–9910.

100. Tiong TS, Herington AC. Ontogeny of messenger RNA for the rat growth hormone receptor and serum binding protein. Mol Cell Endocrinol 1992; 83:133–141.

101. Wallenius K, Sjogren K, Peng XD, et al. Liver-derived IGF-I regulates GH secretion at the pituitary level in mice. Endocrinology 2001; 142:4762–4770.

102. Hinchliffe SA, Lynch MR, Sargent PH, et al. The effect of intrauterine growth retardation on the development of renal nephrons. Br J Obstet Gynaecol 1992; 99:296–301.

103. Hinchliffe SA, Sargent PH, Howard CV, et al. Human intrauterine renal growth expressed in absolute number of glomeruli assessed by the disector method and Cavalieri principle. Lab Invest 1991; 64:777–784.

104. Manalich R, Reyes L, Herrera M, et al. Relationship between weight at birth and the number and size of renal glomeruli in humans: a histomorphometric study. Kidney Int 2000; 58:770–773.

105. Horta BL, Barros FC, Victora CG, Cole TJ. Early and late growth and blood pressure in adolescence. J Epidemiol Community Health 2003; 57:226–230.

106. Law CM, Shiell AW, Newsome CA, et al. Fetal, infant, and childhood growth and adult blood pressure: a longitudinal study from birth to 22 years of age. Circulation 2002; 105:1088–1092.

107. Ramirez SP, Hsu SI, McClellan W. Low body weight is a risk factor for proteinuria in multiracial Southeast Asian pediatric population. Am J Kidney Dis 2001; 38:1045–1054.

108. Pham TD, MacLennan NK, Chiu CT, et al. Uteroplacental insufficiency increases apoptosis and alters p53 gene methylation in the full term IUGR rat kidney. Am J Physiol Regul Integr Comp Physiol 2003; 285:R962–R970.

109. Merlet-Benichou C, Gilbert T, Muffat-Joly M, et al. Intrauterine growth retardation leads to a permanent nephron deficit in the rat. Pediatr Nephrol 1994; 8:175–180.

110. Welham SJ, Wade A, Woolf AS. Protein restriction in pregnancy is associated with increased apoptosis of mesenchymal cells at the start of rat metanephrogenesis. Kidney Int 2002; 61:1231–1242.

111. Vehaskari VM, Aviles DH, Manning J. Prenatal programming of adult hypertension in the rat. Kidney Int 2001; 59:238–245.

112. Schreuder MF, van Wijk JA, Delemarre-van de Waal HA. Intrauterine growth restriction increases blood pressure and central pulse pressure measured with telemetry in aging rats. J Hypertens 2006; 24:1337–1343.

113. Leeson CP, Whincup PH, Cook DG, et al. Flow-mediated dilation in 9- to 11-year-old children: the influence of intrauterine and childhood factors. Circulation 1997; 96:2233–2238.

114. Leeson CP, Kattenhorn M, Morley R, et al. Impact of low birth weight and cardiovascular risk factors on endothelial function in early adult life. Circulation 2001; 103:1264–1268.

115. Halvorsen CP, Andolf E, Hu J, et al. Discordant twin growth in utero and differences in blood pressure and endothelial function at 8 years of age. J Intern Med 2006; 259:155–163.

116. Martin H, Gazelius B, Norman M. Impaired acetylcholine-induced vascular relaxation in low birth weight infants: implications for adult hypertension? Pediatr Res 2000; 47:457–462.

117. Forsyth JS, Reilly J, Fraser CG, Struthers AD. Angiotensin converting enzyme activity in infancy is related to birth weight. Arch Dis Child Fetal Neonatal Ed 2004; 89:F442–F444.

118. Riviere G, Michaud A, Breton C, et al. Angiotensin-converting enzyme 2 (ACE2) and ACE activities display tissue-specific sensitivity to undernutrition-programmed hypertension in the adult rat. Hypertension 2005; 46:1169–1174.

119. Roghair RD, Lamb FS, Bedell KA, et al. Late-gestation betamethasone enhances coronary artery responsiveness to angiotensin II in fetal sheep. Am J Physiol Regul Integr Comp Physiol 2004; 286:R80–R88.

120. Segar JL, Roghair RD, Segar EM, et al. Early gestation dexamethasone alters baroreflex and vascular responses in newborn lambs before hypertension. Am J Physiol Regul Integr Comp Physiol 2006; 291:R481–R488.

121. Payne JA, Alexander BT, Khalil RA. Reduced endothelial vascular relaxation in growth-restricted offspring of pregnant rats with reduced uterine perfusion. Hypertension 2003; 42:768–774.

122. Kajantie E, Phillips DI, Andersson S, et al. Size at birth, gestational age and cortisol secretion in adult life: foetal programming of both hyper- and hypocortisolism? Clin Endocrinol (Oxf) 2002; 57:635–641.

123. Nyirenda MJ, Lindsay RS, Kenyon CJ, et al. Glucocorticoid exposure in late gestation permanently programs rat hepatic phosphoenolpyruvate carboxykinase and glucocorticoid receptor expression and causes glucose intolerance in adult offspring. J Clin Invest 1998; 101:2174–2181.

124. O'Regan D, Kenyon CJ, Seckl JR, Holmes MC. Glucocorticoid exposure in late gestation in the rat permanently programs gender-specific differences in adult cardiovascular and metabolic physiology. Am J Physiol Endocrinol Metab 2004; 287:E863–E870.

125. Geng CD, Pedersen KB, Nunez BS, Vedeckis WV. Human glucocorticoid receptor alpha transcript splice variants with exon 2 deletions: evidence for tissue- and cell type-specific functions. Biochemistry 2005; 44:7395–7405.

126. Turner JD, Schote AB, Macedo JA, et al. Tissue specific glucocorticoid receptor expression, a role for alternative first exon usage? Biochem Pharmacol 2006; 72:1529–1537.

127. Baserga M, Hale MA, McKnight RA, et al. Uteroplacental insufficiency alters hepatic expression, phosphorylation, and activity of the glucocorticoid receptor in fetal IUGR rats. Am J Physiol Regul Integr Comp Physiol 2005; 289:R1348–R1353.

128. Bertram C, Trowern AR, Copin N, et al. The maternal diet during pregnancy programs altered expression of the glucocorticoid receptor and type 2 11beta-hydroxysteroid dehydrogenase: potential molecular mechanisms underlying the programming of hypertension in utero. Endocrinology 2001; 142:2841–2853.

129. Holmes MC, Abrahamsen CT, French KL, et al. The mother or the fetus? 11beta-hydroxysteroid dehydrogenase type 2 null mice provide evidence for direct fetal programming of behavior by endogenous glucocorticoids. J Neurosci 2006; 26:3840–3844.

130. Lucas A, Gore SM, Cole TJ, et al. Multicentre trial on feeding low birthweight infants: effects of diet on early growth. Arch Dis Child 1984; 59:722–730.

131. Clark RH, Thomas P, Peabody J. Extrauterine growth restriction remains a serious problem in prematurely born neonates. Pediatrics 2003; 111:986–990.

132. Lucas A, King F, Bishop NB. Postdischarge formula consumption in infants born preterm. Arch Dis Child 1992; 67:691–692.

133. Hack M, Breslau N, Weissman B, et al. Effect of very low birth weight and subnormal head size on cognitive abilities at school age. N Engl J Med 1991; 325:231–237.

134. Hofman PL, Regan F, Jackson WE, et al. Premature birth and later insulin resistance. N Engl J Med 2004; 351:2179–2186.

135. Bonamy AK, Bendito A, Martin H, et al. Preterm birth contributes to increased vascular resistance and higher blood pressure in adolescent girls. Pediatr Res 2005; 58:845–849.

136. O'Connor DL, Jacobs J, Hall R, et al. Growth and development of premature infants fed predominantly human milk, predominantly premature infant formula, or a combination of human milk and premature formula. J Pediatr Gastroenterol Nutr 2003; 37:437–446.

137. Lucas A, Morley R, Cole TJ, et al. Early diet in preterm babies and developmental status in infancy. Arch Dis Child 1989; 64:1570–1578.

138. Singhal A, Fewtrell M, Cole TJ, Lucas A. Low nutrient intake and early growth for later insulin resistance in adolescents born preterm. Lancet 2003; 361:1089–1097.

139. Singhal A, Cole TJ, Lucas A. Early nutrition in preterm infants and later blood pressure: two cohorts after randomised trials. Lancet 2001; 357:413–419.

140. Singhal A, Farooqi IS, O'Rahilly S, et al. Early nutrition and leptin concentrations in later life. Am J Clin Nutr 2002; 75:993–999.

141. Singhal A, Cole TJ, Fewtrell M, Lucas A. Breastmilk feeding and lipoprotein profile in adolescents born preterm: follow-up of a prospective randomised study. Lancet 2004; 363:1571–1578.

142. Lavrik IN, Golks A, Krammer PH. Caspases: pharmacological manipulation of cell death. J Clin Invest 2005; 115:2665–2672.

143. Green DR, Kroemer G. The pathophysiology of mitochondrial cell death. Science 2004; 305:626–629.

144. Willis SN, Adams JM. Life in the balance: how BH3-only proteins induce apoptosis. Curr Opin Cell Biol 2005; 17:617–625.

145. Gross A, McDonnell JM, Korsmeyer SJ. BCL-2 family members and the mitochondria in apoptosis. Genes Dev 1999; 13:1899–1911.

146. Vousden KH. Switching from life to death: the Miz-ing link between Myc and p53. Cancer Cell 2002; 2:351–352.

147. Okada H, Mak TW. Pathways of apoptotic and non-apoptotic death in tumour cells. Nat Rev Cancer 2004; 4:592–603.

148. Meyer N, Kim SS, Penn LZ. The Oscar-worthy role of Myc in apoptosis. Semin Cancer Biol 2006; 16:275–287.

149. Cain K, Inayat-Hussain SH, Wolfe JT, Cohen GM. DNA fragmentation into 200–250 and/or 30–50 kilobase pair fragments in rat liver nuclei is stimulated by Mg^{2+} alone and Ca^{2+}/Mg^{2+} but not by Ca^{2+} alone. FEBS Lett 1994; 349:385–391.

150. Yoshida A, Pommier Y, Ueda T. Endonuclease activation and chromosomal DNA fragmentation during apoptosis in leukemia cells. Int J Hematol 2006; 84:31–37.

151. Russell M, Berardi P, Gong W, Riabowol K. Grow-ING, Age-ING and Die-ING: ING proteins link cancer, senescence and apoptosis. Exp Cell Res 2006; 312:951–961.

152. Carson DA, Seto S, Wasson DB, Carrera CJ. DNA strand breaks, NAD metabolism, and programmed cell death. Exp Cell Res 1986; 164:273–281.

153. Tanaka Y, Yoshihara K, Itaya A, et al. Mechanism of the inhibition of Ca^{2+}, Mg^{2+}-dependent endonuclease of bull seminal plasma induced by ADP-ribosylation. J Biol Chem 1984; 259:6579–6585.

154. Cohen HY, Miller C, Bitterman KJ, et al. Calorie restriction promotes mammalian cell survival by inducing the SIRT1 deacetylase. Science 2004; 305:390–392.

155. Stewart CE, Rotwein P. Growth, differentiation, and survival: multiple physiological functions for insulin-like growth factors. Physiol Rev 1996; 76:1005–1026.

156. Adashi EY. Growth factors and ovarian function: the IGF-I paradigm. Horm Res 1994; 42:44–48.

157. Baserga M, Bertolotto C, Maclennan NK, et al. Uteroplacental insufficiency decreases small intestine growth and alters apoptotic homeostasis in term intrauterine growth retarded rats. Early Hum Dev 2004; 79:93–105.

158. Ke X, McKnight RA, Wang ZM, et al. Nonresponsiveness of cerebral p53-MDM2 functional circuit in newborn rat pups rendered IUGR via uteroplacental insufficiency. Am J Physiol Regul Integr Comp Physiol 2005; 288:R1038–R1045.

159. Chvojkova Z, Ostadalova I, Ostadal B. Low body weight and cardiac tolerance to ischemia in neonatal rats. Physiol Res 2005; 54:357–362.

160. Van den Hove DL, Steinbusch HW, Bruschettini M, et al. Prenatal stress reduces S100B in the neonatal rat hippocampus. Neuroreport 2006; 17:1077–1080.

161. Hekimi S, Guarente L. Genetics and the specificity of the aging process. Science 2003; 299:1351–1354.

162. Alcendor RR, Kirshenbaum LA, Imai S, et al. Silent information regulator 2alpha, a longevity factor and class III histone deacetylase, is an essential endogenous apoptosis inhibitor in cardiac myocytes. Circ Res 2004; 95:971–980.

163. Holliday R. The inheritance of epigenetic defects. Science 1987; 238:163–170.

164. Morgan HD, Sutherland HG, Martin DI, Whitelaw E. Epigenetic inheritance at the agouti locus in the mouse. Nat Genet 1999; 23:314–318.

165. Wolffe AP, Matzke MA. Epigenetics: regulation through repression. Science 1999; 286:481–486.

166. Ng HH, Bird A. DNA methylation and chromatin modification. Curr Opin Genet Dev 1999; 9:158–163.

167. Bird AP. CpG-rich islands and the function of DNA methylation. Nature 1986; 321:209–213.

168. Ben-Hattar J, Beard P, Jiricny J. Cytosine methylation in CTF and Sp1 recognition sites of an HSV tk promoter: effects on transcription in vivo and on factor binding in vitro. Nucleic Acids Res 1989; 17:10179–10190.

169. Jones PA. The DNA methylation paradox. Trends Genet 1999; 15:34–37.

170. Jenuwein T, Allis CD. Translating the histone code. Science 2001; 293:1074–1080.

171. Turner BM. Cellular memory and the histone code. Cell 2002; 111:285–291.

172. Agalioti T, Chen G, Thanos D. Deciphering the transcriptional histone acetylation code for a human gene. Cell 2002; 111:381–392.

173. Cheung P, Allis CD, Sassone-Corsi P. Signaling to chromatin through histone modifications. Cell 2000; 103:263–271.

174. Ke X, Lei Q, James SJ, et al. Uteroplacental insufficiency affects epigenetic determinants of chromatin structure in brains of neonatal and juvenile IUGR rats. Physiol Genomics 2006; 25:16–28.

175. Lillycrop KA, Phillips ES, Jackson AA, et al. Dietary protein restriction of pregnant rats induces and folic acid supplementation prevents epigenetic modification of hepatic gene expression in the offspring. J Nutr 2005; 135:1382–1386.

176. Fu Q, McKnight RA, Yu X, et al. Uteroplacental insufficiency induces site-specific changes in histone H3 covalent modifications and affects DNA-histone H3 positioning in day 0 IUGR rat liver. Physiol Genomics 2004; 20:108–116.

177. Fu Q, McKnight RA, Yu X, et al. Growth retardation alters the epigenetic characteristics of hepatic dual specificity phosphatase 5. Faseb J 2006; 20:2127–2129.